T0203164

BSAVA Manual of Canine and Feline Ophthalmology

Third edition

Editors:

David Gould
BSc(Hons) BVM&S PhD DVOphthal DipECVO MRCVS
RCVS and European Specialist in Veterinary Ophthalmology
Davies Veterinary Specialists, Manor Farm Business Park,
Higham Gobion, Herts SG5 3HR

and

Gillian J. McLellan
BVMS PhD DVOphthal DipECVO DipACVO MRCVS
European Specialist in Veterinary Ophthalmology
School of Veterinary Medicine, University of Wisconsin-Madison,
2015 Linden Drive, Madison, WI 53706, USA

Published by:

British Small Animal Veterinary Association
Woodrow House, 1 Telford Way, Waterwells Business Park,
Quedgeley, Gloucester GL2 2AB

A Company Limited by Guarantee in England
Registered Company No. 2837793
Registered as a Charity

First published 1993
Second edition 2002
Third edition 2014
Reprinted 2017, 2018, 2019, 2022

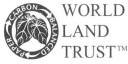

WORLD LAND TRUST™

www.carbonbalancedpaper.com
CBP006075

Carbon Balancing is delivered by World Land Trust, an international conservation charity, who protects the world's most biologically important and threatened habitats acre by acre. Their Carbon Balanced Programme offsets emissions through the purchase and preservation of high conservation value forests.

17269PUBS22

Titles in the BSAVA Manuals series:

For further information on these and all BSAVA publications, please visit our website: **www.bsava.com**

Contents

Contributors

Jim Carter BVetMed DVOphthal DipECVO MRCVS
RCVS and European Specialist in Veterinary Ophthalmology
South Devon Referrals, c/o Abbotskerswell Veterinary Centre, The Old Cider Works,
Abbotskerswell, Newton Abbot, Devon TQ12 5GH

Louise Clark BVMS CertVA DipECVAA MRCVS
RCVS and European Specialist in Veterinary Anaesthesia
Davies Veterinary Specialists, Manor Farm Business Park, Higham Gobion, Herts SG5 3HR

Ruth Dennis MA VetMB DVR DipECVDI MRCVS
RCVS and European Specialist in Veterinary Diagnostic Imaging
Animal Health Trust, Lanwades Park, Kentford, Newmarket, Suffolk CB8 7UU

Emma Dewhurst MA VetMB FRCPath MRCVS
Axiom Veterinary Laboratories Ltd, The Manor House, Brunel Road,
Newton Abbot, Devon TQ12 4PB

David Donaldson BVSc(Hons) DipECVO MRCVS
European Specialist in Veterinary Ophthalmology
Animal Health Trust, Lanwades Park, Kentford, Newmarket, Suffolk CB8 7UU

Laurent Garosi DVM DipECVN MRCVS
RCVS and European Specialist in Veterinary Neurology
Davies Veterinary Specialists, Manor Farm Business Park, Higham Gobion, Herts SG5 3HR

David Gould BSc(Hons) BVM&S PhD DVOphthal DipECVO MRCVS
RCVS and European Specialist in Veterinary Ophthalmology
Davies Veterinary Specialists, Manor Farm Business Park, Higham Gobion, Herts SG5 3HR

Claudia Hartley BVSc CertVOphthal DipECVO MRCVS
RCVS and European Specialist in Veterinary Ophthalmology
Animal Health Trust, Lanwades Park, Kentford, Newmarket, Suffolk CB8 7UU

Christine Heinrich DVOphthal DipECVO MRCVS
RCVS and European Specialist in Veterinary Ophthalmology
Willows Veterinary Centre and Referral Service, Highlands Road, Shirley,
Solihull, West Midlands B90 4NH

Philippa J. Johnson BVSc CertVDI DipECVDI MRCVS
European Specialist in Veterinary Diagnostic Imaging
Animal Health Trust, Lanwades Park, Kentford, Newmarket, Suffolk CB8 7UU

Robert Lowe BVSc DVOphthal MRCVS
Optivet Referrals, 3 Downley Road, Havant PO9 2NJ

Mark Lowrie MA VetMB MVM DipECVN MRCVS
RCVS and European Veterinary Specialist in Neurology
Davies Veterinary Specialists, Manor Farm Business Park, Higham Gobion, Herts SG5 3HR

Sue Manning BVSc(Hons) DVOphthal MRCVS
Pride Veterinary Centre, Riverside Road, Derby, Derbyshire DE24 8HX

Gillian J. McLellan BVMS PhD DVOphthal DipECVO DipACVO MRCVS
European Specialist in Veterinary Ophthalmology
School of Veterinary Medicine, University of Wisconsin-Madison, 2015 Linden Drive, Madison, WI 53706, USA

Natasha Mitchell MVB DVOphthal MRCVS
Crescent Veterinary Clinic, Dooradoyle Road, Limerick, Ireland

Kristina Narfström DVM PhD DipECVO
European Specialist in Veterinary Ophthalmology
Djurakuten Animal Hospital, Kungstensgatan 58, 113 29 Stockholm, Sweden

James Oliver BVSc CertVOphthal DipECVO MRCVS
European Specialist in Veterinary Ophthalmology
Animal Health Trust, Lanwades Park, Kentford, Newmarket, Suffolk CB8 7UU

Simon Petersen-Jones DVetMed PhD DVOphthal DipECVO MRCVS
European Specialist in Veterinary Ophthalmology
Department of Small Animal Clinical Science, Michigan State University, D-208 Veterinary Medical Center, MI 48824-1314, USA

Simon Pot DVM DipACVO DipECVO
European Specialist in Veterinary Ophthalmology
Veterinary Ophthalmology Service, Equine Department, Vetsuisse Faculty, University of Zürich, Winterthurerstrasse 260, CH-8057 Zürich, Switzerland

Peter Renwick MA VetMB DVOphthal MRCVS
Willows Veterinary Centre and Referral Service, Highlands Road, Shirley, Solihull, West Midlands B90 4NH

Rick F. Sanchez DVM DipECVO MRCVS
European Specialist in Veterinary Ophthalmology
The Royal Veterinary College, Hawkhead Lane, North Mymms, Hatfield, Herts AL9 7TA

Emma Scurrell BVSc DipACVP MRCVS
Cytopath Ltd, PO Box 24, Ledbury, Herefordshire HR8 2YD

Kerry Smith BVetMed CertVOphthal DipECVO MRCVS
RCVS and European Specialist in Veterinary Ophthalmology
Davies Veterinary Specialists, Manor Farm Business Park, Higham Gobion, Herts SG5 3HR

Sally Turner MA VetMB DVOphthal MRCVS
RCVS Specialist in Veterinary Ophthalmology
Mandeville Veterinary Hospital, Northolt, Middlesex UB5 5HD
Stone Lion Veterinary Hospital, Wimbledon, London SW19 5AU

Christine Watté DVM DipECVO
European Specialist in Veterinary Ophthalmology
Department of Clinical Veterinary Medicine, Small Animal Clinic, Länggassstrasse 128, CH-3012 Bern, Switzerland

Foreword

The first edition of the *BSAVA Manual of Small Animal Ophthalmology*, published in 1993, was one of the most successful Manuals published by BSAVA and was followed by a second edition in 2002. The third edition is an eagerly anticipated sequel and has been extensively rewritten and updated, as is entirely appropriate, because the latest edition has a new editorial team in place and a veritable Who's Who of talented authors. The editors, Dr David Gould and Dr Gill McLellan, are both veterinary ophthalmologists of international reputation; Dr Gould is a Director at Davies Veterinary Specialists and Dr McLellan is an Assistant Professor of Comparative Ophthalmology at the University of Wisconsin.

The decision to focus this new edition on canine and feline ophthalmology is sensible given the amount of new information available since the last Manual was published. Clearly, concentrating on dogs and cats enables subjects to be covered in greater detail and allows important new contributions, such as the ophthalmic manifestations of systemic disease, to be included.

Veterinary ophthalmology remains a popular and rapidly expanding subject with unique characteristics. Where else is it possible to look at an outpost of the brain, examine blood vessels for normality, or directly visualize pathology in action? The challenge is to produce an attractively laid out, up-to-date book with clear text and excellent illustrations which is used by every member of the general practice team, including those who are keen to develop a deeper insight and understanding of this fascinating subject and those who have already developed specialist interest and expertise. It is clear that the editors, authors and the BSAVA Publications team have succeeded in producing such a desirable book and they are to be congratulated.

Professor Sheila Crispin
MA VetMB BSc PhD DVA DVOphthal DipECVO FRCVS

Preface

In the 12 years that have passed since the last edition of this Manual, there has been significant progress in many areas of veterinary ophthalmology. This new edition has been fully updated and rewritten to encompass all the major advances that have developed over this time.

Despite the increase in complexity within our specialty, the fundamental principles of ocular examination remain unchanged. A thorough guide to examination of the eye is provided in Chapter 1, presenting a logical, step-wise approach for general practitioners. The increased availability of advanced diagnostic imaging modalities since 2002 means that access to MRI and CT scanners is no longer necessarily the preserve of universities or select specialist practices. The imaging chapter has been significantly expanded to include an overview of these advanced techniques, whilst retaining practical advice on the more traditional ophthalmic imaging methods commonly available in general practice.

Of particular note in recent years is the increase in the availability of genetic tests for canine inherited eye diseases. In 2002, a commercial DNA test was available for just one canine inherited eye disease. At the time of writing, more than 50 such tests are now on offer, and this number can expect to increase significantly in the years to come. The ability of DNA testing not only to confirm a clinical diagnosis but also to predict future risk of disease has significant implications for pet owners, breeders and veterinary surgeons alike. Its potential has, however, not yet been fully realized and a new chapter on inherited eye disease has been included in the Manual in an attempt to address this.

Improvements in surgical techniques and equipment have led to a concomitant increase in surgical success rates for many eye surgeries, including those for corneal disease, lens luxation and cataract. Reflecting this, an updated chapter on ophthalmic surgical principles complements expanded surgical sections within other chapters, whilst we have made an effort to ensure that adequate guidance is provided on when to refer.

As in previous editions, recommendations for further reading are provided, but these lists of references are not intended to be exhaustive or exhausting. The Manual is now even more richly illustrated with colour photographs and line drawings than its popular predecessors. We have added new chapters on problem-solving approaches and ocular manifestations of systemic diseases, and expanded or updated all other chapters to reflect the advances in the field over recent years. Regrettably, this expansion of content came at the expense of chapters on rabbit and exotic animal ophthalmology, and practitioners seeking information on specific ophthalmic conditions in these species are directed to chapters in the relevant BSAVA Manuals.

Throughout the Manual, we have paid attention to providing clear, easily understandable text, tables and figures in a format that lends itself to reference 'on the fly' in the consulting room, as well as being an enjoyable read for those who wish to study the subject in greater depth. We sincerely hope that this Manual will provide a useful and practical resource for veterinary surgeons in general practice as well as for those with a special interest in the field of veterinary ophthalmology.

We are most grateful to the authors, all specialists in their field, for the skill and the dedication shown in preparing their contributions to this new Manual. Finally, special thanks must go to the team at BSAVA, without whom this publication would not have seen the light of day.

David Gould
Gill McLellan

The ocular examination

Christine Heinrich

The ocular examination is an extremely rewarding procedure for the examiner because the eye lends itself to visual inspection like no other organ and often allows an instant clinical diagnosis to be made at the time of consultation. The ocular examination can also provide important information about other organ systems. With regard to the nervous system, the ocular examination not only allows assessment of the neuro-ophthalmic reflexes, but the examiner is also able to visually inspect the optic nerve, which is in direct communication with the brain and is surrounded by the meninges and cerebrospinal fluid (CSF). Fundic examination allows visual inspection of veins and arteries and provides important information about the cardiovascular system. Fundoscopy can be a quick and inexpensive way to alert the examiner to the possible presence of systemic hypertension, particularly in elderly cats. By detecting conjunctival or retinal haemorrhages, the examiner may be directed towards a systemic coagulopathy, and many metabolic diseases may present with ocular signs early in the course of disease (e.g. cataract formation in diabetes mellitus and jaundice in liver disease). The health of the corneal surface can be an indicator for many immune-mediated and infectious conditions, and even the position of the globe within the orbit and the position of the third eyelid can give the observant examiner information about the state of the patient's general health.

However, the ability to complete a thorough ocular examination and interpret the findings correctly is not often a 'day one skill' that the newly qualified veterinary surgeon will possess. When assessing the ocular fundus, in particular, there is enormous variation in what is considered physiologically and anatomically normal, and the inexperienced clinician must strive to examine as many patients as possible to build up a rich mental 'reference library'. This allows the experienced examiner to distinguish instantly between normal variations and pathological appearances of ocular structures. The study of textbook chapters on the ocular examination helps to provide a foundation for the practical skills that can only be gained by practice (Martin, 2005; Ollivier et al., 2007; Maggs, 2008). The use of photographic atlases of canine and feline ophthalmology is also highly recommended (Barnett et al., 2002; Crispin, 2004; Ketring and Glaze, 2012).

For this reason it is recommended that the veterinary surgeon should aim to carry out as many eye examinations (particularly examinations of the fundus) as possible. These should be integrated into the routine patient examination. Of course, time constraints and appointment scheduling generally do not allow a complete ocular examination to be performed on every patient. It may, therefore, be a more realistic option for the veterinary surgeon to aim to perform one new task each week, such as looking at the optic nerve in every patient's eye, followed by assessing the non-tapetal fundus in each patient the following week, and so on. In this way, the examiner will gradually gain the skills necessary to carry out an ocular examination in an efficient and prompt manner and interpret the findings with confidence.

Technique

Patient restraint

In general, minimal restraint is required to perform an ocular examination in the dog and cat. A calm and confident approach with patient cooperation is much preferred over manual or chemical methods of restraint, and in most patients it is possible to carry out a complete ocular examination with the help of the owner only. When choosing illumination levels for the different instruments used throughout the ocular examination, the examiner should strive to keep the level of illumination to the minimum required because the use of excessively bright light will be uncomfortable for the patient and result in reduced patient compliance. Ideally, the patient should be placed in a seated position close to the edge of the examination table. The owner should provide gentle support, with one hand reaching over the patient's back towards the chest and the other hand stretched out flat, supporting the patient's chin, elevating the head to a horizontal position (Figure 1.1).

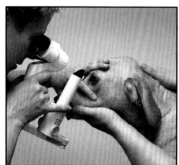

1.1 The patient is seated on a height-adjustable examination table and gently supported by an assistant. Note how the muzzle is elevated and supported by the assistant's palm. (©Willows Referrals)

For fractious and difficult dogs and cats, appropriately trained personnel such as animal care assistants or nurses should assist. A muzzle should be used if indicated. To prevent injury to the examiner, owner and staff, muzzles should be completely enclosed, considering the very close proximity of the examiner's face to the patient's mouth. This rules out the use of most fabric muzzles, which are often open at the front. Cat claw injuries can be avoided either by gently wrapping the patient in a towel or by using a commercially available 'cat bag'. For very fractious or dangerous patients, chemical restraint may have to be employed (see Chapter 5).

- For dogs, a combination of medetomidine/ dexmedetomidine and butorphanol provides immobilization and adequate visualization of the eye.
- In cats, a combination of ketamine and midazolam or medetomidine/ketamine/opioid generally works well.

The doses chosen depend on the temperament of the patient, the underlying condition and the procedure to be undertaken. It should be noted that none of the aforementioned drug combinations result in marked enophthalmia, globe rotation or protrusion of the third eyelid, unlike sedation with acepromazine or general anaesthesia, neither of which are suitable choices to facilitate the ocular examination in fractious patients. The examiner should bear in mind that most drugs that have a sedative effect may negatively influence the eye examination and, specifically, will limit assessment of the ocular reflexes and responses as well as pupil size and vision. Both Schirmer tear test (STT) and intraocular pressure (IOP) readings may be altered in the sedated or anaesthetized patient (Herring *et al.*, 2000; Sanchez *et al.*, 2006; Hofmeister *et al.*, 2008, 2009; Ghaffari *et al.*, 2010). Patients with eyelid anomalies such as entropion must be assessed in their conscious state because the eyelid conformation may dramatically change following sedation or under anaesthesia.

Equipment

The first requisite for the comfortable performance of an ocular examination is a room that is quiet and can be darkened. Ideally, a height-adjustable table should be available so that the patient can be positioned at the eye level of the examiner; whether the examiner is seated or standing depends on personal preference. A focal light source such as a pentorch or Finoff transilluminator (preferred) (Figure 1.2), a direct ophthalmoscope (Figure 1.3) and a 20 or 30 dioptre (D) condensing lens (Figure 1.4) are the minimum equipment that should be at hand in every practice. A number of consumables, including STT strips, fluorescein-impregnated paper strips (Fluorets®), cotton buds and gauze-free swabs, as well as sterile water or artificial tear solution to clean periocular debris or flush away excess fluorescein, should also be available.

Drugs routinely used for an ocular examination include proxymetacaine 0.5% eye drops to induce

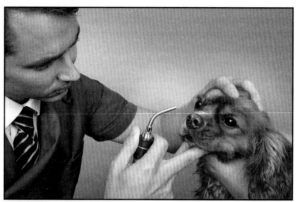

1.2 Finoff transilluminator for mounting on an ophthalmoscope handle. (©Willows Referrals)

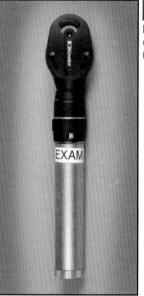

1.3 Hand-held battery-operated direct ophthalmoscope. (©Willows Referrals)

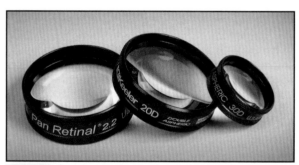

1.4 Condensing lenses for ocular examination: (L–R) Pan-retinal 2.2, 20 D and 30 D. (©Willows Referrals)

local anaesthesia of the ocular surface, tropicamide 0.5–1% to induce short-duration mydriasis and, less frequently, 2.5 or 10% phenylephrine eye drops for pharmacological testing (see Chapter 19). Ideally, every practice should also have an instrument to allow exact measurement of IOP (Schiøtz tonometer, Tono-pen or TonoVet). More advanced diagnostic instruments, such as the slit-lamp biomicroscope, the head-mounted indirect ophthalmoscope, retinoscopes and skiascopy racks, as well as gonioscopy lenses, are recommended for those clinicians who wish to further their knowledge and skills in ophthalmology; these instruments are routinely used by veterinary ophthalmology specialists. There is no doubt that a basic ocular examination sufficient for everyday veterinary practice can be carried out with minimal equipment (including a focal light source, direct ophthalmoscope and a condensing lens); however, many more subtle ocular changes will be missed, especially without the use of a slit-lamp biomicroscope.

Signalment and history

The age, breed and sex of the patient should be noted because these can provide vital clues to the diagnosis. This applies particularly in veterinary ophthalmology, where many conditions are known to be inherited or at least considered 'breed related'. The coat and iris colour of the patient can, in both cats and dogs, give clues about which fundus coloration may be expected and can help to distinguish normal fundus variations from pathological states. For example, the red appearance of the pigment-dilute fundus in a Siamese cat can be mistaken for retinal haemorrhage. A brief but relevant history should be taken, including how long the patient has been in the owner's possession, whether the patient's general health is good and which previous illnesses or accidents the patient has suffered. For cats, it should be established how many other cats live in the same house because being part of a multi-cat household may increase the risk of contracting specific infectious diseases. All recent or current medications should be noted because they may be relevant, not only to the medication that the clinician plans to include in the treatment plan, but also potentially to the aetiology of the ocular problem for which the patient is being presented. Examples include:

- Sudden-onset vision loss in an elderly feline patient who has been receiving a long course of enrofloxacin, a drug that can cause retinal toxicity at only mildly elevated serum levels and which may not be metabolized and excreted adequately in a patient with compromised renal function
- Dry eye in a patient suffering from chronic colitis, which has been managed with sulfasalazine, a drug well known to induce keratoconjunctivitis sicca (KCS).

Only after a full history has been recorded should the client be questioned about the ocular problem that the patient is being presented for. The client should be asked whether there has been any deterioration in their pet's eyesight, for how long this has been the case, whether the change is progressive and whether this is more noticeable in bright or dim lighting conditions. The client should also be asked whether there has been any change in the appearance of one or both eyes, any ocular discharge or any signs of ocular pain. The laterality of conditions should be considered because in bilateral ocular conditions an underlying systemic cause is more likely.

Examination with ambient illumination and without instruments

Distant examination

To begin with, a 'hands-off' approach is taken and the patient's head is observed from a distance. In patients with suspected entropion, trichiasis or facial droop, it is important that the examiner studies the ocular conformation in different head positions and without manual restraint, because the latter may result in worsening of any spastic component of painful adnexal conditions, leading to overestimation of the surgical correction required. Ideally, the examiner should start observing the patient when they enter the examination room and continue throughout history taking, without making the patient aware that attention is being paid to their face and eyes. The blink rate and presence of ocular discharges are noted and facial symmetry and orbital conformation are assessed. If exophthalmos is suspected, it may be helpful to look at the patient's head from above and compare the position of the globes in relation to each other.

Close examination

Following the distant examination, the patient's head can now be manipulated, although this may have to be kept to a minimum if there is a risk to globe integrity (i.e. in the presence of deep corneal ulcers). The head and periocular areas are assessed for symmetry and the position of the globe within the orbit, as well as any signs of strabismus, are noted. Ocular motility can be tested at this point: normal ocular movements should result when the patient's head is moved from side to side and up and down (the so-called 'doll's head reflex' or vestibulo-ocular reflex). Extraocular muscle paralysis or restriction may impair globe movement in different directions, depending upon which nerve/muscle group is involved (see Chapter 19). The periocular area is palpated gently and both globes are lightly retropulsed concurrently with pressure from the index fingers through the closed upper eyelids to check for the possible presence of increased resistance, which could indicate a retrobulbar space-occupying lesion (Figure 1.5). The relationship between globe position and eyelids is examined.

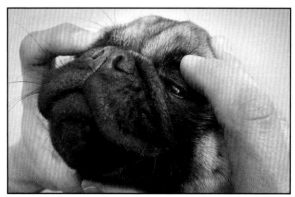

1.5 To assess for possible retrobulbar space-occupying lesions, both globes are gently retropulsed with pressure applied to the closed upper eyelids. (©Willows Referrals)

In patients with facial droop, it is important to assess the palpebral fissure not only when the head is elevated (Figure 1.6ab) but also when the patient's nose is directed to the floor (Figure 1.6cd) because the head will be in the latter position for much of the time that the patient is awake. For this reason, it may be necessary for the examiner to kneel in front of the patient, who is seated or standing on the examination table (Figure 1.6c). The

examiner should also evert both the upper and lower eyelids to inspect the eyelid margins, identify the lacrimal puncta and examine the conjunctival fornices, palpebral conjunctiva and third eyelid. Changes, including conjunctival haemorrhage or variation from the normal pink appearance of the conjunctiva, as a result of jaundice, pallor or cyanosis, will be readily apparent and point the examiner towards a systemic disease. To improve exposure of the third eyelid for examination, this structure can be temporarily protruded by gentle retropulsion of the globe via the closed upper eyelid while the lower eyelid is held everted (Figure 1.7).

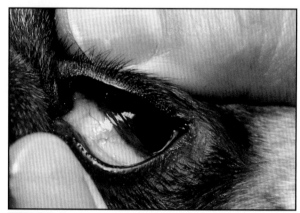

1.7 For improved visualization, the third eyelid can be protruded temporarily by applying pressure on the globe through the upper lid whilst the lower lid is pulled down. (©Willows Referrals)

Schirmer tear test
The Schirmer tear test (STT) quantifies the level of tear production and is an objective diagnostic tool indispensable for the management of canine KCS (see Chapter 10). Two types of STT have been described:

- STT-1, which is carried out before the application of local anaesthetic and measures both basal and reflex tear production. STT-1 is the established procedure in veterinary ophthalmology and is usually referred to as 'STT'
- STT-2, which is carried out following ocular surface anaesthesia and only measures the basal tear level.

Procedure
To perform the STT, a specifically designed strip of filter paper is folded 90 degrees at a pre-set area approximately 5 mm from the tip, which is usually marked with a small notch. The strip should be folded whilst still in the plastic packaging to avoid contamination of the paper with grease and sweat from the examiner's fingers, which could decrease the ability of the paper to absorb tears. The short, folded piece of the STT strip is then inserted between the lower eyelid and globe, approximately at the site of the transition between the middle and lateral third of the lower eyelid. The STT strip should be in contact with the corneal surface; this is intended to cause some reflex tear production

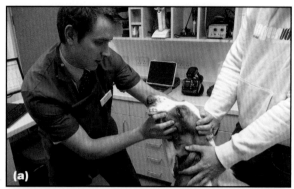

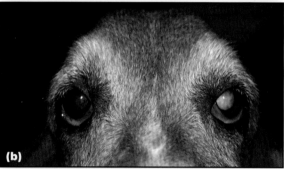

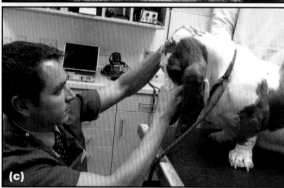

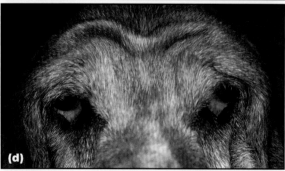

1.6 When examining patients with facial droop or excess facial skin, care must be taken to assess the eyelid conformation not only when **(a–b)** the head is elevated but also **(c–d)** during a time of low head posture because trichiasis associated with facial droop will otherwise not be diagnosed. (©Willows Referrals)

(Figure 1.8). Ideally, the palpebral fissure should be kept at least partially open during STT readings and minimal manual pressure exerted to maintain the strip in position. The strip is left in place for 1 minute and immediately following removal of the strip from the conjunctival fornix, the distance from the notch to the end of the wet part of the strip is measured and recorded in millimetres/minute (mm/min). Most STT strips are impregnated with an indicator dye and have a millimetre scale imprinted upon them to facilitate instant reading of the level of wetting.

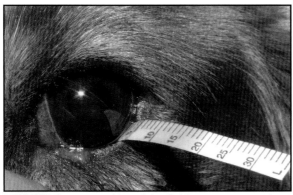

1.8 Correct position of the Schirmer tear test strip. (©Willows Referrals)

Results

In the dog, there is a well documented negative correlation between the STT reading and KCS. Normal dogs are expected to have STT readings of at least 15 mm/min (Maggs, 2008). KCS should be suspected in dogs with STT readings between 10 and 15 mm/min, and disease is confirmed if STT readings <10 mm/min are recorded. To prevent the possible effect of the ocular examination and manipulation of the eye and adnexa on the STT result, it is recommended that the test be carried out early in the course of the examination, preferably immediately after the initial 'hands-off' distant assessment of the patient. The application of any topical drugs, collection of bacteriology or cytology samples and ocular examination with a bright light may falsely elevate STT readings by inducing reflex tear production. Most sedatives and anaesthetics affect STT readings adversely and the test should therefore be carried out in the fully conscious patient (Herring *et al.*, 2000; Sanchez *et al.*, 2006; Ghaffari *et al.*, 2010).

When interpreting STT results in patients with painful ocular conditions, the examiner must consider that, because of the pain, the reflex component of tear production may falsely elevate STT readings in a patient with low basal tear production and thus mask a degree of KCS, which might have been instrumental in the genesis of the problem that the patient presents with. In this instance, it is important that the examiner pays attention to the STT in the contralateral eye, which may only have subtle clinical signs of KCS but may display low STT readings.

The STT can also be performed in the same manner in the cat, but the correlation between the level of tear production and KCS is usually not as clear-cut in this species as in the dog. The reported range of STT in normal cats varies from 3–32 mm/min, with a mean of 17 mm/min. However, some feline patients without any signs of ocular surface disease present with extremely low, or even zero, STT readings and it is likely that, in these patients, tear production has been affected temporarily by stress and associated changes to the autonomic control of tear production (Ollivier *et al.*, 2007).

Sample collection

At this point in the examination, samples may be obtained for a number of different laboratory investigations, including microbiology, cytology and polymerase chain reaction (PCR) testing (see Chapter 3). Ideally, samples should be collected prior to the application of any topical agents to the eye because these can have a negative impact upon the growth of microorganisms in culture or the results of other laboratory tests. For example, the application of fluorescein prior to sampling might interfere with an immunofluorescent assay. An exception to this rule in a clinical setting, and specifically when dealing with painful eyes, is made for the use of topical anaesthetics. It has been shown that a single application of 0.5% proxymetacaine does not have a negative effect on bacteriological culture results (Champagne and Pickett, 1995).

Samples for microbiology are usually obtained with cotton-tipped sterile swabs, which are gently rolled in the ventral conjunctival fornix or on the corneal surface. Swabs with small tips are especially useful for this purpose. For all microbiological samples, the examiner must use the appropriate swab as well as transport container and culture medium; if they are at all uncertain about the requirements, the laboratory should be consulted before the sample is taken. Samples for cytology can be obtained by direct impression smears or with the help of cytobrushes, which are gently rolled across the area and the sample collected is then transferred to a glass slide and stained as appropriate. In the absence of cytobrushes, cytological samples can be harvested using a Kimura spatula or the blunt end of a scalpel blade (Figure 1.9). Both of these instruments are especially useful when collecting samples from the corneal surface. Cells can be harvested for PCR testing either with cotton-tipped sterile swabs or cytobrushes, and these samples should be transported in a plain tube.

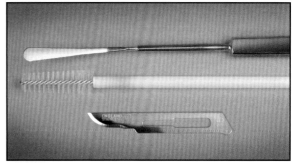

1.9 Kimura spatula, cytobrush and scalpel blade which can be used for collecting cytological samples. (©Willows Referrals)

Vision testing and neuro-ophthalmic reflexes

Vision testing in veterinary patients is complex and routinely involves a number of neuro-ophthalmic and behavioural tests, the results of which must be interpreted in combination. Generally, pupillary light reflexes (PLRs) and dazzle and menace responses are tested before the patient is subjected to visual tracking tests, maze testing at different levels of illumination and visual placing responses. Neuro-ophthalmic testing is described below, as well as in greater detail in Chapter 19.

Pupillary light reflex

The PLR (which should be assessed in a darkened room) has two components: direct and consensual. A bright light shone into one eye causes both pupils to constrict (positive direct and consensual response). The optic nerve (cranial nerve (CN) II) comprises the afferent arm of the reflex, whilst the parasympathetic fibres that run with the oculomotor nerve (CN III) comprise the efferent arm. In the normal patient, parasympathetic stimulation leads to pupillary constriction in both eyes owing to contraction of the iris sphincter muscle and relaxation of the dilator muscle. The consensual response is the result of decussation of nerve fibres at both the optic chiasm and the pretectal area. The PLR arc does not include the cortical visual centres because the pupillomotor fibres branch from the optic tract before the visual fibres. Many factors influence the PLR, including excitement of the patient (a systemic adrenergic state decreases the photomotor response), iridal disease (e.g. iris atrophy, uveitis/synechiae and iridal neoplasia), increased IOP, and reduced retinal, optic nerve or higher centre function. The integrity of both the sympathetic and parasympathetic nerve supply to the iridal musculature is also required for an intact PLR. A positive PLR does not necessarily indicate the presence of vision because the PLR may be unaltered in cases of cortical blindness, and a negative result does not necessarily indicate blindness because the PLR may be absent as a result of iris atrophy or pharmacologically induced pupillary dilation.

Swinging flashlight test

The swinging flashlight test is used to detect prechiasmal defects in the retina or optic nerve of the examined eye. The penlight is used to illuminate one pupil and is then swung rapidly to the opposite eye. If the pupil of the second eye dilates as it is illuminated, this indicates a blinding lesion in that eye, involving the retina or optic nerve (up to the point of the optic chiasm). However, a slight amount of dilation following initial pupillary constriction upon direct stimulation is normal and is known as *pupillary escape.*

Dazzle reflex

A very bright light shone in each eye in turn should result in a reflex blink in both eyes. The dazzle reflex is subcortical (i.e. does not involve the visual cortex) but provides more information about the visual pathways than the PLR alone because it also involves fibres in the nucleus of the facial nerve (CN VII) (i.e. it tests the visual pathways up to the level of the midbrain). Even patients with a complete cataract would still be expected to have a positive dazzle reflex if stimulated with a sufficiently bright light source.

Menace response

The menace response is not a true reflex but a learned response, which can be suppressed voluntarily by veterinary patients. The menace response tests the integrity of the complete visual pathway, up to the cortical level, and also reflects cerebellar function because it is absent in some patients with cerebellar disease. However, the menace response gives only a crude assessment of vision (in humans, a positive menace response is considered just one step above the ability to perceive light). It is elicited by briskly moving a flat hand or single finger towards one of the patient's eyes whilst covering the other eye. Excessive air movement, which could be perceived by the cornea, vibrissae or eyelashes of the patient, should be avoided. Care should be taken to perform menace testing from medial and lateral sides to test both the lateral and medial visual fields.

The afferent arm of the menace response is the optic nerve (CN II), whilst the efferent arm consists of the facial nerve (CN VII) and abducens nerve (CN VI). In the sighted patient, eyelid closure mediated by the orbicularis oculi muscle should occur; the concurrent subtle globe retraction mediated by the retractor bulbi muscle is not generally noted. However, in patients with facial paralysis, where eyelid closure is absent or limited, a positive menace response may be assessed by observing subtle globe retraction and transient third eyelid protrusion. The menace response is not present in dogs and cats under the age of 8–12 weeks and may be absent in anxious or excited patients. To rule out the latter, it may be helpful to perform both palpebral and menace testing repeatedly in rapid succession because this may increase the patient's response to the threatening gesture.

Behavioural testing of vision

Visual tracking, visual placing and maze testing are all techniques employed to assess vision in veterinary patients.

Visual tracking: This requires the patient to focus on an object that is moved or dropped in front of them, following its path (Figure 1.10). This can usually be achieved easily with a biscuit held at an adequate distance to avoid the patient purely following the smell or by dropping a piece of cotton wool (which makes no noise during its fall) 20–30 cm in front of the patient. With cats, a laser pointer directed at the floor or wall and toys such as feathers on a string or a toy mouse may arouse their interest. However, owing to the subjective nature of this test, failure to respond with visual tracking does not necessarily equate to absence of sight.

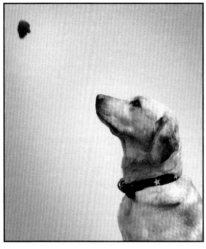

1.10

Visual tracking. (©Willows Referrals)

Visual placing: This can be used to assess vision in nervous or stoic patients of small size (if they have motor control over their limbs). The patient is lifted up from the examination table and slowly moved towards the edge of the table. A normal response for a sighted patient is to extend one or both front legs towards the table, indicating that the object has been seen. Each of the patient's eyes can be covered in turn during this test to assess vision in the individual eyes.

Maze testing: This can be carried out with a variety of obstacles and allows assessment of vision at different lighting levels. A very efficient way to assess vision is to lead dogs up to a set of steps; most patients with marked visual deficits will not be comfortable negotiating steps in an unfamiliar environment and, in particular, will resent going down such steps. The safety of the patient must of course be considered at all times during maze testing, which must be carried out in the most humane way possible.

Additional neuro-ophthalmic tests

Palpebral reflex: The palpebral reflex tests the sensory innervation to the eyelids, which is provided by the first (ophthalmic) and second (maxillary) branches of the trigeminal nerve (CN V). A gentle tap on the periocular skin should result in closure of the eyelids (mediated by the facial nerve) and retraction of the globe (mediated by the abducens nerve). Care should be taken to assess all branches of the trigeminal nerve involved in innervation of the periocular skin and the reflex should be elicited by touching the skin at:

- The centre of the upper lid (supraorbital nerve; branch 1 of CN V)
- The lateral canthus (lacrimal nerve; branch 1 of CN V)
- The centre of the lower lid (zygomatic nerve; branch 2 of CN V)
- The medial canthus (trochlear nerve; branch 1 of CN V).

Corneal reflex: The corneal reflex tests the sensory innervation to the cornea, which is provided by the first branch of the trigeminal nerve. To test corneal sensation, the eyelids are held open with one hand whilst a thin wisp of cotton wool is gently applied to the cornea. This should elicit a blink response (mediated by the facial nerve via the orbicularis oculi muscle) and globe retraction (mediated by the abducens nerve via the retractor bulbi muscle). In patients with chronic facial nerve paralysis (loss of CN VII function), a positive corneal reflex can be assessed simply by observing the subtle globe retraction and resultant brief protrusion of the third eyelid.

Examination with focal illumination ± magnification

In the next step of the ocular examination, the adnexa and ocular surface as well as the anterior segment are examined using a bright focal light source, ideally a Finoff transilluminator (see Figure 1.2). Some examiners also prefer to use a low level of magnification (such as 2–3x) for this part of the examination, which can be provided by a set of head loupes. The eyelid margins are scanned for aberrant lashes such as those seen with distichiasis and it may be possible to see ectopic cilia erupting as small, pigmented dots during examination of the palpebral conjunctiva with the eyelids everted.

The health of the corneal surface is assessed with the help of the Purkinje image of the light source on the cornea. This image represents the reflection of the light source itself and should, in eyes with normal corneal surface health, be sharp and clearly outlined (Figure 1.11a). In eyes with corneal surface disease, such as KCS, corneal ulceration or sequestration, the Purkinje image on the corneal surface will be irregular (Figure 1.11bc); this is a clear indicator of poor corneal surface health and warrants further

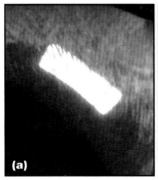

(a)

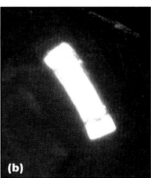

(b)

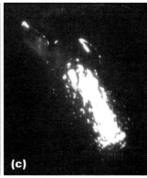

(c)

1.11 The Purkinje image can provide important information about the health of the ocular surface. **(a)** In the healthy eye, the image is sharp and bright. **(b)** In mild cases of KCS, only subtle changes to the edges of the image may be seen. **(c)** In eyes with severe KCS and corneal ulceration, the image is broken up and less bright. (©Willows Referrals)

investigation. However, a Purkinje image of the light source will not only be generated on the corneal surface but also on both the anterior and posterior lens capsule in eyes with clear anterior ocular media. These three Purkinje images can be helpful when determining the depth of a lesion in the anterior segment using the technique of parallax. The Purkinje images on the cornea and anterior lens capsule move away from the examiner and light source, whilst the image on the posterior lens capsule moves towards them, during movement of the examiner.

To gain familiarity with the phenomenon of parallax, the examiner should place three bottles short distances behind each other on an examination table (Figure 1.12). The examiner now holds the focal light source close to their face and moves from side to side in front of the bottles: the first two bottles appear to move to the left as the examiner moves to the right (i.e. away from the examiner), whilst the third and most distant bottle appears to move in the same direction as the examiner (i.e. towards the examiner). Note that the opposite holds true if

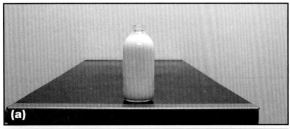

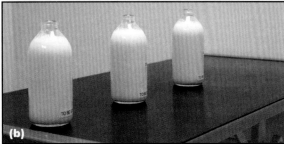

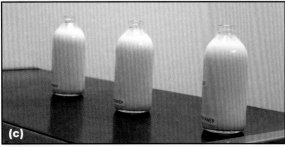

1.12 The phenomenon of parallax can be recreated with three milk bottles placed on a table in front of the examiner, representing the three Purkinje images on the cornea and the anterior and posterior lens capsules. **(a)** When the examiner stands directly in front of the bottles they obscure each other and it is not possible to distinguish them. **(b)** If the examiner moves to the right, the first and second bottles appear to move away from the examiner, whilst the third bottle moves with the examiner. **(c)** When moving in the opposite direction, the same phenomenon occurs. This demonstrates that opacities of the cornea and anterior lens capsule appear to move away from the examiner, whilst those on the posterior lens capsule move with the examiner. (©Willows Referrals)

the observer remains stationary and the animal moves its gaze. More posterior lesions will move in the opposite direction to the patient's eye movement. The use of parallax is especially important in determining the depth of a cataract because the exact position of certain cataracts gives valuable information about their possible aetiology and also their potential for progression. Using the technique of parallax, anterior capsular and anterior cortical cataracts will be moving away from the examiner, whilst posterior cortical or capsular cataracts will appear to be moving with the examiner.

Corneal opacities, pigmentation and active vascularization are readily apparent on examination with a focal light source. Corneal defects may be visible and should be assessed in more detail following the application of fluorescein. The anterior chamber is observed for clarity and depth. Shallow anterior chambers are seen in feline glaucoma associated with aqueous misdirection and with intumescent cataracts. Lesions such as masses, haemorrhage, fibrin and cellular accumulations are noted and recorded, to be assessed in more detail at a later stage. The iris is examined for colour and surface homogeneity and the pupil for symmetry and size. At rest, a relatively wide pupil is to be expected in veterinary patients, compared with humans, and during examination with the focal light source, the pupil may not constrict as much as expected, even in normal patients, given the sympathetic response that they may display. The presence of a small pupil may indicate a degree of uveitis, whilst an abnormally wide pupil is seen in patients with iris hypoplasia or iris atrophy. The PLR is assessed as described above. The iris and pupil margin are inspected for evidence of irregularity, cystic and colour changes, as well as for iris adhesions to the lens (posterior synechiae) or cornea (anterior synechiae). The position of the lens in the patellar fossa is evaluated and the presence of lento- or iridodonesis is ruled out. Lentodonesis (also termed phacodonesis) describes a subtle wobble of the lens during movement of the globe, whilst iridodonesis describes its counterpart in the iris.

Assessment for lens instability should ideally be carried out later in the course of the ocular examination, following the application of a short-acting mydriatic, specifically to rule out more subtle signs of lens instability, including the presence of a peripheral aphacic crescent or peripheral vitreal herniation (see Chapter 16). The presence of lens opacities is noted and their approximate position is determined using both the parallax technique and their clinical appearance. For example, opacities affecting the anterior lens cortex in the region of the suture lines typically appear as an upright Y, whereas opacities in the region of the posterior suture line appear as an inverted Y.

Ophthalmoscopy

Both direct and indirect ophthalmoscopy techniques are suitable for examination of the fundus in dogs and cats, and both are applied routinely in the same patient because they complement each other (Figure

1.13). Indirect ophthalmic assessment allows the examiner to gain a rapid overview of the patient's fundus and to locate areas of concern, which can then be examined in more detail using the higher magnification provided by direct ophthalmoscopy (see also Chapter 18). In addition, distant direct ophthalmoscopy can be a helpful technique in highlighting lesions of the clear ocular structures of the anterior segment and to distinguish nuclear sclerosis from true cataract formation. Ophthalmoscopes are required for examination of the fundus because they provide the necessary alignment of the examiner's visual axis/axes with the light needed to illuminate this structure, which is otherwise dark as a result of the limited influx of ambient lighting through the small pupillary opening. Ideally, ophthalmoscopy should be carried out following pupil dilation to allow assessment of both the central and peripheral fundus. However, a somewhat more limited view can be obtained without the induction of mydriasis, especially if the lowest possible level of illumination is chosen. In general, the examiner should at all times aim to maintain illumination levels as low as possible because bright light will be perceived as uncomfortable by the patient, resulting in reduced compliance with the fundic examination.

Tropicamide (0.5%) is the drug of choice to induce mydriasis in dogs and cats owing to its rapid onset (usually within 20 minutes) and short duration of action. Tropicamide can significantly increase the IOP in the treated eye and its use must therefore be considered carefully in patients predisposed to glaucoma (Grozdanic *et al.*, 2010; McLellan and Miller, 2011). The use of atropine for this purpose is not recommended because of its long duration (a single application can last up to 5 days). In addition, atropine can cause excessive salivation in feline patients. In some dogs with heavy iris pigmentation and in patients with uveitis or microphthalmos, more than one application of tropicamide may be required to achieve mydriasis and the effect may remain suboptimal.

Direct ophthalmoscopy
A direct ophthalmoscope will be available in almost every veterinary clinic because the instrument is usually supplied in a boxed set together with an otoscope. The direct ophthalmoscope consists of a battery handle with a rheostat and a headpiece (Figure 1.14). This provides the light source and aligns the beam, which is reflected by a mirror via an aperture for viewing along the observer's visual axis. A series of positive and negative lenses can be inserted between the viewer and patient, allowing correction of the refractive error of either; however, no lenses are required to examine the fundus if both the examiner and patient are emmetropic. The lenses can also be used to focus on structures in front of or behind the retina. For example, to focus on the lens in a normal canine eye, a positive (black) +8 to +12 D lens is used, whilst for examination of the ocular surface, a +20 D lens is used. Negative (red) lenses have to be inserted to focus on the floor of an optic nerve coloboma, which is depressed in relation to the retina. For the dog and cat, the specific 'dioptre equivalent' has been established as approximately 0.3–0.4 mm, allowing translation of dioptre values into the actual distance (in mm) by which lesions are elevated or depressed in relation to the retina (Murphy and Howland, 1987) (Figure 1.15).

Feature	Direct ophthalmoscopy	Indirect ophthalmoscopy
Image type	Real	Virtual
Image orientation	Upright	Inverted
Level of magnification	High (up to 15x)	Low (1.3–3x)
Field of view	Narrow	Wide
Penetration of cloudy ocular media	Relatively limited	Relatively good

1.13 Comparison of direct and indirect ophthalmoscopy.

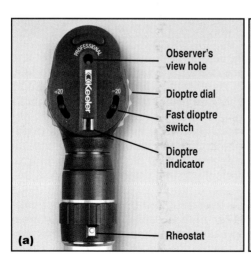
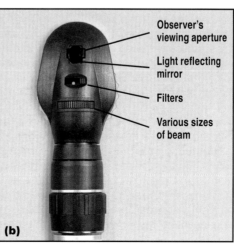

Observer's view hole

Dioptre dial

Fast dioptre switch

Dioptre indicator

Rheostat

(a)

Observer's viewing aperture

Light reflecting mirror

Filters

Various sizes of beam

(b)

1.14
Direct ophthalmoscope headpiece. **(a)** Viewer's side. **(b)** Patient's side with viewing aperture and reflecting mirror, as well as a filter and switches to change the light beam size and shape. (©Willows Referrals)

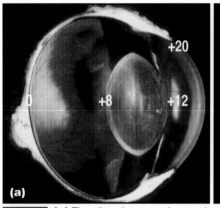
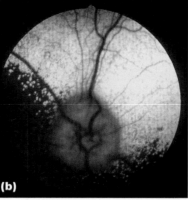
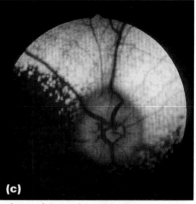

1.15 **(a)** The dioptric strengths required to allow examination of the structures in front of the retina with direct ophthalmoscopy. **(b–c)** In a patient with optic neuritis, the swollen optic nerve head is blurred and the retina is in focus on a setting of 0 D. To focus on the swollen optic nerve head, the examiner must insert positive (black) lenses to move the focus within the eye forward. In this patient, the optic nerve head was in focus at +6 D, which translates into swelling of the optic nerve head of 1.5 mm. (a, Courtesy of J Mould; b–c, ©Willows Referrals)

The examiner should become familiar with both the front and back of the ophthalmoscope head, which usually contains a series of dials or switches to change the size, colour and shape of the light beam as well as a dial to change the lenses that are inserted. For routine fundic examination of patients with pupil dilatation, the widest white light beam is usually chosen, whilst small beams are reserved for patients with small pupils in order to minimize light scattering. The shape of the beam can also be changed to a slit in some models, allowing use of the direct ophthalmoscope as a primitive slit-lamp. The green light beam presents a 'red-free' light, which allows improved visualization of the retinal vasculature and helps distinguish retinal haemorrhage (which appears black) from pigment (which appears brown). The blue light filter on the direct ophthalmoscope can be used to highlight fluorescein staining during corneal assessment.

Distant direct ophthalmoscopy: Initially, the emmetropic examiner should set the direct ophthalmoscope on a full beam at moderate illumination without any lenses inserted. Examiners who wear corrective glasses usually remove these for direct ophthalmoscopy and change the lenses (using the dial on the ophthalmoscope head) according to their prescription. Short-sighted examiners require insertion of negative (red) lenses, whilst long-sighted examiners require insertion of positive (black) lenses. If the examiner does not know their prescription, the dioptre change required to produce emmetropia can be established by trial and error while the ophthalmoscope is directed at a distant object, stopping when the examiner achieves the sharpest image. The examiner then aligns their visual axis with the reflected light by holding the instrument firmly to their temple, looking through the view hole. It is of the utmost importance that the position of the ophthalmoscope in relation to the examiner's head and eye does not change because only in this way can the visual axis and light required for fundic examination be aligned during head movements of the observer. Ideally, the observer's right eye should

be used to examine the patient's right eye, and the observer's left eye should be used to examine the patient's left eye, to prevent the observer's nose being an obstacle.

The patient is gently held by the owner or an assistant and the examiner holds the patient's head at arm's length with their free hand, keeping the eyelids opened. With correct hand position on the patient's head and appropriately low illumination levels, the eyelids can usually be held open by the examiner alone (Figure 1.16); additional opening of the eyelids by an assistant should not be required. The examiner looks for and picks up the bright green or yellow fundic reflex seen in most canine and feline patients; in some pigment-dilute (merle or albino) patients, the fundic reflex is red. Any opacities in the clear ocular media anterior to the retina appear black against the bright background of the fundic reflex.

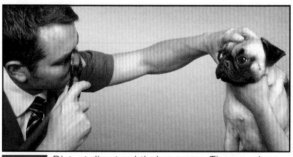

1.16 Distant direct ophthalmoscopy. The examiner picks up the fundic reflex at arm's length. (©Willows Referrals)

The parallax technique can be used to estimate the approximate depth of ocular lesions. With distant direct ophthalmoscopy, it is also possible to distinguish between nuclear sclerosis of the lens (a normal age-related change of the lens with minimal impact on vision) and true cataract formation. A true cataract will stand out as an opacity in front of the fundic reflex (partial cataract) or extinguish it altogether (total or mature cataract), whilst in nuclear sclerosis only subtle ring-shaped refractive changes are visible against the bright fundic reflex (Figure

1.17). At the distance of the outstretched arm, the examiner may be able to pick up the fundic reflection from both eyes at the same time, allowing comparison of pupillary diameters and diagnosis of even subtle degrees of anisocoria.

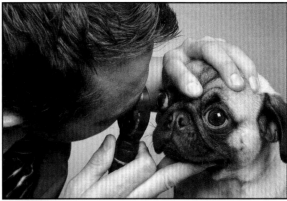

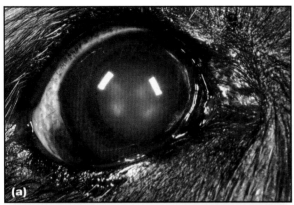

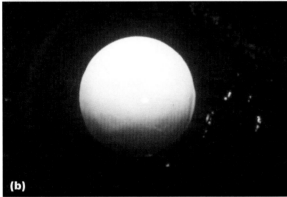

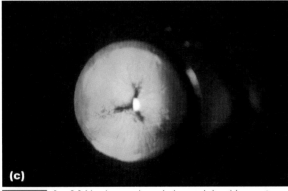

1.17 **(a–b)** Nuclear sclerosis has minimal impact on the visibility of the fundic reflex using distant direct ophthalmoscopy and only subtle concentric rings are visible. **(c)** A cataract stands out as a dark opacity against the fundic reflex. (©Willows Referrals)

Close direct ophthalmoscopy: Having identified the fundic reflex at arm's length with distant direct ophthalmoscopy, the examiner now reduces the light intensity via the rheostat and moves closer to the patient, guided by the fundic reflex, until the ophthalmoscope head almost touches the patient's brow (Figure 1.18). Direct ophthalmoscopy follows the 'key-hole principle', thus the closer the examiner is to the patient's eye, the better and wider the fundic view obtained will be. For the experienced examiner, this will be carried out in one swift motion, whilst for the examiner new to ophthalmoscopy, it may take

1.18 Close direct ophthalmoscopy. The examiner's eye is as close as possible to the patient's eye. (©Willows Referrals)

several attempts to obtain a satisfactory fundic image. The key to success with the procedure is to stop approaching the patient's eye if the fundic reflex has been lost and re-start at arm's length, again picking up the reflex.

Direct ophthalmoscopy provides an upright and magnified fundic image (approximately x15) but only allows assessment of the ocular fundus in small segments. Therefore, the examiner must make every effort not only to assess the optic nerve head and immediate peri-papillary area, but also to move the ophthalmoscope across the retina to obtain a more complete impression of the fundus. It is not important to follow a particular order during fundic assessment, but it is important that the tapetal and non-tapetal fundus, optic nerve head and retinal vasculature are examined in a reproducible and systematic fashion, which is routinely followed by the examiner. Many examiners divide the fundus into segments following initial inspection of the optic nerve head and assess each segment in a clockwise or anticlockwise fashion.

Abnormalities found during the fundic examination should be recorded (either during the assessment or immediately upon completion) on a diagram (Figure 1.19). This also helps the examiner to form a mental composite of the many small images obtained during direct ophthalmoscopy. The Panoptic, a direct ophthalmoscope with unique optics, is preferred by some general practitioners as it combines relative ease of use with a wider field of view and greater magnification than conventional direct ophthalmoscopes.

Following assessment of the fundus and in the absence of a slit-lamp, the examiner may wish to use the direct ophthalmoscope to examine more anterior ocular structures. For this purpose, positive (black) lenses in the region of +8 D to +12 D are inserted for examination of the lens. At a setting of +20 D, examination of the corneal surface, eyelid margins and lacrimal puncta is possible. The level of illumination may need to be increased for examination of the more anterior ocular structures and it must be kept in mind that the level of magnification provided by the direct ophthalmoscope declines rapidly with the insertion of positive (black) lenses, with only x2 magnification provided at the corneal surface.

Date: ....   Owner: ....   Animal: ....   Breed: ....

Client address: ....

....

[ ] Mydriasis   [ ] Gonioscopy   [ ] Other..

Clinical findings:

	Right	Left
PLR – direct		
PLR – consensual	R to L	L to R
Menace response		
Dazzle response		
Tracking		
Maze test		

IOPs (mmHg)   [ ] Tonopen   [ ] Tonovet   R [   ]   L [   ]   STT (mm/min)   R [   ]   L [   ]

Right   Left

P   A   A   P

LENS

FUNDUS

Eye examination record

Photo information	
Owner	
Animal	
Condition	
Date	
Vet	

1.19   Example of an ocular examination chart. (©Willows Referrals)

Indirect ophthalmoscopy

There are two distinct forms of indirect ophthalmoscopy: binocular and monocular. All forms of indirect ophthalmoscopy require a bright focal light source and a hand-held condensing lens. In indirect ophthalmoscopy, a virtual image is formed between the condensing lens and examiner's eye, on which the examiner focuses. The image is inverted and it will take some time for the examiner to get used to the fact that, when determining where a fundic lesion is located, the image has to be mentally turned upside-down and reversed from side-to-side. In contrast to direct ophthalmoscopy, indirect ophthalmoscopy provides a large angle of view of the fundus but little magnification (2–5x). The exact field of view and degree of magnification are dependent on the condensing lens chosen. As a rule of thumb, the higher the dioptre of the lens, the wider the field of view, but the lower the magnification provided (see below).

Binocular indirect ophthalmoscopy: To undertake binocular indirect ophthalmoscopy, a head-mounted indirect ophthalmoscope set is required to bring the visual axis of both the examiner's eyes closer together and align it with light from a halogen or light-emitting diode (LED) source, which is directed towards the fundus of the patient. Light reflected from the fundus is then split via a series of prisms to travel to both of the observer's eyes, thus permitting stereopsis. Modern indirect ophthalmoscopes are head-mounted and wireless (i.e. the battery is included in the head-band) (Figure 1.20). The indirect head-set contains a switch to adjust the intensity of the light level, allows adjustment of the examiner's inter-pupillary distance and has levers to vary the size and quality of the light beam. Some models include a light diffuser, which broadens the illumination beam for enhanced viewing of the peripheral retina. Whilst the visual axis of both eyes must be narrowed optically to allow splitting of the image to provide stereopsis, most head-mounted models strike a balance at the basic setting to preserve as much distance between the visual axes as possible, thus maximizing the degree of stereopsis. However, in some models it is possible to adjust this setting to a minimum to allow examination of the fundus in eyes with small pupils where mydriasis cannot be induced, whilst at the same time retaining some stereopsis. In addition, adaptors can be added to the optics of the head-mounted ophthalmoscope to allow teaching, either via a mirror or digital video; the latter is possible in some models via wireless connections.

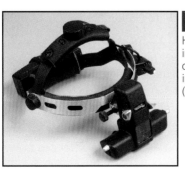

1.20

Head-mounted indirect ophthalmoscope with integrated battery. (©Willows Referrals)

To perform binocular indirect ophthalmoscopy, the examiner adjusts the position of the indirect ophthalmoscope head-set on their head and ensures that the light beam is aligned with their visual axes by observing the projection of light upon a wall. Not having to hold the light source, the examiner has the use of both hands and will usually use one hand to hold and move the patient's head, whilst the other hand is used to hold the condensing lens (Figure 1.21). The examiner picks up the patient's fundic reflex at arm's length with both eyes and then briskly inserts a condensing lens approximately 3–5 cm in front of the patient's eye being examined. The fundic image should now become visible and the lens is gently moved forwards and backwards to allow focusing of the image. Unwanted reflections are eliminated by slightly tilting the lens.

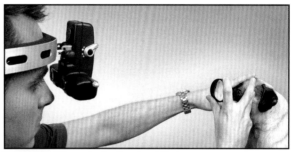

1.21 Binocular indirect ophthalmoscopy. (©Willows Referrals)

Similar to direct ophthalmoscopy, the examiner should halt the procedure if the fundic image is lost, briefly remove the lens, re-focus on the fundic reflex and then reposition the condensing lens in front of the eye. As in direct ophthalmoscopy, the fundus should be assessed in a systematic manner and any anomalies noted should be recorded. To facilitate the correct documentation of retinal lesions in the presence of an inverted image, it may help the examiner to note findings on an examination chart which has been turned upside down. Upon completion of the examination, the chart can be turned upright again and will contain any lesions noted in the correct fundus location.

Monocular indirect ophthalmoscopy: This technique allows fundic examination with minimal investment in ophthalmic equipment because it can be carried out with a simple and cheap plastic condensing lens and a pentorch (Figure 1.22). The image obtained is similar to that observed with binocular

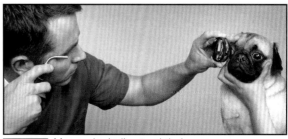

1.22 Monocular indirect ophthalmoscopy. (©Willows Referrals)

indirect ophthalmoscopy, but, in the absence of stereopsis, depth perception will be reduced.

To perform monocular indirect ophthalmoscopy, the observer must first align their visual axis in the eye being used for the examination with that of the light source. This is best achieved by the examiner pressing the light source with one hand against the temple on the side of the eye being used for the examination. This leaves the other hand free to hold the condensing lens, but the examiner will have to rely on the owner or an assistant to steady the patient's head for the procedure. As in binocular ophthalmoscopy, the examiner locates the fundic reflection of the eye to be examined and inserts the condensing lens approximately 3–5 cm in front of the patient's eye.

Condensing lenses: A great variety of condensing lenses for the purpose of indirect ophthalmoscopy are commercially available. The price of a lens is generally governed by the material it is made of (i.e. cheap plastic lenses *versus* expensive glass lenses) and, with regard to glass lenses, by the standard to which it is finished. Advanced lenses are coated to minimize reflections that can hamper fundic examination. Lenses are available with varying dioptric strengths, and 20 or 30 D lenses are most commonly used in veterinary ophthalmology (see Figure 1.4). The refractive power of a lens determines the field of view and level of magnification it provides in a given species; the field of view increases with dioptric strength whilst the level of magnification decreases. In canine and feline patients where mydriasis has been induced successfully, a 20 D lens is suitable, whilst the use of a 30 D lens is recommended for use in patients with small pupils, kittens and puppies. The 2.2 pan-retinal lens provides a maximally enhanced field of view whilst maintaining the level of magnification usually only provided by lower dioptre lenses (Snead *et al.*, 1992).

Slit-lamp examination

The slit-lamp is the most versatile instrument for the veterinary ophthalmologist, allowing detailed examination of the anterior ocular segment with 12–40x magnification under a series of different forms of illumination (Martin, 1969abc; Martonyi *et al.*, 2007). With the help of gonioscopy lenses, the slit-lamp can be used to observe a greatly magnified image of the iridocorneal angle and, with the use of condensing lenses, the slit-lamp can also be used for fundic examination. The slit-lamp is a combination of a biomicroscope with a versatile light source; these are co-pivotal (i.e. they swing on the same axis), confocal (i.e. they focus on the same point) and isocentric (i.e. they centre on the same point). The light beam of the slit-lamp can be modified from a broad, round beam into a thin slit of light, with which the clear anterior ocular media (cornea, anterior chamber, lens and anterior vitreous) can be optically sectioned and examined in great detail.

Hand-held slit-lamps (Figure 1.23) are preferable to table-mounted models for use in veterinary practice and routinely offer levels of magnification

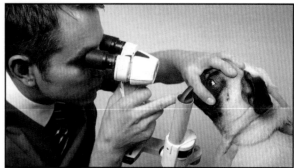

1.23 Hand-held slit-lamps are extremely versatile for the examination of veterinary patients. (©Willows Referrals)

between 10x and 16x. Table-mounted slit-lamps generally include a beam splitter and photographic attachment ports to allow photograph and video documentation, although most newer hand-held models provide the option of digital documentation. Unfortunately, owing to their high cost, slit-lamps are not available in most general practices.

Direct illumination

Full beam: Using a full beam on the slit-lamp with direct illumination provides the examiner with a generalized view of the adnexal and anterior segment structures. The degree of obliquity of the incident light can be varied to enhance the detection of three-dimensional (3D) structures (a similar effect to that seen when viewing features in a landscape – their ease of detection varies depending upon the position of the sun in the sky). The full beam with moderate to high magnification is used to examine for distichiasis and ectopic cilia, as well as punctal anomalies and corneal foreign bodies. Used at high levels of illumination, the slit-lamp is also a useful instrument to test the dazzle reflex (see above).

Slit beam: The slit beam is used to provide more focal illumination and to give an optical section through the clear ocular media of the anterior ocular segment. This allows smaller areas to be concentrated upon in detail and also gives an indication of the depth of lesions within transparent structures such as the cornea or lens. For example, it is possible to determine whether a corneal opacity lies within the stroma or on the endothelium, to estimate the exact depth of a corneal ulcer (which helps determine whether medical or surgical therapy is required) and to pinpoint the location of a lens opacity (which may be important in determining whether the condition is likely to be inherited).

In general, deflection of the slit beam towards the examiner indicates a raised lesion (e.g. an iris mass; Figure 1.24), whereas deflection of the slit beam away from the examiner indicates a defect (e.g. a corneal ulcer; Figure 1.25). The slit beam also enables an estimation of distance and, with practice, the experienced examiner will be able to form a mental reference library of ocular distances in the healthy eye, allowing detection of abnormal distances in the diseased eye. The use of a slit beam, ideally a short

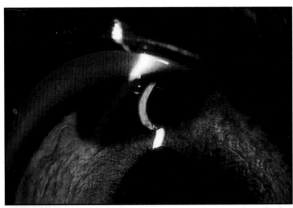

1.24 Slit image deflected towards the examiner in the case of an iris melanoma. (Courtesy of the Animal Health Trust)

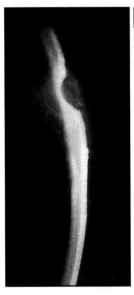

1.25

Slit image deflected away from the examiner in a patient with a stromal corneal ulcer. The degree of slit deflection allows accurate assessment of corneal ulcer depth. (Courtesy of N Wallin Hakansson)

one, is also useful for the detection of aqueous flare because any cells and protein within the normally optically clear aqueous show as a bluish tinge within the slit beam (the Tyndall effect) (Figure 1.26). At high levels of magnification, the examiner may also see cells within the aqueous. Both of these findings can be very helpful when assessing the integrity of the blood–aqueous barrier, for example in the diagnosis and monitoring of uveitis.

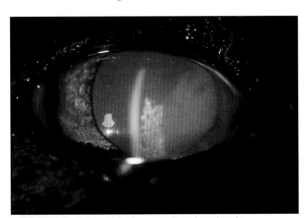

1.26 Protein within the anterior chamber is highlighted by the slit beam of light, showing the Tyndall effect. (Courtesy of the Animal Health Trust)

Retro-illumination

This can be very useful when performing slit beam examination of the eye to observe structures slightly to one side of the slit. These structures are illuminated by light reflected back from intraocular structures such as the iris or fundus. Often very subtle abnormalities (e.g. ghost vessels within the cornea, lens vacuoles) can be seen more readily using this technique (Figure 1.27). In addition, it is useful for assessing the thickness of structures such as the iris or the wall of a potentially cystic lesion (e.g. an iris cyst will be transilluminated by light directed near it and can, therefore, be distinguished from a solid neoplastic lesion such as a melanoma; Figure 1.28). To perform the technique, a thin slit beam is shone through the pupil and the iris or lesion is observed away from the light beam: thin areas can be seen to transilluminate.

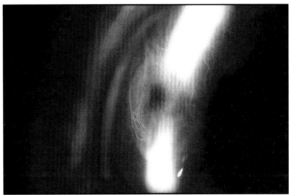

1.27 Subtle corneal lesions are best highlighted with indirect illumination. Note how the corneal ghost vessels are visible in the area adjacent to the directly illuminated cornea. (Courtesy of the Animal Health Trust)

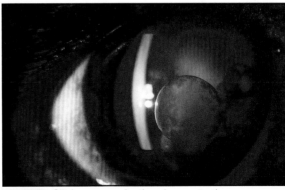

1.28 Slit-lamp examination demonstrating transillumination of iris cysts. (Courtesy of the Animal Health Trust)

External staining techniques

Fluorescein

Fluorescein is an orange water-soluble dye that changes to green in slightly alkaline solutions (i.e. if in contact with the pre-corneal tear film) and fluoresces if excited by blue light. It will adhere to and stain hydrophilic tissues (such as the exposed corneal stroma), but will not adhere to and be washed off hydrophobic tissues (including the intact corneal epithelium or Descemet's membrane).

Fluorescein is widely used in the evaluation of corneal surface health, not only in the detection of frank corneal ulceration but also in the assessment of the tear film break up time (TFBUT) and the Seidel test (see below). In addition, fluorescein is employed to test nasolacrimal system patency in the Jones test (see below).

Fluorescein can be obtained in the form of impregnated strips or in single-use fluid vials, sometimes in combination with local anaesthetic. The strips are preferred because they are less likely to 'overload' the eye with a deluge of fluorescein. Fluorescein in vials is formulated for single-use application because fluorescein solution can harbour serious ocular pathogens such as *Pseudomonas* spp. (Cello and Lasmanis, 1958). The fluorescein strip is wetted with the application of a drop of saline (Figure 1.29) (false tear preparations can be used, but may alter the TFBUT) and then applied carefully to the conjunctiva of the dorsal fornix (the lid is elevated) (Figure 1.30). The strip should *not* touch the cornea itself because this may lead to false-positive areas of stain uptake. Following the application of fluorescein to the conjunctiva, the eyelids are closed in a 'forced' blink motion a couple of times, to distribute the fluorescein over the corneal surface. Fluorescein stain will only be retained by the corneal stroma (Figure 1.31) and not by the epithelium or Descemet's membrane. It is best if viewed when excited with a cobalt blue light (e.g. a Wood's lamp, pentorch, ophthalmoscope or slit-lamp with a blue filter).

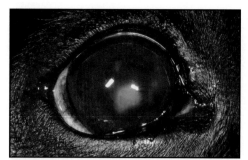

1.31 Exposed corneal stroma taking up the fluorescein stain in a case of superficial ulceration. Note the loose epithelial edges, which indicate the presence of a spontaneous chronic corneal epithelial defect. (©Willows Referrals)

Examination of the corneal surface can now be carried out and any fluorescein staining should be assessed and documented. As a rule of thumb, superficial lesions stain slightly less intensely then stromal lesions (Figure 1.32). In cases of severe stromal degeneration (i.e. melting ulceration), diffusion of the stain throughout large areas of the stroma may be apparent (Figure 1.33). Under-running of the epithelium adjacent to a superficial lesion suggests non-adherence of this epithelium, which is the hallmark of a spontaneous chronic corneal epithelial defect (SCCED) (see Chapter 12). If a visibly deep lesion is present (a crater or an obvious defect with visible walls), care must be taken to assess whether pooling of fluorescein gives the false impression of staining at the bottom of the ulcer. To remove any pooled fluid, the corneal surface should be flushed carefully

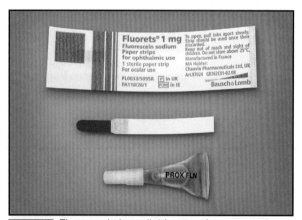

1.29 Fluorescein is available as an impregnated paper strip (top and middle) or as a ready-made solution in a single-use vial (bottom). Note that the paper strip has been wetted with saline and is ready to use. (©Willows Referrals)

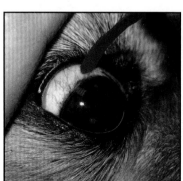

1.30 Fluorescein is applied to the conjunctiva overlying the dorsal sclera. Contact between the strip and cornea should be avoided because this may result in false-positive stain uptake. (©Willows Referrals)

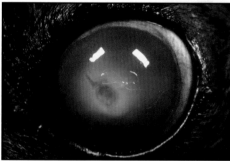

1.32 With this stromal ulcer, fluorescein stain is seen diffusing from the exposed stroma into areas of the cornea which have not yet lost their epithelium. (©Willows Referrals)

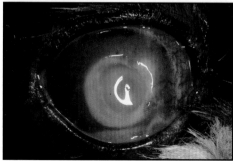

1.33 With melting ulcers, large amounts of fluorescein are retained by the degenerate stromal tissue and the ulcer stains strongly. (©Willows Referrals)

with approximately 5 ml of sterile saline (Figure 1.34). The absence of staining at the bottom of a deep defect indicates the presence of a descemetocele (Figure 1.35). A ring of fluorescein stain uptake around the walls of the lesion is often still present; however, this may be absent in a descemetocele that has epithelialized but remains very fragile.

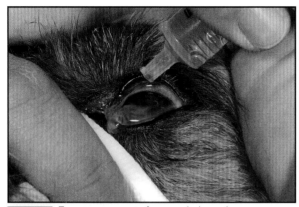

1.34 For assessment of corneal ulceration, particularly deep ulcers where stain might pool and be interpreted as positive stain uptake at the bottom of the ulcer, the stain is flushed out with saline solution. (©Willows Referrals)

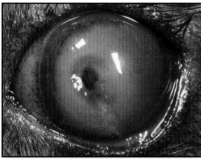

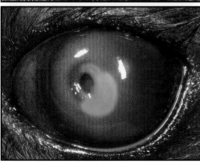

1.35

Descemet's membrane does not retain fluorescein stain, which identifies the deep part of this ulcer as a descemetocele. (©Willows Referrals)

Seidel test: The Seidel test is used to assess whether a full-thickness corneal perforation is leaking aqueous humour or has self-sealed. For this purpose, a generous amount of fluorescein is applied to the affected eye and distributed by a 'forced' blink motion, so that the entire corneal surface is covered with a thin film of green stain. The corneal wound will retain fluorescein, but any aqueous that leaks out of the corneal wound will dilute the film of green stain on the ocular surface as a gradually expanding dark rivulet (Figure 1.36). Gentle pressure can be applied to the globe via the upper eyelid, if the test is initially negative, to determine whether the wound is stable or whether it will open and leak if the IOP increases.

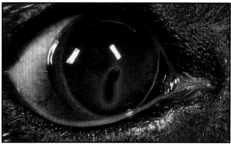

1.36 Fluorescein on the ocular surface is diluted (seen as a dark rivulet) by the aqueous humour escaping from the full-thickness focal corneal perforation in this patient. (©Willows Referrals)

Tear film break up time: Assessment of the TFBUT provides important information about the quality of the pre-corneal tear film. Specifically, conditions that result in poor Meibomian gland function or reduced ocular mucin production have a negative impact on the TFBUT and result in an unstable tear film, which predisposes to the development of corneal ulceration. To measure the TFBUT, fluorescein is applied to the globe and distributed over the ocular surface with a couple of 'forced' blink motions. The eyelids are then held open and the seconds are counted until the uniform layer of stain on the corneal surface starts to break up. The breaking up of the tear film is visible as dark spots on the corneal surface in the area being observed (usually the dorsolateral quadrant is chosen). The TFBUT in the dog has been reported to be on average 20 seconds and in the cat about 17 seconds (Ollivier et al., 2007).

Jones test: The Jones or nasolacrimal passage test is used to test the patency of the nasolacrimal drainage system. A generous amount of fluorescein is applied to the ocular surface and its appearance at the nares is noted (Figure 1.37). In most patients, fluorescein is expected to be visible at the nares within 5–14 minutes (Binder and Herring, 2010). A negative Jones test does not necessarily imply that the nasolacrimal system is blocked because, in some brachycephalic dogs and cats, the nasolacrimal duct has accessory openings in the oropharynx. In such patients it may be helpful to examine the mouth and throat for the presence of fluorescein, which is not always simple to achieve but is aided by the use of a blue light.

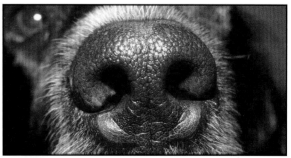

1.37 A negative Jones test result is the failure of fluorescein to appear at the nostril on the ipsilateral side of a nasolacrimal duct blockage, which may indicate lacrimal drainage obstruction. (©Willows Referrals)

Rose Bengal

Rose Bengal stains dead and devitalized cells and is retained in subtle cases of corneal surface disease where the corneal epithelium is only partially eroded and fluorescein would not be retained. The use of Rose Bengal is particularly helpful in conditions such as herpesvirus keratitis, in which, in early dendritic lesions, affected and possibly devitalized cells are still retained in the epithelium and the underlying stroma is not exposed. Rose Bengal is also helpful in the diagnosis of early KCS and qualitative tear film deficiencies, specifically those involving reduced levels of mucins in the tear film.

Fluorescein angiography

This technique is used to highlight fundic lesions that are not visible on ophthalmoscopic examination. Fluorescein dye, which is injected as an intravenous preparation, is imaged as it passes through the fundus and associated ocular tissues: the initial and most diagnostically significant phases occur in a matter of seconds. The fundus is illuminated during this time with light of a specific wavelength that excites fluorescence, which is photographed using a fundus camera (frame rate of 1 photograph/second). The camera is modified with barrier filters so that effectively only the fluorescein is visualized.

Five different phases of fluorescein angiography have been described:

- A choroidal phase
- An arteriolar phase
- An arteriovenous phase
- A venous phase
- A late phase.

In the normal eye, fluorescein does not penetrate the endothelium of retinal or choroidal vessels, but does penetrate the choriocapillaris. In diseased eyes, such as those with hypertensive retinopathy or uveitis, there may be excessive leakage of fluorescein dye, whilst filling defects presenting as hypofluorescence have been described for certain forms of inherited retinal disease. In human medicine, fluorescein angiography is a widely used technique for the diagnosis and monitoring of conditions such as macular degeneration and diabetic retinopathy.

Apart from rare incidences of an anaphylactic reaction to fluorescein, the procedure is established as routine and safe. However, the technique presents several technical difficulties for veterinary ophthalmologists because the tapetum and pigmentation can make recording of the findings challenging. In addition, the patient must be immobile for the crucial first few seconds and the camera must be focused firmly on the fundus during this time. In general, this means that the patient has to undergo sedation or general anaesthesia for the procedure. It is also questionable whether the findings on fluorescein angiography would be likely to have a significant impact on the clinical management of the veterinary patient, given that most dogs and cats with retinal disease are presented late in the course of the condition. At this point, the lesions are rarely so subtle that fluorescein angiography would be required to detect them. Considering these facts and the cost of the necessary equipment, it is likely that fluorescein angiography will remain largely restricted to research in veterinary ophthalmology.

Tonometry

Measurement of IOP is essential in the detection and management of canine and feline glaucoma, as well as a helpful tool in the management of uveitis in these species. Accurate assessment of IOP is only possible with tonometry; manual estimation is not reliable in veterinary patients. The IOP in the majority of non-glaucomatous canine and feline patients measures between 10 and 25 mmHg (mean values of 15–18 mmHg and 17–19 mmHg have been reported for the dog and cat, respectively) (Gum *et al.*, 2007; McLellan and Miller, 2011). A variety of different tonometers are available to measure IOP.

Schiøtz tonometry

A Schiøtz tonometer is the minimum that should be available in any clinic to assess IOP. This instrument is relatively cheap, but it has to be assembled and is cumbersome to use. Unfortunately, this often results in it rusting away in a cupboard. In addition, if its use has not been practised with normal eyes, it may be hard to obtain meaningful readings in the stressful situation when a patient presents with acute glaucoma. The Schiøtz tonometer works by indenting the corneal surface with a small plunger that protrudes from a footplate, which is rested gently and repeatedly on the corneal surface. The measurements are carried out under topical anaesthesia, but the cornea must be in a horizontal position to obtain readings (Figure 1.38). This usually requires elevation of the patient's head and it is of the utmost importance that no pressure is placed on the jugular veins, because this results in spuriously high readings. The plunger indenting the cornea is connected to an indicator, which points at a scale. These scale readings are not actual IOP measurements, but can be converted using a chart into actual IOP measurements in mmHg. The Schiøtz tonometer is of limited use in patients with severely ulcerated corneas or corneas with extensive surface pathology (e.g. granulation tissue formation).

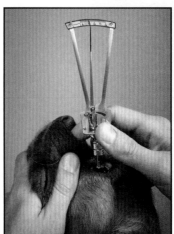

1.38
Schiøtz tonometry. Note how the head of the patient is held by the assistant to maintain the cornea in a horizontal plane without excessive pressure on the neck. (©Willows Referrals)

Applanation tonometry

The Tono-pen XL™/Tono-pen Vet is a digital applanation tonometer, which converts the force required to applanate (i.e. flatten) a small area of cornea into a digital IOP value. The instrument is easy to use and owing to its small footplate it is suitable for both small and large animals (Ollivier *et al.*, 2007). Physiological IOP ranges measured with the Tono-pen have been reported for many species. The Tono-pen is also hardwearing and reliable; the only practical drawbacks are its price and its possible negative effect on corneal health, especially if used too frequently or roughly. The Tono-pen can be used to measure IOP with the animal in any position (elevation of the head is not required to bring the cornea into a horizontal position), but an effort must still be made to not place pressure on the neck, eyelids or globe of the patient because this could result in a falsely high reading. A small disposable rubber tip cover, which must be changed between patients, protects the fine electronic footplate of the Tono-pen from corrosion and contamination, and also helps to prevent the transfer of infectious agents between patients. The tip cover must be neither too tight nor too loose, to ensure that the tonometer works correctly (Figure 1.39).

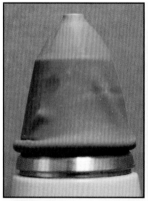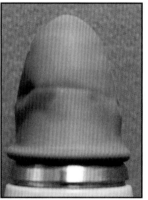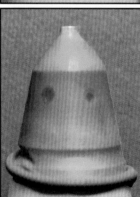

1.39 Incorrect placement of the rubber tip cover on the Tono-pen can make it difficult to obtain reproducible measurements. The cover should be a snug fit (top left) but not be too loose (top right) or too tight (bottom left). (©Willows Referrals)

The Tono-pen must be calibrated at least once daily and this is usually recommended prior to initial use. For this procedure, the instrument is activated (the black button is pressed quickly three times) whilst being held vertically with the tip down and, when prompted by the display, turned upwards until the digital display shows 'good'. The appearance of 'bad' during use of the instrument does not indicate an abnormal IOP but rather indicates that re-calibration is required. Prior to use of the Tono-pen, topical anaesthetic (proxymetacaine) is applied to the eye. The instrument is activated by a short push on the black button and the tip is then gently touched in small and rapid movements on the surface of the cornea to achieve a light contact (Figure 1.40). The corneal surface should not be indented. A short 'beep' indicates that a reading has been successfully obtained. A number of successful readings (indicated by short 'beeps') are registered and displayed as a final averaged result, indicated by a long 'beep'. Together with the averaged reading of IOP, the Tono-pen displays the statistical reliability of the measurement: only readings with a coefficient of variation of <10% should be considered.

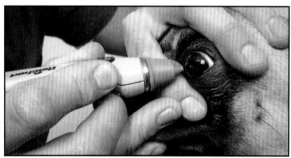

1.40 To obtain IOP measurements, the Tono-pen is gently touched in small and rapid movements on the surface of the cornea, following the application of local anaesthetic. Care must be taken not to apply pressure to the globe when keeping the eyelids open as this could result in falsely elevated IOP readings. (©Willows Referrals)

Rebound tonometry

The TonoVet™ is another digital tonometer, which measures the speed with which a small, magnetized probe that is 'shot' out of a sleeve towards the corneal surface is decelerated upon impact before returning back to its sleeve (rebound tonometry) (Figure 1.41). Eyes with a higher IOP have a faster deceleration and more rapid return of the probe into the sleeve than eyes with a low IOP. The measurement is converted into a digital reading in mmHg.

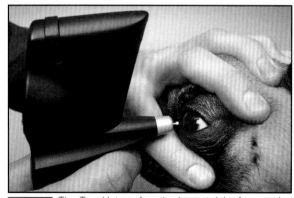

1.41 The TonoVet confers the lowest risk of corneal damage, which may be of importance in brachycephalic patients and those with corneal disease. As with the Tono-pen, care must be taken not to apply pressure to the globe when opening the eyelids. (©Willows Referrals)

To use the TonoVet, the instrument is activated by pressure on the 'measurement button', a species calibration is chosen ('d' for both dogs and cats) and a disposable probe is inserted into the opening at the tip. The button is pressed again, magnetizing the tip, visible as several short oscillations, which prevents it from falling out. The instrument is then held at a distance of approximately 4–8 mm from the central cornea and a series of six readings is taken by briefly pressing the measurement button, which results in the tip being 'shot' at the central cornea. Each successful measurement is accompanied by a short audible beep, whilst erroneous readings are accompanied by a double beep. After the sixth successful reading has been obtained, a prolonged beep is emitted as an audible indication that the test is completed.

This instrument is extremely easy to use, has minimal potential to cause corneal injury and can be used in a range of small and large animals but, to date, only calibrations for the eyes of dogs/cats and horses are available. The disadvantage is that it must be held in an upright position with the probe propelled horizontally, which makes its use in recumbent animals difficult. The TonoVet might be more accurate than other methods in determining IOP in cats and its advantages include the fact that the application of topical anaesthetic is not required prior to use (Rusanen *et al.*, 2010; McLellan and Miller, 2011).

Gonioscopy

Gonioscopy is the procedure used to assess the physical appearance of the entrance to the iridocorneal angle. In the dog, it is not possible to visualize the iridocorneal angle with the naked eye because it is obscured by the scleral shelf. To overcome this, a gonioscopy lens is applied to the corneal surface under topical anaesthesia, changing the cornea-to-air interface to a cornea-to-lens interface, which in turn changes the refractive index slightly and allows light rays from the iridocorneal angle to pass into the examiner's eye. In addition to making visualization of the iridocorneal angle possible, direct gonioscopy lenses (which include the commonly used Koeppe and Barkan lenses) provide x2–3 magnification. The examiner usually uses a slit-lamp or a direct ophthalmoscope to illuminate and magnify the area to be examined.

Gonioscopy reveals whether the entrance to the iridocorneal angle is open, narrow or closed, and the examiner can assess both the pectinate ligament, which spans the angle, and the width of the angle opening. Gonioscopy is an essential tool for the diagnosis and management of canine glaucoma. However, often the procedure cannot be carried out in the affected eye because of corneal pathology. In these cases, information about the state of the iridocorneal angle in the contralateral eye is obtained to allow inferences to be made about the aetiology of the glaucomatous state on the affected side. Dysplasia of the pectinate ligament is a commonly used marker for inherited forms of glaucoma and the identification of goniodysgenesis is a firm part of the BVA/KCS/ISDS scheme, which aims to reduce the incidence of inherited forms of closed-angle glaucoma (see Chapters 4 and 15).

In the cat, it is possible to visualize the iridocorneal angle without the use of a lens by observing the eye at an angle with a bright light. However, glaucoma due to goniodysgenesis is a rare occurrence in the cat. Gonioscopy is a challenging procedure and substantial experience is required to ensure accurate interpretation of the findings. For this reason, gonioscopy is largely reserved for ophthalmic specialist practice (see Chapter 15).

Retinoscopy

Retinoscopy is the technique employed to objectively determine the refractive state of the eye. The procedure allows the examiner to evaluate whether a patient is:

* Emmetropic (normal sighted)
* Myopic (near- or short-sighted)
* Hyperopic (far- or long-sighted)
* Astigmatic (has variation in refraction between different corneal quadrants).

Retinoscopy is carried out in the conscious patient using a retinoscope (which has a similar appearance to a hand-held direct ophthalmoscope) and a set of positive and negative lenses of varying dioptric power (termed a skiaskopy rack) (Figure 1.42). Most normal dogs have been found to be within 1 D of emmetropia (Kubai *et al.*, 2008), although myopia has been reported with a familial incidence in some large working breeds, including the Rottweiler, Labrador Retriever and German Shepherd Dog (Murphy *et al.*, 1992; Black *et al.*, 2008).

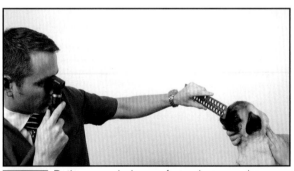

1.42 Retinoscopy being performed on a canine patient. (©Willows Referrals)

With foldable lens replacements being used routinely following phacoemulsification in both dogs and cats, assessment of the refractive state of the phacic and pseudo-phacic patient is now an established part of the ocular examination process in veterinary ophthalmic referral practice (Gift *et al.*, 2009). Retinoscopy can also be used to investigate reported visual deficits in otherwise ophthalmoscopically normal patients and to evaluate performance problems in working dogs (Murphy *et al.*, 1997). Retinoscopy is not a tool that would be expected to be employed in general practice, but the practitioner should be aware of its availability.

Electroretinography

Electroretinography is used to study light potentials produced by the retina and provides a measure of retinal function (Komaromy *et al.*, 1998ab; Narfstrom *et al.*, 2002). Electroretinography is commonly performed in specialist referral practice prior to cataract surgery because it can confirm the existence of retinal function in patients where fundic assessment is not possible due to the extent of lens opacification. Electroretinography is also used to investigate cases of blindness (often of sudden onset) where the fundus is ophthalmoscopically normal (e.g. sudden acquired retinal degeneration syndrome and optic neuritis). The value of electroretinography in the early detection of inherited forms of retinal degeneration, such as generalized progressive retinal atrophy, is diminishing with the rapidly increasing availability of DNA tests to diagnose specific conditions.

To record an electroretinogram, electrodes are placed at set positions on and around the eye, the patient is acclimatized to pre-defined lighting conditions and the retina is subjected to a variety of light stimuli, which differ in intensity, frequency and duration. The resultant electrical potentials are amplified and recorded as waves, which can be stored electronically and interpreted according to their amplitudes and implicit times. A crude assessment of photopic retinal function can be obtained in most patients with electroretinography performed under only light sedation, but more detailed electroretinographic studies (e.g. those required to detect early cases of retinal degeneration) necessitate deep sedation or anaesthesia.

Different forms of electroretinography are available to test specific structures of the fundus:

- Flash electroretinography is used to quantify photoreceptor function
- Pattern electroretinography can be used to investigate the function of retinal ganglion cells in the inner retina in glaucomatous conditions
- With the placement of additional electrodes in the skin over areas of the visual cortex and the use of specifically designed stimulation protocols, the central visual pathways can also be assessed by recording visual evoked potentials (VEPs).

However, the latter two techniques remain largely reserved for research purposes (for further details on electroretinography, the reader is referred to Chapter 18).

Nasolacrimal system patency

In addition to the Jones test, the patency of the nasolacrimal duct system can be assessed by cannulation and flushing via both the upper and lower nasolacrimal puncta. This procedure is described in more detail in Chapter 10.

Ocular centesis

The analysis of aqueous and vitreous samples can provide vital clues in the investigation of ocular conditions for which the examiner has not been able to establish a diagnosis by other clinical means. Aqueous and vitreous samples can be submitted for protein level assessment, cytology, culture, antibody testing and DNA analysis (as discussed in greater detail in Chapter 3). These tests can be instrumental in differentiating neoplastic conditions (e.g. ocular lymphoma), infectious diseases (e.g. bacterial endophthalmitis or toxoplasmosis) and sterile inflammatory conditions (e.g. uveodermatological syndrome). In addition, therapeutic drugs such as fibrinolytics and steroids can be delivered to the anterior or vitreal chamber.

However, the removal of a small sample of aqueous (termed aqueocentesis) or vitreous (termed vitreocentesis or hyalocentesis) is a highly invasive procedure with potentially severe complications if performed incorrectly. Even when performed by experienced veterinary ophthalmologists, these procedures routinely cause breakdown of the blood–aqueous barrier and result in at least temporary uveal inflammation, which could complicate an existing case of uveitis (Allbaugh *et al.*, 2011). Inflamed eyes can respond to centesis with spontaneous intraocular haemorrhage. Inadvertent injury to the lens can result in cataract formation and phacoclastic uveitis. To perform aqueocentesis or vitreocentesis, bright illumination and magnification must be available. The patient must be deeply sedated or anaesthetized because inadvertent movement when the needle has entered the eye could have catastrophic results.

Aqueocentesis

The patient is usually placed in lateral recumbency with the eye from which the sample is to be obtained uppermost. The head of the patient is positioned so that the ocular surface is approximately horizontal, the eye is aseptically prepared with a 1:50 preparation of povidone–iodine solution, draped and 2–3 drops of local anaesthetic are applied over 1–2 minutes. The surgeon's hands should be scrubbed and sterile gloves should be worn. A speculum is placed to keep the eyelids open and the conjunctiva is grasped with fine-toothed forceps. Usually, the dorsolateral quadrant is chosen for the procedure because access to the globe here is the least restricted by the eyelids and orbital bones.

Using a 27 or 30 gauge needle on a 1 ml syringe, in which the plunger has been mobilized and primed, the globe is entered 1–2 mm posterior to the limbus through the conjunctiva and sclera in a transverse, slightly tunnelling fashion. The needle tip enters the anterior chamber just 1–2 mm on the corneal side of the limbus. The needle tip should be positioned in front of the iris and advanced in a plane parallel to it, avoiding contact with and damage to the iris and lens (Figure 1.43). Once the position of the needle tip within the anterior chamber has been ascertained, the plunger is very slowly drawn back until 0.1–0.2 ml of aqueous appears in the syringe.

For this procedure, it may be helpful to have an assistant who watches the position of the syringe plunger and updates the surgeon on the volume of aqueous that has been aspirated, so that the

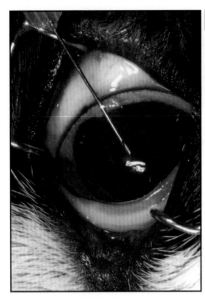

1.43

Correct placement of the needle for aqueocentesis. (©Willows Referrals)

surgeon does not have to move their eyes from the tip of the needle within the anterior chamber. Once an adequate volume of aqueous has been obtained and any therapeutic drugs have been delivered, the needle is slowly withdrawn from the eye and the conjunctiva overlying the scleral perforation site is pinched with the forceps and compressed briefly to give stability to the needle tract, which should be self-sealing.

Vitreocentesis

The patient and surgeon are prepared and positioned as described for aqueocentesis. When entering the globe to obtain a vitreous sample, the needle puncture site must be accurately located at the pars plana of the ciliary body to minimize damage to the posterior segment. If the needle is placed too far forward (towards the limbus) the lens may be injured, resulting in cataract formation and possibly phacoclastic uveitis, or the pars plicata of the ciliary body may be damaged, leading to potentially severe intraocular haemorrhage. If the needle is placed too far posteriorly, the retina can be damaged. Guides to the position of the pars plana of the ciliary body have been published for the dog and in the dorsolateral quadrant they are located 7 mm posterior to the limbus (Smith *et al.*, 1997). Using a 25–27 gauge needle, which has been attached firmly to a 1 ml syringe, the vitreal cavity is entered using a slight 'drilling' motion. The tip of the needle must be directed towards the posterior pole to avoid the large canine lens. Once within the vitreal cavity, 0.1–0.3 ml of liquefied vitreous is withdrawn, any therapeutic drugs are delivered, and the needle is then slowly withdrawn. This technique is usually restricted to globes that have been therapy-resistant and carry little hope for vision. Vitreocentesis should under ideal circumstances only by carried out by veterinary ophthalmologists.

Sample processing

Aqueous and vitreous samples are placed either into a pipette for cytospin or into a plain sterile container for direct smears, serology, culture or PCR analysis. Aqueous and vitreous humours are considered to be fluids of low cellularity and are unlikely to clot even in conditions that result in increased protein content. It is not recommended to place aqueous samples into containers containing ethylene diamine tetra-acetic acid (EDTA), with the possible exception of paediatric EDTA tubes, because the samples are usually much smaller than required for the amount of EDTA in the tube and cellular damage might result. EDTA tubes are also not suitable for samples intended for microbiological culture.

References and further reading

Allbaugh RA, Roush JK, Rankin AJ and Davidson HJ (2011) Fluorophotometric and tonometric evaluation of ocular effects following aqueocentesis performed with needles of various sizes in dogs. *American Journal of Veterinary Research* **72**, 556–561

Barnett KC, Sansom J and Heinrich C (2002) Examination of the eye and adnexa. In: *Canine Ophthalmology: An Atlas and Text,* ed. KC Barnett *et al.*, pp. 1–8. Saunders Ltd, London

Binder DR and Herring IP (2010) Evaluation of nasolacrimal fluorescein transit time in ophthalmically normal dogs and non-brachycephalic cats. *American Journal of Veterinary Research* **71**(5), 570–574

Black J, Browning SR, Collins AV and Phillips JR (2008) A canine model of inherited myopia: familial aggregation of refractive error in Labrador Retrievers. *Investigative Ophthalmology and Visual Science* **49**, 4784–4789

Cello RM and Lasmanis J (1958) *Pseudomonas* infection of the eye of the dog resulting from the use of contaminated fluorescein solution. *Journal of the American Veterinary Medical Association* **132**, 297–299

Champagne ES and Pickett JP (1995) The effect of topical 0.5% proparacaine HCl on corneal and conjunctival culture results. *Transactions of the American College of Veterinary Ophthalmology* **26**, 144–145

Crispin SM (2004) Examination of the eye and adnexa. In: *Equine Ophthalmology: An Atlas and Text, 2nd edn,* ed. KC Barnett *et al.,* pp. 1–13. Saunders Ltd, London

Ghaffari MS, Malmasi A and Bokaie S (2010) Effect of acepromazine or xylazine on tear production as measured by Schirmer tear test in normal cats. *Veterinary Ophthalmology* **13**, 1–3

Gift BW, English RV, Nadelstein B, Weigt AK and Gilger BC (2009) Comparison of capsular opacification and refractive status after placement of three different intraocular lens implants following phacoemulsification and aspiration of cataracts in dogs. *Veterinary Ophthalmology* **12**, 13–21

Grozdanic SD, Kecova H, Harper MM, Nilaweera W, Kuehn MH and Kardon RH (2010) Functional and structural changes in a canine model of hereditary primary angle-closure glaucoma. *Investigative Ophthalmology and Visual Science* **51**, 255–263

Gum GG, Gelatt KN and Esson D (2007) Physiology of the eye. In: *Veterinary Ophthalmology,* ed. KN Gelatt, pp. 14–182. Blackwell Publishing, Iowa

Herring IP, Pickett JP, Champagne ES and Marini M (2000) Evaluation of aqueous tear production in dogs following general anesthesia. *Journal of the American Animal Hospital Association* **36**, 427–430

Hofmeister EH, Weinstein WL, Burger D *et al.* (2009) Effects of graded doses of propofol for anesthesia induction on cardiovascular parameters and intraocular pressures in normal dogs. *Veterinary Anaesthesia and Analgesia* **36**, 442–448

Hofmeister EH, Williams CO, Braun C and Moore PA (2008) Propofol *versus* thiopental: effects on peri-induction intraocular pressures in normal dogs. *Veterinary Anaesthesia and Analgesia* **35**, 275–281

Ketring KL and Glaze MB (2012) *Atlas of Feline Ophthalmology, 2nd edn.* Wiley & Sons, West Sussex

Komaromy AM, Smith PJ and Brooks DE (1998a) Electroretinography in dogs and cats. Part I. Retinal morphology and physiology. *Compendium on Continuing Education for the Practicing Veterinarian* **20**, 343–345 and 348–350

Komaromy AM, Smith PJ and Brooks DE (1998b) Electroretinography in dogs and cats. Part II. Technique, interpretation, and indications. *Compendium on Continuing Education for the Practicing Veterinarian* **20**, 355–359 and 362–366

Kubai MA, Bentley E, Miller PE, Mutti DO and Murphy CJ (2008) Refractive states of eyes and association between ametropia and breed in dogs. *American Journal of Veterinary Research* **69**, 946–951

Maggs DJ (2008) Basic diagnostic techniques. In: *Slatter's Fundamentals of Veterinary Ophthalmology, 4th edn*, ed. DJ Maggs *et al.*, pp. 81–106. Saunders Elsevier, St Louis

Martin CL (1969a) Slit lamp examination of the normal canine anterior ocular segment. I. Introduction and technique. *Journal of Small Animal Practice* **10**, 143–149

Martin CL (1969b) Slit lamp examination of the normal canine anterior ocular segment. II. Description. *Journal of Small Animal Practice* **10**, 151–162

Martin CL (1969c) Slit lamp examination of the normal canine anterior ocular segment. III. Discussion and summary. *Journal of Small Animal Practice* **10**, 163–169

Martin CL (2005) Anamnesis and the ophthalmic examination. In: *Ophthalmic Disease in Veterinary Medicine*, ed. CL Martin CL, pp.11–10. Manson Publishing Ltd, London

Martonyi CL, Bahn CF and Meyer RF (2007) *Clinical Slit Lamp Biomicroscopy and Photo Slit Lamp Biomicrography.* Time One Ink, Michigan

McLellan GJ and Miller PE (2011) Feline glaucoma – a comprehensive review. *Veterinary Ophthalmology* **14**(Suppl 1), 15–29

Murphy CJ and Howland HC (1987) The optics of comparative ophthalmoscopy. *Vision Research* 27, 599–607

Murphy CJ, Mutti DO, Zadnik K and ver Hoeve J (1997) Effect of optical defocus on visual acuity in dogs. *American Journal of Veterinary Research* **58**, 414–418

Murphy CJ, Zadnik K and Mannis MJ (1992) Myopia and refractive error in dogs. *Investigative Ophthalmology and Visual Science* **33**, 2459–2463

Narfstrom K, Ekesten B, Rosolen SG *et al.* (2002) Guidelines for clinical electroretinography in the dog. *Documenta Ophthalmologica* **105**, 83–92

Ollivier FJ, Plummer CE and Barrie KP (2007) Ophthalmic examination and diagnostics. Part 1: The eye examination and diagnostic procedures. In: *Veterinary Ophthalmology*, ed. KN Gelatt, pp. 438–483. Blackwell Publishing, Iowa

Rusanen E, Florin M, Hassig M and Spiess BM (2010) Evaluation of a rebound tonometer (Tonovet) in clinically normal cat eyes. *Veterinary Ophthalmology* **13**, 31–36

Sanchez RF, Mellor D and Mould J (2006) Effects of medetomidine and medetomidine-butorphanol combination on Schirmer tear test 1 readings in dogs. *Veterinary Ophthalmology* **9**, 33–37

Smith PJ, Pennea L, Mackay EO and Mames RN (1997) Identification of sclerotomy sites for posterior segment surgery in the dog. *Veterinary and Comparative Ophthalmology* **7**, 180–189

Snead MP, Rubinstein MP and Jacobs PM (1992) The optics of fundus examination. *Survey of Ophthalmology* **36**, 439–445

2

Diagnostic imaging of the eye and orbit

Ruth Dennis, Philippa J. Johnson and Gillian J. McLellan

The first step in clinical evaluation of the eye involves direct ophthalmic examination (see Chapter 1). However, there are occasions when significant extraocular disease or opacification of ocular media prevent direct visualization of intraocular structures. In addition, orbital disease often gives rise to ocular signs and this area cannot be directly visualized. Under these circumstances, diagnostic imaging provides valuable information about the extent and character of the disease process. Some indications for diagnostic imaging of the eye and orbit are given in Figure 2.1.

Indications for ocular imaging
• Eyelid and periocular swelling obscuring the eye • Opacity of ocular media (cornea, aqueous humour, lens, vitreous) • Assessment of globe integrity (suspected rupture) • Congenital abnormality (e.g. multiple ocular defects) • Measurement of globe dimensions (biometry) • Localization of ocular foreign body
Indications for orbital imaging
• Exophthalmos • Strabismus • Enophthalmos • Third eyelid protrusion • Orbital trauma • Pain on opening the mouth • Known or suspected orbital foreign body • Suspected optic nerve disease • Chronic or recurrent epiphora • Suspected involvement in nasal, maxillary, dental or frontal sinus disease • Facial deformity (e.g. swelling, involving the periocular region)

2.1 Indications for diagnostic imaging of the eye and orbit.

Imaging tools available to veterinary clinicians include radiography (plain and contrast), ultrasonography, magnetic resonance imaging (MRI) and computed tomography (CT). Each of these modalities has advantages and limitations (Figure 2.2), and often the combined findings of two or more modalities are of greater diagnostic value than those from a single technique alone. Whilst ultrasonography is usually the logical choice for ocular diseases, deciding which technique to employ first for the investigation of orbital disease can be challenging and there is no definitive sequence of work-up that is universally applicable. Factors to consider include the ease, accessibility and cost of the technique, the most likely diagnosis, the treatment choices, the animal's temperament and the owner's wishes. For example, in an older dog with slowly progressive and non-painful exophthalmos in which neoplasia is a likely cause, radiography of the skull may be the most practical initial study in a general practice setting and also permits a thoracic metastasis check. In contrast, in a young animal with acute onset of painful exophthalmos and periocular swelling, findings of an ultrasonographic examination may support a diagnosis of retrobulbar abscess when radiographs would probably be normal. Advanced cross-sectional imaging techniques (CT and MRI) are increasingly available via referral, even if not available on-site, and are likely to yield far more information than radiography or ultrasonography. Whilst diagnostic imaging may not provide a definitive diagnosis, imaging findings may aid in the formulation of a ranked list of differential diagnoses and allow planning for further investigation or treatment, when taken into consideration along with the signalment of the patient, their clinical history and concurrent clinical signs.

Radiography	
Advantages	**Limitations**
• Readily accessible • Relatively cheap • Familiarity with use • Shows orbital bony changes • Shows other areas of the head • Thoracic and abdominal metastasis check	• Usually requires general anaesthesia or heavy sedation (although it can then be combined with other procedures, e.g. biopsy or nasolacrimal duct flushing) • Can be time-consuming • Superimposition of structures and conformational variability of this area complicate radiographic interpretation • Provides little or no information about soft tissues or precise extent of lesions involving bone. Cannot differentiate between solid soft tissue and fluid (e.g. in frontal sinus) • Of no value for evaluation of the eye itself • Contrast studies can be technically demanding

2.2 Advantages and limitations of different imaging modalities. (continues) ▶

Ultrasonography	
Advantages	*Limitations*
• Often available • Relatively cheap • Quick to perform • Can usually be performed in conscious patients • Versatile – many ocular and orbital indications • Permits ultrasound-guided techniques (e.g. biopsy) • Abdominal metastasis check possible	• Operator-dependent; requires practice and skill • High-quality transducers required • Diffuse pathology may be hard to recognize (compared with focal lesions) • May be non-specific (e.g. intraocular neoplasia and blood clots can have identical appearance) • Images are confined to globe and orbit and do not show other areas of the head • Static saved images are often less useful than those of other imaging techniques (although, when available, the ability to save dynamic sequences may be advantageous)

Magnetic resonance imaging	
Advantages	*Limitations*
• Superb soft tissue definition and contrast with considerable information about bone; ready differentiation between fluid and solid tissue • 'Slice' images can be obtained in any plane, yielding three-dimensional (3D) information and abolishing superimposition • Provides information about the nature of the tissues (e.g. fluid, fat) • Accurate patient positioning is not crucial • Shows other areas of the head and the brain in excellent detail • Contrast studies are easily performed and provide excellent information about the vascularity of tissues • Allows 3D treatment planning for surgery or radiotherapy • Usually the technique of choice for orbital disease	• May not be readily accessible to practitioners • Requires general anaesthesia and, with high field systems, requires MRI-compatible anaesthetic equipment • Expensive • Time-consuming, especially with low field magnets • Difficult to design set protocols due to the variability of lesions • Can be challenging to interpret • Non-diagnostic or even contraindicated in the presence of ferrous metallic foreign bodies; may be non-diagnostic with certain ocular or orbital prostheses • Does not provide metastasis check • Guided biopsy requires specialist equipment

Computed tomography	
Advantages	*Limitations*
• Superb bony detail and provides fair soft tissue information (superior to radiography) • Quicker than MRI and radiography and thus safer for trauma patients • Can be performed under sedation and general anaesthesia is not necessarily required • Slice images can be obtained, primarily in the transverse plane • Contrast studies are easily performed • Allows 3D treatment planning for surgery or radiotherapy; reconstructed 3D images are very helpful for evaluation of bone • Shows other areas of the head, beyond the orbit • Guided biopsy may be possible • Metastasis check possible and more sensitive than radiography	• May not be readily accessible • Usually requires heavy sedation or general anaesthesia • Expensive • Exposure to higher doses of ionizing radiation than with radiography means that personnel should not usually be present in the CT room during the study • Accurate patient positioning is necessary as images are only acquired transverse to the gantry • Images reconstructed in other planes are inferior • Inferior to MRI for information on the soft tissues, including the brain • Diffuse inflammation may be hard to detect • Streak artefacts arise with metallic foreign bodies • Can be challenging to interpret

2.2 (continued) Advantages and limitations of different imaging modalities.

Radiography

Radiography is unhelpful for the investigation of eye disease, other than for suspected radiopaque ocular foreign bodies, but may be useful in cases of orbital disease (see Figure 2.1). When other imaging techniques are not readily available, radiography is often the first line of investigation. Orbital clinical signs may arise from primary orbital disease processes or as a result of extension of lesions from the nasal cavity, frontal sinuses, calvarium, maxillae, teeth or temporomandibular joints, and all of these areas are amenable to radiographic investigation. However, there are a number of important limitations of plain film radiography of this area (see Figure 2.2), not least that pathology confined to the soft tissues of the orbit will not result in any radiographic changes other than possible soft tissue swelling.

General anaesthesia or heavy sedation is usually required to permit accurate positioning and eliminate the need for manual restraint, although in a patient with marked deformity of the area, a lesion-oriented oblique view may be possible in a conscious patient. Thoracic radiographs should also be obtained in cases of suspected orbital or ocular neoplasia and for trauma patients. A thorough metastasis check also requires abdominal imaging.

Radiographic views

Several radiographic views are useful for the evaluation of the orbit and surrounding areas. These include the dorsoventral (DV) or ventrodorsal (VD), laterolateral, right and left lateral oblique, rostrocaudal (RCd), open-mouth angled VD, intraoral of the nasal cavities and special views for the temporomandibular joints and teeth. For further detailed description of positioning and interpretation, readers are referred to the *BSAVA Manual of Canine and Feline Radiography and Radiology: A Foundation Manual.*

Normal radiographic appearance

Radiographic atlases should be consulted for the normal appearance of the orbital area on lateral and DV radiographs (bordered mainly by the frontal, zygomatic, maxillary and palatine bones).

Radiographic interpretation

Radiographs of the orbital area can be complex to interpret due to the superimposition of structures and the wide variation in conformation of the head, especially in dogs. Knowledge of radiographic anatomy and variants is necessary and is aided by bone specimens, radiographic atlases and a library of previous radiographic studies. It is helpful to compare the two sides in order to detect deviation from normal anatomy. The absence of radiographic changes is a useful sign since it may help to rule out some potential diagnoses and supports the use of advanced imaging as a further diagnostic tool.

Radiographic findings in orbital disease include:

- Soft tissue swelling (non-specific)
- Osteolysis (frontal bone, maxilla, zygoma, cribriform plate, calvarium, sphenoid bones, temporomandibular joint). This feature suggests an aggressive disease process such as malignant neoplasia or advanced osteomyelitis
- Opacification of normally air-filled spaces (e.g. nasal cavity and frontal sinus; opacificaton of the latter is often due to trapped fluid, rather than a specific indicator of primary sinus disease)
- Fractures
- New bone production and hyperostosis
- Soft tissue mineralization
- Radiopaque foreign material
- Maxillary dental disease (e.g. periapical lucency)
- Soft tissue emphysema.

Contrast radiography

Dacryocystorhinography

Dacryocystorhinography is a valuable technique in the investigation of nasolacrimal disease. It is used to demonstrate the patency or otherwise of the nasolacrimal duct, the presence of any nasolacrimal duct filling defects and the involvement of the nasolacrimal duct in nasal and maxillary disease, all of which can lead to ocular clinical signs (see below and Chapter 10). However, dacryocystorhinography can be difficult to perform and challenging to interpret, although no special equipment is required other than lacrimal cannulae and appropriate contrast medium.

Indications:

- Chronic, recurrent or intractable epiphora and conjunctivitis due to suspected dacryocystitis.
- Fluctuant swellings in the region of the medial canthus.
- Suspected congenital atresia of the duct.
- For detection of involvement of the nasolacrimal duct in nasal and maxillary disease.
- To identify the location of a nasolacrimal duct lesion if corrective surgery is planned (e.g. for stenosis, foreign body or cyst).

Technique: The technique detailed below is after Gelatt *et al.* (1972):

1. Anaesthetize the patient and obtain plain radiographs for comparison with the subsequent contrast study. Orthogonal views are required (i.e. a lateral view together with an open-mouth VD view or an intraoral DV view of the nasal cavity).
2. Place the patient in lateral recumbency with the side to be investigated uppermost and the nose tilted down slightly to avoid retrograde flow of contrast medium into the nasal cavity from the rostral opening of the nasolacrimal duct.
3. Cannulate the upper (usually) punctum with a fine lacrimal cannula (e.g. 21 gauge for dogs and 26 gauge for cats).
4. Flush with sterile saline.
5. Inject 0.5–2 ml of iodinated contrast medium slowly whilst occluding the other punctum with a swab and digital pressure or with fine toothed forceps, until a few drops appear at the nostril. Non-ionic contrast medium of ≥300 mg I/ml is preferable as its low osmotic pressure is less irritant to the tissues than ionic media; warming the contrast medium to body temperature reduces its viscosity and makes it easier to inject.
6. Obtain a lateral radiograph as quickly as possible and, if necessary, DV and oblique views as well.
7. In some cases, it may be helpful to perform a bilateral study, for comparison of the two sides.

Normal radiographic appearance:

- The canaliculi and nasolacrimal sac may be visible.
- The normal nasolacrimal duct is smooth and well defined. It runs rostroventrally along the medial aspect of the maxilla to terminate behind the nares at the junction of the lateral wall and floor of the nasal cavity.
- The proximal third of the nasolacrimal duct may be narrower than the distal two-thirds, as it is enclosed in the maxillary bone.

Radiographic abnormalities of the nasolacrimal duct:

- Partial or complete obstruction.
- Agenesis.
- Filling defects due to debris or foreign material (Figure 2.3).
- Irregularity of the duct wall.

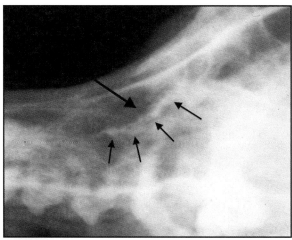

2.3 Abnormal dacryocystorhinogram in a 7-year-old English Springer Spaniel with chronic dacryocystitis. The nasolacrimal duct is dilated and the contrast medium filling of the duct is uneven (arrowed) due to the presence of filling defects, which suggest the presence of inflammatory debris or foreign material.

- Dilatation.
- Displacement.
- Extravasation of contrast medium into the nasal cavity or into a cystic lesion.

Problems:

- The radiographic images may be challenging to interpret.
- Inability to catheterize the punctum.
- Iatrogenic trauma to the canaliculi or nasolacrimal sac.
- Duct rupture and spread of infection.
- Leakage of contrast medium around the eye or reflux into the nasal cavity.

Zygomatic sialography

Indications:

- Investigation of zygomatic salivary gland involvement in orbital disease, particularly in cases in which a space-occupying lesion is suspected within the ventral orbit (see Chapter 8).

Technique:

1. Anaesthetize the patient and obtain plain lateral and DV radiographs for comparison with the subsequent contrast study.
2. Place the patient in lateral recumbency with the side to be investigated uppermost and cannulate the opening of the salivary duct with a 25–26 gauge catheter; the opening is on a ridge of buccal mucosa approximately level with the second upper molar tooth, 1 cm caudal to the opening of the parotid duct.
3. Inject 0.5–2 ml of warmed, non-ionic, iodinated contrast medium.
4. Obtain lateral and DV radiographs as quickly as possible.
5. In some cases, it may be helpful to perform a bilateral study, for comparison of the two sides.

Normal radiographic appearance:

- The main duct is short and runs caudodorsally.
- The gland itself is a large, single-lobed structure lying ventromedial to the rostral end of the zygomatic arch.

Radiographic abnormalities of the zygomatic salivary gland and duct:

- Displacement or compression.
- Enlargement or irregularity of the gland.
- Salivary duct dilatation.
- Filling defects.
- Contrast medium extravasation or fistulation.

Problems:

- Iatrogenic damage to the soft tissues.

Ultrasonography

Ultrasonography is an extremely useful technique for ocular and orbital examination and is generally performed without the use of chemical restraint, using only topical anaesthesia. It is used to examine structures that are not visible with a slit-lamp or ophthalmoscope and in cases in which opacity of normally transparent structures prevents visual inspection, as well as for the investigation of orbital disease. Several different forms of ultrasonography are used in veterinary ophthalmology.

B-mode ultrasonography

This provides a real-time two-dimensional (2D) image of the eye and is the most commonly used form of ocular ultrasonography, allowing assessment of both the globe and orbit. Transducers used for B-mode ocular ultrasonography should have a relatively high frequency of around 10 MHz (range typically 7.5–13 MHz), which provides both good resolution and evaluation of the deeper structures of the posterior segment of the globe and orbit.

Technique

Patient preparation:

- Preferably patients are either conscious or minimally sedated, since heavy sedation and general anaesthesia may cause the globe to become enophthalmic and rotate ventrally. This reduces image quality as the globe is no longer aligned with the ultrasound beam and complicates the acquisition of truly axial scans.
- Topical local anaesthetic should be applied to both eyes at least 2 minutes prior to the examination and again immediately prior to scanning.
- Sterile ultrasound coupling gel that is approved for ocular use should be used to improve contact between the transducer and tissue surface.

Procedure: The globe and orbit can be scanned via the transcorneal, transpalpebral and temporal windows.

- Transcorneal ultrasonography requires the eyelids to be held open manually and the transducer to be applied directly to the cornea, using gel or a fluid-filled glove as a stand-off, or, alternatively, a commercially available stand-off (Figure 2.4a). This method provides optimal resolution of the globe but is not recommended in the presence of globe fragility or ulcerative corneal lesions.
- The transpalpebral approach involves scanning the globe through the eyelids. This method results in greatly reduced image quality due to artefacts generated from the interposing skin layers and hair, but applies less pressure to the globe and is less likely to cause further damage to a compromised corneal surface. This approach may also be better tolerated in fractious patients.
- The temporal approaches are performed by applying the transducer caudolateral to the eye either dorsal or ventral to the zygomatic arch. Images obtained dorsal to the zygomatic arch are useful for evaluation of the orbital cone and retrobulbar space, whereas an approach ventral to the zygomatic arch provides a useful window for assessment of the zygomatic salivary gland (Figure 2.4bc).

The globe and orbit should be scanned by fanning the ultrasound beam slowly in dorsal, sagittal and (where applicable) transverse planes. Oblique planes may be useful to delineate certain lesions. Views obtained with the transducer centrally aligned to an axial plane of the globe ('axial views') allow the globe and lens size to be measured.

When describing the eye, the terms 'anterior' and 'posterior' are generally used instead of 'rostral' and 'caudal', and 'superior' and 'inferior' for 'dorsal' and 'ventral', respectively (as in humans). The use of a clock face analogy around the central axis of the globe can be helpful when describing the location of ocular lesions.

Normal ultrasonographic appearance
The normal ultrasonographic appearance of the eye and orbit is shown in Figure 2.5.

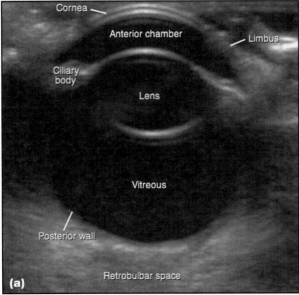

2.4 Ocular ultrasonography techniques. **(a)** The transcorneal scan, in which the transducer is placed directly on to the cornea following the application of topical anaesthetic. **(b)** The temporal scan, in which the transducer is placed caudodorsal to the globe. **(c)** The zygomatic scan, in which the transducer is placed ventral to the zygomatic arch.

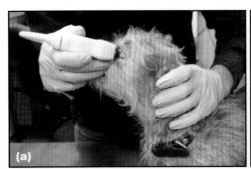
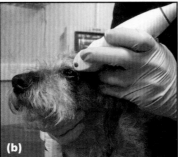
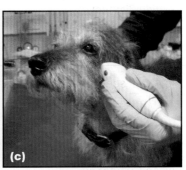
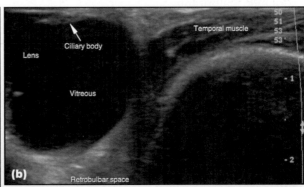
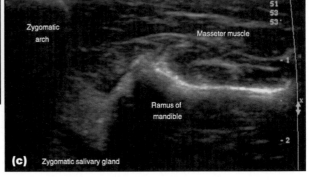

2.5 Ultrasonograms acquired using the techniques shown in Figure 2.4: **(a)** the transcorneal approach, **(b)** the temporal approach and **(c)** the zygomatic approach. The anatomical structures visible in these images obtained from normal dogs are annotated.

Globe: The globe measures approximately 20–22 mm along its central axis in the dog (18–20 mm in the cat) and its wall has a smooth, regular surface. Normal aqueous and vitreous humours are anechoic. A remnant of the hyaloid artery may be observed in neonatal animals, although in the normal dog complete atrophy of this vessel should occur before the eyelids open.

Cornea and sclera: The cornea is seen as two parallel, curvilinear echogenic interfaces representing its anterior and posterior surfaces. Only the axial region of the cornea perpendicular to the ultrasound beam is visible on ultrasonography, as echoes from the corneal periphery do not return to the transducer. Between these interfaces is hypoechoic corneal stroma. Anatomically, the normal canine cornea measures approximately 600 μm in thickness, but conventional B-mode ultrasonography tends to overestimate thicknesses and a mean corneal thickness of 1 mm has been identified in normal dogs using this modality (Boroffka *et al.*, 2006). The sclera is diffusely echogenic and can be identified extending posteriorly from the corneoscleral junction (limbus) around the periphery of the globe.

Uveal tract: The iris is seen as a distinct, echogenic line, but has a slightly variable appearance due to its ability to contract and relax, altering the size of the pupil (as seen in transverse plane images of the globe). The iris is contiguous with the ciliary body posteriorly. The latter provides the zonular attachments of the lens and can be seen as a plump, echogenic structure posterior to the iris around the margin of the lens. The choroid cannot be distinguished ultrasonographically from the adjacent retina or external echogenic sclera in the normal eye.

Lens: The normal lens is anechoic with curvilinear acoustic interfaces on its anterior and posterior margins. It is circular in transverse section and ellipsoidal in dorsal and sagittal sections with an axial thickness in the dog of approximately 7 mm (range: 5.7–7.7 mm), which increases slightly with age (Williams, 2004). Lens thickness should be measured as part of a routine ultrasonographic examination. The lens should appear stable during eye movement.

Retina and optic nerve: The normal retina is ultrasonographically indistinct from the adjacent choroid and sclera of the posterior globe wall. The optic nerve head lies inferior to the posterior pole of the globe and may sometimes be seen as a small indentation within the posterior wall. The optic nerve may be identified extending from the optic nerve head into the orbital cone; it is hypoechoic compared with the adjacent orbital fat and has a slightly undulating course.

Orbit and retrobulbar soft tissues: The osseous borders of the orbit are identified ultrasonographically as smooth, convex, hyperechoic interfaces with distal acoustic shadowing. The floor of the orbit is bordered by the zygomatic salivary gland, which can be visualized via a window through the masseter muscle, ventral to the zygomatic bone. It has a lobulated appearance on ultrasonography (see Figure 2.5c). The orbital soft tissues create a symmetrical, elongated cone behind the globe. The extraocular muscles have a smooth, spindle shape and are hypoechoic relative to the adjacent orbital fat. The ophthalmic arteries and veins can be seen with colour Doppler or contrast ultrasonography (see below).

Ultrasonographic interpretation

The acquisition and interpretation of images can be challenging and requires experience. In most cases, however, the contralateral globe and orbit can be used as a control. In the globe, many lesions are seen as increases in echogenicity contrasted against the normally anechoic structures of the cornea, lens, aqueous or vitreous humour. Important features to note are the location and nature of any increase or decrease in echogenicity; whether these changes are diffuse or focal; whether these changes are heterogeneous or homogeneous; and whether a mass effect (with displacement of the adjacent tissues and/or indentation of the globe) can be observed. Depending on their nature and the character of the surrounding ocular media, lesions may appear fixed or demonstrate 'after-movement', continuing to move or swirl within the aqueous or vitreous following movement of the globe. In the retrobulbar space, loss or distortion of the normal conical (triangular) delineation of the orbital soft tissues is suggestive of pathology. Although focal orbital lesions may be readily identified, diffuse change is much more difficult to detect. Larger areas of frontal bone osteolysis can be recognized as disruption of the normally smooth outline of this echogenic structure. Ultrasonographic features that may be associated with selected common ocular and orbital disease processes are listed in Figure 2.6 and are described in greater detail later in the chapter. For further information on specific disease conditions, the reader is directed to the appropriate chapters in the Manual.

Condition	Ultrasonographic features	Examples
Globe size changes (increase in buphthalmos or decrease in microphthalmos or phthisis bulbi)	Changes in globe size are most accurately measured by A-mode ultrasonography, but estimates of axial length and globe diameter may be obtained from B-mode scans	
Ruptured globe	Reduced globe size; lack of continuity of outer echogenic eye wall (sclera)	Figure 2.11a

2.6 Ultrasonographic findings in ocular and orbital diseases. (continues) ▶

Condition	Ultrasonographic features	Examples
Uveitis/panophthalmitis	Thickening of the iris and ciliary body may be evident. Diffuse increase in echogenicity or multiple small echogenic points within otherwise hypoechoic anterior and vitreous chambers	Figure 2.17c
Cataract	Hyperechoic; may be seen as an increase or decrease in the size of the lens	Figures 2.8, 2.14, 2.15 and 2.16
Ruptured lens	Altered lens size and contour. Liberated lens cortex may appear as hyperechoic material adjacent to the lens	Figure 2.16
(Sub)luxated lens	Altered anterior chamber depth and lens position; increased lens mobility/instability evident with eye movement	
Ocular or orbital foreign body	Appearance depends on the extent of the related disease (e.g. uveitis, globe rupture, retrobulbar abscess) and nature of foreign body (e.g. metallic foreign bodies have very pronounced acoustic shadowing, whereas plant material may not be visible)	Figures 2.12ab and 2.21
Ocular haemorrhage	May be diffusely hyperechoic and fill the anterior or vitreous chambers, or appear as small to large areas that are hyperechoic, or have a mixed echogenicity that mimics intraocular tumours. May demonstrate 'after-movement'	
Vitreal degeneration	Small echogenic foci within the vitreous cavity; may be fixed in the centre of the vitreous (asteroid hyalosis) but often demonstrate 'after-movement' if the vitreous is liquefied (syneresis, synchisis scintillans). Larger echogenic structures may also be seen ('floaters')	Figure 2.14
Retinal detachment	Curvilinear echogenic structures that can be traced to the optic nerve head. A complete detachment has a 'gull-wing' appearance	Figure 2.17abc
Vitreal detachment	Thin echogenic linear structure; typically seen at the posterior pole of the eye	
Optic nerve head changes	Focal protuberance and increased echogenicity may be seen in the region of the optic nerve head in patients with optic nerve swelling/neoplasia	Figure 2.18
Intraocular neoplasia	Mass effect may distort adjacent intraocular structures (e.g. the lens). Relatively fixed position, with no or less 'after-movement' than blood clots. Variable echogenicity and echotexture	Figure 2.13
Retrobulbar cellulitis/abscess	May be a diffuse increase in echogenicity or may have a hypoechoic centre (cavitary lesion) if the lesion is an abscess. The latter may demonstrate a mass effect	Figure 2.20a
Orbital neoplasia	Mass effect may be observed; generally hyperechoic, although can be hypoechoic in some instances. There may be irregularity of the medial, echoic, bony orbital wall	Figures 2.23a and 8.8
Extraocular muscle myositis	Enlargement of the extraocular muscles, particularly the medial rectus muscle, may be evident and is typically bilateral	Figure 8.16

2.6   (continued) Ultrasonographic findings in ocular and orbital diseases.

A-mode ultrasonography

This form of ultrasonography is used primarily for obtaining precise length or depth measurements of the eye (biometry) and for longitudinal monitoring of changes in size of ocular lesions. It does not provide images of the eye and orbit and requires specialist equipment, which may be included in dedicated ophthalmic ultrasonography units.

High-frequency ultrasonography and ultrasound biomicroscopy

High-frequency ultrasonography and ultrasound biomicroscopy are specific ocular techniques which use transducers with frequencies of around 20 MHz and 60 MHz, respectively. These high frequency transducers provide greatly improved resolution of the superficial structures and are ideal for assessment of the anterior segment, providing exquisite resolution and permitting accurate measurement of the various anterior segment structures, such as estimates of the depth of corneal lesions or thickness of iris tissue, as illustrated in Figure 2.7 (Aubin *et al.,* 2003; Bentley *et al.,* 2003).

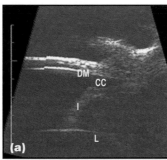
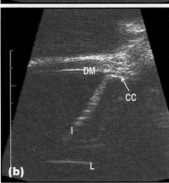

2.7

High-resolution ultrasonograms of the anterior segment acquired using a 20 MHz transducer. **(a)** Appearance of the aqueous outflow pathways in a normal cat. **(b)** A cat with congenital glaucoma and extreme narrowing and collapse of the ciliary cleft. CC = ciliary cleft; DM = Descemet's membrane; I = iris; L = lens. (continues) ▶

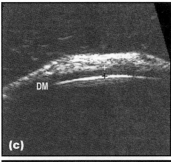

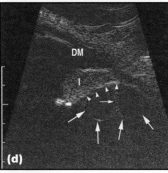

2.7 (continued) High-resolution ultrasonograms of the anterior segment acquired using a 20 MHz transducer. **(c)** A cat with a corneal sequestrum. The posterior surface of the echogenic sequestrum (white cross) and well defined posterior corneal echo corresponding to Descemet's membrane (black cross) allow the depth of the sequestrum to be estimated. **(d)** Thin-walled iridociliary cysts (arrowed) in the posterior chamber of a 2-year-old Golden Retriever are causing forward bowing of the posterior iris epithelium (arrowheads). DM = Descemet's membrane; I = iris. (c–d Courtesy of E Bentley)

However, these specialized high frequency transducers are relatively costly and these techniques have not yet been widely adopted in veterinary clinical ophthalmology. High-frequency ultrasonography is clinically useful in the assessment of the iridocorneal angle and ciliary cleft in glaucoma patients (Gibson *et al.,* 1998; Tsai *et al.,* 2012). Unlike gonioscopy it can be performed without the use of light, which alters the relationship between the anatomical structures of the anterior segment. High-frequency ultrasonography provides information on the ciliary processes and ciliary cleft and can still be performed even if there is opacification of the cornea or ocular media. However, the technique is operator-dependent, with measurements being subjective and reproducibility sometimes poor (Bentley *et al.,* 2005). In order to obtain the most accurate measurements, consistent probe orientation and scan location is essential and indentation of the anterior segment should be avoided. In dogs it is recommended to scan superiorly, and in cats superior-temporally, as these provide the most consistent measurements (Bentley *et al.,* 2005; Gomes *et al.,* 2011).

Colour flow and spectral Doppler ultrasonography

These forms of ultrasonography are used to evaluate vascular flow in and around the globe and orbit. Doppler ultrasonography may be helpful in the detection of blood flow through patent hyaloid vasculature (Figure 2.8). Special measurements, known as resistive and pulsatility indices, can provide information on vascular impedance through a structure, and normal values for these indices have been described for blood vessels of the eye and orbit in normal non-sedated and sedated dogs and in dogs with glaucoma (Gelatt-Nicholson *et al.,* 1999ab; Gelatt *et al.,* 2003; Novellas *et al.,* 2007ab), but are not typically evaluated in a clinical setting.

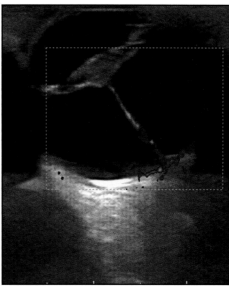

2.8 Colour Doppler ultrasonogram of a 7-month-old Miniature Schnauzer with persistent hyperplastic primary vitreous and cataract. The characteristic Doppler signal at the posterior pole and within the vitreous cavity is consistent with blood flow in a patent hyaloid artery in the affected eye. (Courtesy of D Gould and G Gent)

Contrast ultrasonography

This form of ultrasonography uses stabilized microbubble contrast agents to demonstrate vascularity within the organs. This technique can be used in the eye for various ocular structures and pathologies, including differentiation of vitreous membranes and posterior vitreous detachment from retinal detachment, assessment of the vascularity of ocular masses and detection of blood flow within persistent hyaloid arteries (Labruyère *et al.,* 2011). As the retina is a vascular structure, microbubble contrast agents can be observed entering the vessels within the retina during contrast studies, although the flow is often slow and tortuous, making the Doppler signal variable.

Magnetic resonance imaging

MRI is a well established tool for the investigation of ocular and orbital diseases in humans and its value in small animal ophthalmology was recognized soon after the introduction of MRI to veterinary medicine (Morgan *et al.,* 1994, 1996). Its main indication in ophthalmology is the investigation of orbital disease, although useful information about conditions affecting the globe may also be provided in certain cases.

In addition, it is the best imaging technique for examining the optic nerves, optic chiasm and brain in patients with neurological signs or central blindness. Its value compared with radiography and ultrasonography for the investigation of orbital disease has been assessed very favourably; in a series of 25 cases, MRI alone gave the correct diagnosis of inflammatory or neoplastic disease in 22 instances, producing detailed images which yielded more information about the nature and extent of the pathology than did the other imaging techniques (Dennis, 2000). MRI is strongly recommended for patients in which radiography and ultrasonography fail to result in a confident diagnosis or for which surgery is proposed. However, if MRI is readily available and cost is not an issue, it is highly recommended as a first-line diagnostic tool. The use of MRI in a further series of small animal ophthalmology patients with a variety of conditions has been described (Armour *et al.,* 2011).

The advantages and disadvantages of MRI are summarized in Figure 2.2. MRI is superior to other techniques for orbital imaging because it provides images with high soft tissue definition and contrast, giving more information about the nature of many disease processes than radiography, ultrasonography or CT. The ability to obtain primary images in any plane is of great benefit, since image slices may be oriented to the oblique plane of the orbits and their contents, and the use of a combination of different planes provides valuable three-dimensional (3D) information, which is of particular value if surgery is proposed. Intravenous paramagnetic contrast media are used to demonstrate the vascularity of a lesion, which is particularly helpful in the orbit to delineate abscesses and foreign bodies and in the eye to differentiate blood clots from vascular masses. MRI has the added benefit of permitting investigation of the brain in cases with neurological signs (e.g. central visual deficits or ophthalmoplegia) and is vastly superior to CT for this purpose. Other areas of the head which may be involved in orbital disease are also readily evaluated. Fine bone detail is inferior to that seen with CT, but this is compensated for by the greatly increased sensitivity for soft tissue changes. Indeed, osteolysis is usually readily recognized by extension of soft tissue pathology beyond the confines of the orbit. Although MRI requires general anaesthesia (usually of about 45 minutes duration to permit a sufficiently thorough investigation), the technique itself is non-invasive and safe for the patient.

Technique
The detailed physical principles which underlie MRI are well described elsewhere and are beyond the scope of this chapter (Gavin, 2009). MRI uses a combination of an external magnetic field and the energy of radiowaves, which are a type of electromagnetic radiation, produced by radiofrequency (RF) coils that surround the area to be imaged. The magnetic field is provided by the scanner itself, which is often referred to as 'the magnet'. Magnets vary in strength, from low field systems of about 0.2 Tesla to high field systems of ≥1.5 Tesla. Both types

are commonly used in veterinary MRI. Protons in the tissues of the patient align with the magnetic field, but are then disoriented by RF pulses. RF signals re-emitted by the protons as they realign themselves in the magnetic field (by a process known as 'relaxation') are then detected and converted by a computer into cross-sectional images. These greyscale image pixels are composed of many tiny volumes of tissue (or 'voxels').

Radiofrequency pulse sequences
These are commonly used for ophthalmic imaging and include:

- **T1-weighted** – fluid and hydrated areas are dark (hypointense) and fat is bright (hyperintense). Other soft tissues have an intermediate grey shade. T1-weighted images have high anatomical resolution
- **Contrast-enhanced T1-weighted** – MRI contrast media are mostly compounds of the element gadolinium. Following intravenous injection, the gadolinium enters the tissues to an extent depending on their vascularity and makes these areas appear brighter on subsequent scans. This effect is known as 'contrast enhancement'. Within the central nervous system (CNS), contrast enhancement also reflects damage to the blood–brain barrier, and this is an essential technique for imaging brain pathology which might result in visual deficits, such as neoplasia and inflammatory disease
- **Subtraction** – this is a post-processing manoeuvre in which the digital information from pre-contrast T1-weighted images is removed from that of an identical sequence of post-contrast images. The resulting images are very sensitive for areas of contrast enhancement, especially those close to fat (such as in the orbit). This technique is especially important in systems where fat suppression (see below) cannot be applied
- **T2-weighted** – both fluid/hydrated areas and fat are hyperintense and other soft tissues are hypointense. T2-weighted images are of high contrast and, therefore, sensitive for pathology, since most disease processes result in increased water content of the affected area. However, anatomical detail is poorer than with T1-weighted images on low field machines
- **STIR** (short T1 inversion recovery) – this is a T2-weighted sequence but with suppression of the normally bright signal from fat. Thus, areas of pathology near fat are readily seen as hyperintense regions
- **Fat suppression** – pulse sequences that suppress the normally high signal from fat may be used with high field magnets. These sequences have the advantage that, following contrast medium administration, any area which is hyperintense is solely due to contrast enhancement, reflecting vascularity. This gives a more accurate reflection of the extent of the primary disease than does a STIR sequence, in

which hyperintensity reflects both the underlying lesion and the surrounding oedema and inflammation

- *Gradient echo (GRE)* or field echo sequences – a number of sequences use a technique known as gradient echo, which can also be T1-weighted or T2-weighted. They can be used to create very thin slices or 3D images, which can be viewed in different planes. A sequence known as GRE T2* ('T2 star') results in images that are very sensitive for haemorrhage, calcification, bone and some types of foreign material, and these produce areas of very low signal or 'signal void'
- *FLAIR* (fluid-attenuated inversion recovery) – this is a T2-weighted sequence with suppression of the hyperintense signal from free fluid such as normal cerebrospinal fluid (CSF). Areas of pathology remain hyperintense. This technique is widely used for brain imaging due to its sensitivity for inflammatory disease, and should be part of the imaging protocol for patients with central visual deficits. FLAIR is also susceptible to contrast enhancement
- *MR angiography (MRA)* – this is a complex technique which utilizes the flow of blood to demonstrate vessels, either with or without contrast media. In the orbit it is of value for vascular anomalies such as varices.

Slice thickness

Generally, for small animal orbital MRI, slice thicknesses of 2–3 mm are used as they provide the optimum combination of high signal intensity and fine detail. For extensive lesions in larger dogs, 4–5 mm slices may be adequate.

Image planes

Standard imaging planes for the head are transverse, dorsal and sagittal. Symmetrically positioned transverse and dorsal images permit comparison between the two sides, which is of great value in interpretation. However, the oblique orientation of the orbit means that images aligned parallel or transverse to the orbital soft tissues, especially the optic nerve, may be helpful.

Protocol

Due to the large number of sequences and planes available, it is not practical to perform every sequence in every plane. Some operators prefer to use a set protocol for consistency, but a more flexible approach is recommended for orbital MRI as lesions can vary widely. A practical approach may be to perform several sequences in the same plane (e.g. dorsal) and then to scan in other planes using the sequences which would be expected to be the most sensitive for the lesion.

Normal MRI appearance

The normal MRI appearance of the eye and orbit is shown in Figure 2.9. The globes are very distinctive since both the aqueous and vitreous humours are predominantly composed of water, making them hypointense on T1-weighted images and hyperintense on T2-weighted images. The lens is of low to void signal, as is the sclera, on all pulse sequences. On T1-weighted images, the iris, ciliary body, lens capsule, choroid and retina are moderately hyperintense and can be recognized, although the choroid and retina cannot be distinguished from each other. All vascularized structures show contrast

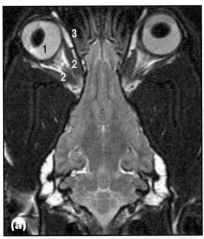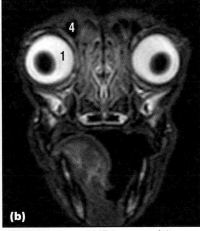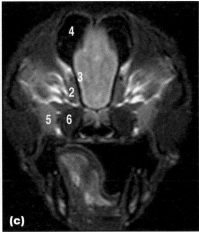

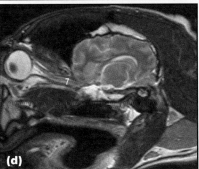

2.9 Normal MR images of the eyes and orbits. **(a)** Dorsal T2-weighted image. **(b)** Transverse T2-weighted image at the level of the globes. **(c)** Transverse T2-weighted image immediately posterior to the globes. **(d)** Sagittal oblique T2-weighted image aligned for the optic nerve. 1 = globe; 2 = extraocular muscles; 3 = medial orbital wall; 4 = frontal sinus; 5 = zygomatic salivary gland; 6 = medial pterygoid muscle; 7 = optic nerve.

enhancement. On T2-weighted images, the iris and ciliary body are seen as hypointense structures relative to the bright signal of the aqueous and vitreous, but the lens capsule and choroid/retina cannot be identified as separate structures as they are isointense to the vitreous humour. Ocular misalignment, with asymmetry of globe position, is often apparent as an effect of anaesthesia, although movement artefact is not usually a problem.

In the retrobulbar space, the extraocular muscles are seen as slender, spindle-shaped structures of medium signal intensity, similar to that of other head muscles, interspersed with hyperintense fat converging towards the orbital apex. The optic nerve is of similar signal intensity to the muscles and can be hard to identify, especially since its course is usually slightly undulant, so it is rarely seen in its entirety on a single image. The optic nerve is best recognized on T2-weighted sequences due to the surrounding hyperintense CSF, as a tract of the brain enclosed within the meninges. The optic canal and orbital fissure are also seen and the optic chiasm is readily identified. MRI technique and the appearance of the optic nerve have been described in detail elsewhere (Boroffka et al., 2008).

Other structures surrounding the orbital cone and forming the margins of the retrobulbar space can be easily identified. These include the zygomatic salivary gland ventrally, the medial pterygoid muscle ventromedially, the bony medial and dorsomedial orbital wall (mainly frontal bone) and the temporal muscle, coronoid process and zygomatic arch laterally. Cortical bone contains protons which are bound tightly and do not resonate, hence it appears as a signal void. With careful evaluation the orbital ligament can also be identified as a signal void band.

Metallic objects affect the local magnetic field and result in signal loss and image distortion, an effect known as 'susceptibility artefact'. Thus, MRI is not suitable for imaging patients with metallic ocular or orbital foreign bodies and, if the object is of ferrous metal, there is also the risk that it may move under the effect of the magnetic field. The same effect is seen in post-enucleation scans if metal staples are present. In addition, the pigment in brown globe prostheses has been found to cause severe susceptibility artefacts, necessitating removal of the prostheses for brain imaging, whereas black prostheses cause no artefacts (Dees et al., 2012).

MRI interpretation

Interpretation of MR images relies on the detection of deviations from normality and the recognition of the location, size, shape, signal intensity, and the degree and pattern of any contrast enhancement of lesions. It requires a thorough knowledge of cross-sectional anatomy and, in the case of unilateral disease, is assisted by comparing the two sides. Subtle alterations in globe position are more easily seen on dorsal and transverse images than they are clinically. The globe may also be seen to be compressed or distorted, and if this is seen the cause must be identified. In the case of focal lesions, such as tumours or abscesses, this is straightforward.

Diffuse pathology, such as cellulitis or myositis, may be hard to recognize as a structural change and in these cases detection of signal alteration on STIR and contrast studies is important.

The anatomical areas surrounding the orbit should be examined carefully, since aggressive disease may extend outwards from the orbit or, conversely, arise elsewhere and secondarily invade the orbit. These areas include the caudal nasal cavity, frontal sinuses, maxillae, sphenoid bones, cribriform plate, cranial fossa and temporomandibular joints. Osteolysis may be recognized as a loss of the normal signal void line, which represents cortical bone (provided there is soft tissue or fluid abutting it), or by changes in the bone marrow signal intensity and/or contrast enhancement in the case of medullary bone.

Computed tomography

CT is also a good imaging modality for the investigation of orbital disease, and its value in this area was recognized soon after its introduction to veterinary medicine (LeCouteur et al., 1982; Fike et al., 1984). Relatively large case series have been described (Calia et al., 1994; Boroffka et al., 2007). The tomographic nature of CT images is ideal for understanding processes in complex areas, such as the skull, and results in excellent bony detail, which is of particular value in cases of trauma and neoplasia involving bone, with reasonably good soft tissue detail due to the contrast between the retrobulbar fat and soft tissues. Certain types of foreign body are recognized, depending on their nature. Although overall MRI is superior for imaging the eye and orbit, CT provides an adequate alternative if MRI is not available. The advantages and disadvantages of CT are summarized in Figure 2.2.

Technique

CT images can be considered as thin, cross-sectional radiographs. The degree of attenuation of the X-ray beam by the tissues is manipulated by a computer to create images with far greater contrast resolution than conventional radiographs, permitting, for example, discrimination between fluid and soft tissue and revealing differences in tissue density that are too small to be detected radiographically. The images acquired primarily are in the transverse plane and images in other planes are produced by reformatting, although this results in a slight loss of resolution with the axial mode. Three-dimensional reconstruction is also possible and is especially useful for the depiction of orbital fractures or for treatment planning for orbital tumours.

CT images are composed of pixels (as for MRI), each representing the absorption of the X-ray beam within a tiny volume of tissue. The pixels are assigned a number, or Hounsfield unit (HU), and are displayed on a greyscale relative to water. Water is assigned a HU of 0 with air at −1000, cortical bone at +1000, and contrast media and metals in excess of this. The greyscale can be manipulated to optimize viewing of different structures by selecting a window level (WL) and a window width (WW) of HUs corresponding to the tissues of interest. Above and below the WW, the tissues appear white and black, respectively, and within the window the range of grey shades is expanded to increase the contrast resolution. For the orbit, images should be reviewed using both the bone and soft tissue windows (the latter using a narrow WW in order to discriminate between the different types of orbital soft tissue).

CT almost always requires chemical restraint of the patient (either general anaesthesia or, in some cases, heavy sedation). For transverse orbital images, the patient is placed in dorsal or ventral recumbency; special positioning of the patient and/or angling of the gantry allows acquisition of images in the oblique dorsal and sagittal planes, aligned with the optic nerve (Boroffka and Voorhout, 1999).

CT-guided biopsy

Percutaneous CT-guided fine-needle aspiration or core biopsy of orbital lesions can be helpful in the diagnosis of orbital neoplasia and is most often performed using a 'free-hand' technique (Tidwell and Johnson, 1994). Lesions are first localized on initial diagnostic CT scans and, after noting table position and utilizing the laser line of the gantry to help identify the site and optimal angle for needle entry, the needle tip position within the tissue of interest is verified by additional scans prior to biopsy.

Normal CT appearance

The CT appearance of normal ocular and orbital structures has been described (Fike *et al.*, 1984; Boroffka and Voorhout, 1999) and is shown in Figure 2.10. Structures which may be identified include the lens, optic nerve, extraocular muscles, orbital fat, zygomatic salivary gland, orbital ligament, surrounding masticatory muscles and the nasal cavity, frontal sinuses and cranial vault.

CT interpretation

The principles of interpretation are similar to those described for MRI. The HU of regions of interest may be measured and this can provide information about the nature of the tissue being examined. Areas of increased and decreased X-ray attenuation are referred to as 'hyperdense' and 'hypodense', respectively. Subtle osteolysis and mineralization are more readily detected on CT than MRI, but soft tissue resolution and contrast are inferior.

Contrast CT

Radiographic contrast media may be administered intravenously, and, as with MRI, contrast enhancement reflects vascularity of the lesion or breakdown of the blood–brain barrier. However, CT is less sensitive to contrast enhancement than MRI. The use of cisternography (injection of myelographic contrast medium into the cisterna magna followed by deliberate head positioning to encourage the contrast medium to migrate rostrally) to fill the optic nerve sheaths has been described (Boroffka and Voorhout, 1999), but is not without risk to the patient.

CT dacryocystography

The technique for CT dacryocystography has been described in dogs (Nykamp *et al.*, 2004; Rached *et al.*, 2011) and cats (Schlueter *et al.*, 2009), and is similar to that for a radiographic study, using iodinated radiographic contrast medium. The technique reliably depicts small structures such as the canaliculi and lacrimal sac, as well as the bone surrounding the duct, and is superior to radiographic dacryocystorhinography. Reconstructed 3D images are helpful for understanding the relationship between the duct and other structures when planning for surgery.

CT zygomatic sialography

The use of CT may be very helpful in cases where zygomatic salivary gland disease is suspected. Cannulation of the zygomatic papilla and the administration of iodinated contrast media is as previously described for radiographic contrast studies.

Imaging features of ocular disease

Ultrasonography is the principal imaging modality used for the investigation of intraocular disease, although MRI (and possibly CT) may be of value in selected cases, such as the detection of posterior globe perforations or tumour extension. Ultrasonographic features of specific ocular conditions are summarized in Figure 2.6. However, it must be recognized that although diagnostic imaging provides structural information, this is usually non-specific for the histological nature of the underlying pathology. For specific information on the clinical presentation and management of these conditions, the reader should refer to the appropriate chapters.

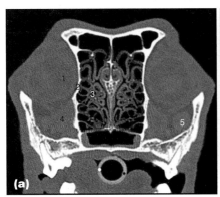
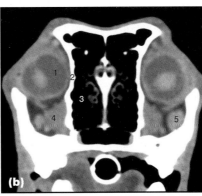

2.10 CT images of the normal orbit of a dog seen via **(a)** a bone window and **(b)** a soft tissue window. 1 = globe; 2 = medial orbital wall; 3 = nasal cavity; 4 = medial pterygoid muscle; 5 = zygomatic salivary gland.

Globe

Assessment of size

B-mode ultrasonography can provide approximate measurements of globe size, which may be helpful for differentiating glaucoma from exophthalmos and for assessment of the degree of microphthalmos associated with congenital abnormalities of the eye (Boroffka *et al.,* 2006). Several measurements should be obtained, aiming for axial scans to provide the most reproducible representation of globe dimensions. As previously discussed, A-mode ultrasonography is considered a more accurate means of measuring ocular dimensions, but this modality is less widely available.

Rupture

Detection of globe rupture is an important prognostic indicator, but is often accompanied by other signs of ocular and periocular trauma which prevent direct visualization, such as swelling and hyphaema. Ultrasonographically, anterior globe rupture appears as thickening of the cornea or sclera around the region of the defect. Displacement of the iris anteriorly towards the site of the defect is often observed. Posterior scleral rupture is primarily identified as loss of the normal contour and continuity of the echogenic posterior wall of the globe (Figure 2.11). There may be evidence of complete distortion of the posterior segment with accompanying changes consistent with vitreous haemorrhage and inflammation (described later). MRI is an excellent investigative tool in these cases, particularly if the ultrasonographic findings are equivocal (if MRI is not available, CT is an alternative but will provide less soft tissue information). T2-weighted MR images are usually the most helpful, as the high signal intensity of the vitreous humour helps to delineate the distortion and area of discontinuity (see Chapter 13). Post-contrast T1-weighted MR images demonstrate contrast enhancement of vascularized soft tissues, delineating hypointense vitreous. Damage to the surrounding tissues can also be seen.

Ocular foreign bodies

Radiopaque foreign bodies are evident radiographically, but even with multiple views it is generally not possible to determine whether the foreign body is located within or outside the globe. Radiolucent foreign bodies cannot be detected with radiography. Ultrasonography can be used to identify the location of larger foreign objects. However, small and/or linear foreign bodies may be impossible to differentiate ultrasonographically from tracks of abnormal tissue created by transient penetration of a sharp object, even when no foreign material remains. Foreign material appears hyperechoic compared with the surrounding ocular tissues (Figure 2.12) and denser materials also create distal acoustic shadowing, a helpful diagnostic sign. The use of MRI and CT for the diagnosis of intraocular foreign bodies has not been described in veterinary patients; in theory they might be detectable, but, as with ultrasonography, could be difficult to distinguish from tissue reaction. MRI should not be used in cases in which there is a suspicion of metallic foreign bodies, due to the risk of movement of ferrous material and the inevitable image distortion.

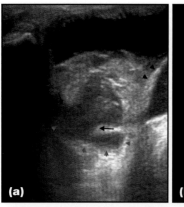
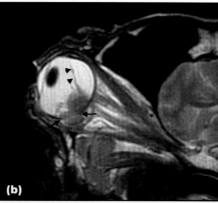

2.11 Globe rupture in a 12-year-old Labrador Retriever.
(a) Ultrasonogram: discontinuity of the posterior globe wall and vitreous can be observed extending into the retrobulbar space. There is also complete retinal detachment, which can be seen as a curvilinear echogenic structure.
(b) Corresponding MR image. The black arrows highlight the defect in the posterior globe wall. The red arrowheads depict the leakage of the vitreous through the defect into the retrobulbar space. The black arrowheads show the retinal detachment present.

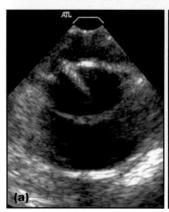
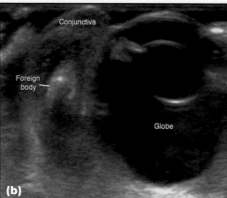

2.12 Ultrasonographic appearance of ocular foreign bodies.
(a) Transcorneal image of the globe in a 4-year-old Domestic Shorthaired cat showing a linear, echogenic foreign body extending into the lens. The foreign body was confirmed as a thorn.
(b) A 12-week-old English Cocker Spaniel with echogenic material present within a thickened conjunctiva, adjacent to the globe. The foreign body was confirmed as a grass seed.

Neoplasia

Ultrasonography is helpful for identifying the presence of ocular masses in globes with common secondary complications, which may lead to opacification of the ocular media. Concurrent ultrasonographic features of intraocular haemorrhage, uveitis, glaucoma and retinal detachment may also be evident. Neoplastic masses involving the eye may be primary ocular tumours, metastases or invasive extraocular tumours. Ultrasonography is helpful in evaluating the location, size and invasiveness of ocular masses, but gives no indication as to their histological nature. Ocular tumours can have a variable echogenicity and echotexture and are usually broad-based at their attachment to normal tissue. The characteristic features of specific ocular and orbital neoplasms are detailed in the sections on ultrasonographic features of uveal disease and orbital disease, respectively.

Differentiation of tumours from haematomas, clotted blood and serous fluid can be problematic with conventional ultrasonography, but the vascularity of the former can be demonstrated using colour Doppler or contrast ultrasonography as a useful distinguishing feature. Determining the extent of the mass is important for treatment planning and so, if there is any suggestion of extraocular extension of a mass, or significant orbital involvement, MRI is recommended. However, with the exception of pigmented melanoma (see below), MRI is also non-specific for histological type.

Cornea

Keratitis

Although corneal disease is best assessed using slit-lamp biomicroscopy, imaging may be helpful in the evaluation of corneal disease associated with pronounced opacification. Conventional B-mode ultrasonography is less sensitive for the assessment of corneal disease than high-frequency ultrasonography. Keratitis appears ultrasonographically as thickening of the cornea, increase in echogenicity, and uneven thickness and disruption of the normal regular, lamellar architecture. Endothelial disease may result in severe oedema with pockets of fluid accumulation, leading to bullous keratopathy or hydrops, which appear as hypoechoic cavitations within the stroma. Ultrasonography can be used to locate corneal foreign bodies and, in particular, the use of high-resolution ultrasonography can help determine the depth of corneal foreign bodies and sequestra (see Figure 2.7c).

Iris and ciliary body

Anterior uveitis

Animals with anterior uveitis may have no detectable ultrasonographic changes, although thickening and enlargement of the iris and ciliary body may be evident in severe cases. Multiple small echogenic foci may be detected within the anterior chamber, associated with accumulations of particulate inflammatory debris and cell clumps. In severe cases, exudates may appear more diffusely hyperechoic.

Anterior uveitis may be complicated by cataract formation, hyphaema, glaucoma or retinal detachment (the ultrasonographic features of which are described in the sections that follow). Alterations in iris contour associated with iris bombé due to extensive posterior synechiae are also readily visualized on ultrasonography.

Iridociliary cysts

Single or multiple iridociliary cysts may be an incidental finding on ultrasonography. They may also be seen in association with uveitis and glaucoma. Ultrasonographically, they appear as rounded anechoic structures with thin echogenic margins (see Figure 2.7d). As they are formed from the epithelium of the iris and ciliary body, they may be attached to these sites or within the posterior chamber, but they can break free and have been identified floating in the anterior chamber, adherent to the cornea or lens capsule and, rarely, within the vitreous cavity.

Neoplasia

The general ultrasonographic features and secondary complications of intraocular tumours are described above. Ocular neoplasms involving the iris and ciliary body appear ultrasonographically as either focal or diffuse thickening, or as a distinct mass extending from these structures (Figure 2.13). In both dogs and cats, the most common primary ocular neoplasm is uveal melanoma. In dogs, this usually appears as a focal, hyperechoic mass lesion; whereas in cats, ocular melanocytic neoplasms are more malignant in behaviour and typically associated with diffuse, progressive iris thickening and pupil distortion. High-frequency ultrasonography may be particularly valuable in the assessment of suspected early anterior uveal melanoma, but is not yet widely available in clinical veterinary practice. On MRI, pigmented melanomas usually have a characteristic signal intensity due to the presence of melanin (hyperintense on T1-weighted images and hypointense to void on T2-weighted images); this

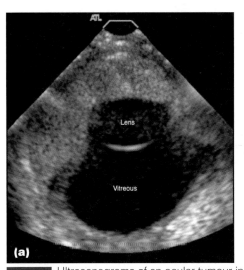

2.13 Ultrasonograms of an ocular tumour in a 9-year-old Golden Retriever. **(a)** A large echogenic uveal mass can be seen displacing the lens and extending into the anterior chamber. (continues) ▶

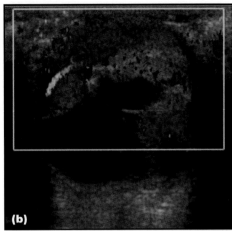

2.13 (continued) Ultrasonograms of an ocular tumour in a 9-year-old Golden Retriever. **(b)** A large blood vessel extending into the mass is identifiable with colour Doppler ultrasonography.

may be more obvious with high field scanners than with low field systems. The most common secondary ocular neoplasm in dogs and cats is lymphoma, which is often associated with diffuse infiltrates, and is seen as thickening of the iris and ciliary body.

Glaucoma

As glaucoma commonly occurs secondary to other serious ocular disorders, including neoplasia and uveitis (see Chapter 15), ultrasonography is indicated in all glaucoma patients in which corneal oedema or other opacities within the ocular media preclude thorough evaluation of the intraocular structures. The cross-sectional information provided by ultrasonography may aid in determining the pathogenesis and most appropriate management plan for the glaucoma (e.g. by identifying features consistent with underlying intraocular masses, lens luxation or evidence of intraocular haemorrhage, uveitis and retinal detachment).

Iridocorneal angle: High-frequency ultrasonography can be used to evaluate the iridocorneal angle and ciliary cleft in cases of glaucoma (see Figure 2.7b). The ability to evaluate the ciliary cleft is a major advantage over gonioscopy (see Chapters 1 and 15). Whilst high-resolution ultrasonographic measurements have been found to be comparable with gonioscopic measurements, and are more quantitative than the subjective assessments provided by gonioscopy, reproducibility between observers remains a problem (Aubin *et al.*, 2003; Bentley *et al.*, 2005). The longitudinal evaluation of ciliary cleft dimensions in the second eye of dogs previously diagnosed with primary glaucoma is currently under investigation. Although not yet widely available in clinical practice, this technique shows promise as a means of predicting the onset of acute angle closure glaucoma following cataract surgery or in the second eye of dogs with primary glaucoma (Rose *et al.*, 2008; E Bentley and P Miller, personal communication). For example, ultrasonographic features may indicate the need for surgical rather than medical therapy in an effort to prevent acute glaucomatous crises.

Lens

Cataracts

Assessment of patients with cataracts is one of the most common uses for B-mode ultrasonography in veterinary ophthalmology. Opacification of the lens prevents ophthalmoscopic assessment of the posterior segment of the eye, but ultrasonography permits evaluation of the lens and the structures behind it. Vitreal degeneration (see below) is commonly seen in association with cataracts and may predispose the eye to retinal detachment. Retinal detachment is not an uncommon finding in dogs with long-standing resorbing cataracts and may be identified on ultrasonography (van der Woerdt *et al.*, 1993).

Cataract formation results in the development of acoustic interfaces within the normally anechoic lens, rendering it echogenic on ultrasonography. As with slit-lamp biomicroscopy, the location and extent of the cataract within the lens can be classified on ultrasonography as anterior or posterior capsular, subcapsular, cortical or nuclear (see Chapters 1 and 16). Globes with congenital cataracts may demonstrate reduced axial length and diameter of the globe and reduced axial thickness of the lens. These eyes may also show evidence of other congenital ocular anomalies such as concurrent persistent hyaloid artery or persistent hyperplastic primary vitreous.

Lenses with hypermature cataracts may have a wrinkled capsule and may be reduced in thickness due to cortical resorption. Eyes with hypermature cataracts may show evidence of ultrasonographic findings consistent with uveitis, vitreous degeneration or retinal detachment and are also more prone to lens luxation or subluxation (see below). In patients with diabetic cataracts, affected lenses often demonstrate an increase in axial thickness and diameter due to water imbibition with a corresponding reduction in the depth of the anterior chamber (Figure 2.14). Diabetic cataracts may also undergo spontaneous capsular rupture due to rapid increases in lens size and intumescence.

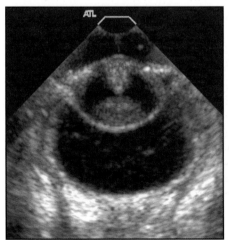

2.14 Ultrasonogram of a diabetic cataract in a 6-year-old West Highland White Terrier showing increased echogenicity of the lens nucleus, cortex and capsule. The intumescent lens is enlarged and rounded in shape. Within the vitreous there are multiple echogenic foci, consistent with vitreal degeneration.

Lens malformations, such as posterior lenticonus and lentiglobus (Figure 2.15), have also been associated with cataract formation (see Chapters 16 and 17). In addition, other related ocular abnormalities such as microphthalmos, persistent hyaloid artery and persistent hyperplastic primary vitreous (see later) may be evident ultrasonographically (see Figures 2.8 and 2.15). It is important to recognize the presence of these malformations during preoperative evaluation of cataract patients as they can increase the risk of surgical complications.

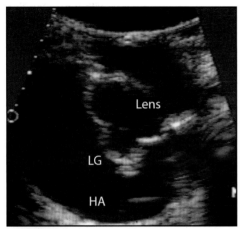

2.15 Ultrasonographic appearance of posterior lentiglobus (LG), with distortion of the posterior lens capsular echo, in a Golden Retriever with persistent hyperplastic primary vitreous. In this dog, the lens cortex was sufficiently clear to allow the distortion of the posterior lens capsule, hyaloid artery (HA) remnant and a posterior lens capsular plaque to be identified on slit-lamp biomicroscopy. The opposite eye presented with a complete cataract and intralenticular haemorrhage.

Lens capsule rupture

Lens capsule rupture can occur spontaneously or secondary to trauma. Ultrasonographically, extruded lens cortex associated with capsular rupture appears as echogenic material extending from the lens capsule (Figure 2.16). The lens proteins released may cause uveitis, retinal detachment, fibroplasia and secondary glaucoma, which can all lead to additional ultrasonographic findings.

Traumatic rupture most commonly involves the anterior lens capsule. A focal or diffuse increase in lens echogenicity is observed, depending on the degree of the insult and the time elapsed since the injury occurred. There are often concurrent signs of trauma, such as penetrating foreign bodies, corneal lesions, hyphaema or inflammatory debris within the anterior or posterior segments (see Figure 2.12).

Spontaneous rupture occurs most often in relation to diabetic cataract formation, due to rapid lens enlargement and intumescence, although it can occur with any cataract with a rapid onset and progression or with a hypermature cataract. Spontaneous ruptures often occur at the junction of the thick anterior and thin posterior capsule at the lens equator. The anterior chamber may appear uneven in depth with asymmetrical shallow regions. The contour of lens capsular echoes may be altered due to the loss of capsular integrity and may be difficult to

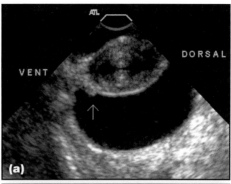

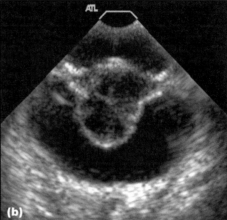

2.16 Ultrasonograms of lens rupture. **(a)** Equatorial lens rupture in an 8-year-old Jack Russell Terrier. An echogenic nodule of material (arrowed) extends from the ventral equator of the lens. The lens itself is echogenic, consistent with cataract formation. **(b)** Posterior lens capsule rupture in a 2-year-old Border Terrier with a cataract. A large volume of echogenic material is seen extending from the posterior lens into the vitreous.

distinguish from adjacent echogenic lens material or inflammatory debris. Detection of lens rupture during ultrasonographic cataract evaluation is important as it may impact the recommended treatment course and prognosis (Wilkie *et al.*, 2006).

Lens luxation

Lens luxation may be primary or secondary to trauma, glaucoma, uveitis, cataracts or neoplasia, and can result in ultrasonographic changes. Corneal opacification, due directly to lens luxation or resulting from an underlying condition, may render ultrasonography essential for accurate diagnosis. In subluxation, the lens remains in the hyaloid (patellar) fossa, whereas complete luxation results in posterior or anterior displacement of the lens. The latter, in particular, is important to identify as it is considered an ophthalmic emergency. An early sign of lens subluxation is the presence of phacodonesis, in which the lens has a characteristic oscillating motion with ocular movement on ultrasonographic evaluation.

Vitreous

Vitreal degeneration and detachment

Vitreal degeneration may take one of several different forms (see Chapter 17):

- Syneresis (vitreous liquefaction)
- Vitreal floaters (condensation of collagen fibrils within a variably liquefied vitreous)
- Asteroid hyalosis (suspended calcium phospholipid)
- Synchysis scintillans (cholesterol particles in a liquefied vitreous).

Mild vitreal degeneration is common in normal dogs (Labruyère *et al.,* 2008). Syneresis and vitreal floaters appear ultrasonographically as multiple, small, pinpoint or linear echoes, which are mobile and settle dependently within the vitreous (see Figure 2.14). The particles in synchysis scintillans, in particular, are highly mobile and can be observed swirling around the vitreous on ultrasound examination.

Asteroid hyalosis creates multiple, highly reflective, triangular echoes within the centre of the vitreous. As these particles are attached to the collagen framework, they have a fixed position and limited movement with globe movements. Unlike other forms of vitreal degeneration, these highly-reflective particles remain visible when the ultrasonographic gain is lowered.

As part of the degenerative process, posterior detachment may occur. This creates a curvilinear echogenic line parallel to the posterior wall of the globe. Posterior vitreous detachment can mimic retinal detachment and caution should be exercised when interpreting curvilinear echoes in the vitreous cavity. Although the former generally results in a thinner echogenic line, it can be distinguished from retinal detachment by its lack of attachment to the region of the optic nerve head and, if necessary, use of contrast techniques described previously.

Vitreal haemorrhage
Vitreal haemorrhage can occur secondary to a broad range of disease processes, including trauma, neoplasia, coagulopathies, hypertension, uveitis, chronic glaucoma, neovascularization and persistent hyaloid artery, as well as following ocular surgery. Haemorrhage can take several days to become apparent ultrasonographically. When visible, vitreal haemorrhage may be recognized as multiple, highly mobile echogenic foci or as a focal echogenic mass when there is clot formation. Contrast ultrasonography can be used to differentiate blood clots from neoplastic lesions, which can otherwise be very challenging to distinguish. Over time, vitreal haemorrhage may form linear, echogenic vitreal membranes that can mimic retinal detachment (Gallhoefer *et al.,* 2013).

Vitreal membranes
Intravitreal membrane formation can occur as a primary degenerative process or secondary to trauma, glaucoma, uveitis or vitreal haemorrhage. Vitreal membranes and condensations can contribute to tractional retinal detachment. Thus, ultrasonographic features associated with underlying conditions or complications may be seen concurrently. Ultrasonographically, vitreal membranes appear as irregular, linear echoic strands. They can have a

similar appearance to retinal detachment, but generally do not attach in the region of the optic nerve head. As with posterior vitreous detachment (described above), vitreal membranes may be differentiated from retinal detachment with the use of contrast ultrasonography as vitreal membranes are avascular (Labruyère *et al.,* 2011), although concurrent retinal detachment may be present.

Vitreal inflammation
Vitreal inflammation occurs as an extension of inflammation in other posterior segment tissues, penetrating foreign bodies or infectious endophthalmitis. Ultrasonographically, echogenic foci form within the vitreous, but this a non-specific finding. Ultrasonographic features of the underlying lesion (e.g. evidence of globe perforation) may also be present, depending on the aetiology.

Persistent hyperplastic primary vitreous
Ultrasonographically, persistent hyperplastic primary vitreous (PHPV) may be seen as a variably sized, echogenic, linear or cone-shaped structure, extending from the posterior pole of the lens to the region of the optic nerve head (see Figure 2.8). PHPV can be associated with other ocular lesions, including increased lens echogenicity due to cataract formation, distortion of the posterior lens capsule echo due to fibrous plaque or posterior lenticonus (see Figure 2.15) and microphthalmos. PHPV may be unilateral or bilateral and can result in retinal detachment and vitreal haemorrhage. It is important to assess whether the hyaloid artery is patent, as this will have implications for surgery. Colour Doppler and contrast ultrasonography can be used to detect patent vasculature within a persistent hyaloid artery (Boroffka *et al.,* 1998).

Retina

Retinal detachment
The retina has firm peripheral attachments at the ora ciliaris retinae, where it is continuous with the ciliary body epithelium, and at the optic nerve head. As a result, when the retina detaches, it moves away from the wall of the globe but maintains attachment sites anteriorly and adjacent to the optic nerve head. Ultrasonographically, total retinal detachment appears as echogenic curvilinear strands extending across the vitreous cavity between the ora ciliaris retinae and posterior pole of the globe, often in a V shape (likened to a cartoon seagull wing) (Figure 2.17). These linear strands are often immobile with ocular movement and have a smooth, even course and structure. Partial retinal detachment often precedes complete detachment and appears as a focal, convex, curvilinear echo with separation from the echogenic posterior eye wall.

Vitreal membrane formation and vitreal detachment can have a similar appearance to partial retinal detachment. However, contrast ultrasonography can be used to differentiate these conditions as the retina is a vascular structure and microbubbles can be observed travelling through the echogenic

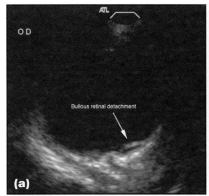
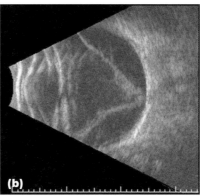
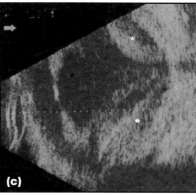

2.17 Ultrasonograms of retinal detachment. **(a)** Focal bullous retinal detachment in a 6-year-old crossbred dog. A thick curvilinear echo extends into the vitreous from the posterior wall of the globe. **(b)** Complete retinal detachment in a 15-year-old crossbred dog. A thick, echogenic, curvilinear structure extends from the location of the optic nerve head to the ora ciliaris retinae. The subretinal space is hypoechoic in this dog with systemic hypertension. **(c)** Complete retinal detachment in a 4-year-old Labrador Retriever with endophthalmitis due to blastomycosis. An echogenic, highly cellular exudate fills the subretinal space (*) underlying a total retinal detachment in this patient and indicates a very poor prognosis for restoration of vision in the affected eye.

strands (Labruyère *et al.*, 2011). The echogenicity of the subretinal space can have prognostic importance in retinal detachment. Subretinal haemorrhage or dense cellular exudates and infiltrates that are associated with a poor visual prognosis appear as hyperechoic material, whereas the subretinal space is relatively anechoic with serous detachments that carry a more favourable prognosis for retinal reattachment and restoration of vision. Concurrent imaging features indicative of intraocular or obital masses, haemorrhage or choroidal thickening may be present. Retinal detachment may also be visible on MRI, where it appears as a V-shaped hypointense line highlighted against the hyperintense vitreous on T2-weighted scans.

Choroid

Posterior uveitis
Ultrasonographically, severe posterior uveitis is seen as gross thickening and an abnormal layered appearance of the posterior wall of the globe, often accompanied by retinal detachment. The middle choroidal layer is diffusely thickened and hypoechoic compared with the adjacent retina and sclera. If choroidal inflammation is part of a more generalized endophthalmitis, pinpoint echogenic foci may be present within the vitreous and anterior chamber, and thickening of the iris and ciliary body may also be seen. Uveal inflammation may be seen on MRI as an increase in contrast enhancement on T1-weighted images. This is a subjective finding, but comparison between the two eyes is helpful if the condition is unilateral.

Neoplasia
General principles of interpretation apply (see above). Choroidal melanoma is rare in dogs and cats, but may result in characteristic signal changes on MRI.

Optic nerve
For further information on the aetiopathogenesis and clinical signs of disease processes affecting the optic nerve, the reader is referred to Chapter 18.

Optic neuritis
Radiographs are normal; in severe cases, swelling of the optic nerve head and enlargement of the optic nerve may be evident on ultrasonography (Figure 2.18a). Suspected optic neuritis is best evaluated

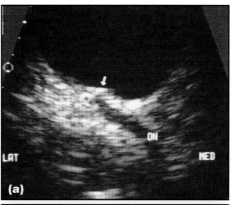

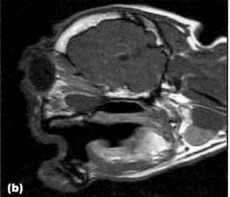

2.18 Imaging findings in optic neuritis. **(a)** Transcorneal ultrasonogram showing the enlarged optic nerve (ON) as a tortuous, hypoechoic band, with swelling of the echogenic optic nerve head (arrowed) seen against the anechoic vitreous in a Cavalier King Charles Spaniel. **(b)** Sagittal oblique post-contrast T1-weighted MR image aligned to the orbit in a Lhaso Apso. The optic nerve is thickened and shows an increased degree of contrast enhancement. CSF samples from both dogs suggested a probable diagnosis of granulomatous meningoencephalitis.

using MRI: the optic nerve(s) and often the optic chiasm may be swollen and hyperintense on T2-weighted images and show increased contrast enhancement on sagittal oblique and dorsal T1-weighted images (Figure 2.18b). These structures are best detected on fat suppression or subtraction images. Lesions suggestive of multifocal inflammatory disease are often seen in the brain and/or spinal cord. These manifest as ill defined areas of hyperintensity on T2-weighted and FLAIR images, some of which may show mild contrast enhancement. A mass effect may be present. Very severe cases may also be detectable on CT.

Neoplasia

The most common optic nerve neoplasm is meningioma. Optic nerve neoplasia is most readily diagnosed using MRI, in which a well defined, intraconal mass is seen in association with the optic nerve. The mass is usually spindle-shaped with tapering margins, hypointense on T1-weighted images and with marked homogeneous contrast enhancement (Figure 2.19). Intracranial extension may occur following the path of the nerve. Ultrasonography and CT both demonstrate intraconal masses, but the relationship of the mass to the optic nerve may be less clear; although, as they arise within the centre of the extraocular muscle cone, peripheral displacement of the extraocular muscles may be identified. Other histological types of optic nerve tumour are rare and are likely to be indistinguishable from meningioma.

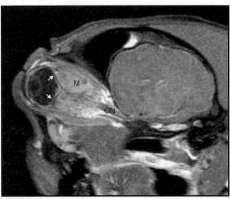

2.19 A sagittal oblique, fat-suppressed, post-contrast T1-weighted MR image of an optic nerve meningioma in an 8-year-old crossbred dog. A large mass (M) with tapering margins surrounds the optic nerve (ON), displacing the extraocular muscles peripherally and compressing and indenting the posterior globe (arrowed). The mass is hyperintense and therefore more contrast enhancing than the adjacent optic nerve.

Imaging features of orbital disease

For further information on the aetiopathogenesis and clinical signs of specific orbital diseases, the reader is referred to Chapter 8.

Inflammatory diseases

Orbital cellulitis

Orbital cellulitis is usually unilateral, which allows comparison with the unaffected orbit. Images should be examined carefully for any possible underlying cause, such as dental, nasal or frontal sinus disease. When the pathology is confined to the soft tissues of the orbit, radiographs are unremarkable except for non-specific evidence of local soft tissue swelling. When inflammation has extended into the orbit from adjacent areas, bony or dental changes and opacification of the nasal cavity and/or frontal sinus may be evident radiographically (see Chapter 8).

Orbital inflammation can result in either diffuse cellulitis or focal lesions (such as granulomas). Diffuse cellulitis may be overlooked as it is often difficult to detect on ultrasonography. However, in some cases, a disturbance and loss of visualization of the normal orbital structural features may be observed, as they are replaced by a heterogeneous appearance or an overall increased echogenicity. In severe cases, the posterior aspect of the globe may be deformed. Focal inflammation is more easily detected and appears as a discrete, hypoechoic or complex mass. This appearance is similar to that of orbital neoplasia and an ultrasound-guided fine-needle aspirate, tissue biopsy sample (e.g. taken under CT guidance) or even orbitotomy may be required for diagnosis.

Diffuse orbital cellulitis is better detected on MRI than CT, although both techniques show general swelling of the orbital soft tissues and globe displacement and/or distortion. Lack of a discrete mass is helpful to rule out focal neoplasia, although the possibility of diffusely infiltrative neoplasia cannot be definitively excluded. Inflammation is evident as diffuse hyperintensity of the affected tissues on T2-weighted and STIR images, and both CT and MRI show evidence of abnormal contrast enhancement. With MRI, fat-suppressed, post-contrast T1-weighted and subtraction images are especially helpful. As with ultrasonography, focal inflammatory lesions may appear similar to tumours, but evidence of involvement of the surrounding tissues (such as the temporal, masseter and medial pterygoid muscles) is highly suggestive of an inflammatory process.

Minor osteolysis and new bone production are occasionally seen with orbital inflammatory diseases, especially if adjacent areas such as the nasal cavity or frontal sinus are also affected. Although the bony changes are better seen with CT, the underlying disease process (such as aggressive sinusitis or rhinitis) can be readily detected on MRI. Careful examination of the caudal maxillary teeth should be performed in order to identify occult dental disease. Inflammatory orbital disease can occasionally extend into the cranial cavity and may cause severe osteolysis and mimic neoplasia, or be associated with more subtle extension of inflammation through the bony orbital foramina (Kneissl *et al.*, 2007).

Orbital abscesses

Orbital abscesses are relatively common (see Chapter 8). Associated imaging changes may provide evidence of foreign bodies, penetrating trauma or extension from infections in structures surrounding the orbit (e.g. maxillary dental disease or sinus disease). Apart from the soft tissue swelling, radiographs are normal and relatively uninformative unless radiopaque foreign bodies are present.

Ultrasonography usually identifies orbital abscesses, although the procedure may be painful for the patient, necessitating sedation or general anaesthesia. On ultrasonography, abscesses appear as well defined, hypoechoic areas with thick echogenic walls (Figure 2.20a). The contents of the abscess may be so thick and echogenic as to mimic a solid mass, such as a tumour, and a mass effect with globe indentation is possible. However, gentle pressure on the transducer results in slight movement of the small echogenic foci within the abscess, confirming its fluid nature (Dennis, 2000). Ultrasonography can be helpful for guiding aspiration of the lesion for sampling or drainage, but may fail to show the full extent of complex abscessation.

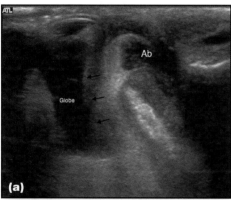

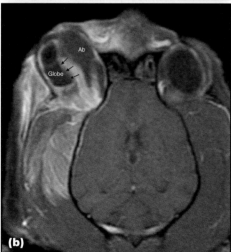

2.20 A retrobulbar abscess in a 10-year-old Border Terrier bitch. **(a)** Ultrasonogram showing a complex cavitated mass (Ab) medial to the globe, compressing and displacing it (arrowed). **(b)** Dorsal, fat-suppressed, post-contrast T1-weighted MR image showing a large, hypointense cavity (Ab) with surrounding contrast-enhancing tissue, located medial to the globe and severely deforming it (arrowed).

With CT, abscesses are seen as hypodense cavities with a rim of contrast-enhancing soft tissue. Displacement or distortion of the globe may be evident. MRI is the preferred imaging modality for orbital abscesses as it shows the full extent of the abscessation and any surrounding inflammation.

Often several abscess cavities are present, which may interconnect, and this knowledge is important for planning treatment. Abscess contents appear hyperintense on T2-weighted and STIR images and hypointense on pre-contrast T1-weighted images. Contrast enhancement of a well defined inflammatory abscess margin is usually dramatic and subtraction images confirm that the centre of the lesion is avascular (Figure 2.20b). Orbital abscesses are always surrounded by extensive, diffuse soft tissue inflammation, seen as areas of soft tissue swelling, hyperintensity on T2-weighted images and contrast enhancement. As with orbital cellulitis, inflammation associated with orbital abscesses may extend into the cranial cavity via the skull foramina, resulting in imaging features consistent with meningitis and/or osteomyelitis (Kneissl *et al.*, 2007).

Orbital foreign bodies

The imaging appearance of orbital foreign bodies depends on the nature of the foreign material, the presence of infection and the extent of any reaction provoked in the local soft tissues. A combination of radiography and ultrasonography is often a practical first line of investigation (Sansom and Labruyère, 2012). Radiography demonstrates the presence of radiopaque foreign material, although it may be impossible to determine whether the objects are ocular or retrobulbar, even with multiple radiographic views. Radiolucent foreign bodies cannot be detected radiographically. The use of fluoroscopy with image intensification has been described for the removal of a sewing needle from the orbit of a cat (Kim *et al.*, 2011).

Ultrasonography may be used to identify larger foreign bodies, but will often miss smaller fragments of plant material and may fail to demonstrate multiple structures; even when a foreign body is identifiable, its size may be grossly underestimated (Hartley *et al.*, 2007). Foreign material is usually seen as a strongly reflective linear or curved surface with distal acoustic shadowing; in the case of metallic foreign bodies, characteristic distal reverberations known as 'comet tail artefacts' are also seen (Figure 2.21a). Associated changes which may be recognized include surrounding, reactive, hyperechoic orbital fat, abscessation and globe distortion or indentation. Some foreign bodies may also penetrate the globe causing intraocular changes (see above). Ultrasound-guided removal of grass awns via a suprascleral approach has been described in dogs (Stades *et al.*, 2003).

CT and MRI can be used in the search for suspected orbital foreign bodies, either as a primary imaging study or to provide more detailed information following a tentative ultrasonographic diagnosis. CT is useful for the detection of metallic objects, for which the risk of movement of ferrous items and the image distortion caused by susceptibility artefacts make MRI inappropriate. Although beam hardening artefacts occur with CT, special software programmes can be used to minimize these. Wooden foreign bodies are seen as hyperdense structures with surrounding contrast enhancement.

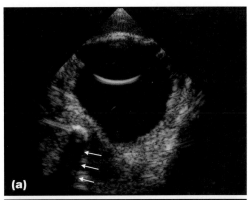

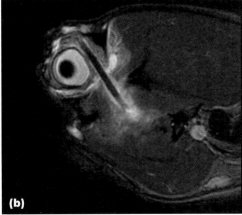

2.21 Orbital foreign body (stick) in a 7-year-old Golden Retriever. **(a)** Transcorneal ultrasonogram showing the tip of the stick as a curvilinear echogenic structure with distal acoustic shadowing (arrowed). The adjacent globe wall is distorted. Although the presence of a retrobulbar foreign body is confirmed, its precise dimensions and orientation are unclear. **(b)** Sagittal STIR image showing the extent of the foreign body, which was >5 cm in length. Surrounding soft tissue inflammation is also evident in this fat-suppressed image. The size of the foreign body was grossly underestimated on ultrasonography.

MRI is the technique of choice for the detection of non-metallic foreign bodies. Most are seen as geometric hypointense or signal void structures due to their dehydrated nature (e.g. dry wood and grass awns), although small fragments of hydrated 'green' wood may be missed (Woolfson and Wesley, 1990; Hoyt *et al.*, 2009). Even when the foreign material is not clearly identifiable, MRI shows the surrounding soft tissue reaction, most clearly via contrast enhancement, which may delineate an otherwise obscure fragment (Figure 2.21b). Foreign body associated abscesses are also evident and the full extent of pathology is demonstrated, providing the best chance of successful treatment.

Orbital myositis

With extraocular muscle myositis, ultrasonography may show enlargement of the medial rectus muscle, in particular, although often the individual muscles cannot be distinguished (see Chapter 8). MRI reveals diffuse swelling and increased contrast enhancement of the affected muscles and excludes focal pathology. CT may also show enlargement of the extraocular muscles.

Exophthalmos may also result from severe masticatory myositis affecting the temporalis, masseter and pterygoid muscles. In acute cases, T2-weighted MR images reveal multifocal, ill defined areas of hyperintensity in the affected muscles, which show marked contrast enhancement, reflecting inflammation. In chronic cases, muscle wastage with fat infiltration is readily apparent.

Reactive strabismus may result from chronic myositis, leading to fibrosis and a reduction in size of the affected muscles, and may be detected on MRI (Morgan *et al.*, 1996). CT may also be useful in such cases as the muscles are clearly delineated by orbital fat.

Zygomatic sialadenitis

The imaging features seen with ultrasonography, MRI and CT in 11 dogs with zygomatic sialadenitis have been described (Cannon *et al.*, 2011). Ultrasonographic findings are consistent with a mass lesion in the inferior orbit and, in some cases, its origin in the salivary gland is evident. MRI shows gland enlargement, heterogeneous hyperintensity on T2-weighted images and hypointensity with increased contrast enhancement on T1-weighted images; these are non-specific findings which reflect inflammation. The surrounding soft tissues may also show evidence of inflammation, a feature which may be considered to reduce the likelihood of salivary gland neoplasia. CT reveals gland enlargement and hypodensity.

In some dogs, fluid pockets suggestive of associated salivary mucoceles (see below) are evident on ultrasonography, MRI and CT. Radiographic and CT zygomatic sialography show gland enlargement and irregularity, as well as extravasation or collection of contrast material within the tissues of animals with salivary mucoceles.

Osteomyelitis of the sphenoid bone

Osteomyelitis of the sphenoid bone has been described as a cause of visual impairment in dogs and cats (Busse *et al.*, 2009). MR images showed thickening and distortion of the sphenoid bone, loss of normal bone marrow signal and diffuse contrast enhancement of the bone and adjacent meninges. Contrast enhancement is suggestive of an inflammatory rather than a neoplastic process, although differentiation may not be certain. Such bony changes would also be expected to be visible on CT and possibly even on radiography if severe enough. CSF analysis may reveal abnormalities.

Neoplasia

Many histological types of tumour can affect the orbit, but most are malignant (see Chapter 8). Tumours may arise primarily within the orbit or may extend into it from adjacent areas such as the frontal sinuses or nasal cavity. Those lesions arising within the orbit may remain confined or may extend outwards into the surrounding tissues. Orbital metastases occur occasionally and orbital infiltration with multicentric neoplasia, particularly lymphoma, is not uncommon. Imaging features of orbital tumours are usually non-specific with reference to histological type, although assessment of the aggressiveness of the tumour can be made from first principles. The appearance of an orbital tumour on imaging depends upon its size, margination, architecture and extent. Imaging features from case studies of orbital disease comprising partly or entirely neoplastic conditions have been published (Gilger *et al.,* 1992; Dennis, 2000; Mason *et al.,* 2001; Boroffka *et al.,* 2007).

Radiography

Right and left lateral thoracic radiographs should be obtained prior to skull radiography as a metastasis check if neoplasia is clinically suspected. Skull radiographs are normal (except for soft tissue swelling and exophthalmos) when tumours are confined to the orbit or have relatively minor extension beyond it. However, if a tumour has extended significantly beyond the orbital margins or has originated in the surrounding tissues, especially in a normally air-filled area such as the frontal sinus or nasal cavity, radiographs will be abnormal. Extension is harder to detect radiographically if it involves the cranial cavity (Dennis, 2000).

Radiographic features of aggressive orbital neoplasia include thinning or irregularity of the medial orbital wall and soft tissue opacity in the adjacent part of the nasal cavity and/or frontal sinus (Figure 2.22a). In the latter case, this is often due to trapped fluid rather than tumour tissue, but nevertheless is a grave sign. In advanced cases, obvious osteolysis of the bones surrounding the orbit, the sphenoid bones or the cribriform plate may be evident. Occasionally, bone-producing tumours arise within the orbital region (e.g. osteomas and multilobular bone tumours or osteochondrosarcomas). Such lesions are seen as dense masses of unstructured bone, often with a 'broccoli-like' appearance; osteolysis is variable and in many cases is absent. Wispy new bone may be seen with aggressive bone-producing tumours such as osteosarcomas.

Ultrasonography

The ultrasonographic appearance of orbital tumours is very variable. Most are hypoechoic relative to orbital fat, but some are hyperechoic; likewise echotexture can vary from homogeneous to heterogeneous. Smaller tumours are often easily detected as focal, well defined masses causing deformation of the orbital cone, but more extensive neoplasms are harder to recognize and may simply cause loss of normal orbital soft tissue architecture (see Chapter 8). Distortion and indentation of the globe may be present, although this is not a specific sign of neoplasia. Other occasional ultrasonographic features include disruption of the medial orbital wall if severe osteolysis is present (Mason *et al.*, 2001) and foci of mineralization causing acoustic shadowing (Dennis, 2000). Neoplasms with necrotic centres may mimic abscesses. Ultrasound-guided fine-needle aspiration performed under general anaesthesia is often possible and is a very valuable technique.

MRI and CT

Both MRI (Figure 2.22b) and CT (Figure 2.22c) are excellent imaging modalities for the diagnosis of orbital neoplasia and the detection of tumour extension beyond the orbit, which is usually the hallmark of malignancy (see also Chapter 8). These imaging modalities also clearly identify whether a mass is intraconal or extraconal in origin. Subtle exophthalmos may be easier to recognize on MRI than on clinical examination and indentation of the globe may also be evident, although this is a non-specific finding. Whilst CT is better at showing small areas of osteolysis or new bone production, MRI provides more detailed soft tissue information. Extensive bony lesions are easily recognized using either technique. In addition, CT is a valuable technique for a thoracic metastasis check and is more sensitive for small lesions than radiography.

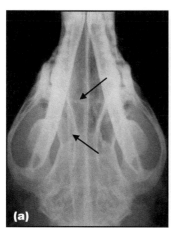 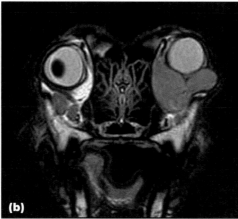 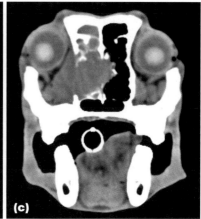

2.22 Orbital neoplasia. **(a)** DV radiograph of a 13-year-old crossbred dog with exophthalmos. There is diffuse opacification of the adjacent part of the nasal cavity and frontal sinus (arrowed), which suggests a neoplasm eroding through the medial orbital wall. **(b)** Transverse T2-weighted MR image of the head of a 9-year-old Staffordshire Bull Terrier with exophthalmos. The globe is displaced by a homogeneous soft tissue mass which fills the orbit, contacting, but not eroding, its bony margins. The mass appears to be confined to the orbit and the nasal cavity and frontal sinus are unaffected. **(c)** CT image (soft tissue window) of the head of a 9-year-old Belgian Shepherd Dog with left-sided epistaxis, reverse sneezing and mild exophthalmos. A soft tissue mass is present in the nasal cavity, which has eroded through the medial wall of the orbit and displaced the normal orbital soft tissues. The final diagnosis was nasal carcinoma. (c, Courtesy of S Boroffka)

Neoplasms are generally seen as mass lesions that displace and distort other orbital structures. Most lesions are solid, although some demonstrate cystic or necrotic areas. Inflammation of the adjacent soft tissue structures is often absent and this is a useful feature to distinguish neoplasia from inflammatory orbital disease. Signal intensity on MRI is inconsistent, although tumours are usually hypointense to orbital fat. Contrast-enhanced images are helpful in demonstrating the vascularity of the lesion and for detecting intracranial extension. As with other imaging techniques, the appearance of neoplasms is typically non-specific for histological type.

Types of neoplasm
Several neoplastic conditions which affect the orbit do have particular imaging features, including:

- Orbital lipoma
- Orbital myxosarcoma
- Sphenoid bone neoplasia
- Feline restrictive orbital myofibroblastic sarcoma (orbital 'pseudotumour').

Orbital lipoma: Fat has a characteristic appearance on CT (hypodense) and MRI (hyperintense; confirmed using fat suppression techcniques) and can be readily recognized. Similarly, MRI and CT are helpful for the investigation of orbital fat prolapse.

Orbital myxosarcoma: The imaging features of orbital myxosarcoma in five dogs have been described (Dennis, 2008). Myxosarcomas are characterized by abundant, mucinous stroma and these orbital lesions were found to be predominantly fluid-filled complex cavities. All extended to the temporomandibular joint along fascial planes and osteolysis of various bones was evident in some dogs. Although the full extent of the lesions was only seen using MRI, CT would also be expected to be helpful, and ultrasonography clearly demonstrated the complex, fluid-filled, hypoechoic cavities within the orbital tissues, whilst radiography showed large areas of osteolysis (Figure 2.23). A solid ocular and orbital myxosarcoma with major intracranial extension has also been described (Richter *et al.*, 2003).

Sphenoid bone neoplasia: Various types of tumour may arise within, or infiltrate, the sphenoid bones, which lie ventral to the brain and enclose the optic nerves. On MRI, the bones are seen to be expanded and distorted with loss of normal bone architecture and marrow signal, along with replacement by heterogeneous contrast-enhancing tissue; concurrent meningitis is common. These MRI features are non-specific and may mimic sphenoid osteomyelitis, although the mass effect is likely to be larger with neoplasia (Figure 2.24). CT demonstrates the bony changes and, if severe enough, they may also be detectable on a lateral skull radiograph.

Feline restrictive orbital myofibroblastic sarcoma: Diagnostic findings in a series of cats with an uncommon condition, previously referred to as

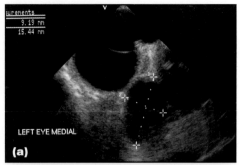
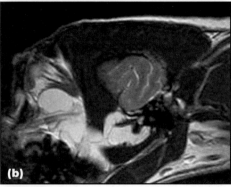

2.23 Myxosarcoma in a 14-year-old crossbred dog with severe but non-painful exophthalmos. **(a)** Ultrasonogram showing a hypoechoic cavity in the lateral aspect of the orbit, which measured >9 cm x 15 cm in this orientation. **(b)** Sagittal T2-weighted MR image showing the complex nature of the cystic structure, which extends caudally to the temporomandibular joint.

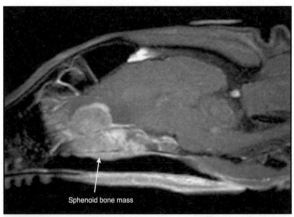

2.24 Parasagittal, fat-suppressed, post-contrast MR image in a 12-year-old crossbred dog with sphenoid bone neoplasia, bilateral blindness and mild exophthalmos. The presphenoid bone is markedly expanded and distorted, compressing the brain and obliterating the optic chiasm. The mass has expanded anteriorly into the apices of both orbits, disrupting both optic canals.

orbital 'pseudotumour', have been described (Bell *et al.*, 2011). Histology showed an invasive but low-grade malignancy and the condition was renamed feline restrictive orbital myofibroblastic sarcoma. Cross-sectional imaging features include thickening of the sclera, episcleral tissues and eyelids, swelling of the retrobulbar tissues with indistinct delineation of fat and muscles and, where contrast medium has been administered, contrast enhancement. Osteolysis may also occur. The use of ultrasonography to diagnose this condition has not been reported, but it would be expected to show non-specific changes.

Orbital trauma

Diagnostic imaging is valuable in cases of trauma involving the orbit and is essential for determining whether surgical intervention is required. Specific features of ocular trauma have been considered above. CT is the ideal technique for assessment of fractures and displaced fragments (Figure 2.25); radiography is satisfactory, but even with multiple views it may be hard to understand the conformation of any fractures. CT also shows intracranial and extracranial haematomas as hyperdense areas. MRI is ideal in cases of head trauma, since it combines acceptable demonstration of bony lesions with excellent soft tissue detail, including that of any associated intracranial pathology. Air within the

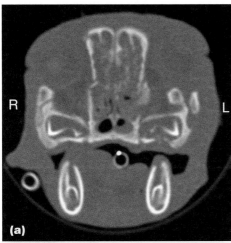

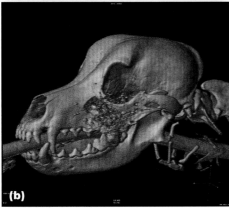

2.25 CT findings in cases of orbital trauma. **(a)** CT image (bone window) of a Labrador puppy that had suffered bite injuries. There are multiple displaced fractures affecting the right frontal bone and both right and left palatine bones. Fluid (blood) is present in the frontal sinuses and ethmoturbinate regions and there is unilateral dorsal and lateral globe displacement. **(b)** 3D reconstruction of CT images (bone window) of a 6-year-old Beagle which sustained a gunshot wound to the face. An entry wound was observed in the right maxilla but the more extensive exit wound on the left side of the face is shown here. This case illustrates the utility of this technique in locating multiple bone fragments in the orbital region. (a, Courtesy of S Boroffka; b, Courtesy of C Snyder and the University of Wisconsin-Madison Diagnostic Imaging Service)

orbit, arising from either a penetrating injury or due to extension from the frontal sinus or nasal cavity as a result of fractures involving these structures, may be visible with any of these techniques. Ultrasonography is generally unhelpful in patients with orbital trauma, except for the detection of globe rupture. Where indicated, imaging of the thorax and/or abdomen should be carried out in trauma patients.

Miscellaneous orbital and periocular cavitary lesions

Zygomatic salivary mucoceles

Plain radiography is unrewarding as it only shows soft tissue swelling, but zygomatic sialography may be helpful. Ultrasonography depicts a well defined, anechoic structure with deep acoustic enhancement. However, although a location in the inferior orbit may be suggestive of a salivary mucocele, the origin of the salivary gland is likely to be overlooked and only a general diagnosis of a cystic orbital lesion can be made. CT and MRI are both useful and reveal a cystic structure in the inferior orbit, in the region of the salivary gland, although its origin may still not be certain. Both modalities show the full extent of the lesion and contrast sialography may be readily performed in conjunction with CT, but MRI will provide considerably more information about the nature of the structure and any associated surrounding inflammation.

Cystic lesions

Cystic lesions in the periorbital region may arise from, or in the region of, the proximal nasolacrimal duct or from the adjacent nasal cavity or frontal sinus. Diagnostic imaging, whether ultrasonography, CT or MRI, is of value in establishing the cystic nature of the lesions. Dacryocystography, or the injection of contrast medium directly into the cyst, may identify their association or lack of communication with the nasolacrimal system (Ota *et al.*, 2009). These uncommon cystic lesions include dacryops, canaliculops, dermoid and epidermoid cysts, as well as microphthalmos with cyst formation and other congenital cysts of neural origin.

Benign frontal bone lesions

Thickening of the orbital portion of the frontal bone may lead to exophthalmos and strabismus. There are case reports of several benign pathologies in this area, including craniomandibular osteopathy (CMO), idiopathic calvarial hyperostosis (ICH), feline osteochondromatosis and bacterial osteomyelitis. There are clinical and histological similarities between CMO and ICH, which are probably different manifestations of the same condition; they may both be bilateral on imaging with unilateral clinical signs. Since the imaging features of these conditions are all similar they are considered together.

Radiography shows marked thickening of the frontal bone, mainly at its orbital surface, with a reduction in, or obliteration of, the normally air-filled sinus lumen (Figure 2.26a). The new bone may be smooth or irregular in appearance without evidence of osteolysis. Ultrasonography may show this bony thickening as a strongly echogenic curved structure with deep acoustic shadowing in the dorsomedial aspect of the orbit, and globe indentation may be present (Dennis *et al.*, 1993). CT and MRI demonstrate the bony changes readily; the orbital part of the frontal bone is markedly thickened and irregular, and vascularized soft tissue is present within it (Figure 2.26b). Compression and displacement of the orbital soft tissues result. Adjacent soft tissue inflammation is best shown on MRI.

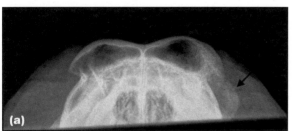
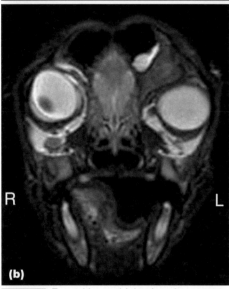

2.26 Frontal bone thickening due to osteomyelitis in a 6-month-old Jack Russell Terrier with frontal area swelling and ventral deviation of the globe. **(a)** Rostrocaudal radiograph of the frontal area. The affected frontal bone is thickened laterally and a smooth mass of mineralized tissue protrudes into the orbit (arrowed). **(b)** Transverse T2-weighted MR image showing ventral strabismus due to thickening of the outer surface of the frontal bone. The tissue is of low signal due to mineralization. There is hyperintense fluid in the ipsilateral frontal sinus (sinusitis).

Vascular malformations

Orbital vascular malformations are rare in domestic animals. Clinical and imaging signs depend on whether the lesion is an arteriovenous fistula or a venous aneurysm (varix) without arterial contribution. Radiographic arteriography can be used to demonstrate the presence of an arteriovenous communication and venography (or contrast medium injection directly into the vascular structure, if accessible) can be used to demonstrate the extent of a venous anomaly. Ultrasonography shows the enlarged vascular structures as tubular or complex anechoic cavities and colour flow Doppler ultrasonography demonstrates the direction and nature of the blood flow. Angiography with 3D reconstruction may be performed with both CT and MRI.

Advances in imaging technology

Optical coherence tomography

Optical coherence tomography (OCT), first developed in the 1990s, has been widely adopted for the evaluation and monitoring of retinal and optic nerve diseases in humans. The principle of operation of OCT, 'low coherence interferometry', is broadly comparable with ultrasonography, except that it uses light rather than sound and thus relies on clear ocular media. By laterally combining a large series (tens of thousands) of A-mode images acquired over a few seconds, the technique allows the acquisition of data sets that provide exquisitely detailed cross-sectional and 3D images, approaching *in vivo* 'histopathology' (Figure 2.27). Distinct layers within the tissues, visible as alternating bright and dark signals in cross-sectional images of the retina obtained by OCT *in vivo*, can be correlated with layers that are histologically identifiable on light microscopy.

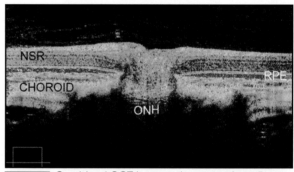

2.27 Combined OCT images demonstrating <5 μm resolution of the fine structural detail of the retinal layers, choroid and optic nerve head (ONH) in a normal cat, which approaches *in vivo* 'histopathology'. NSR = neurosensory retina; RPE = retinal pigment epithelium.

Modifications in OCT technology have subsequently been made that allow high resolution imaging of anterior segment structures, including the cornea and anterior chamber angle. Unlike ultrasonography, which requires direct contact between the transducer, coupling media and tissues, OCT does not require any contact with the surface of the eye. This limits the potential for tissue distortion and trauma.

Although these techniques have been described in the veterinary literature, they remain largely within the research domain at present due to high cost and the need for heavy sedation or general anaesthesia, but are likely to become more widely available to veterinary clinicians as the technology becomes more affordable (Rosolen *et al.*, 2012; Almazan *et al.*, 2013; Famose, 2013). Further description of this technique is outwith the scope of this chapter and the use of OCT in animals has been reviewed elsewhere (McLellan and Rasmussen, 2012).

References and further reading

Almazan A, Tsai S, Miller PE *et al.* (2013) Iridocorneal angle measurements in mammalian species: normative data by optical coherence tomography. *Veterinary Ophthalmology* 16, 163–166

Armour MD, Broome M, Dell'Anna G, Blades NJ and Esson DW (2011) A review of orbital and intracranial magnetic resonance imaging in 79 canine and 13 feline patients (2004–2010). *Veterinary Ophthalmology* 14, 215–226

Aubin ML, Powell CC, Gionfriddo JR and Fails AD (2003) Ultrasound biomicroscopy of the feline anterior segment. *Veterinary Ophthalmology* 6, 15–17

Bell CM, Schwarz T and Dubielzig RR (2011) Diagnostic features of feline restrictive orbital myofibroblastic sarcoma. *Veterinary Pathology* 48, 742–750

Bentley E, Miller PE and Diehl KA (2003) Use of high-resolution ultrasound as a diagnostic tool in veterinary ophthalmology. *Journal of the American Veterinary Medical Association* 223, 1617–1622

Bentley E, Miller PE and Diehl KA (2005) Evaluation of intra- and interobserver reliability and image reproducibility to assess usefulness of high-resolution ultrasonography for measurement of anterior segment structures of canine eyes. *American Journal of Veterinary Research* 66, 1775–1779

Boroffka SAEB, Görig C, Auriemma E *et al.* (2008) Magnetic resonance imaging of the canine optic nerve. *Veterinary Radiology and Ultrasound* 49, 540–544

Boroffka SAEB, Verbruggen AM, Boevé MH and Stades FC (1998) Ultrasonographic diagnosis of persistent hyperplastic tunica vasculosa lentis/persistent hyperplastic primary vitreous in two dogs. *Veterinary Radiology and Ultrasound* 39, 440–444

Boroffka SAEB, Verbruggen AM, Grinwis GCM, Voorhout G and Barthez PY (2007) Assessment of ultrasonography and computed tomography for the evaluation of unilateral orbital disease in dogs. *Journal of the American Veterinary Medical Association* 230, 671–680

Boroffka SAEB and Voorhout G (1999) Direct and reconstructed multiplanar computed tomography of the orbits of healthy dogs. *American Journal of Veterinary Research* 60, 1500–1507

Boroffka SAEB, Voorhout G, Verbruggen AM and Teske E (2006) Intraobserver and interobserver repeatability of ocular biometric measurements obtained by means of B-mode ultrasonography in dogs. *American Journal of Veterinary Research* 67, 1743–1749

Busse C, Dennis R and Platt SR (2009) Suspected sphenoid bone osteomyelitis causing visual impairment in two dogs and one cat. *Veterinary Ophthalmology* 12, 71–77

Calia CM, Kirschner SE, Baer KE and Stefanacci JD (1994) The use of computed tomography scan for the evaluation of orbital disease in cats and dogs. *Veterinary and Comparative Ophthalmology* 4, 24–30

Cannon MS, Paglia D, Zwingenberger AL *et al.* (2011) Clinical and diagnostic imaging findings in dogs with zygomatic sialadenitis: 11 cases (1990–2009). *Journal of the American Veterinary Medical Association* 239, 1211–1218

Dees DD, Knollinger AM, Simmons JP, Seshadri R and MacLaren NE (2012) Magnetic resonance imaging susceptibility artifact due to pigmented intraorbital silicone prosthesis. *Veterinary Ophthalmology* 15, 386–390

Dennis R (2000) Use of magnetic resonance imaging for the investigation of orbital disease in small animals. *Journal of Small Animal Practice* 41, 145–155

Dennis R (2003) Advanced imaging: indications for CT and MRI in veterinary patients. *In Practice* 25, 243–263

Dennis R (2008) Imaging features of orbital myxosarcoma in dogs. *Veterinary Radiology and Ultrasound* 49, 256–263

Dennis R, Barnett KC and Sansom J (1993) Unilateral exophthalmos and strabismus due to craniomandibular osteopathy. *Journal of Small Animal Practice* 34, 457–461

Famose F (2013) Assessment of the use of spectral domain optical coherence tomography (SD-OCT) for evaluation of the healthy and pathological cornea in dogs and cats. *Veterinary Ophthalmology* doi: 10.1111/vop.12028

Fike JR, LeCouteur RA and Cann CE (1984) Anatomy of the canine orbit: multiplanar imaging by CT. *Veterinary Radiology* 25, 32–36

Gallhoefer NS, Bentley E, Ruetten M *et al.* (2013) Comparison of ultrasonography and histologic examination for identification of ocular diseases of animals: 113 cases (2000–2010). *Journal of the American Veterinary Medical Association* 243, 376–388

Gavin PR (2009) Physics. In: *Practical Small Animal MRI*, ed. PR Gavin and RS Bagley, pp. 1–22. Wiley Blackwell, Oxford

Gelatt KN, Cure TH, Guffy MM and Jessen C (1972) Dacryocystorhinography in the dog and cat. *Journal of Small Animal Practice* 13, 381–397

Gelatt KN, Miyabayashi T, Gelatt-Nicholson KJ and MacKay EO (2003) Progressive changes in ophthalmic blood velocities in Beagles with primary open angle glaucoma. *Veterinary Ophthalmology* 6, 77–84

Gelatt-Nicholson KJ, Gelatt KN, MacKay E, Brooks DE and Newell SM (1999a) Doppler imaging of the ophthalmic vasculature of the normal dog: blood velocity measurements and reproducibility. *Veterinary Ophthalmology* 2, 87–96

Gelatt-Nicholson KJ, Gelatt KN, MacKay E, Brooks DE and Newell SM (1999b) Comparative Doppler imaging of the ophthalmic vasculature in normal Beagles and Beagles with inherited primary open-angle glaucoma. *Veterinary Ophthalmology* 2, 97–105

Gibson TE, Roberts SM, Severin GA, Steyn PF and Wrigley RH (1998) Comparison of gonioscopy and ultrasound biomicroscopy for evaluating the iridocorneal angle in dogs. *Journal of the American Veterinary Medical Association* 213, 635–638

Gilger BC, McLaughlin SA, Whitley D and Wright JC (1992) Orbital neoplasms in cats: 21 cases (1974–1990). *Journal of the American Veterinary Medical Association* 201, 1083–1086

Goh PS, Gi MT, Charlton A *et al.* (2008) Review of orbital imaging. *European Journal of Radiology* 66, 387–395

Gomes FE, Bentley E, Lin TL and McLellan GJ (2011) Effects of unilateral topical administration of 0.5% tropicamide on anterior segment morphology and intraocular pressure in normal cats and cats with primary congenital glaucoma. *Veterinary Ophthalmology* 14(Suppl.), 75–83

Hartley C, McConnell JF and Doust R (2007) Wooden orbital foreign body in a Weimaraner. *Veterinary Ophthalmology* 10, 390–393

Holloway A and McConnell F (2013) *BSAVA Manual of Canine and Feline Radiography and Radiology: A Foundation Manual.* BSAVA Publications, Gloucester

Hoyt L, Greenberg M, MacPhail C, Eichelberger B, Marolf A and Kraft S (2009) Imaging diagnosis – magnetic resonance imaging of an organizing abscess secondary to a retrobulbar grass awn. *Veterinary Radiology and Ultrasound* 50, 646–648

Kim SE, Park YW, Ahn JS *et al.* (2011) C-arm fluoroscopy for the removal of an intraorbital foreign body in a cat. *Journal of Feline Medicine and Surgery* 13, 112–115

Kneissl S, Konar M, Fuchs-Baumgartinger A and Nell B (2007) Magnetic resonance imaging features of orbital inflammation with intracranial extension in four dogs. *Veterinary Radiology and Ultrasound* 48, 403–408

Labruyère JJ, Hartley C and Holloway A (2011) Contrast-enhanced ultrasonography in the differentiation of retinal detachment and vitreous membrane in dogs and cats. *Journal of Small Animal Practice* 52, 522–530

Labruyère JJ, Hartley C, Rogers K *et al.* (2008) Ultrasonographic evaluation of vitreous degeneration in normal dogs. *Veterinary Radiology and Ultrasound* 49, 165–171

LeCouteur RA, Fike JR, Scagliotti RH and Cann CE (1982) Computed tomography of orbital tumors in the dog. *Journal of the American Veterinary Medical Association* 180, 910–913

Mason DR, Lamb CR and McLellan GJ (2001) Ultrasonographic features in 50 dogs with retrobulbar disease. *Journal of the American Animal Hospital Association* 37, 557–562

McLellan GJ and Rasmussen CA (2012) Optical coherence tomography for the evaluation of retinal and optic nerve morphology in animal subjects: practical considerations. *Veterinary Ophthalmology* 15(Suppl. 2), 13–28

Moore D and Lamb C (2007) Ocular ultrasonography in companion animals: a pictorial review. *In Practice* 29, 604–610

Morgan RV, Daniel GB and Donnell RL (1994) Magnetic resonance imaging of the normal eye and orbit of the dog and cat. *Veterinary Radiology and Ultrasound* 35, 102–108

Morgan RV, Ring RD, Ward DA and Adams WH (1996) Magnetic resonance imaging of ocular and orbital disease in 5 dogs and a cat. *Veterinary Radiology and Ultrasound* 37, 185–192

Noller C, Henninger W, Grönemeyer DHW, Hirschberg RM and Budras KD (2006) Computed tomography anatomy of the normal feline nasolacrimal drainage system. *Veterinary Radiology and Ultrasound* 47, 53–60

Novellas R, Espada Y and Ruiz de Gopegui R (2007a) Doppler ultrasonographic estimation of renal and ocular resistive and pulsatility indices in normal dogs and cats. *Veterinary Radiology and Ultrasound* 48, 69–73

Novellas R, Ruiz de Gopegui and R Espada Y (2007b) Effects of sedation with midazolam and butorphanol on resistive and pulsatility indices in normal dogs and cats. *Veterinary Radiology and Ultrasound* 48, 276–280

Nykamp SG, Scrivani PV and Pease AP (2004) Computed tomography dacryocystography evaluation of the nasolacrimal apparatus. *Veterinary Radiology and Ultrasound* 45, 23–28

Ota J, Pearce JW, Finn MJ, Johnson GC and Giuliano EA (2009) Dacryops (lacrimal cyst) in three young Labrador Retrievers. *Journal of the American Animal Hospital Association* 45, 191–196

Penninck D, Daniel GB, Brawer R and Tidwell AS (2001) Cross-sectional imaging techniques in veterinary ophthalmology. *Clinical Techniques in Small Animal Practice* 16, 22–39

Rached PA, Canola JC, Schlüter C *et al.* (2011) Computed tomographic-dacryocystography (CT-DCG) of the normal canine nasolacrimal drainage system with three-dimensional reconstruction. *Veterinary Ophthalmology* **14**, 174–179

Richter M, Stankeova S, Hauser B, Scharf G and Spiess BM (2003) Myxosarcoma in the eye and brain in a dog. *Veterinary Ophthalmology* **6**, 183–189

Rose MD, Mattoon JS, Gemensky-Metzler AJ, Wilkie DA and Rajala-Schultz PJ (2008) Ultrasound biomicroscopy of the iridocorneal angle of the eye before and after phacoemulsification and intraocular lens implantation in dogs. *American Journal of Veterinary Research* **69**, 279–288

Rosolen SG, Rivière ML, Lavillegrand S *et al.* (2012) Use of a combined slit-lamp SD-OCT to obtain anterior and posterior segment images in selected animal species. *Veterinary Ophthalmology* **15**(Suppl. 2), 105–115

Sansom J and Labruyère J (2012) Penetrating ocular gunshot injury in a Labrador Retriever. *Veterinary Ophthalmology* **15** 115–122

Schlueter C, Budras KD, Ludewig E *et al.* (2009) CT and anatomical study of the relationship between head conformation and the nasolacrimal system. *Journal of Feline Medicine and Surgery* **11**, 891–900

Stades FC, Djajadiningrat-Laanen SC, Boroffka SAEB and Boevé MH (2003) Suprascleral removal of a foreign body from the retrobulbar muscle cone in two dogs. *Journal of Small Animal Practice* **44**, 17–20

Tidwell AS and Johnson KL (1994) Computed tomography-guided percutaneous biopsy in the dog and cat: description of technique and preliminary evaluation in 14 patients. *Veterinary Radiology and Ultrasound* **35**, 445–456

Tsai S, Bentley E, Miller PE *et al.* (2012) Gender differences in iridocorneal angle morphology: a potential explanation for the female predisposition to primary angle closure glaucoma in dogs. *Veterinary Ophthalmology* **15** (Suppl. 1), 60–63

van der Woerdt A, Wilkie DA and Myer CW (1993) Ultrasonographic abnormalities in the eyes of dogs with cataracts: 147 cases (1986–1992). *Journal of the American Veterinary Medical Association* **203**, 838–841

Whatmough C and Lamb CR (2006) Computed tomography: principles and applications. *Compendium on Continuing Education for the Practicing Veterinarian* **28**, 789–800

Wilkie DA, Gemensky-Metzler AJ, Colitz CM *et al.* (2006) Canine cataracts, diabetes mellitus and spontaneous lens capsule rupture: a retrospective study of 18 dogs. *Veterinary Ophthalmology* **9**, 328–334

Williams DL (2004) Lens morphometry determined by B-mode ultrasonography of the normal and cataractous canine lens. *Veterinary Ophthalmology* **7**, 91–95

Woolfson JM and Wesley RE (1990) Magnetic resonance imaging and computed tomographic scanning of fresh (green) wood foreign bodies in dog orbits. *Ophthalmic Plastic and Reconstructive Surgery* **6**, 237–240

3

Laboratory investigation of ophthalmic disease

Emma Dewhurst, Jim Carter and Emma Scurrell

Laboratory investigation is an important diagnostic tool in veterinary ophthalmology and covers techniques such as microbiological culture, haematology, serum biochemistry, serology, polymerase chain reaction (PCR) testing, cytology and histopathology. As well as being the primary target for many diseases, the eye is also often involved in systemic disease processes, including infectious, neoplastic and immune-mediated conditions. Laboratory investigation can be the gateway to the accurate diagnosis of such diseases, which in turn plays a fundamental role in patient care and management.

Not only is it useful for the clinician to be familiar with the techniques used for laboratory investigation, it is also beneficial to have a good relationship with the diagnostic laboratory processing the samples. If there is any confusion regarding the results and interpretation, it is always worth contacting the laboratory for a discussion as additional clinical details may help determine the diagnosis.

This chapter describes some of the techniques used for sample collection and submission, and discusses which investigations are possible within the practice environment and which samples should be sent to a commercial laboratory. The appropriate investigation is then considered and the choices available explained. The reader is also directed to the relevant chapters in the Manual which deal with the individual disease processes.

Sample collection and handling

Correct sample collection is paramount if the clinical investigation is going to achieve reliable results. There are several different types of sample that may be submitted:

- Swabs for microbiological culture (bacterial, viral or fungal)
- Blood samples for haematology, serum biochemistry and serology
- Samples for PCR testing
- Cytological samples (including impression smears, scrapes and hair plucks, fine-needle aspirates and aqueocentesis and vitreocentesis samples)
- Biopsy samples and globe submission for histopathology.

When investigating an infectious process, the risk to the health of personnel both in the clinic and in the laboratory should be considered, particularly if there is concern regarding a zoonotic agent. Labelling any submission forms or slide boxes with the possible agent of concern (e.g. *Mycobacterium*) is good practice.

Microbiological investigation

Bacterial culture

Conjunctival swabs can be collected from a conscious patient with only the occasional need for topical local anaesthesia. It must be remembered that there is a normal conjunctival flora in domestic animal patients, so the fornix is not sterile (Prado *et al.*, 2005; Wang *et al.*, 2008). Samples for investigation of conjunctival or corneal infection should be taken avoiding contact with the lid margin or skin of the face, which may lead to sample contamination. Small tip swabs are best for sample collection and may be marketed as urethral swabs or mini-tip swabs, depending on the supplier.

The transport medium present in the swab (normally Amies transport medium) should help prevent loss or overgrowth of the organism whilst in transit to the laboratory, thus avoiding distortion of the clinical picture of the extent of the infection. Survival of fastidious bacteria can be prolonged by the addition of charcoal to the Amies medium. As different diagnostic testing laboratories may have a preference for submission of samples either in charcoal-enriched or plain Amies medium, it may be of benefit to contact them to determine which samples work best with their submission criteria and laboratory techniques. If chlamydial culture is required, samples must be submitted in chlamydial transport medium, which can be supplied by the diagnostic testing laboratory.

In cases of infectious conjunctivitis, there is often a mucopurulent discharge adherent to the globe, lid margin and conjunctiva. If possible, this should be sampled prior to cleaning the site for ocular examination. It is vital for the clinician to record where the sample was collected from because this may influence the antibiotics used in the sensitivity panel. It may be worth asking the laboratory to set up a specific panel for conjunctival and corneal bacteriology, so that sensitivity is ascertained according to the topical preparations available in the practice.

Recent antimicrobial therapy will affect the recovery of any organisms present, as will insufficient material collected from the site sampled; the larger the amount of material submitted for culture, the greater the chances of recovering any organisms. Although material is usually submitted on a transport swab, if ample material is recovered it can be sent to the laboratory in a plain pot, providing there is no expected delay in transit that may lead to tissue desiccation. Preferably, material should not be stored in the refrigerator because this may increase the possibility of false-negative culture results.

Virus isolation

Virus isolation is rarely used nowadays, owing to the development of PCR testing. Virus isolation requires the collection of sufficient viable organisms to cause a cytopathic effect in cell culture. Problems with acquiring sufficient viable organisms lead to false-negative results, which are a potential drawback with this methodology. Swabs taken for virus isolation must be transported in viral transport medium, which can be supplied by the diagnostic laboratory offering the service.

Fungal culture

Collection of sufficient material is a potential limiting factor for the culture of fungi from ocular samples. Material should be collected from the periphery of the lesions, where it is more likely that viable fungal elements may be recovered. Samples can be submitted to the diagnostic testing laboratory on standard bacteriology swabs (containing Amies medium). Alternatively, whole tissue samples can be submitted in a plain pot, as long as they do not desiccate during transportation.

Serology

The most commonly performed serological tests for the diagnosis of infectious disease are the immunofluorescent assay (IFA) and the enzyme-linked immunosorbent assay (ELISA). These assays are used to detect pathogen-specific antibodies or antigens.

For IFA antibody detection, test serum is incubated with plates or slides containing immobilized antigen. If antibodies to the antigen are present within the test serum, they will bind to it and can be detected by incubation with a secondary antibody, which targets the antigen-bound antibody. This secondary antibody is labelled with a fluorescent marker that can then be visualized. The results are given as an antibody titre and represent the lowest dilution of the sample which shows fluorescence.

However, it should be noted that the presence of an antibody only gives an indication of exposure and seroconversion, and is not a direct marker of active disease. For example, around 30% of healthy dogs and cats have positive *Toxoplasma gondii* titres (Dubey and Lappin, 2006) and, therefore, the presence of a positive *Toxoplasma* immunoglobulin (Ig) G titre in a dog or cat with uveitis is not necessarily proof of a causal link. For this reason, many laboratories also offer measurement of *Toxoplasma* IgM titres, which are relatively short-lived and thus indicative of recent infection.

Polymerase chain reaction

PCR testing (the various techniques are summarized in Figure 3.1) involves the exponential amplification of very small amounts of DNA to detectable levels. In theory, a specific section of DNA can be amplified $>5 \times 10^8$ times during the 30 cycles of a typical PCR amplification cycle, and it is this exquisite sensitivity and specificity that has revolutionized diagnostic testing for infectious and inherited

Methodology	Advantages and disadvantages
Conventional PCR	
Using a series of heating and cooling cycles, a temperature-dependent DNA polymerase with code-specific primers is used to detect and amplify tiny quantities of DNA	The DNA detected does not need to be intact, therefore, the organism does not need to be viable. Unexpected pieces of DNA may be amplified if the primers bind to a different part of the target DNA than expected
Nested PCR	
Conventional PCR but using two sets of primers. First run as above, then a second set of primers is directed against a segment of code from the first product	Using two sets of primers reduces amplification of inappropriate DNA segments and increases sensitivity and specificity. However, the technique is laborious and non-quantitative
Quantitative real-time PCR (qRT-PCR)	
After every PCR cycle, the amount of product formed is measured and displayed in fluorescence units. The greater the amount of target DNA in the submitted sample, the more quickly product (and therefore fluorescence) is formed. Once a certain threshold of fluorescence is reached, the sample is deemed to be positive, and the number of cycles taken to reach that threshold allows a quantitative measurement of DNA in the original sample	Allows a quantitative estimate of the amount of DNA associated with a given pathogen that is present in the submitted sample and thus an interpretation of its clinical significance
Reverse transcriptase PCR (RT-PCR)	
A reverse transcriptase is added to produce complementary DNA (cDNA) from an RNA sequence. This cDNA is then amplified as for qRT-PCR	As for qRT-PCR. Used in the detection of RNA viruses (e.g. feline immunodeficiency virus)

3.1 Polymerase chain reaction (PCR) techniques.

diseases. However, in the case of infectious disease, this strength is also its weakness, in that PCR may amplify small, clinically insignificant, amounts of DNA, leading to the risk of false-positive results. This may lead to problems in interpreting the test results for some diseases, most notably feline herpesvirus-1 (FHV-1).

Cytological evaluation

Sample collection

When sampling the conjunctiva or cornea for cytology, it is important to remove any gel or lubricant prior to taking the sample because the presence of such material can obscure the cells and interfere with staining and evaluation. Cytological samples from the conjunctiva and cornea can be made either via direct impression, by applying asymmetrical strips of Millipore filter on to the ocular surface (Bolzan *et al.*, 2005), or with the aid of a cytology brush or swab (Tsubota *et al.*, 1990). The results from cytological samples obtained using a swab will be improved if the swab has been moistened using transport medium or saline. It is important for the swab to be rolled over the conjunctival surface and then rolled in the opposite direction on the slide to prevent smearing or excessive damage to the cells collected. Sample collection with a cytobrush (a small nylon bristled brush) is undertaken by rubbing the brush in the conjunctival fornix and then gently rolling it on a cytology slide to air dry. The cellularity of the submission is generally very good with this technique, although the cellular volume of the sample may be lower.

If a larger sample is required for submission, a scraping technique for superficial cell collection may be used. This can be achieved using topical local anaesthesia and the handle end of a No. 11 or 15 Bard Parker scalpel blade. When conducted properly, this technique is safe and can release a significant volume of tissue for cytological evaluation. In order for this technique to work well, the blunt, handle end of the scalpel blade should be held at an acute angle to the tissue surface and gently dragged backwards, collecting a sample within the acute angle. The sample can then be gently placed on a slide for submission and, if necessary, smeared with another slide using the crush technique. Very slight force only is applied to the slides as they are placed together and pulled apart in a parallel direction (Figure 3.2).

Cytological samples from ocular lesions can be made using impression smears, scrapes or aspirates (Figure 3.3). Scrapes and smears tend to sample more superficial tissue than aspiration. If an inflamed area is sampled, scrape or impression smear cytology may only reflect that which was already known. In these instances, aspiration may be a better tool, if applicable to the site of the lesion. Irrespective of the technique used, the most important process is to ensure that a smear is made from the material collected. Spraying material on to a slide from an aspirate will often only yield a few dense droplets of material, which then provides very

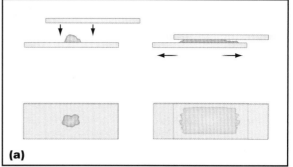

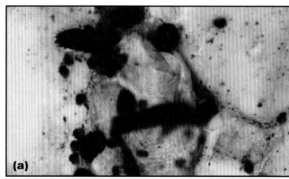

3.2 **(a)** Technique for preparing a cytology smear. Note that the slides can also be held perpendicular to each other, rather than parallel, before smearing. **(b)** A scrape of material from a region of chronic superficial keratitis (pannus) in a German Shepherd Dog, which has been correctly smeared. A mixture of non-degenerate neutrophils and the occasional lymphocyte can be seen. (Wright–Giemsa stain; original magnification x1000)

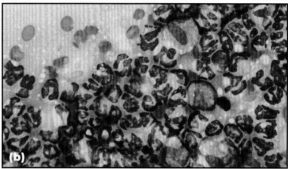

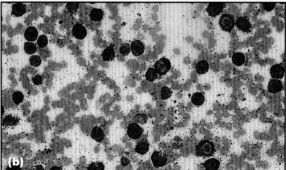

3.3 **(a)** Impression smear of a third eyelid lesion showing a mixture of anucleated keratinized squames, keratin scrolls and a low number of granulocytes. (Wright–Giemsa stain; original magnification x100) **(b)** Fine-needle aspirate of the same lesion. A background of red blood cells can be seen, through which is scattered a moderate number of variably granulated mast cells. (Wright–Giemsa stain; original magnification X400)

few individual cells for good microscopic examination. Gentle smearing of any material collected, particularly from an aspirate, is often more rewarding. The material must be rapidly air dried. If the sample is bloody, drying should be facilitated by waving the slide in the air in order to decrease drying time and reduce cell deterioration.

Fine-needle aspiration

Fine-needle aspiration can be a very rewarding technique, when used in the correct diagnostic situation, for the evaluation of adnexal, globe and orbital masses. With adequate sampling technique, the vast majority of neoplasms and inflammatory lesions (e.g. adenomas, adenocarcinomas, squamous cell carcinomas, melanomas, sarcomas, mast cell tumours, lymphomas, abscesses and pyogranulomas) can provide a diagnostic cell yield that can at least allow differentiation of inflammatory and neoplastic lesions. Exceptions include lesions of low cellularity, which often have a predominant collagenous component (e.g. collagenous hamartomas). Cystic masses can be challenging, but the examination of aspirated fluid may still be rewarding. However, more often than not, aspiration of cystic fluid simply reveals nonspecific inflammation and therefore aspiration of any associated solid material is ideal.

Conjunctival and eyelid lesions may be aspirated using techniques identical to those used in other cutaneous regions. Aspiration of objects within the orbit is best conducted under ultrasound guidance. Prior to the aspiration of lesions within the orbit, an understanding of orbital anatomy is important in order to minimize trauma to other orbital structures. Typically, a 23 gauge needle is inserted, either via the conjunctiva or transcutaneously through the upper or lower lid, and directed away from the globe to prevent trauma. A spinal or retrobulbar needle (see Chapter 5) may be required to allow access to deeper tissues. For medial orbital masses, the needle may be gently 'walked' around the medial bony orbital wall, under ultrasound guidance, until the desired lesion is located.

Alternatively, it may be preferable to insert the needle via the oral cavity, posterior to the last maxillary molar tooth, or via the supraorbital fossa caudal to the orbital rim. Both of these locations require the use of imaging techniques such as ultrasonography or, occasionally, computed tomography (CT) in order to ensure that the needle is inserted in the correct location without inadvertent trauma to the globe or orbital structures. A sample can be aspirated using a 2 ml or, rarely, a 5 ml syringe and a smear made.

Aqueocentesis

Aqueocentesis is a sampling technique in which aqueous humour is aspirated from the anterior chamber of the eye. The fluid collected can be submitted for cytological and serological evaluation or microbiological culture. This technique may also be used to aspirate cells from masses in the anterior segment or on the iridal surface. This technique is usually conducted under general anaesthesia, or at least deep sedation with topical local anaesthesia,

because incorrect placement of the needle or movement of the patient once the needle has been inserted may result in potentially catastrophic intraocular damage. Thus, referral to a specialist is strongly recommended. Occasionally, in a very compliant patient and with an experienced clinician, this can be performed with just topical local anaesthesia and gentle manual restraint.

Patient positioning and preparation: Positioning of the patient is paramount for quick accurate sampling. The patient is placed in lateral recumbency with the globe facing upwards and the ocular surface oriented horizontally. The eyelids are held open with a lid speculum of the correct size to prevent excessive pressure being placed on the globe, causing an increase in intraocular pressure. A speculum that is too long will stretch the lid margins laterally and medially, reducing the size of the palpebral aperture, subsequently reducing globe exposure and making the procedure more difficult.

Procedure: It is normally recommended that the procedure is performed in as sterile a manner as possible, with the operator using sterile gloves, drapes and instruments. The use of magnification and illumination provided by operating loupes with a light source or operating microscope makes this procedure significantly more accurate and reduces the risk of incorrect needle placement or trauma to intraocular structures such as the iris or lens. Inadvertent lens perforation or trauma may result in uncontrolled phacoclastic uveitis or traumatic cataract formation.

The site of entry is usually superio-temporal to the limbus because exposure of the eye is better in that area. A 1 ml syringe with a 27 or 30 gauge needle is most commonly used. Insulin syringes with swaged-on 28 gauge needles can work well and are often available in only 0.5 ml volumes. The conjunctiva and fornix are flushed with a 1:50 dilute solution of povidone–iodine to reduce the risk of intraocular contamination. The globe is then treated with 2–3 sterile drops of topical proxymetacaine over 1–2 minutes to provide sufficient analgesia and anaesthesia of the cornea.

With one hand, the conjunctiva and episclera adjacent to the desired location are grasped using small conjunctival or St Martins rat-toothed forceps. The tissue is held firmly so that the globe does not move during insertion of the needle. Prior to insertion of the needle, the plunger on the syringe is depressed to release the friction on the plunger within the syringe barrel. With the other hand, the needle is inserted just rostral to the limbus (approximately 0.5 mm into clear cornea). The angle of insertion is at approximately 45 degrees to the conjunctival surface and almost parallel with the iridal surface, providing a reasonably flat long tract that will seal after the needle has been removed. Care must be taken not to puncture the iris during needle insertion, especially in the region of the major arterial circle.

Once the needle is in place, approximately 0.1–0.2 ml of fluid can be removed for serological or cytological evaluation. It is always worth contacting the laboratory before collecting the sample for advice on how they would prefer to have the sample submitted. If in any doubt, the following information should help:

- Fluid is best submitted in paediatric tubes because they are of a lower overall volume and small samples will not get lost within the tube by adhesion to the walls
- Submission of fluid is better than a swab because it allows the laboratory a greater opportunity for plating the sample out than if a cellulose or rayon swab has been used
- If the fluid is intended for culture, then submission in a plain tube is better than submission in an ethylene diamine tetra-acetic acid (EDTA) tube
- For cytological evaluation, EDTA tubes should be used. However, whilst EDTA helps to preserve cell morphology, the high concentration in a routine 1 ml haematology blood tube may cause cell lysis because the volume of aqueous collected is only 0.1–0.2 ml. To help reduce this risk:
  - If a paediatric EDTA tube is not available, a plain tube can be used
  - If a cytospin machine is present on site, this can be used to prepare an air dried, unstained sediment smear. Otherwise, a direct smear of the fluid can be made at the time of sampling and submitted alongside the remaining fluid in a paediatric EDTA tube
  - With smears made from fluid-rich samples, drying artefacts are a common problem, causing cell shrinkage and interfering with cytological evaluation. In order to avoid this, any smears should be air dried as quickly as possible (the use of a hairdryer on a cool setting can be helpful) and submitted unstained to the laboratory.

Complications: Aqueocentesis is not without risk. Acute hypotony of the eye and haemorrhage are amongst the potential complications. Note that in experienced hands there are seldom complications. It is important that relatively large volumes of aqueous are not removed too rapidly or the subsequent severe hypotony could potentially lead to choroidal effusion and retinal detachment. Haemorrhage is most likely to occur during the aspiration of masses or if the iris stroma is accidently punctured with the needle.

Findings: Normal findings for aqueous humour analysis are:

- No cells on cytological evaluation
- Total protein concentration of 21–37 mg/dl
- Negative microbiological culture.

Alterations in this appearance or positive serological values are indicative of clinical disease (Figure 3.4).

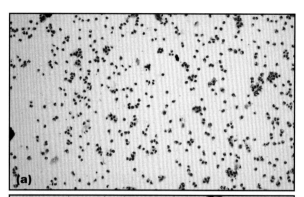

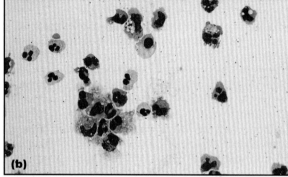

3.4 Aqueous humour collected 10 days following phacoemulsification from a dog with endophthalmitis. **(a)** Cellularity is increased and the population is mixed with non-degenerate neutrophils and mononuclear cells evident. (Wright–Giemsa stain; original magnification x100) **(b)** Magnified view. A mixed population of non-degenerate neutrophils, macrophages and the occasional lymphocyte is visible. The macrophages contain a dark green–black pigment, which may be melanin. The granular material throughout the background is stain, not bacteria. (Wright–Giemsa stain; original magnification x400)

Vitreocentesis

This technique is performed as for aqueocentesis, except that a 25–27 gauge needle is inserted approximately 7 mm behind the limbus through the pars plana, aiming towards the optic nerve head. Microscopic observation through the pupil, if dilated, can help the surgeon to visualize the posterior lens capsule anterior to the needle, preventing trauma. Approximately 0.1–0.25 ml of vitreous may be aspirated. This technique should only be performed under general anaesthesia and by experienced ophthalmologists. It is also preferable to use this technique only in non-visual globes for the diagnosis of potential infectious diseases (e.g. cryptococcosis or blastomycosis).

Sample labelling, submission and staining

Once the sample has been collected, it is important to label the slide clearly with the patient's identification number or name and the site from which the sample was collected. If multiple slides are to be submitted, a written note should be supplied with a key for the cytologist, in order for them to report what is on each specific slide and its location. Slides with a ground-glass end are preferable, for ease of labelling. Pencil should be used because this is not removed by the cytological preparation stains and fixatives (unlike ink). Correct labelling of the slide will also help the laboratory to identify which side of the slide has material on it. Drawing a circle with a wax marker around material not visible to the naked eye is also useful because it will guide the laboratory technicians to stain the correct side of the slide.

Slides are then safe to store in boxes, out of direct light and at room temperature. Slides must not be put in the refrigerator, especially not in boxes, because condensation may form on the slides and affect cell morphology. Slides must not be stored or sent in the same submission package as formalin pots. The presence of formaldehyde fumes will adversely affect staining if a Romanowsky stain is to be used.

Cytological preparations are most commonly stained with a Romanowsky stain or modification, including Wright–Giemsa and Diff-Quik. These stains contain variable combinations of acidic and basic dyes, which stain nuclear and cytoplasmic material. Diff-Quik is simply a quick in-house modification of the Wright–Giemsa stain. If the Diff-Quik is used for other purposes in the clinic (e.g. staining skin scrapes) this can lead to contamination of the stain with debris and bacteria, which can easily be transferred to any ocular cytology slides (Figure 3.5). Another source of artefacts to consider when examining cytology smears from corneal scrapes, especially ultrasound-guided aspirates, is lubricating gel (Figure 3.6).

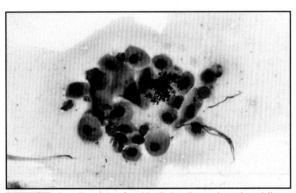

3.5 A collection of epithelial cells and eosinophils from a patient with eosinophilic keratitis. The large pool of blue–purple granular material is stain deposit and should not be confused with bacteria. (Wright–Giemsa stain; original magnification x400)

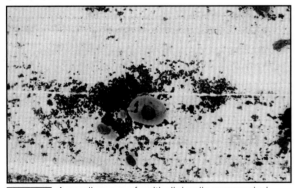

3.6 A small group of epithelial cells surrounded by lubricating gel. The lubricating gel appears as dark purple amorphous granular material. (Wright–Giemsa stain; original magnification x400)

Direct slide examination

Slides are best examined with a well maintained and serviced light microscope with multiple objective lenses (x10, x40 and a x100 oil objective). Micro-organisms may be visualized on cytological specimens from ocular samples. However, this is a relatively insensitive means of detecting the presence of infectious agents. False-negative results may occur because, although an infectious agent is present *in vivo*, it is not present in sufficient quantities to be identified in the material collected. Fungi may be identified by the direct examination of slides containing material from hair plucks, eyelid or ocular surface scrapes, fluid or biopsy samples. Unstained slides should be submitted to the diagnostic testing laboratory, where they are examined following staining with Romanowsky-type stains such as Leishman's, Giemsa, Wright's or Diff-Quik.

Direct slide examination may also be useful in the investigation of bacterial infections. Although accurate identification of specific bacterial pathogens is not possible without culture, direct slide examination can prove useful in certain circumstances (e.g. when dealing with a case of acute stromal infiltrates collagenolysis or 'melting' corneal ulcer). A swab, scrape or cytobrush sample taken from the edge of a corneal ulcer (following application of topical anaesthetic) is rolled on to a slide, which is then air dried and stained with Diff-Quik. Examination of the slide under high power magnification may allow the identification of intracellular rods or cocci within keratocytes and inflammatory cells, thus allowing a presumptive diagnosis of bacterial keratitis and aid the selection of appropriate antibiotic therapy.

Histopathological examination

Biopsy

Biopsy can be incisional or excisional; the former is often most helpful in cases of diffuse eyelid/conjunctival disease or in the presence of a large mass where a diagnosis is important for the formulation of a therapeutic approach. Full-thickness lid biopsy should only be performed under general anaesthesia and, for accurate closure, some level of magnification is beneficial. Closure of the biopsy site may be complicated, depending on the location and nature of the disease. Following biopsy, it is recommended that the use of topical anti-inflammatory medications (e.g. dexamethasone and prednisolone) be delayed for approximately 5 days to allow sufficient healing of the wound. Conjunctival biopsy is straightforward and can be performed under local anaesthesia, with a simple snip technique, using a pair of curved Westcott scissors and conjunctival or St Martins rat-toothed forceps.

For deeper samples, it may be necessary to perform a Tru-cut biopsy rather than a deep excisional biopsy. This must be undertaken with extreme caution because of the many delicate structures that lie within the orbit, in order to avoid inadvertent globe perforation, pronounced haemorrhage or neurological damage. This procedure has been reported for large orbital masses in conjunction with advanced imaging techniques to guide placement of the Tru-cut needle (CT or ultrasonography; Hendrix and Gelatt, 2000). Tru-cut biopsy sampling may be a good prequel to exenteration or orbitotomy in the case of a large, apparently aggressive, neoplasm (Boston, 2010).

Samples should be fixed in 10% neutral buffered formalin (NBF) and submitted accompanied by a record of the signalment, clinical history and clinical diagnosis. If appropriate, tissue margins of concern should be tagged with a suture or inked and indicated using a simple diagram to aid orientation of the specimen. Keratectomy specimens are prone to folding and can be mounted flat on a non-absorbent surface (e.g. plastic). Alternatively, keratectomy specimens or very small biopsy samples can be placed in a biopsy capsule (Figure 3.7a), which in turn is placed in a formalin-filled container (Figure 3.7b). It should be remembered that ophthalmic tissue is very delicate and substantial handling prior to submission (i.e. during sampling) may result in a macerated sample of minimal diagnostic use.

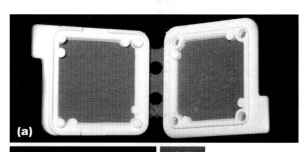
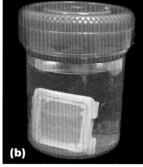

3.7 **(a)** A biopsy capsule can be useful, particularly for small specimens. **(b)** The biopsy capsule containing the specimen is then placed in a formalin-filled container.

The globe

Histopathological evaluation of an enucleated or eviscerated globe is often valuable to confirm the clinical diagnosis and, in some cases, to report important additional information which may have implications for the remaining eye and systemic health of the patient. In addition, routine submission of diseased ocular tissue contributes to the recognition of diagnostically significant trends and emerging disease entities.

Indications for removal

The most common reasons for enucleation include intractable glaucoma (for which there is a multitude of possible causes), neoplasia, inoperable structural disruption of the globe and ocular infection which is unresponsive to treatment. Surgical placement of an intrascleral prosthesis is sometimes used as an alternative to enucleation, where chronic painful diseases such as glaucoma and uveitis have caused irreversible blindness. In such cases, the intraocular contents (including the aqueous, uveal tract, lens, vitreous and retina) are removed and routinely submitted for histopathology as an evisceration sample. This is particularly important to rule out intraocular neoplasia, as tumour recurrence will lead to failure of the intrascleral prosthesis.

Preparation of the globe

To aid scleral penetration of the fixative, it is advisable to remove all non-diseased extraocular tissue, including the eyelids, periocular fat and muscle prior to fixation (Figure 3.8). If a transconjunctival technique has been used for enucleation then very little, if any, tissue will need to be removed. Although the sclera is a dense outer fibrous tunic, the inner uveal tract and retina are prone to rapid deterioration, and removal of any extraneous tissue is important. An exception to this is when there is involvement of the adnexal or orbital tissues (Figure 3.9); in these cases, the extraocular tissue should remain intact and be submitted with the globe to help the pathologist with orientation and assessment of surgical margins. If there is a particular surgical margin of concern, this can be tagged with a suture or inked and indicated on a diagram. In all cases, the optic nerve should be retained with the globe. The globe

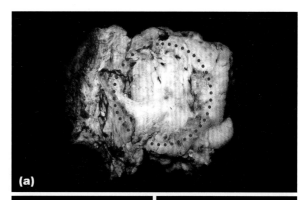
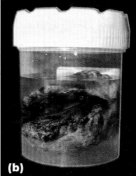
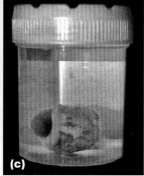

3.8 **(a)** Non-diseased extraocular tissue should be trimmed off the globe prior to immersion in fixative. The dotted line marks the approximate position of the globe. **(b)** The extraocular tissue has not been removed. This is a common error and results in the tissue:formalin ratio being too large. **(c)** This globe has been properly prepared and fixed. The eyelids, extraocular muscles and fat have been removed and the attached optic nerve has been left intact.

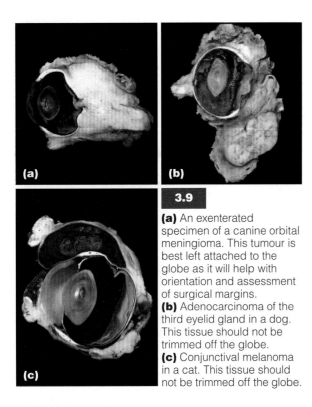

3.9

(a) An exenterated specimen of a canine orbital meningioma. This tumour is best left attached to the globe as it will help with orientation and assessment of surgical margins. **(b)** Adenocarcinoma of the third eyelid gland in a dog. This tissue should not be trimmed off the globe. **(c)** Conjunctival melanoma in a cat. This tissue should not be trimmed off the globe.

should not be transected or incised in an attempt to enhance the rate of fixation because this will severely distort the globe and hinder orientation and pathological examination.

Selection of the fixative: The choice of fixative depends predominantly on what disease process is suspected, what technique is going to be used to examine the eye (e.g. routine histopathology, immunohistochemistry and/or electron microscopy) and the preference of the pathologist. For the majority of routine diagnostic cases, 10% NBF is perfectly adequate for histopathological and immunohisto-pathological examination. It is not ideal for electron microscopy, but ultrastructural evaluation may still be possible. Buffered solutions are best as these prevent pigment deposition (e.g. acid haematin derived from haemoglobin) within the tissue sections.

A tissue:fixative ratio of at least 1:10 and up to 1:20 is recommended. If a large amount of tissue requires fixation, it may be best to fix the tissue over 48 hours in the appropriate amount of formalin at the clinic and then transfer the fixed specimen to a smaller amount of formalin prior to submission. Formalin is inexpensive, widely available and easy to ship, preserves macroscopic detail and colour, and carries little danger of overfixation. However, formalin fixation results in poor globe rigidity and scleral penetration is relatively slow, hence retinal detachment and autolysis are common artefacts, even if the globe is placed in the fixative immediately post-enucleation. An intravitreal injection of 0.25–0.5 ml of formalin through the sclera near the optic nerve using a 25 gauge needle is advocated by some to enhance retinal preservation; however, in the authors' opinion this is not necessary for routine diagnostic tests.

In cases where the preservation of retinal detail is paramount to the diagnosis, fixatives such as Davidson's, Bouin's and Zenker's can be used. These fixatives generally offer rapid globe penetration, good globe rigidity and excellent retinal preservation; however, stricter adherence to fixation times is required and the tissue discoloration (Figure 3.10) associated with these fixatives can interfere with macroscopic examination and photography. Fixation with Davidson's (formaldehyde, ethanol and acetic acid) or Bouin's (picric acid, formaldehyde and acetic acid) solution is good for both routine histopathology and immunohistochemistry, but will render tissues unsuitable for electron microscopy. In addition, Bouin's solution discolours the ocular tissue yellow and dry picric acid is explosive. Zenker's solution is the least desirable because of its mercury content. Glutaraldehyde is the fixative of choice for electron microscopy, but the tissue will be rendered unsuitable for immunohistochemistry.

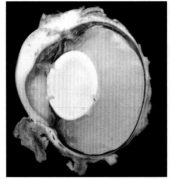

3.10

A globe from a dog with anterior scleritis that has been fixed with Davidson's solution. Note the generalized white opacification of the tissue, which can make macroscopic examination and photography difficult.

Submission of the globe

The globe is typically placed in a non-glass rigid container with fixative, inserted into a second rigid container, wrapped in sufficient absorbent material to absorb all leakage in the event of damage, and finally placed in a leak-proof plastic bag. When submitting a globe for histopathology, it is important to provide the pathologist with a complete signalment, clinical history and clinical diagnosis or differential diagnoses. This is because reaching the correct diagnosis in many cases relies on correlating the pathological findings with the age and breed of the patient, as well as pertinent clinical features of the disease. The pathologist can provide a morphological diagnosis, which is an aetiologically non-specific summation of the basic pathological process, but to translate this into a more useful clinical disease entity diagnosis, knowledge of the clinical setting is required.

When completing the submission form, any focal lesions that may be of interest should be indicated (usually with the aid of a diagram) as identification may be difficult once the globe has been fixed due to tissue opacification (particularly the cornea). The individual submitting the globe should be familiar with the regulations governing the submission of pathological specimens, which vary depending on country, fixative used and method of submission (e.g. mail *versus* courier).

Routine processing at the laboratory

Macroscopic examination of the globe (Figure 3.11a), together with knowledge of the clinical history, is important to ensure orientation and embedding of the globe in such a way that the lesion(s) will be included in the histopathological sections. Once the globe has been sectioned, the calotte of interest (usually half of the globe) is placed in a cassette (Figure 3.11bc) and undergoes routine processing. Routine processing involves dehydration of the tissue using alcohol, permeation of the tissue with a clearing agent (solvent) and then replacement of the solvent with a wax. This paraffin wax hardens and the embedded tissue (Figure 3.11d) is then amenable to sectioning: 4 μm thick sections are cut, mounted on a glass slide, stained with routine haematoxylin and eosin (H&E) (Figure 3.11e) and finally examined under the microscope (Figure 3.11f).

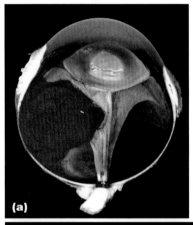

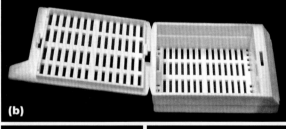

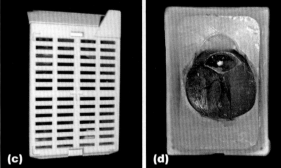

3.11 **(a)** The submitted globe is macroscopically examined and then sectioned adjacent to the optic nerve to reveal an extensive pigmented mass that proved to be a choroidal melanoma. **(b)** Half the globe is then placed in a cassette. **(c)** The cassette undergoes routine processing, which involves dehydration of the tissue, permeation with a clearing agent (solvent) and then replacement of the solvent with a wax. **(d)** The processed part of the globe is embedded in a firm wax block from which 4 μm sections can be cut. (continues) ▶

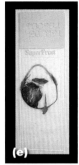
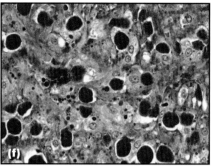

3.11 (continued) **(e)** The 4 μm section is mounted on a glass slide and routinely stained with H&E. **(f)** Histopathological examination reveals neoplastic melanocytes. (H&E stain; original magnification x400)

Additional diagnostic techniques

For the majority of cases, microscopic examination of routine H&E stained sections will be sufficient to achieve a diagnosis. The most common additional diagnostic techniques include special stains, immunohistochemistry and PCR. Special stains are used to identify suspected pathogens or to demonstrate specific cell components or products. For example, if a fungal infection is suspected but no fungi are visible on routine H&E stained sections, a new section can be cut and stained with either a Gomori methenamine silver (GMS) or periodic acid–Schiff (PAS) stain, which highlight fungal walls that are rich in polysaccharides (Figure 3.12a). Other commonly used special stains for pathogens include the Gram stain and the acid–fast Ziehl–Neelson (ZN) stain for bacteria (Figure 3.12b).

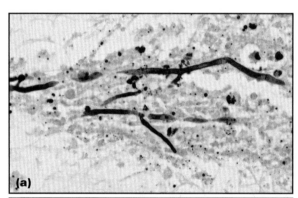

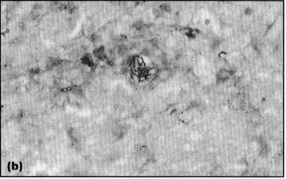

3.12 **(a)** GMS stain highlights fungal hyphae, which stain black. (Original magnification x400) **(b)** ZN stain confirms the presence of acid–fast organisms, which stain bright red (typical of *Mycobacterium* spp.) (Original magnification x1000)

Fundamentally, immunohistochemistry is used to demonstrate antigen(s) within tissue sections using specific antibodies. The antigen–antibody binding complex is visualized using a coloured histochemical reaction. Routine uses of immunohistochemistry include immunophenotyping and prognostication for neoplasia (Figure 3.13), further characterization of cellular infiltrates and identification of pathogens (Figure 3.14). PCR is a technique which uses amplification of a DNA sequence and its many applications include further characterization of neoplasms and detection of genetic mutations and pathogens.

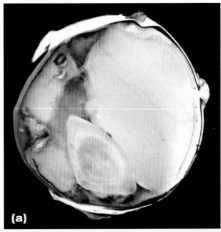

(a)

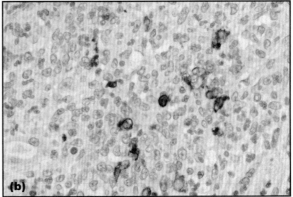

(b)

3.14 **(a)** A feline globe with extensive proteinaceous exudation in the anterior chamber and vitreous, highly suspicious for feline infectious peritonitis (FIP). The dislocated lens is artefactual. **(b)** Immunohistochemistry confirms the presence of feline coronavirus (FCoV) antigen within the macrophages, which is demonstrated by the brown immunopositive staining. (Diaminobenzidine chromogen stain; original magnification x200)

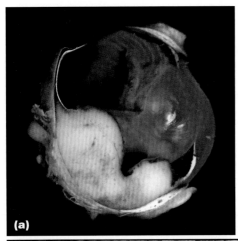

(a)

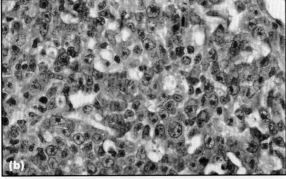

(b)

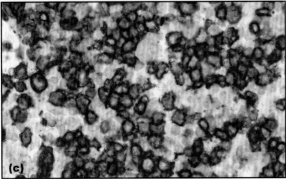

(c)

3.13 **(a)** Macroscopic examination of a feline globe showing a solid white intraocular mass, which partially replaces the uveal tract. **(b)** Histopathological examination reveals sheets of large neoplastic lymphocytes, indicative of lymphoma. (H&E stain; original magnification x400) **(c)** Immunohistochemistry indicates that this is a T-cell lymphoma. The neoplastic lymphocytes are immunopositive for the T-cell marker CD3. Immunopositivity is characterized by the brown staining. (Diaminobenzidine chromogen stain; original magnification x200)

References and further reading

Bolzan AA, Brunelli AT, Castro MB *et al.* (2005) Conjunctival impression cytology in dogs. *Veterinary Ophthalmology* **8**, 401–405

Boston SE (2010) Craniectomy and orbitectomy in dogs and cats. *The Canadian Veterinary Journal (La Revue Veterinaire Canadienne)* **51**, 537–540

Dubey JP and Lappin MR (2006) Toxoplasmosis and neosporosis. In: *Infectious Diseases of the Dog and Cat, 3rd edn*, ed. CE Greene, pp. 754–775. Saunders Elsevier, St Louis

Dubielzig RR, Ketring KL, McLellan GJ and Albert DM (2010) The principles and practice of ocular pathology. In: *Veterinary Ocular Pathology: a comparative review*, pp. 2–5. Saunders Elsevier, St Louis

Grahn BH and Pfeiffer RL (2007) Fundamentals of veterinary ophthalmic pathology. In: *Veterinary Ophthalmology, 4th edn*, ed. KN Gelatt, pp. 355–359. Blackwell Publishing, Iowa

Hendrix DV and Gelatt KN (2000) Diagnosis, treatment and outcome of orbital neoplasia in dogs: a retrospective study of 44 cases. *The Journal of Small Animal Practice* **41**, 105–108

Prado MR, Rocha MF, Brito EH *et al.* (2005) Survey of bacterial microorganisms in the conjunctival sac of clinically normal dogs and dogs with ulcerative keratitis in Fortaleza, Ceara, Brazil. *Veterinary Ophthalmology* **8**, 33–37

Tsubota K, Kajiwara K, Ugajin S *et al.* (1990) Conjunctival brush cytology. *Acta Cytologica* **34**, 233–235

Wang L, Pan Q, Zhang L *et al.* (2008) Investigation of bacterial microorganisms in the conjunctival sac of clinically normal dogs and dogs with ulcerative keratitis in Beijing, China. *Veterinary Ophthalmology* **11**, 145–149

Wilcock BP (2007) Eye and ear. In: *Jubb, Kennedy, and Palmer's Pathology of Domestic Animals, vol. 1, 5th edn*, ed. G Maxie, pp. 460–461. Saunders Elsevier, St Louis

4

Diagnosis and control of inherited eye disease

Simon Petersen-Jones and David Gould

This chapter reviews the UK, European and North American eye disease control schemes and gives an overview of genetic testing for hereditary eye diseases in dogs and cats. For information on the clinical aspects of these diseases, the reader should refer to the appropriate chapters elsewhere in this manual.

Hereditary eye disease control schemes

The British Veterinary Association/Kennel Club/ International Sheep Dog Society (BVA/KC/ISDS) scheme was established in 1966 in order to reduce the incidence of inherited eye diseases in pedigree dogs. Some 9 years later, in the USA, the Canine Eye Registration Foundation (CERF) scheme was formed and at a similar time the Swedish Panel for Eradication of Hereditary Eye Disease was established. When the European College of Veterinary Ophthalmologists (ECVO) was founded in the mid-1990s, it established a Hereditary Eye Disease screening scheme (ECVO HED scheme) in an attempt to standardize the testing of dogs across Europe. These schemes are summarized in the following sections. The reader is advised to refer to the respective websites for up-to-date information on these continuously evolving schemes.

BVA/KC/ISDS scheme

The purpose of the BVA/KC/ISDS scheme (www.bva.co.uk) is to ensure that there is no evidence of hereditary eye disease in dogs used for breeding. At the time of writing, the scheme covers 10 hereditary eye diseases (Figure 4.1) in over 50 breeds of dog. The scheme is primarily used for pedigree and working breeds, although any dog can be submitted for eye testing as long as they have permanent identification in the form of a microchip or tattoo. Owners of KC or ISDS registered dogs must also present their original registration document at the time of eye testing. Puppies up to the age of 12 weeks can be examined as part of a litter (litter screening) in order to test for the congenital hereditary eye conditions listed in Figure 4.1. At present, and in contrast to the situation in adult dogs, there is no requirement for permanent identification for litter screening.

An up-to-date list of hereditary eye diseases and breeds affected can be found on the BVA website. Schedule A lists those breeds and conditions that are

Congenital conditions
• Collie eye anomaly
• Congenital hereditary cataract
• Goniodysgenesis
• Multifocal retinal dysplasia
• Persistent hyperplastic primary vitreous
• Total retinal dysplasia

Non-congenital conditions
• Retinal pigment epithelial dystrophy
• Generalized progressive retinal atrophy
• Hereditary cataract
• Primary lens luxation
• Primary open-angle glaucoma

4.1 Hereditary eye diseases currently certified under the BVA/KC/ISDS scheme.

currently certified under the scheme, whilst Schedule B lists those conditions and/or breeds that are not yet certified but are under investigation. If increased numbers of a particular inherited eye condition are recorded within a particular breed listed in Schedule B, it may then be transferred to Schedule A.

The BVA website lists names and contact details of BVA registered eye panellists. These are veterinary ophthalmologists who, following assessment of their clinical diagnostic skills by practical and slide examination, are appointed by the BVA to carry out eye examinations under the scheme. Owners who wish their dog to undergo an eye test under the scheme must contact a BVA eye panellist directly, who will then schedule an examination. As some inherited eye diseases develop later in life, breeders are generally advised to submit dogs for annual eye tests.

At the eye examination, once the eye panellist has confirmed the identity of the dog and, for KC or ISDS registered dogs, checked its registration certificate details, the examination is performed and the eye certificate is completed. The certificate has three sections:

• The upper section details the dog's KC/ISDS registered name and number, breed, colour, sex, date of birth and permanent identification number, along with details of the owner and eye panellist
• The middle section is used to record any ocular or periocular abnormalities identified by the panellist, regardless of whether these are due to inherited disease

- The bottom section lists the 10 certified hereditary eye diseases alongside boxes marked 'clinically unaffected' and 'clinically affected'. The panellist ticks the appropriate box (unaffected or affected) only for those conditions that are specified for the breed being examined (i.e. only those on Schedule A).

Eye certificates comprise four copies. Following completion of the eye test, the copies are distributed as follows:

- The white (top) copy is given to the owner or agent
- The blue copy is sent to the BVA
- The yellow copy is retained by the panellist
- The pink copy is sent to the owner's veterinary surgeon.

For KC registered dogs, the KC publishes the results of individual eye examinations quarterly in the KC Breed Records Supplement (excluding multifocal retinal dysplasia for which it operates an open registry). The ISDS publishes the unaffected and affected results of ISDS registered Border Collies annually in the ISDS Stud Book.

ECVO HED scheme

An ECVO HED (www.ecvo.org) examination may be undertaken by practising ECVO Diplomates or by Eye Scheme Examiners. The latter are veterinary surgeons within national eye panels that have been examined and accepted as examiners for the scheme by the ECVO. Countries in which the HED scheme operates generally form a national panel to oversee eye testing in that country. Alternatively, the HED Committee of the ECVO may act in its place.

The main purpose of the scheme is to identify signs of presumed inherited eye disease in breeding dogs and cats (its inclusion of feline eye examinations makes the ECVO scheme unique). As with the BVA/KC/ISDS scheme, permanent identification (microchip or tattoo) is mandatory in adult animals undergoing an eye examination under the scheme. However, in contrast to the BVA/KC/ISDS scheme, permanent identification is also required for litter screening.

Following the eye examination, a certificate is issued which is valid for 1 year from the date of examination. Annual re-examinations are recommended. Copies of the certificate are also sent to the appropriate kennel club or national panel and to the appropriate breed club where applicable. In addition, the results may be published.

CERF scheme

The CERF was founded by a group of collie breeders from Seattle. The organization coordinates the screening of dogs by Diplomates of the American College of Veterinary Ophthalmologists (ACVO). The list of conditions and the breeding advice and guidelines are established and updated by the Genetics Committee of the ACVO. Following examination of the dog by an ACVO Diplomate, a CERF form is completed. The owner receives a copy of the form, a copy is sent to the CERF by the ophthalmologist and a copy is kept by the ophthalmologist. The forms can be read automatically at the CERF and the results entered into the breed database maintained by the Veterinary Medical Database (VMDB). If a dog achieves a clear examination, the owner, for an additional fee, can register the dog with the CERF as being clear of hereditary eye disease. The CERF monitors the recording of eye conditions on the submitted CERF forms. When the incidence of a condition in a particular breed detected during CERF examinations reaches 1%, the Genetics Committee of the ACVO is notified. The Committee reviews the information and decides whether the condition should be added to the list of hereditary eye diseases for that breed. The list of breeds and conditions used to be published in a book, but more recently the information has been made available electronically. The advice given to breeders, in relation to the various eye conditions that are assumed or proven to be inherited, is:

- NO BREEDING – there is substantial evidence to show heritability of the trait and/or it is a serious condition that may compromise vision or other ocular function
- BREEDER OPTION – the condition is suspected to be inherited but is not likely to compromise vision or other ocular function.

In 2012, the ACVO took the decision to move their hereditary eye disease control scheme to the Orthopedic Foundation for Animals (www.offa.org/), although the move means no change to the existing examination protocols or interpretation/classification of results.

Genetic testing for hereditary eye diseases

In recent years there has been a revolution in testing for hereditary eye diseases, as the identification of the underlying causal genetic mutations has allowed the development of specific genetic tests (Clements *et al.*, 1993; Suber *et al.*, 1993; Aguirre *et al.*, 1998; Petersen-Jones *et al.*, 1999; Mellersh *et al.*, 2006; Zangerl *et al.*, 2006; Menotti-Raymond *et al.*, 2007; Parker *et al.*, 2007; Farias *et al.*, 2010; Menotti-Raymond *et al.*, 2010; Downs *et al.*, 2011). The number of DNA-based tests available for hereditary eye diseases is rapidly increasing with new tests being offered as the gene mutations underlying eye diseases are identified. By taking advantage of the available tests, breeders have the opportunity to eliminate the disease under test from their stock. There are a number of important features of genetic testing of which breeders and dog owners should be aware.

Genetic testing *versus* ophthalmic examination

Genetic tests are not a substitute for ophthalmoscopic screening because they only test for known specific gene mutations. Certain conditions may show genetic heterogeneity and tests can only be run for those traits for which the underlying genetic cause has been identified. Furthermore, each DNA test only checks for a single inherited condition, whereas an ophthalmoscopic examination screens for a wide range of eye diseases. These include genetic diseases for which the gene mutation has been identified and can be tested, genetic diseases for which the gene mutation has not been identified (including new and emerging hereditary conditions) and also acquired eye diseases (i.e. those conditions which do not have a genetic cause). A comparison of genetic testing *versus* ophthalmic examination is given in Figure 4.2.

However, genetic tests do have some important advantages over ophthalmoscopic screening:

- The genetic test identifies the *genotype* of the animal, whereas the ophthalmoscopic examination identifies the *phenotype*. The genotype is the genetic make-up that the animal is born with. DNA testing to identify the genotype is possible from any age at which a DNA sample can be collected from the animal. The phenotype is the physical manifestation of the genotype and may not be apparent until the animal is several years old (depending on the age of onset of the condition). If phenotypic diagnosis is relied upon to identify conditions of late onset, the animal may have already been bred from before the diagnosis is made; whereas genetic testing can always be performed prior to breeding age
- Some genetic conditions may present diagnostic challenges. An example is collie eye anomaly (see also Chapter 18): choroidal hypoplasia (the diagnostic lesion for collie eye anomaly) may be ophthalmoscopically detectable in puppies at 6–7 weeks of age, but can be masked in as many as 50–60% of animals by development of pigmentation in the fundus (Bjerkas, 1991; Beuing and Erharft, 2002). The development of this pigmentation means that the lesions of choroidal hypoplasia can no longer be seen when the animal is examined later in life. This is described as the 'go normal' phenomenon, which is a misnomer because the animal is not normal; it is still genetically affected with collie eye anomaly. A genetic test for choroidal hypoplasia

performed at any age will detect the presence of the causal gene mutation
- Identification of phenocopies. A phenocopy is an environmentally induced condition that mimics a hereditary condition. An example might be a dog with sudden acquired retinal degeneration that eventually develops generalized retinal thinning. Ophthalmoscopically, this generalized retinal degeneration may be indistinguishable from generalized retinal degeneration resulting from a hereditary condition such as progressive retinal atrophy (PRA) (although the history might distinguish them). An ophthalmoscopic examination identifies the phenotypic appearance and then infers the genotype. Thus, if retinal degeneration is detected on ophthalmoscopic examination, the ophthalmologist might describe it as typical for PRA, but because the DNA is not examined with the ophthalmoscope this cannot definitively be proven (although there may be a high probability). DNA testing can distinguish animals with phenocopies from those with genetic diseases
- Identification of carriers of recessive disease. For recessive conditions, carrier animals (those heterozygous for the condition) do not have an identifiable disease phenotype. This means that carriers cannot be identified by clinical examination. The presence of carriers makes elimination of a recessive condition from a breed very difficult because, without a genetic test, carriers may only be identifiable by pedigree analysis (e.g. if a parent was affected) or by test breeding. In contrast, genetic tests will identify carrier animals.

In summary, both genetic testing and ophthalmoscopic screening are required in the attempts to eradicate genetic disease.

Specificity of genetic tests

DNA-based genetic tests will only identify the presence or absence of the gene mutation being tested for. Thus, they are highly specific, which for conditions with genetic heterogeneity may potentially lead to confusion. An example of this could be PRA in the Golden Retriever; at the time of writing it appears that there are at least four separate genetic causes

Genetic testing	Ophthalmic examination
100% accurate (excluding sampling or laboratory error)	Some subjectivity in clinical interpretation (e.g. choroidal hypoplasia in collie eye anomaly, retinal folds in multifocal retinal dysplasia)
Only tests for a single specific gene mutation	Screens for a wide range of ophthalmoscopically visible inherited conditions and also identifies non-inherited ocular diseases
Identifies carrier animals for recessive diseases	Unable to identify carriers
Identifies genetically clear animals that can then be used safely in breeding programmes	Cannot distinguish unaffected from carrier animals, and animals affected with late-onset disease may not be identified prior to breeding
Identifies affected animals before onset of ophthalmoscopic signs	Unable to identify affected animals until ophthalmoscopic signs become apparent

4.2 Comparison of genetic testing *versus* ophthalmic examination.

for PRA in the breed. It is known that they have the progressive rod–cone degeneration form of PRA, which is caused by a mutation in the *PRCD* gene (Zangerl *et al.*, 2006), and Downs *et al.* (2011) reported a second form of PRA in the breed that was due to a mutation in the *SLC4A3* gene. However, the latter study identified Golden Retrievers with clinical signs of PRA that had normal versions of the *PRCD* and *SLC4A3* genes, indicating that there was at least one more form of PRA in this breed for which the underlying gene mutation had, at that time, not yet been identified. A third genetic cause of PRA in the Golden Retriever (*TTC8*) has since been identified, for which a genetic test is available (see Figure 4.3), but there is strong evidence that a fourth form, as yet unidentified, is also present in this breed (Downs *et al.*, 2014). This genetic heterogeneity means that a breeder could have an animal cleared for the *PRCD*, *SLC4A3* and *TTC8* forms of PRA by DNA-based tests only to be told later at an eye screening examination that their dog, in fact, does have PRA.

Sample collection

DNA can be isolated from many types of tissue sample. For DNA-based genetic tests either a blood sample or a brushing of cells from the buccal mucosa (cheek swab) is generally utilized. Before collecting samples it is important to find out what type of sample the diagnostic laboratory requires and how that sample should be collected, handled and shipped.

Blood samples

DNA is isolated from nucleated blood cells (i.e. white blood cells). Samples are typically collected into an ethylenediamine tetra-acetic acid (EDTA) or citrate (ACD) blood tube (after checking the requirements of the laboratory). Although DNA-based tests can be run on a very small sample, laboratories typically request a minimum sample size. The sample must be collected using a new sterile syringe for each animal and must be checked to ensure that it has not clotted. If a sample clots it should be discarded and a fresh sample collected. The sample should be kept cold (e.g. refrigerated) and sent to the laboratory ensuring that packaging instructions and regulations are followed. The sample should not be frozen or spun down.

Cheek swabs

Cytology brushes or sterile cotton-tipped brushes are used to rub against the oral mucosa (inside the cheeks) to collect a sample of surface epithelial cells. The requirements of the laboratory conducting the test should be checked carefully prior to collecting the sample. There is a greater chance of contamination of a cheek swab than a blood sample with DNA from other animals or from the person collecting the sample. For this reason, the brush or swab should be sterile and care must be taken not to contaminate it by touching the tip. It is usually recommended that the animal not be given food or drink for an hour prior to sample collection, to avoid contamination, and some laboratories recommend separating the dog from other animals for a similar period.

To collect the sample, the swab/brush is held between the cheek and gum and rotated or brushed against the inside of the cheek to collect cells from the surface mucosa. The laboratory may request more than one swab per animal be submitted for examination. Following collection, the swab is allowed to air dry (without touching anything, to avoid contamination) and placed back in the packaging. The package must be labelled clearly and accurately. Cheek swabs should not be put in plastic containers because the humidity may lead to the growth of contaminating organisms and possibly destruction of the DNA. Paper envelopes are ideal. The quantity and quality of DNA samples collected from cheek swabs are not as good as those from blood samples. For that reason, it may not be possible to perform some tests on cheek swab samples.

Identification of the sample

Some certifying agencies may require that the origin of the sample is verified by a veterinary surgeon and that the animal from which the sample has been obtained is permanently identifiable (e.g. microchipped). The requirements should be checked prior to sampling.

How genetic tests allow selective breeding choices

Many genetic diseases of pure-bred dogs show recessive inheritance. The presence of phenotypically normal carrier animals (those heterozygous for the gene mutation) in the breed population makes it difficult to eliminate such conditions using selective breeding. An example is PRA in the Irish Setter in the UK: breeders used test breeding to identify carrier animals and eliminate them from breeding programmes. This usually involved breeding the test animal to a known affected animal. The resultant offspring were then tested at an early age using electroretinography to determine whether they had PRA, or monitored ophthalmoscopically. If an affected puppy was produced, then it meant that the test animal was a carrier. To be confident that the test animal was unlikely to be a carrier, several normal puppies had to be produced; the more normal puppies produced, the lower the odds of the test animal being a carrier (depending on litter size, more than one test litter may be required). The UK Irish Setter breeders had not reported a case of PRA in the breed for many years and the general assumption was that the condition had been eradicated. Once the underlying gene mutation for PRA in the Irish Setter was identified, a genetic test was developed (Clements *et al.*, 1993; Suber *et al.*, 1993). This test was used to screen a cross-section of the UK Irish Setters and it showed that carrier animals were still present in the population (Petersen-Jones *et al.*, 1995). This study showed that carrier animals can remain undetected in a population at a low frequency for many generations. Genetic testing allows carrier animals to be identified and removed from the gene pool.

However, genetic testing does allow the use of animals that are carriers of a recessive disease to be used in breeding programmes, whilst still preventing the birth of any affected animals. To avoid production of affected animals, the carrier animal must be mated with a genetically clear animal. The resultant offspring will be a mixture of carriers and genotypically normal animals (with an expected ratio of 50:50). The continued use of carrier animals in breeding programmes is particularly important if the carrier animal has characteristics that would be desirable to save for the next generation, or if the incidence of the genetic disease in the breed is high. In breeds with a high incidence of a recessive condition, there may be a relatively small number of genetically clear animals. For example, if a population is in Hardy–Weinberg equilibrium and the incidence of a recessive condition is just 1%, then approximately 18% of the population are predicted to be carriers. Allowing only genetically normal animals to breed would narrow the gene pool, reducing genetic diversity, and run the risk of losing desirable characteristics from the breed. It may also allow another recessive disease to be expressed that is currently at a low level in the breed, perhaps cannot

be tested for, and might be more serious than the condition being eliminated.

An example of this is primary lens luxation (PLL) in the Miniature Bull Terrier. This is a numerically small breed, yet estimates of the frequency of the PLL mutation indicate that up to 15% of the breed is affected, and around 47% of individuals are carriers (Gould *et al.*, 2011). Simply eliminating all affected and carrier animals from the breeding stock would be disastrous for long-term survival of the breed. Gradually eliminating the hereditary condition over several generations would be the most sensible approach, and can be considered as genetic testing can be used to make breeding choices to separate the 'good' genes from the 'bad' genes.

Genetic tests currently available

Figure 4.3 lists the hereditary eye diseases that can be tested for at the time of writing. However, because the field of companion animal genetics is so dynamic, readers should refer to the websites of DNA testing laboratories for the latest information regarding DNA testing.

Breed	Disease	Gene	Laboratory
Abyssinian, Somali, Ocicat, Siamese and related cat breeds	arPRA – *RdAc*	*CEP290*	Laboklin; CatDNAtest.org; UC Davis VGL
Abyssinian and Somali cat breeds	adPRA – *Rdy*	*CRX*	UC Davis VGL
Alaskan Malamute	Cone degeneration (achromatopsia)	*CNGB3*	Optigen
American Cocker Spaniel	arPRA – *prcd*	*PRCD*	Optigen
American Eskimo Dog	arPRA – *prcd*	*PRCD*	Optigen
American Pit Bull	crd2	Not yet published	Optigen
Australian Cattle Dog	arPRA – *prcd*	*PRCD*	Optigen
	PLL	*ADAMTS17*	Animal Health Trust
Australian Shepherd	CEA–CH	Intronic mutation in *NEHJ1*	Optigen
	Cone degeneration (achromatopsia)	*CNGB3*	Optigen
	cmr-1	*BEST1*	Optigen
	arPRA – *prcd*	*PRCD*	Optigen
	Hereditary cataract	Heat shock factor 4 (*HSF4*)	Animal Health Trust
Australian Stumpy Tail Cattle Dog	arPRA – *prcd*	*PRCD*	Optigen
Basenji	arPRA – (Bas_PRA1)	S-antigen	Optigen
Beagle	POAG	*ADAMTS10*	Not commercially available
Border Collie	CEA–CH	Intronic mutation in *NEHJ1*	Optigen

4.3 Genetic tests that are currently available. adPRA = autosomal dominant progressive retinal atrophy; arPRA = autosomal recessive progressive retinal atrophy; CEA–CH = collie eye anomaly–choroidal hypoplasia; CKCSID = congenital keratoconjunctivitis sicca and ichthyosiform dermatosis; *cmr-1* = canine multifocal retinopathy type 1; *cmr-2* = canine multifocal retinopathy type 2; *cord1* = cone–rod dystrophy 1; CRD = cone–rod dystrophy; crd2 = cone–rod dystrophy 2; crd3 = cone–rod dystrophy 3; CSNB = congenital stationary night blindness; *drd1* = dwarfism with retinal dysplasia type 1; *drd2* = dwarfism with retinal dysplasia type 2; *erd* = early retinal degeneration; GR_PRA1 = Golden Retriever PRA type 1, GR_PRA2 = Golden Retriever PRA type 2; LOPRA = late-onset PRA; OSD = oculoskeletal dysplasia; PLL = primary lens luxation; POAG = primary open angle glaucoma; PRA = progressive retinal atrophy; *prcd* = progressive rod–cone degeneration; *rcd1* = rod–cone dysplasia type 1; *rcd1a* = rod–cone dysplasia type 1a; *rcd2* = rod–cone dysplasia type 2; *rcd3* = rod–cone dysplasia type 3; *rcd4* = rod–cone degeneration type 4; *RdAc* = retinal degeneration in Abyssinian cats; *Rdy* = retinal dystrophy; xlPRA = X-linked progressive retinal atrophy. (continues)

Breed	Disease	Gene	Laboratory
Boston Terrier	Hereditary cataract (early-onset form only)	HSF4	Animal Health Trust
Boykin Spaniel	CEA–CH	Intronic mutation in *NEHJ1*	Optigen
Briard	CSNB	RPE65	Animal Health Trust; Optigen
Bull Mastiff	adPRA	*rhodopsin*	Optigen
	cmr-1	*bestrophin 1 (BEST1)*	Optigen
Cane Corso	*cmr-1*	BEST1	Optigen
Cardigan Welsh Corgi	arPRA – *rcd3*	PDE6A	Optigen
Cavalier King Charles Spaniel	Curly coat dry eye/CKCSID	FAM83H	Animal Health Trust
Chesapeake Bay Retriever	arPRA – *prcd*	PRCD	Optigen
Chinese Crested	arPRA – *prcd*	PRCD	Optigen
	PLL	ADAMTS17	Animal Health Trust
Coton du Tulear	*cmr-2*	BEST1	Optigen
Dogue de Bordeaux	*cmr-1*	BEST1	Optigen
English Cocker Spaniel	arPRA – *prcd*	PRCD	Optigen
English and Bull Mastiff	*cmr-1*	BEST1	Optigen
English Springer Spaniel	PRA – *cord1*	RPGRIP1	Animal Health Trust
Entlebucher Sennenhund	arPRA – *prcd*	PRCD	Optigen
Finnish Lapphund	arPRA – *prcd*	PRCD	Optigen
French Bulldog	Hereditary cataract	HSF4	Animal Health Trust
German Shorthaired Pointer	Cone degeneration (achromatopsia)	CNGB3	Optigen
Glen of Imaal Terrier	*crd3*	ADAM9	Optigen
Golden Retriever	arPRA – *prcd*	PRCD	Optigen
	arPRA (GR_PRA1)	SLC4A3	Animal Health Trust
	arPRA (GR_PRA2)	TTC8	Animal Health Trust; Optigen
Gordon Setter	Late-onset PRA (LOPRA) – *rcd4*	C2orf71	Animal Health Trust
Great Pyrenees (Pyrenean Mountain Dog)	*cmr-1*	BEST1	Optigen
Irish Red and White Setter	arPRA – *rcd1*	PDE6B	Animal Health Trust; Optigen
Irish Setter	arPRA – *rcd1*	PDE6B	Animal Health Trust; Optigen
	Late-onset PRA (LOPRA) – *rcd4*	C2orf71	Animal Health Trust
Jack Russell Terrier	PLL	ADAMTS17	Animal Health Trust
Jagdterrier	PLL	ADAMTS17	Animal Health Trust
Karelian Bear Dog	arPRA – *prcd*	PRCD	Optigen
Kuvasz	arPRA – *prcd*	PRCD	Optigen
Labrador Retriever	arPRA – *prcd*	PRCD	Optigen
	OSD – *drd1*	COL9A2	Optigen

4.3 (continued) Genetic tests that are currently available. adPRA = autosomal dominant progressive retinal atrophy; arPRA = autosomal recessive progressive retinal atrophy; CEA–CH = collie eye anomaly–choroidal hypoplasia; CKCSID = congenital keratoconjunctivitis sicca and ichthyosiform dermatosis; *cmr-1* = canine multifocal retinopathy type 1; *cmr-2* = canine multifocal retinopathy type 2; *cord1* = cone–rod dystrophy 1; CRD = cone–rod dystrophy; crd2 = cone–rod dystrophy 2; crd3 = cone–rod dystrophy 3; CSNB = congenital stationary night blindness; *drd1* = dwarfism with retinal dysplasia type 1; *drd2* = dwarfism with retinal dysplasia type 2; *erd* = early retinal degeneration; GR_PRA1 = Golden Retriever PRA type 1; GR_PRA2 = Golden Retriever PRA type 2; LOPRA = late-onset PRA; OSD = oculoskeletal dysplasia; PLL = primary lens luxation; POAG = primary open angle glaucoma; PRA = progressive retinal atrophy; *prcd* = progressive rod–cone degeneration; *rcd1* = rod–cone dysplasia type 1; *rcd1a* = rod–cone dysplasia type 1a; *rcd2* = rod–cone dysplasia type 2; *rcd3* = rod–cone dysplasia type 3; *rcd4* = rod–cone degeneration type 4; *RdAc* = retinal degeneration in Abyssinian cats; *Rdy* = retinal dystrophy; xlPRA = X-linked progressive retinal atrophy. (continues) ▶

Breed	Disease	Gene	Laboratory
Lancashire Heeler	CEA–CH	Intronic mutation in *NEHJ1*	Optigen
	PLL	*ADAMTS17*	Animal Health Trust
Lapponian Herder	*cmr-3*	*BEST1*	Optigen
	arPRA – *prcd*	*PRCD*	Optigen
Longhaired Whippet	CEA–CH	Intronic mutation in *NEHJ1*	Optigen
Markiesje	arPRA – *prcd*	*PRCD*	Optigen
Miniature Bull Terrier	PLL	*ADAMTS17*	Animal Health Trust
Miniature Longhaired, Smooth-haired and Wirehaired Dachshund	PRA – *cord1*	*RPGRIP1*	Animal Health Trust
Miniature Wirehaired Dachshund	CRD	*NPHP4*	Animal Health Trust
Miniature and Toy Poodle	arPRA – *prcd*	*PRCD*	Optigen
Miniature Schnauzer	arPRA – type A	*Phosducin*	Optigen
Norwegian Elkhound	arPRA – *prcd*	*PRCD*	Optigen
	arPRA – *erd*	*STK38L*	Not available
Nova Scotia Duck Tolling Retriever	CEA–CH	Intronic mutation in *NEHJ1*	Optigen
	arPRA – *prcd*	*PRCD*	Optigen
Old English Mastiff	adPRA	*rhodopsin*	Optigen
	cmr-1	*BEST1*	Optigen
Papillon	arPRA – (Pap_PRA1)	*CNGB1*	Optigen
Parson Russell Terrier	PLL	*ADAMTS17*	Animal Health Trust
Patterdale Terrier	PLL	*ADAMTS17*	Animal Health Trust
Perro de Presna Canario	*cmr-1*	*BEST1*	Optigen
Portuguese Water Dog	arPRA – *prcd*	*PRCD*	Optigen
Rat Terrier	PLL	*ADAMTS17*	Animal Health Trust
Rough and Smooth Collie	*rcd2*	*c1orf36*	Optigen
	CEA–CH	Intronic mutation in *NEHJ1*	Optigen
Samoyed	xlPRA	*RPGR*	Optigen
	OSD – *drd2*	*COL9A3*	Optigen
Schapendoes	arPRA	*CCDC66*	Not available
Sealyham Terrier	PLL	*ADAMTS17*	Animal Health Trust
Shetland Sheepdog	CEA–CH	Intronic mutation in *NEHJ1*	Optigen
Siberian Husky	xlPRA	*RPGR*	Optigen
Silken Windhound	CEA–CH	Intronic mutation in *NEHJ1*	Optigen
Silky Terrier	arPRA – *prcd*	*PRCD*	Optigen
Sloughi	arPRA – *rcd1a*	*PDE6B*	Optigen
Spanish Water Dog	arPRA – *prcd*	*PRCD*	Optigen
Staffordshire Bull Terrier	Hereditary cataract	*HSF4*	Animal Health Trust

4.3 (continued) Genetic tests that are currently available. adPRA = autosomal dominant progressive retinal atrophy; arPRA = autosomal recessive progressive retinal atrophy; CEA–CH = collie eye anomaly–choroidal hypoplasia; CKCSID = congenital keratoconjunctivitis sicca and ichthyosiform dermatosis; *cmr-1* = canine multifocal retinopathy type 1; *cmr-2* = canine multifocal retinopathy type 2; *cord1* = cone–rod dystrophy 1; CRD = cone–rod dystrophy; crd2 = cone–rod dystrophy 2; crd3 = cone–rod dystrophy 3; CSNB = congenital stationary night blindness; *drd1* = dwarfism with retinal dysplasia type 1; *drd2* = dwarfism with retinal dysplasia type 2; *erd* = early retinal degeneration; GR_PRA1 = Golden Retriever PRA type 1; GR_PRA2 = Golden Retriever PRA type 2; LOPRA = late-onset PRA; OSD = oculoskeletal dysplasia; PLL = primary lens luxation; POAG = primary open angle glaucoma; PRA = progressive retinal atrophy; *prcd* = progressive rod–cone degeneration; rcd1 = rod–cone dysplasia type 1; *rcd1a* = rod–cone dysplasia type 1a; rcd2 = rod–cone dysplasia type 2; rcd3 = rod–cone dysplasia type 3; rcd4 = rod–cone degeneration type 4; *RdAc* = retinal degeneration in Abyssinian cats; *Rd*y = retinal dystrophy; xlPRA = X-linked progressive retinal atrophy. (continues) ▶

Breed	Disease	Gene	Laboratory
Standard Wirehaired Dachshund	crd	NPHP4	Animal Health Trust
Swedish Lapphund	arPRA – prcd	PRCD	Optigen
Tenterfield Terrier	PLL	ADAMTS17	Animal Health Trust
Tibetan Spaniel	arPRA – PRA3	FAM161A	Animal Health Trust
Tibetan Terrier	PLL	ADAMTS17	Animal Health Trust
	arPRA – PRA3	FAM161A	Animal Health Trust
	Late-onset PRA (LOPRA) – rcd4	C2orf71	Animal Health Trust
Toy Fox Terrier	PLL	ADAMTS17	Animal Health Trust
Volpino Italiano	PLL	ADAMTS17	Animal Health Trust
Welsh Terrier	PLL	ADAMTS17	Animal Health Trust
Wirehaired Fox Terrier	PLL	ADAMTS17	Animal Health Trust
Yorkshire Terrier	PLL	ADAMTS17	Animal Health Trust
	arPRA – prcd	PRCD	Optigen

4.3 (continued) Genetic tests that are currently available. adPRA = autosomal dominant progressive retinal atrophy; arPRA = autosomal recessive progressive retinal atrophy; CEA–CH = collie eye anomaly–choroidal hypoplasia; CKCSID = congenital keratoconjunctivitis sicca and ichthyosiform dermatosis; cmr-1 = canine multifocal retinopathy type 1; cmr-2 = canine multifocal retinopathy type 2; cord1 = cone–rod dystrophy 1; CRD = cone–rod dystrophy; crd2 = cone–rod dystrophy 2; crd3 = cone–rod dystrophy 3; CSNB = congenital stationary night blindness; drd1 = dwarfism with retinal dysplasia type 1; drd2 = dwarfism with retinal dysplasia type 2; erd = early retinal degeneration; GR_PRA1 = Golden Retriever PRA type 1; GR_PRA2 = Golden Retriever PRA type 2; LOPRA = late-onset PRA; OSD = oculoskeletal dysplasia; PLL = primary lens luxation; POAG = primary open angle glaucoma; PRA = progressive retinal atrophy; prcd = progressive rod–cone degeneration; rcd1 = rod–cone dysplasia type 1; rcd1a = rod–cone dysplasia type 1a; rcd2 = rod–cone dysplasia type 2; rcd3 = rod–cone dysplasia type 3; rcd4 = rod–cone degeneration type 4; RdAc = retinal degeneration in Abyssinian cats; Rdy = retinal dystrophy; xlPRA = X-linked progressive retinal atrophy.

References and further reading

Aguirre GD, Baldwin V, Pearce-Kelling S et al. (1998) Congenital stationary night blindness in the dog: common mutation in the RPE65 gene indicates founder effect. Molecular Vision **4**, 23

Beuing G and Erharft G (2002) Influences on the frequency of estimated Collie Eye Anomaly (CEA) in Collies and Shelties in preventive examination – results of a breeding club organization. Kleintierpraxis **47**, 407–413

Bjerkås E (1991) Collie eye anomaly in the rough collie in Norway. Journal of Small Animal Practice **32**, 89–92

Clements PJM, Gregory CY, Petersen-Jones SM, Sargan DR and Bhattacharya SS (1993) Confirmation of the rod cGMP phophodiesterase α-subunit (PDEα) nonsense mutation in affected rcd-1 Irish Setters in the UK and development of a diagnostic test. Current Eye Research **12**, 861–866

Downs LM, Hitti R, Pregnolato S and Mellersh CS (2014) Genetic screening for PRA-associated mutations in multiple dog breeds shows that PRA is heterogeneous within and between breeds. Veterinary Ophthalmology **17**, 126–130

Downs LM, Wallin-Hakansson B, Boursnell M et al. (2011) A frameshift mutation in Golden Retriever dogs with progressive retinal atrophy endorses SLC4A3 as a candidate gene for human retinal degenerations. PLoS One **6**, e21452

Farias FH, Johnson GS, Taylor JF et al. (2010) An ADAMTS17 splice donor site mutation in dogs with primary lens luxation. Investigative Ophthalmology and Visual Sciences **51**, 4716–4721

Gould D, Pettitt L, McLaughlin B et al. (2011) ADAMTS17 mutation associated with primary lens luxation is widespread among breeds. Veterinary Ophthalmology **14**, 378–384

Mellersh CS (2012) DNA testing and domestic dogs. Mammalian Genome **23**, 109–23

Mellersh CS, Pettitt L, Forman OP, Vaudin M and Barnett KC (2006) Identification of mutations in HSF4 in dogs of three different breeds with hereditary cataracts. Veterinary Ophthalmology **9**, 369–378

Mellersh CS and Sargan D (2011) DNA testing in companion animals – what is it and why do it? In Practice **33**, 442–453

Menotti-Raymond M, David VA, Schäffer AA et al. (2007) Mutation in

CEP290 discovered for cat model of human retinal degeneration. Journal of Heredity **98**, 211–220

Menotti-Raymond M, Deckman KH, David V et al. (2010) Mutation discovered in a feline model of human congenital retinal blinding disease. Investigative Ophthalmology and Visual Sciences **51**, 2852–2859

Parker HG, Kukekova AV, Akey DT et al. (2007) Breed relationships facilitate fine-mapping studies: a 7.8-kb deletion cosegregates with Collie eye anomaly across multiple dog breeds. Genome Research **17**, 1562–1571

Petersen-Jones SM, Clements PJM, Barnett KC and Sargan DR (1995) Incidence of the gene mutation causal for rod-cone dysplasia type 1 in Irish Setters in the UK. Journal of Small Animal Practice **36**, 310–314

Petersen-Jones SM, Entz DD and Sargan DR (1999) cGMP phosphodiesterase-alpha mutation causes progressive retinal atrophy in the Cardigan Welsh Corgi Dog. Investigative Ophthalmology and Visual Sciences **40**, 1637–1644

Suber ML, Pittler SJ, Quin N, et al. (1993) Irish Setter dogs affected with rod-cone dysplasia contain a nonsense mutation in the rod cGMP phosphodiesterase beta-subunit gene. Proceedings of the National Academy of Sciences of the United States of America **90**, 3968–3972

Zangerl B, Goldstein O, Philp AR et al. (2006) Identical mutation in a novel retinal gene causes progressive rod-cone degeneration in dogs and retinitis pigmentosa in humans. Genomics **88**, 551–563

Useful websites

Information on the testing laboratories can be found at the following websites:

Antagene (www.antagene.com)
CatDNAtest.org (www.catdnatest.org)
Animal Health Trust (AHT) (www.aht.org.uk)
Laboklin (www.laboklin.co.uk)
Optigen (www.optigen.com). Antagene also process blood samples for Optigen tests submitted in Europe
University of California Davis VGL (www.vgl.ucdavis.edu/services)

5

Ophthalmic analgesia and anaesthesia

Louise Clark

Pain is a component of many ophthalmic diseases and the provision of adequate analgesia is an ethical obligation for all veterinary clinicians. Anaesthesia may be required in the management of a variety of cases, from simple immobilization of patients for non-invasive imaging or electrophysiological testing, to minor surgical procedures in healthy patients, through to patients with multiple comorbidities undergoing complex intraocular surgery. This chapter considers the anaesthetic approach to the ophthalmic patient, and encompasses the following aspects:

- Analgesia
- Relevant aspects of ocular physiology
- Pre-anaesthetic assessment
- Formulation of an anaesthetic plan
- Intraoperative monitoring
- Postoperative care
- Special techniques, including provision of neuromuscular blockade.

Analgesia

If pain is managed inappropriately or inadequately the consequences for the animal are severe:

- Activation of the stress response impairs wound healing
- Recovery from anaesthesia may be poor
- Postoperative complication risk is higher
- Increased risk of self-trauma.

Ocular pain

The ophthalmic division of the trigeminal nerve provides sensory innervation to the eye. The centre of the cornea is richly innervated. The corneal epithelium and the more superficial stromal layers have a higher density of nociceptors than does the deeper stroma. Thus, a superficial central ulcer may be more painful than a deeper, more peripheral one, despite the difference in clinical severity. Brachycephalic breeds of cat and dog have fewer nociceptors and exhibit less corneal pain than dolichocephalic breeds with the same pathology.

The deeper corneal stroma contains mechanoreceptors sensitive to pressure. High pressure can be considered a noxious stimulus. These receptors are activated when intraocular pressure (IOP) is raised and contribute to the extreme pain associated with this condition. Ocular surface pain may be temporarily relieved with topical local anaesthesia, whereas pain of intraocular origin, as in patients with glaucoma or intraocular inflammation, is not relieved by topical local anaesthesia and often presents with systemic signs that include depression and dullness.

Pain management – practical considerations

The cause of the pain must be determined and, where possible, eliminated. This may require surgical intervention, e.g. enucleation for irreversible glaucoma, or more limited action directed at dealing with the pathology causing the pain, e.g. anti-inflammatory therapy and cycloplegics in uveitis. Analgesic provision can be planned on the basis of the severity of the clinical signs and the management of the individual case. Where surgery is planned, pre-emptive and polymodal analgesia is appropriate.

Pre-emptive and polymodal analgesia

The basic concept of pre-emptive analgesia is that providing analgesia before the noxious stimulus (e.g. surgery) means that the analgesic drugs will be more effective. Although unconscious animals cannot perceive pain, physiological changes within the CNS can still occur, leading to both peripheral and central sensitization. Pre-emptive analgesia aims to minimize these changes and potentially reduce postoperative analgesic requirements. A polymodal approach means using more than one analgesic simultaneously to capitalize on their different sites of action within the pain pathway. Thus, analgesia will be more effective and the total dose of each drug (and hence its side effects) can be reduced.

Surgical considerations

Meticulous tissue handling to minimize surgical trauma (as described in Chapter 6) may reduce analgesic requirements and postoperative pain.

Nursing considerations

Patients may have comorbidity, unrelated to the ophthalmic complaint but worsened by hospitalization and immobility. For example, frequent mobilization of older patients can reduce the clinical signs associated with painful osteoarthritis.

Analgesic agents

Opioids

Opioid receptors are located throughout the central nervous system (CNS) and the peripheral nervous system. Opioids (Figure 5.1) can be administered in a multitude of ways to target these sites. Pure mu (μ) (OP3) receptor agonists such as morphine and methadone are potent analgesics. Partial mu receptor agonists such as buprenorphine are less potent and less suitable for management of severe pain in dogs. In cats, however, buprenorphine may be a more effective analgesic than morphine: cats are unable to convert morphine to its active metabolites because of a lack of certain liver enzymes. Methadone also has demonstrable efficacy in cats. Buprenorphine is also efficacious in cats when administered by the oral transmucosal route at intramuscular or intravenous doses.

The administration of a partial agonist after a pure agonist can partially antagonize the pure agonist. When administered systemically, opioids have a number of side effects that may be relevant in ophthalmic patients. They may cause marked mydriasis in cats and miosis in dogs. Morphine and papaveretum cause vomiting, which should be avoided in animals with elevated IOP or compromised globe integrity. Pethidine, methadone and buprenorphine are not associated with vomiting. Tramadol has become a popular oral analgesic, because it can be administered 'at home' and thus avoids hospitalization for patients that would otherwise require systemic opioids. However, its pharmacokinetics have yet to be fully determined. There is limited information regarding the efficacy of oral tramadol for corneal pain (Clark *et al.*, 2011). Although it may be an effective analgesic, oral administration is poorly tolerated in cats (Pypendop *et al.*, 2009).

Both mu and delta receptors are localized on nerve fibres within the cornea, which are accessible for topical opioid treatment. Initial studies of the efficacy of topical morphine for ocular analgesia appeared positive, but recent work has failed to demonstrate a beneficial effect (Stiles *et al.*, 2003; Thomson *et al.*, 2010). Another topical opioid, nalbuphine, also proved to be relatively ineffective (Clark *et al.*, 2011).

Non-steroidal anti-inflammatory drugs

Non-steroidal anti-inflammatory drugs (NSAIDs) (Figure 5.2) inhibit the cyclo-oxygenase isoenzymes COX 1 and COX 2, which are involved in prostaglandin synthesis. Prostaglandins are mediators of inflammation in the periphery, and serve as neurotransmitters in the CNS. As well as being analgesic, NSAIDs are anti-inflammatory and antipyretic. They may also affect platelet function, although this is agent dependent.

NSAIDs are highly protein bound and metabolized in the liver. Clearance is slower in cats than in dogs. Gastrointestinal toxicity is the most common side effect, especially with chronic administration. Nephrotoxicity, particularly in the face of hypotension

Drug	Species	Dose	Duration
Methadone*	Dog	0.1–0.5 mg/kg i.m., i.v., s.c.	3–4 hours
	Cat	0.1–0.3 mg/kg i.m., i.v., s.c.	3–4 hours
Buprenorphine*	Dog	0.01–0.02 mg/kg i.v., i.m., s.c.	6–8 hours
	Cat	0.01–0.02 mg/kg i.v., i.m., s.c., OTM	6–8 hours
Butorphanol*	Dog	0.2–0.4 mg/kg i.v., i.m., s.c.	1–2 hours
	Cat	0.2–0.4 mg/kg i.v., i.m., s.c.	1–2 hours
Fentanyl CRI	Dog	3–5 μg/kg bolus + 3–6 μg/kg/h i.v.	
Fentanyl CRI	Cat	2–3 μg/kg bolus + 2–3 μg/kg/h i.v.	
Morphine CRI	Dog	0.3 mg/kg + 0.12 mg/kg/h i.v.	

5.1 Opioid doses for dogs and cats. * = authorized veterinary product. (Reproduced from the *BSAVA Manual of Canine and Feline Anaesthesia and Analgesia*)

Drug	Species	Dose	Notes
Meloxicam	Dog	0.2 mg/kg i.v., s.c.	
	Cat	0.3 mg/kg s.c.	0.2 mg/kg if followed by oral suspension
Carprofen	Dog	4 mg/kg i.v., s.c.	
	Cat	4 mg/kg i.v., s.c.	Once only dose
Robenacoxib	Dog	2 mg/kg s.c.	
	Cat	2 mg/kg s.c.	
Firocoxib	Dog	5 mg/kg orally	
Cimicoxib	Dog	2 mg/kg orally	
Tolfenamic acid	Dog	4 mg/kg i.m., s.c.	

5.2 Non-steroidal anti-inflammatory drugs authorized for perioperative use in dogs and cats (Gurney, 2012).

(shock, anaesthesia) is also a concern. The NSAIDs currently authorized for systemic use in dogs in the UK include carprofen, meloxicam, tepoxalin, firocoxib, mavacoxib and robenacoxib, while meloxicam, robenacoxib and carprofen are authorized in cats. The International Society of Feline Medicine (ISFM) and American Association of Feline Practitioners (AAFP) Consensus Guidelines (2010) on the long-term use of NSAIDs in cats are recommended reading, as they provide detailed practical information.

Local anaesthetics

Local anaesthetics block sodium ion transport, preventing the generation of an action potential and thus the conduction of nerve impulses. They provide total analgesia by completely blocking ascending nociception. They are also used as anti-arrhythmics, but an overdose can cause CNS toxicity and cardiac toxicity. Local anaesthetics are metabolized in the liver and toxicity is more likely in patients with hepatic failure or low cardiac output states. Lidocaine has a low therapeutic index in cats and should not be administered by constant rate infusion. Bupivacaine must **never** be administered intravenously, because it is associated with refractory cardiac arrest. Bupivacaine is, however, a very useful drug when administered using local and regional techniques such as the retrobulbar block. Lidocaine is authorized in dogs and cats, while bupivacaine is not authorized but is widely used.

In a pilot study, Smith *et al.* (2004) demonstrated that intraoperative lidocaine (1.0 mg/kg i.v. followed by an infusion of 0.025 mg/kg/min) provided analgesia similar to morphine for intraocular surgery in dogs. Whilst this study has not been replicated in a larger sample, lidocaine delivered by constant rate infusion has been shown to markedly reduce the requirement for volatile agents (based on reduction in minimum alveolar concentration) in a number of studies.

Regional and topical anaesthesia: Topical local anaesthetics, including proxymetacaine and amethocaine, are considered in detail in Chapter 7. Retrobulbar injection of local anaesthetic provides globe akinesia and analgesia that may be useful during and following enucleation surgery (Myrna *et al.*, 2010).

A combination of rapidly acting lidocaine (~1 mg/kg) with longer acting bupivacaine (1 mg/kg) can be employed to improve postoperative comfort. Bupivacaine 0.5% (5 mg/ml) and lidocaine 2% (20 mg/ml) administered at the above doses results in a total injectate volume of 1.5 ml/10 kg, which should distribute adequately over the retrobulbar space.

Complications include orbital trauma, haemorrhage, globe perforation, anaesthetic myotoxicity and brainstem anaesthesia. Brainstem anaesthesia has recently been reported in a cat that received a retrobulbar block with appropriate doses of local anaesthetic. Following supportive treatment, the animal recovered completely (Oliver and Bradbrook, 2012). A retrobulbar block is ideally performed using a curved retrobulbar needle designed for humans

(Figure 5.3). Alternatively, 22 gauge spinal needles have been used for this technique (Accola *et al.*, 2006). The author does not use spinal needles because of the long bevel and extremely sharp point.

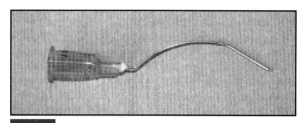

5.3 Retrobulbar needle.

Alpha-2 adrenoceptor agonists

Alpha-2 adrenoceptor agonists are potent sedatives and also analgesics. They may be appropriate for use in pre-anaesthetic medication in aggressive or excitable patients, but due care should be exercised because of their profound cardiovascular side effects. Very low doses of medetomidine are a useful adjunct to sedation and can be used to smooth recovery from anaesthesia. Anecdotally, medetomidine (1 µg/kg diluted in 0.9% saline and administered slowly intravenously) provides effective sedation of short duration in dogs. Dexmedetomidine may be used in a similar manner. Theoretically the dose of the latter should be half that of medetomidine; however, practical experience suggests that it is not twice as potent, and doses greater than 0.5 µg/kg may be required. In very excited or stressed dogs, higher doses (medetomidine 2–3 µg/kg) may be required, but should always be administered diluted, slowly and to effect. Cats may be sedated in a similar manner, but require drug doses 2–3 times those for dogs. These techniques constitute unauthorized use of alpha-2 agonists.

Ketamine

Ketamine is a potent analgesic with effects at the *N*-methyl-D-aspartate (NMDA) receptor in the spinal cord, modulating nociceptive transmission. There is, as yet, limited information pertaining to its analgesic efficacy in dogs and cats specific to ocular procedures. Ketamine does offer the advantage for procedures such as imaging of the retina or electrophysiological assessment of providing a central eye position and mydriasis.

Relevant aspects of ocular physiology

Aspects of ocular physiology are important in the management of certain cases and are likely to be greatly influenced and perturbed by anaesthesia. These include IOP, tear production and cardiac reflexes associated with ocular manipulation.

Intraocular pressure

Inappropriate pre- or perioperative management can result in the rupture of a fragile globe. Ideally the IOP should not increase during patient handling or anaesthesia. Clinical procedures and other physiological factors that may directly or indirectly influence IOP include:

- Venous pressure
- Arterial pressure
- Direct pressure on the globe
- Arterial blood gas tensions (P_aCO_2 and P_aO_2)
- Drugs
- Surgery.

Venous pressure
An increase in venous pressure may increase IOP by reducing venous drainage and aqueous humour outflow from the eye. Collars and neck leads both serve to occlude the jugular veins and increase venous pressure. Jugular occlusion for blood sampling will have a similar effect, as will bandaging or poor positioning during anaesthesia. Jugular compression should be avoided and the head should be elevated slightly to avoid increases in venous pressure due to hydrostatic effects.

Airway obstruction will have a marked effect on venous pressure. It is most likely to occur when the neck is profoundly ventroflexed for positioning for corneal or intraocular surgery. Careful positioning and monitoring should be employed. The capnograph trace and ventilator pressures are often useful indicators of early airway obstruction. Armoured or guarded endotracheal (ET) tubes are also available and their use is recommended for ocular procedures that require neck ventroflexion for positioning.

Arterial pressure
Whilst IOP is stable over a wide range of arterial blood pressures, profound and acute changes in arterial blood pressure will cause transient changes in IOP. Where acute changes in arterial blood pressure are due to inadequate analgesia or an inadequate depth of anaesthesia, administration of potent opioids such as fentanyl may be desirable.

Direct pressure on the globe
Careless placement of facemasks during induction of anaesthesia, and handling during positioning of the anaesthetized patient, can result in pressure on the globe and should be avoided. Pressure on the globe can also cause damage and particular care should be taken with the contralateral eye, which will often be the healthy eye in unilateral procedures. Self-trauma should also be avoided. Bandaging feet may be preferable to overly tight, rigid Elizabethan collars, although opinions differ among veterinary ophthalmologists with regard to the routine use of Elizabethan collars. Good analgesia and, where necessary, sedation may also reduce self-trauma.

Drugs
Vomiting, gagging and coughing all increase IOP. Emetic drugs such as morphine and medetomidine may be best avoided, although low doses of medetomidine rarely result in vomiting. Endotracheal intubation at an inappropriately light plane of anaesthesia may result in coughing, and an increased IOP. Laryngeal manipulation should be avoided. The use of fentanyl (~2 µg/kg) as part of the anaesthetic induction technique may reduce laryngeal reflexes. Topical anaesthesia of the larynx with lidocaine is useful in cats, and intravenous lidocaine (1 mg/kg) may be beneficial in dogs, although evidence is contradictory (Jolliffe *et al.*, 2007).

Tear production
Anaesthesia reduces tear production for up to 24 hours in dogs (Herring *et al.*, 2000; Shepard *et al.*, 2011). Many drugs are administered during anaesthesia, and different pharmacological classes have different effects on tear production:

- Opioids, including butorphanol, fentanyl, pethidine and buprenorphine, reduce tear production
- Whilst the effect of alpha-2 agonists varies with the agent (e.g. xylazine has little effect, whereas medetomidine has a substantial effect), when opioids are combined with alpha-2 agonists, there is a marked decrease in tear production
- Atropine markedly reduces tear production
- Previous studies have also implicated acepromazine, although a more recent study suggested it had no effect on tear production (Mouney *et al.*, 2011).

Ketamine-based anaesthesia also tends to result in a central and 'open' eye, so corneal desiccation may occur. The same concerns are applicable to neuromuscular blocking agents (NMBAs). Tear substitutes (see Chapter 7) should be applied regularly in all cases undergoing sedation or anaesthesia and where opioid analgesia is being administered. Particular care should be taken in brachycephalic patients, and in those who have received NMBA- or ketamine-based anaesthesia.

Cardiac reflexes associated with ocular manipulation
The oculocardiac reflex (OCR) is traditionally considered to be associated with ocular traction or manipulation. Receptors transmit the stimulus via the ciliary nerves and the ophthalmic branch of the trigeminal nerve, to the trigeminal sensory nucleus and the visceral motor nucleus, to the vagus nerve. Vagal stimulation results in profound bradycardia and, in extreme cases, asystole. However, in clinical veterinary practice, the OCR is of limited importance because it is rarely documented in dogs and cats. Pre-emptive use of parenteral parasympatholytics (anticholinergics) prior to ocular procedures is no longer recommended. These drugs have deleterious effects including arrhythmias and their duration of action may not be sufficient. Retrobulbar blocks have also been advocated as a preventive measure, but retrobulbar injection of local anaesthetic can itself elicit the OCR.

Appropriate monitoring and a timely response to bradycardia associated with ocular manipulation are recommended. The initiating stimulus should be removed, for example by releasing traction on the globe, and parasympatholytics administered intravenously if required.

Pre-anaesthetic assessment

Pre-anaesthetic assessment aims to evaluate factors that might influence the course and management of the perianaesthetic period. Ideally this assessment should be undertaken in advance of elective procedures. Whilst it is beyond the scope of this chapter to cover pre-anaesthetic assessment for all patients, some salient points related to specific cases and a strategy for approaching cases are presented below.

History

A full medical history should be obtained, including previous drug administration and anaesthetics. It is important to determine whether the animal has any concurrent diseases likely to influence anaesthesia.

Concurrent medication

Limited attention is paid to drug interactions in veterinary medicine. Many commonly prescribed ophthalmic and non-ophthalmic drugs either interact with anaesthetic drugs or cause physiological changes that may influence anaesthesia (Figures 5.4 and 5.5).

Further diagnostic tests

The value of pre-anaesthetic blood tests remains controversial and many studies have shown that 'random' testing of all animals undergoing anaesthesia does not affect morbidity. However, where a disease is suspected from the history or clinical examination, pertinent tests should be undertaken and the results obtained and assessed prior to anaesthesia.

Type of drug	Examples	Clinical interaction
Antibiotics	Aminoglycosides	Nephrotoxicity; interaction with NMBAs
Cardiac drugs	Beta-blockers	Decreased cardiac contractility; bradycardia
	Angiotensin-converting enzyme (ACE) inhibitors	Vasodilation; potential for hypotension
	Cardiac glycosides (digoxin)	Profound sensitivity to electrolyte abnormalities; avoid parasympatholytics
	Diuretics (various classes)	Potential for hypovolaemia and hypotension; electrolyte abnormalities
Analgesics	Opioids	Synergism with pre-anaesthetic medication
	Non-steroidal anti-inflammatory drugs (NSAIDs)	Avoid concomitant corticosteroid use; caution in hypovolaemia, hypoproteinaemia, hypotension, renal and hepatic disease
Systemic corticosteroids		Chronic administration can lead to iatrogenic hyperadrenocorticism; avoid concomitant use of NSAIDs; corticosteroid supplementation will be required in perioperative period if prior chronic administration; avoid in diabetic patients; may have profound effects on wound healing
Behaviour-modifying drugs	Selegiline/clomipramine	Increase serotonin levels via different mechanisms; theoretically avoid pethidine and tramadol – risk of serotonin syndrome
Incontinence drugs	Phenylpropanolamine	Clinical hypertension (noradrenaline); avoid tramadol because this inhibits noradrenaline reuptake
Anticonvulsants	Phenobarbital	May reduce anaesthetic agent requirement
Antihypertensives	Amlodipine	Potential for hypotension
Chemotherapeutic agents		Organ toxicity; delayed wound healing; myelosuppression; consider operator safety

5.4 Systemic medications that may interact with anaesthetic and analgesic drugs.

Drug	Use	Class	Route	Systemic effects and relevance to anaesthesia
Adrenaline (epinephrine)	Mydriasis	Alpha and beta adrenergic agonist	Intra-cameral	Tachycardia and hypertension. Dilute to 1:10,000 prior to injection. Irrigation solution with low concentrations rarely associated with clinical effects. (Bronchodilation)
Phenylephrine	Mydriasis; haemostasis	Alpha-1 adrenergic agonist	Topical	Profound hypertension, bradycardia and arrhythmias reported. Avoid 10% solutions. Effects may be worse where already vasoconstricted, e.g. with medetomidine. Vasodilation, e.g. use of acepromazine, may ameliorate effects
Atropine	Mydriasis; cycloplegia	Parasympatholytic (anticholinergic)	Topical	Tachycardia and arrhythmias. Reduced tear production. Bitter taste leads to hypersalivation. (Bronchodilation)
Acetazolamide	Intraocular pressure (IOP) reduction	Carbonic anhydrase inhibitor	Systemic	Metabolic acidosis, hypokalaemia and hyperchloraemia. Effects compounded if respiratory acidosis occurs during anaesthesia. Vomiting, diarrhoea, anorexia, weakness and diuresis

5.5 Topical and systemic ophthalmic medications that may interact with anaesthetic and analgesic drugs. Conditions within parentheses have questionable clinical relevance. (continues) ▶

Drug	Use	Class	Route	Systemic effects and relevance to anaesthesia
Timolol Betaxolol	IOP reduction	Beta-1 selective beta-blocker	Topical	Bradycardia and bronchoconstriction
Mannitol	IOP reduction	Osmotic diuretic	Systemic	Acute increase in circulating volume followed by hypovolaemia/ dehydration, plasma hyperosmolarity and electrolyte abnormalities. Care in cardiac disease and renal disease
Glycerol	IOP reduction	Osmotic diuretic	Systemic	Hyperglycaemia and glucosuria. Avoid in diabetics. Nausea and vomiting during administration
Pilocarpine	IOP management; keratoconjunctivitis sicca	Parasympathomimetic (cholinergic)	Topical; oral	Bradycardia and bronchoconstriction (other cholinergic effects including vomiting and diarrhoea)
Acetylcholine	IOP management	Parasympathomimetic (cholinergic)	Intra-cameral	Bradycardia and bronchoconstriction (other cholinergic effects including vomiting and diarrhoea)
Carbachol	IOP management	Parasympathomimetic (cholinergic)	Intra-cameral	Bradycardia and bronchoconstriction (other cholinergic effects including vomiting and diarrhoea)

5.5 (continued) Topical and systemic ophthalmic medications that may interact with anaesthetic and analgesic drugs. Conditions within parentheses have questionable clinical relevance.

Formulation of an anaesthetic plan

In addition to a thorough pre-anaesthetic assessment, specific patient factors, pre-existing disease and ophthalmic presentation are vital considerations when formulating an anaesthetic plan.

Patient factors

Figure 5.6 summarizes some important patient factors that influence anaesthetic management.

Factor	Clinical examples
Age	Neonates metabolize drugs differently as they have immature cardiovascular, respiratory, hepatic and renal function. Geriatrics may have reduced cardiac reserve and reduced cardiac output, decreased functional residual capacity, possibly reduced generalized hepatic and renal function and neuronal degeneration, perhaps without overt clinical signs
Temperament	Fearful and stressed animals require more sedation, which is almost always preferable to excessive physical restraint. Theoretical drug advantages and disadvantages become much less significant if the patient is difficult to handle. **Never** use the scruff to restrain patients with ocular damage. Immediate chamber induction of anaesthesia is contraindicated owing to the negative cardiovascular effects. Even if chamber induction is required, some form of sedation to reduce anxiety and stress levels is indicated
Breed sensitivities	Sight hounds do not metabolize barbiturates effectively, hence prolonged recovery times are common, and these drugs are probably best avoided. Giant breeds may exhibit sensitivity to acepromazine, thus a maximum dose of 1 mg may be prudent
Breed morphology	Brachycephalic breeds need appropriate airway management, especially during recovery
Body condition score	Obesity is common, influences drug distribution and often results in hypoventilation

5.6 Patient factors that influence anaesthetic and analgesic selection.

Pre-existing disease

In the trauma patient, damage to other body systems may be immediately life-threatening (e.g. pneumothorax) and must be prioritized. Many animals presenting for ophthalmological procedures are geriatric with extensive comorbidity, which must be investigated and managed appropriately and adequately.

Diabetes mellitus is a common concurrent disease in animals presented for phacoemulsification surgery. A period of hospitalization, medication and surgery will destabilize most stable diabetics. There is limited information on how best to proceed with these patients but it is sensible to aim for moderate stabilization prior to surgery, the assessment of which can be based on clinical history, serum fructosamine concentrations and serial blood glucose curves. It is prudent to avoid anaesthetizing a ketoacidotic animal. Thus, preoperative urinalysis is useful, as is venous blood gas analysis. Procedures should be performed in the morning to avoid prolonged starvation and to facilitate observation in recovery. There is no consensus as to what is an appropriate preoperative insulin dose. Clinical experience suggests that administration of half the normal insulin dose, provided that the pre-insulin blood glucose concentration is not low, coupled with serial blood glucose evaluation (every 30–45 minutes) is acceptable. Where intraoperative blood glucose is >16 mmol/l, some authors recommend soluble insulin, but there is little evidence of its effect on morbidity (Oliver et al., 2010). Where blood glucose is less than approximately 5 mmol/l, glucose supplementation in the form of a glucose/saline infusion is required. Generally, 2 ml/kg/h of a 4–5% glucose/saline solution is used, coupled with frequent (~15 minutes) assessment of blood glucose to ensure that hypoglycaemia is avoided. In practice, intraoperative hypoglycaemia is uncommon.

Ketoacidosis can develop in the early postoperative period if strict attention is not paid to ▶

glycaemic management. Animals are fed as soon as possible and blood glucose monitoring continued as required. Most patients receiving twice-daily insulin return to their normal regimen on the evening following surgery. Recent work suggests that diabetic patients are more prone to intraoperative systemic hypotension (Oliver *et al.*, 2010). Therefore, appropriate monitoring and adequate fluid therapy are necessary.

In all cases attempts should be made to correct or manage the following before anaesthesia:

- Severe hypovolaemia
- Severe dehydration
- Hypoproteinaemia (albumin <15 g/l), and consider further support
- Anaemia (packed cell volume <20%, depending upon chronicity and cardiovascular status)
- Pneumothorax
- Oliguria/anuria
- Congestive heart failure
- Cardiac arrhythmias
- Acid–base disturbances (pH <7.2)
- Electrolyte disturbances (potassium <2.5–3.0 or >6 mmol/l, hypoglycaemia, hypercalcaemia, severe hypo- or hypernatraemia).

Ophthalmic presentations and management factors

Figure 5.7 gives examples of particular ophthalmic presentations that will have a bearing on anaesthetic management.

Anaesthetic drugs and their effects on the eye

- Opioids have effects on the pupil; the magnitude and effect varies with drug and species but is probably insignificant in the presence of topically administered mydriatics.
- Any drug that induces emesis, e.g. morphine, will increase IOP during vomition.
- Volatile agents generally decrease or have minimal effects on IOP. Sevoflurane has been shown to have minimal effects on IOP in the dog, as has desflurane/nitrous oxide (Almeida *et al.*, 2004).
- Ketamine *alone* will increase IOP through its effects on the extraocular muscles, but ketamine in combination with midazolam does not affect IOP (Ghaffari *et al.*, 2010).
- Propofol has been shown to decrease IOP in many human studies but may increase IOP in the dog (Hofmeister *et al.*, 2008).
- Vecuronium and atracurium have minimal effects on IOP in the dog.
- Familiarity provides a margin of safety. For most cases, the use of 'routine' pre-anaesthetic medication, induction agents and volatile agents is preferable to the use of novel agents in compromised animals.
- Overall, the approach to anaesthesia and the management of the case are more important than the drugs themselves.

Intraoperative monitoring

Selected aspects of good management

Intravenous access

It may be appropriate to place an intravenous catheter in a saphenous vein to allow easy access during surgery and to avoid increases in IOP caused by restraint.

Airway

- Due care should be taken to avoid increases in IOP during induction of anaesthesia and endotracheal intubation.

Clinical example	Management strategies
Blind patient	
Bilateral cataracts	The patient may be frightened or nervous in a strange environment and require considerate and thoughtful handling. Harnesses allow easier handling and are mandatory in cases with raised intraocular pressure (IOP) or fragile eyes. Care during handling to avoid iatrogenic or self-trauma. The animal may panic during recovery from anaesthesia; plan appropriate analgesia, sedation and nursing care
Fragile eye	
Deep corneal ulcer; corneal foreign body/ corneal or intraocular surgery	Aim to avoid increases in IOP. Care with jugular blood sampling. Provide adequate pre-anaesthetic medication; well sedated animals require less restraint. Care with restraint; avoid 'scruffing' or neck restraint for intravenous catheterization. Consider saphenous catheter. Avoid emesis, barking or crying; supply adequate analgesia. Care during intubation; ensure no gagging/coughing. Avoid mask induction; excitement increases IOP and risks trauma to globe. Care when moving animal under anaesthesia; do not compress abdomen. Use appropriate drugs. Keep head slightly elevated with respect to the body. Maintain end-tidal CO_2 within physiological limits; use intermittent positive pressure ventilation (IPPV) if necessary. Maintain mean arterial blood pressure at 65–100 mmHg. Aim for a smooth recovery from anaesthesia. Many of these cases will be brachycephalic; extreme care warranted during recovery owing to pre-existing airway compromise
Painful eye	
	Multimodal analgesia. Address primary problem if possible
Requirement for neuromuscular blockade	
Phacoemulsification	Facilities for IPPV, capnography, monitoring neuromuscular function and reversal required

5.7 Ophthalmic presentations influencing anaesthetic planning.

- **Never** use red rubber ET tubes in cats. They have high pressure–low volume cuffs that predispose to tracheal damage; even if this only manifests as a cough it is not ideal in a case with a fragile eye.
- Where neck flexion is required, there is a risk of ET tube obstruction due to kinking. The use of armoured ET tubes should be considered and the capnograph trace should be monitored carefully.
- Ninety-degree connectors are useful but do increase dead space (Figure 5.8).
- Brachycephalic patients generally have compromised airways. Good airway management is fundamental to successful anaesthesia. The clinician should be aware of the increased risk and allocate early surgery slots, if possible. Investment in a good laryngoscope and intubation aids is prudent. Good analgesia and anxiolysis will calm the animal such that intravenous catheter placement, pre-oxygenation and induction of anaesthesia can be carried out with minimal stress. Background sedation promotes a smooth recovery. Patients should be allowed to recover on oxygen and undisturbed, with the aim to allow them to recover consciousness with the ET tube in place. Many animals will only start to swallow as they move to stand up. Patients should be observed constantly until they are ambulatory.

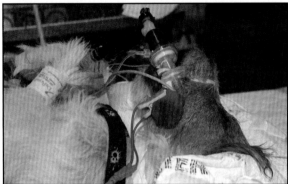

5.8 Positioning for corneal surgery. Note the ventral neck flexion and the monitoring devices attached.

Tear production
Both eyes should be protected during the procedure. Anaesthetic and analgesic drugs decrease tear production, and this is exacerbated by circulating warm air blankets, incubators and lights. Lubrication of vulnerable eyes should be continued postoperatively (see Chapter 7).

Analgesia
The specific types of pain relevant to each case should be addressed. Other considerations include IOP regulation and management, corneal healing, concurrent disease, concurrent drug administration, the degree of pain and corneal sensitivity.

Monitoring procedures
Anaesthesia dramatically perturbs homeostasis, with potentially deleterious consequences. In a well managed anaesthetic procedure there should be appropriate monitoring, so that problems can be detected in a timely manner and strategies to resolve them implemented immediately. The purpose of the circulation is to deliver oxygen to tissues and remove carbon dioxide and other waste products from them. Tissue oxygen delivery should never be compromised. The occipital lobes are particularly sensitive to hypoxia and post-anaesthetic cortical blindness is occasionally reported. This has been associated with intraoperative hypotension, cardiac arrest and the use of mouth gags. In a recent study investigating post-anaesthetic blindness in 20 cats, 3 had a cardiac arrest, 7 had documented hypotension and 7 had no blood pressure monitoring. Thus, in 17 of 20 cases, cerebral hypoperfusion was documented or suspected. In 16 of the 20 cases a mouth gag was also used, which may have compromised maxillary artery blood flow (Stiles *et al.*, 2012). The extent of anaesthesia-related morbidity in small animals is unknown but it is not uncommon to see renal damage apparently induced by poor anaesthetic management. These problems highlight the importance of effective and appropriate anaesthetic monitoring.

The implementation of extensive monitoring has resulted in a marked reduction in anaesthetic morbidity in human medical practice. The correct use of blood pressure monitoring, capnography and pulse oximetry together may allow the detection of over 90% of anaesthesia-related problems. The lack of access to the head impairs assessment of the depth of anaesthesia in ophthalmic patients and prevents early detection of equipment disconnection. For this reason, capnography is highly recommended. It is also useful to detect partial obstruction of the ET tube during neck flexion, to assess the adequacy of spontaneous or mechanical ventilation, and to provide early warning of cardiovascular problems. Pulse oximetry is extremely useful as long as its limitations are understood. It may be most beneficial during the recovery period where oxygen support is removed and the animal has to breathe room air. Arterial blood pressure should be monitored in order to ensure an adequate 'driving pressure' to the tissues. Oscillometric devices are adequate for larger patients, whereas Doppler flow probes are better for small dogs and cats. In severely compromised patients, direct arterial access is ideal. Monitoring of the electrocardiogram (ECG) is also recommended and is required in any animal with preoperative arrhythmias. Body temperature should also be measured and supported, preferably with active warming systems. Hypothermia has multiple deleterious effects and should be avoided.

Postoperative care

Recovery can be the most critical phase of anaesthesia especially after intraocular procedures. Self-trauma may cause irreparable damage. An animal that could see prior to the procedure and is blind postoperatively may panic, as may an animal that was previously blind and has had its sight restored.

Always plan adequately for recovery, especially in brachycephalic cases (as already discussed). Additional analgesia and/or sedation may be required, especially in the early postoperative period. If an otherwise healthy dog is having a poor recovery from anaesthesia, low dose medetomidine or dexmedetomidine intravenously (see Analgesia section) will provide additional sedation and analgesia, and rarely needs to be repeated. Foot bandages or Elizabethan collars may be used but are not a substitute for adequate nursing care and analgesia. Where there is significant coexisting disease, this must also be managed.

Special techniques for ophthalmology patients

Neuromuscular blockade

This is a brief overview of the use of neuromuscular blockade in ophthalmic surgery. Non-depolarizing NMBAs are the drugs of choice for ophthalmic patients and the current discussion is entirely limited to this class of drugs. Readers are directed to the *BSAVA Manual of Canine and Feline Anaesthesia and Analgesia* for comprehensive information on neuromuscular blockade. Muscle relaxation with neuromuscular blockade is useful for the following reasons:

- Providing a centrally positioned eye without stay sutures or deep planes of anaesthesia
- Relaxing extraocular muscles and reducing IOP, thus providing better surgical conditions
- Preventing small movements that could jeopardize surgery (e.g. fighting the ventilator or nystagmus).

Mechanism of action

Non-depolarizing NMBAs bind to postsynaptic acetylcholine (ACh) receptors, effectively competing with ACh, and thus causing muscular paralysis. NMBAs are neither analgesic nor anaesthetic. Thus, adequate anaesthesia and analgesia must be provided and the depth of anaesthesia monitored closely. Inappropriate NMBA administration can result in a paralysed but conscious patient.

Muscles have variable sensitivity to NMBAs; the diaphragm tends to be paralysed last and its function returns first. However, NMBAs paralyse all skeletal muscles, and facilities for controlled ventilation must be available. The use of low doses of NMBAs to try to 'spare' the diaphragm is not recommended because it results in hypercapnia, which tends to increase IOP, and can be dangerous.

Monitoring the blockade

Assessment of the function of the neuromuscular junction is important to ensure adequate neuromuscular function at the end of the procedure. A peripheral nerve stimulator is most commonly used, which delivers a small current via two electrodes placed across a nerve that supplies a large muscle group. The peroneal nerve is often used in ophthalmic procedures, and the motor response in the cranial tibial muscle is evaluated (Figure 5.9). Evaluation is com-

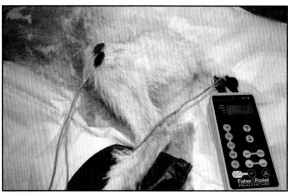

5.9 Nerve stimulator in position on the peroneal nerve.

monly visual and tactile only. Where an acceleromyograph is used, there is objective measurement of the motor response. The current applied is large enough to recruit all the available nerve fibres.

Several stimulation patterns are used to assess neuromuscular blockade and readers are directed to the *BSAVA Manual of Canine and Feline Anaesthesia and Analgesia* for further detail. The two most useful patterns in monitoring neuromuscular blockade are probably train of four (TOF) and double burst stimulation (DBS).

Train of four: Four pulses are delivered over a 2-second period. In a normal neuromuscular junction, this results in four twitches of equal strength, which are referred to as T1 to T4. Following administration of a non-depolarizing NMBA, there is a progressive loss of these twitches, starting with T4 and progressing to T1, in the presence of an adequate NMBA dose. This progressive loss of neuromuscular function is known as 'fade'.

During the recovery period, there is a gradual return of the twitches, starting with T1 and progressing to T4. When T4 is apparently identical to T1 (or is 90% of T1 if using an acceleromyograph) neuromuscular function is deemed to be adequate. Tactile assessment is a very insensitive method of detecting 'fade' (residual neuromuscular blockade). The observer can often only determine whether T4 is just 40% of T1.

Double burst stimulation: Two bursts, each consisting of two or three short pulses, are delivered 0.75 seconds apart. The resultant response is two muscle contractions. DBS is used because it is easier to detect 'fade' (residual neuromuscular blockade) compared with TOF, but it is still less reliable than the use of objective monitoring with an acceleromyograph.

It is important that the animal is also assessed clinically to detect signs of residual neuromuscular blockade. The presence of a normal tidal volume (and normal end-tidal CO_2) demonstrates that diaphragmatic and intercostal muscle function are nearly normal. However, the upper airway muscles are more sensitive to neuromuscular blockade and airway obstruction during recovery can occur if these muscles are not of normal strength.

Monitoring depth of anaesthesia: Animals must be adequately anaesthetized prior to and during neuromuscular blockade. Assessment of the depth of anaesthesia may be more difficult because cranial nerve function is no longer present. There will be no palpebral reflex and the globe will be central in position. Signs that are suggestive of inadequate anaesthesia include tachycardia and hypertension. Changes may be visible on the capnograph trace. On occasion, salivation, pupillary dilation and isolated pharyngeal muscle twitching are seen.

Neuromuscular blocking agents
Many agents have been used for neuromuscular blockade in dogs and cats. These include pancuronium, mivacurium, vecuronium, rocuronium, atracurium and *cis*-atracurium. Atracurium and vecuronium are in common use in the UK. None of the NMBAs is authorized for use in domestic animals.

Atracurium: This is a benzylisoquinoline that is metabolized by non-specific esterases and by spontaneous breakdown (Hofmann degradation). It is generally the drug of choice in severe hepatic or renal disease. It may cause histamine release if administered rapidly intravenously.

In dogs and cats 0.25 mg/kg i.v. provides approximately 30 minutes of neuromuscular blockade. Additional doses are administered to maintain neuromuscular blockade if required. The duration of action is variable between individuals.

Vecuronium: This is an amino steroid that has negligible effects on the cardiovascular system. It undergoes some hepatic metabolism and biliary excretion. It should be avoided in severe hepatopathy.

In dogs and cats 0.1 mg/kg provides 20–25 minutes of neuromuscular blockade, with some variation between patients. Additional doses are administered to maintain neuromuscular blockade if required.

Antagonizing neuromuscular blockade
The neuromuscular blockade is terminated when the concentration of ACh is adequate to resume neuromuscular function. It should be noted that 70% of ACh receptors may still be blocked when the TOF ratio is 0.9. Thus, recovery will occur spontaneously but can be hastened by the use of an anticholinesterase, which prevents degradation of ACh. Anticholinesterases also have some muscarinic effects and may cause bradycardia, salivation and bronchoconstriction. Thus, a parasympatholytic is administered concurrently. Common combinations of drugs include neostigmine with glycopyrrolate and edrophonium with atropine. Readers are directed to the *BSAVA Manual of Canine and Feline Anaesthesia and Analgesia* for more detail on the safe use of NMBAs.

References and further reading

Accola PJ, Bentley E, Smith LJ, *et al.* (2006) Development of a retrobulbar injection technique for ocular surgery and analgesia in dogs. *Journal of the American Veterinary Medical Association* **229**(2), 220–225

Almeida DE, Rezende ML, Nunes N, *et al.* (2004) Evaluation of intraocular pressure in association with cardiovascular parameters in normocapnic dogs anesthetized with sevoflurane and desflurane. *Veterinary Ophthalmology* **7**(4), 265–269

Clark JS, Bentley E and Smith LJ (2011). Evaluation of topical nalbuphine or oral tramadol as analgesics for corneal pain in dogs: a pilot study. *Veterinary Ophthalmology* **14**, 358–364

Flaherty D and Auckburally A (2007) Muscle relaxants. In: *BSAVA Manual of Anaesthesia and Analgesia*, ed. C Seymour and T Duke-Novakovski, pp. 156–166. BSAVA Publications, Cheltenham

Ghaffari MS, Rezaei MA, Mirani AH, *et al.* (2010) The effects of ketamine-midazolam anesthesia on intraocular pressure in clinically normal dogs. *Veterinary Ophthalmology* **13**(2), 91–93

Gurney M (2012) Analgesia in small animal practice: an update. *Journal of Small Animal Practice* **53**(7), 377–386

Herring IP, Pickett JP, Champagne ES and Marini M (2000) Evaluation of aqueous tear production in dogs following general anesthesia. *Journal of the American Animal Hospital Association* **36**, 427–430

Hofmeister EH, Williams CO, Braun C, *et al.* (2008) Propofol versus thiopental: effects on peri-induction intraocular pressures in normal dogs. *Veterinary Anaesthesia and Analgesia* **35**(4), 275–281

ISFM and AAFP (2010) Consensus Guidelines on the long term use of NSAIDS in cats. *Journal of Feline Medicine and Surgery* **12**, 519, www.catvets.com/public/PDFs/PracticeGuidelines/NSAIDSGLS.pdf

Jolliffe CT, Leece EA, Adams V, *et al.* (2007) Effect of intravenous lidocaine on heart rate, systolic arterial blood pressure and cough responses to endotracheal intubation in propofol-anaesthetized dogs. *Veterinary Anaesthesia and Analgesia* **34**(5), 322–330

McMurphy RM, Davidson HJ and Hodgson D (2004) Effects of atracurium on intraocular pressure, eye position, and blood pressure in eucapnic and hypocapnic isoflurane-anesthetized dogs. *American Journal of Veterinary Research* **65**(2), 179–182

Mouney MC, Accola PJ, Cremer J, *et al.* (2011) Effects of acepromazine maleate or morphine on tear production before, during, and after sevoflurane anesthesia in dogs. *American Journal of Veterinary Research* **72**, 1427–1430

Myrna KE, Bentley E and Smith LJ (2010). Effectiveness of injection of local anesthetic into the retrobulbar space for postoperative analgesia following eye enucleation in dogs. *Journal of the American Veterinary Medical Association* **237**(2), 174–177

Oliver JA and Bradbrook C (2013) Suspected brainstem anesthesia following retrobulbar block in a cat. *Veterinary Ophthalmology* **16**(3), 225–226

Oliver JA, Clark L, Corletto F and Gould DJ (2010) A comparison of anesthetic complications between diabetic and nondiabetic dogs undergoing phacoemulsification cataract surgery: a retrospective study. *Veterinary Ophthalmology* **13**(4), 244–250

Pypendop BH, Siao KT and Ilkiw JE (2009) Effects of tramadol hydrochloride on the thermal threshold in cats. *American Journal of Veterinary Research* **70**(12), 1465–1470

Sanchez RF, Mellor D and Mould J (2006) Effects of medetomidine and medetomidine-butorphanol combination on Schirmer tear test 1 readings in dogs. *Veterinary Ophthalmology* **9**(1) 33–37

Shepard MK, Accola PJ, Lopez LA, *et al.* (2011). Effect of duration and type of anesthetic on tear production in dogs. *American Journal of Veterinary Research* **72**, 608–612

Smith LJ, Bentley E, Shih A, *et al.* (2004) Systemic lidocaine infusion as an analgesic for intra-ocular surgery in dogs. *Veterinary Anaesthesia and Analgesia* **31**(1), 53–63

Stiles J, Honda CN, Krohne SG and Kazacos EA (2003) Effect of topical administration of morphine sulphate solution on signs of pain and corneal wound healing in dogs. *American Journal of Veterinary Research* **64**, 813–818

Stiles J, Weil AB, Packer RA and Lantz GC (2012) Post-anesthetic cortical blindness in cats: Twenty cases. *The Veterinary Journal* **193**(2), 367–373

Thomson S, Oliver JA, Gould DJ, *et al.* (2010) Preliminary investigations into the analgesic efficacy of topical ocular morphine in dogs and cats. *Proceedings of the British Small Animal Veterinary Association Congress*

6

Principles of ophthalmic surgery

Sally Turner

It might appear on first consideration that, aside from the matter of scale, there is not much difference between general veterinary surgery and ophthalmic surgery. There are, however, several factors which differ quite significantly and need to be addressed specifically. A thorough understanding of ocular anatomy and physiology (including how this might differ between breeds and species), and attention to detail regarding positioning of both patient and surgeon, correct use of magnification, and careful instrument selection and use are all of vital importance if the best surgical outcome is to be achieved. General principles of ophthalmic surgery are considered in detail in this chapter, and the reader is directed to subsequent chapters for descriptions of specific surgical procedures involving different ocular tissues.

Anatomy and physiology

As with all surgical procedures, a thorough knowledge of the anatomy of the area in question is essential to ensure the best surgical outcome and to avoid any inadvertent damage to structure or function. Although an in-depth discussion of ocular anatomy is beyond the scope of this chapter, the most pertinent points are briefly outlined below.

The different structures which make up the eye and periorbital area (i.e. the orbit, adnexa and globe itself) are composed of a variety of tissue types. These tissues vary widely with respect to the origin of their blood supply and degree of vascularity, differ in their healing rates, and can have diverse inflammatory responses to surgical trauma. These are all issues of which the surgeon must be aware. One common feature, however, is the relative sensitivity of ocular tissues, because all are well innervated with sensory fibres. Thus, an adequate depth of anaesthesia for the procedure, and provision of sufficient analgesia postoperatively are essential (see Chapter 5). Patients that are free from both pain and irritation are far less likely to cause damage as a result of self-trauma following the procedure, thus reducing the risk of wound breakdown and infection and limiting the need for Elizabethan collars.

The orbit
The surgical procedures most commonly performed by general practitioners that involve the orbit include enucleation and exenteration, along with replacement of proptosed globes. Knowledge of the bony components of the orbit and their association with the rest of the skull is important, and is discussed in greater detail in Chapter 8. In dogs and cats the bony orbit is incomplete, with the masseter, temporal and pterygoid muscles contributing to the boundaries of the orbit. In particular, there is only soft tissue separation between the oral and retrobulbar spaces. There are several foramina in the orbital bones, through which nerves and blood vessels pass; the largest of these are the optic foramen and the orbital fissure, and there is direct communication between the tissues of the orbit and the central nervous system (CNS) via the optic nerve. The lacrimal duct can allow passage between the orbit, oropharynx and, potentially, the nasal cavity and paranasal sinuses. The blood supply to the orbit can be increased during infectious, inflammatory or neoplastic conditions, and in glaucomatous eyes, so careful haemostasis is required.

When performing any ocular surgery, especially procedures involving the orbit, it is important to avoid excessive pressure or traction on the globe. Too much force on the optic nerve during enucleation, for example, can result in damage to the contralateral optic nerve via the chiasm, particularly in cats, and permanent blindness can result. The necessity for gentle tissue handling during all ophthalmic surgical procedures cannot be overemphasized. Surgeons must also be aware of the potential to elicit an oculocardiac reflex (see Chapters 5 and 8).

The eyelids
The eyelids protect the globe, especially the corneal surface, and help to spread the tear film. Thus, a normal anatomical relationship between the lid margins and the tear film should be preserved or provided by surgery. Surgical procedures to correct entropion or ectropion, repair lacerations, remove tumours and treat aberrant cilia are all commonly undertaken in general practice. Eyelid tissues are highly vascular and must be handled gently and minimally to avoid the oedema and hyperaemia that occur as rapid inflammatory responses to surgical trauma. Appropriate use of pre- or perioperative systemic anti-inflammatory drugs can limit these acute responses. A major advantage of the good vascular supply is the rapid healing of the eyelid tissue.

Important anatomical features associated with the eyelids are the openings of the meibomian glands on the lid margin, which can serve as useful landmarks for the placement of sutures (see later), and the junction between haired and hairless skin adjacent to the eyelid margin, which serves as the usual site for the initial incision when performing entropion surgery, for example. Careful suture placement should ensure that no rubbing can be caused by sutures along the lid or cornea, and the use of a figure-of-eight suture pattern at the lid margin is preferred (see section on Principles of ophthalmic surgery).

The conjunctiva

The conjunctiva is a multi-layered mucous membrane and is anatomically divided into four regions: the bulbar, palpebral, nictitans and forniceal conjunctiva. The conjunctiva is loosely attached to the underlying tissue, apart from along the limbus and at the transition to the eyelid margin. Therefore, conjunctival tissue requires stabilization if it is to be incised with a surgical blade, and often it is easier to use blunt-tipped scissors. The mobility and good blood supply of the conjunctiva make it a very useful bandage tissue (e.g. conjunctival grafts may be used to treat corneal ulcers). Small incisions in the conjunctiva (e.g. following the removal of an embedded grass seed foreign body) do not require suturing because they heal very rapidly.

The third eyelid

Surgery on the third eyelid (nictitating membrane) is commonly performed in both general and specialist ophthalmic practice owing to the frequency of scrolling of the third eyelid cartilage and prolapse of the third eyelid gland (see Chapter 11). The gland contributes a significant percentage of the aqueous portion of the tear film, whilst the membrane itself helps to spread the tear film and removes debris. The third eyelid acts like a windscreen wiper in this role; therefore, the maintenance of a normal leading edge is an important consideration during any surgical procedure on the third eyelid.

The nasolacrimal system

The nasolacrimal system, consisting of secretory components (lacrimal and third eyelid glands, meibomian glands and conjunctival goblet cells) and excretory components (nasolacrimal puncta, canaliculi and ducts), is considered in greater detail in Chapter 10. Prior to any surgery close to the medial canthus, it is prudent to cannulate the lacrimal puncta with coloured nylon (Figure 6.1) to prevent inadvertent damage during surgery, which can result in chronic epiphora, especially if the ventral punctum is damaged, thus compromising the surgical outcome.

The cornea

Magnification is essential for any corneal surgery. As the cornea of the dog and cat is only about 0.5–0.6 mm thick, without careful dissection and meticulous attention to detail iatrogenic perforation could easily occur. In addition, the normal cornea is

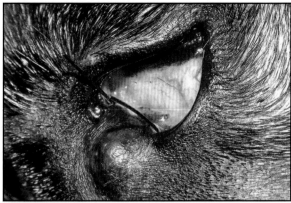

6.1 The placement of coloured suture material within the lacrimal puncta and canaliculi is recommended prior to any procedure close to the medial canthus to help avoid inadvertent damage to these structures, as in this case where the dog is about to undergo surgery to remove a cyst at the medial canthus.

in a somewhat stressed metabolic state owing to the lack of blood vessels, reduced number of cellular organelles and relative lack of immunological cells. As such, the cornea is relatively slow to heal and is susceptible to microbial infection. These factors can contribute to the relatively frequent need for surgical intervention for infected corneal ulcers, for which a combination of keratectomy to remove damaged or infected tissue, along with conjunctival grafts to provide support and rapidly bring a blood supply to the affected area, is commonly performed. In addition to achieving healing, the importance of maintaining a clear visual axis with corneal optical clarity should always be considered because a major goal of the ophthalmic surgeon is not just to salvage the globe but to preserve vision wherever possible. Unfortunately, inexperienced surgeons and those who attempt corneal procedures without suitable instrumentation can fail to achieve a truly successful outcome if they ignore these aims.

Intraocular structures

Intraocular surgery should be considered a specialist procedure, requiring appropriate microsurgical instrumentation and technical proficiency that is outwith the realm of general veterinary practice, so it will not be discussed further in this section.

Patient and surgeon positioning

The positioning of both surgeon and patient is very important for ophthalmic surgery. The surgeon must be comfortable; their movements during the procedure are usually limited to the hands and wrists, which can prove to be surprisingly tiring. Most ophthalmic surgeons prefer to sit with their forearms resting, ideally, on the arm rest of a specially designed surgical chair, or alternatively against rolled up towels positioned at the edge of the surgical site (Figure 6.2). The surgeon should take the time to ensure that they will be positioned comfortably before scrubbing for surgery. The following sequence is suggested:

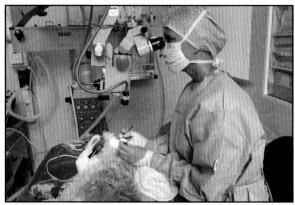

6.2 Surgeon positioned with their arms resting on a folded towel because the chair does not have an integral arm rest. The surgeon should ensure that both they and the patient are appropriately positioned prior to scrubbing for surgery.

- Assuming the surgeon will be seated, the height of the seat should be adjusted; it should not be so low that the knees are cramped, and the feet should rest comfortably on the floor or on the foot pedal of the operating microscope
- The operating table, with the patient, can then be adjusted to fit the height of the surgeon's chair
- If surgical loupes are being used, they should be worn during patient positioning because it is essential that the surgeon is comfortable with the fixed focal length of the loupes
- Once the chair and table are at the right height, the positioning of the patient can be fine tuned. For most procedures the patient will be in lateral recumbency, with the head supported and stabilized on vacuum pillows, with additional beanbags used if necessary. For bilateral procedures where it is necessary to compare both sides for symmetry, sternal or dorsal recumbency may be employed. Dorsal recumbency is generally the preferred patient position for bilateral intraocular surgery
- Normally, the patient's face is parallel to the table-top for adnexal procedures, whilst for corneal surgery the aim is to have the cornea horizontal (Figure 6.3). For some breeds, this will

require the nose to be elevated, and care should be taken to avoid restriction of the endotracheal tube and compromise of the patient's airway as the neck is bent to achieve the surgeon's preferred patient position (as discussed in Chapter 5).

Sterile preparation of the eye and adnexa

Protocols for anaesthesia and perioperative analgesia for ophthalmic surgery are addressed in detail in Chapter 5.

Clipping

Once anaesthetized, the patient can be prepared for surgery. This should be undertaken outside the operating theatre in the preparation room. If the procedure is unilateral, the contralateral eye should be protected with a lubricating gel or ointment (e.g. carbomer gel or soft white paraffin ointment). This may also be applied to the eye to be operated on to protect it from damage by careless clipping and to reduce deposition of hair in the conjunctival sac. However, if corneal rupture or a perforating corneal foreign body are suspected, gels and ointments should not be used due to the risk of intraocular penetration.

The eyelashes should be very carefully trimmed with small sharp scissors. Applying a water-based ophthalmic lubricant to the blades prior to use will encourage the lashes to adhere to the scissors (Figure 6.4). Some surgeons do not clip further for corneal surgery because any clipper rash that may develop might cause the animal to rub the eye. If the area is not clipped, it is essential to use adherent drapes for the surgical procedure, tucking them under the eyelids to provide a sterile operating field. Obviously, clipping is essential for lid surgery. Water-based lubricant can be applied to the fur that is to be removed so that it sticks to the clipper blades; these will need more frequent cleaning as a result, but the production of stray hairs is markedly reduced. Sharp fine clipper blades (no bigger than No. 40) are required; a separate blade dedicated to ophthalmic use is advised. The area clipped should

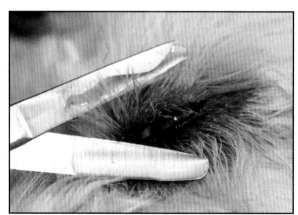

6.4 Small sharp, blunt-tipped, scissors can be coated with a water-soluble lubricant to trap lashes and periocular hairs during trimming, so that they do not contaminate the conjunctival sac.

6.3 Patient positioning for corneal surgery. Note that a vacuum positioning bag has been used to ensure that the cornea is horizontal.

extend 2 cm beyond the expected surgical site. The lateral canthus should be clipped for any procedures that might require a canthotomy. The periocular skin is usually quite loose and can be difficult to clip without snagging by the clipper blades, unless it is pulled tight during the clipping procedure. Care should be taken to clip only in the direction of fur growth because this will reduce the risk of irritation, and attention to neatness will be appreciated by owners concerned about the cosmetic appearance of their animal after the surgery. Following clipping, the stray hairs should be removed; light suction with a handheld vacuum cleaner can be used, but care must be taken to avoid damage to the eye. A lint-roller can be gently moved over the area or, alternatively, lint-free swabs with sterile saline can be used to wipe the area to remove any remaining hairs.

Skin preparation

Clean examination gloves should be worn during surgical preparation to limit contamination of the field. The material used to cleanse the area needs consideration. Standard cotton gauze swabs are too abrasive for the delicate periocular area and, as with cotton wool, can leave lint and threads of material which could be irritating. Thus, neither is advised. Instead, soft woven (i.e. non-gauze) lint-free swabs are recommended. The conjunctival sac is an external body surface with a normal microbial flora that generally consists of a mixed population of bacteria, mainly Gram-positive, but may also include viruses and fungi. This fact, along with the need for gentle handling during patient preparation to prevent swelling, bruising, corneal damage or chemical injury, should be considered when choosing appropriate ocular surface disinfectants. Solutions of povidone–iodine are used to disinfect the surgical site; the dilutions are made in sterile saline (Figure 6.5). Scrub solutions containing alcohol or detergent **must not** be used for preparation of the periocular area or ocular surface because they will damage the ocular surface epithelia of the conjunctiva and cornea. Solutions containing alcohol are particularly damaging and must never be used near the eyes. Chlorhexidine solutions should also be avoided because they are irritant and can damage the cornea and conjunctiva.

Technique

The following steps are suggested for surgical preparation:

1. Clip the required area using fine clippers. A water-based lubricant can be applied to the clipper blades and/or the fur to aid removal of the hairs.
2. Cleanse the periocular skin with a 1:10 dilution of povidone–iodine solution using lint-free swabs. Care should be taken to ensure that the solution does not come into contact with the cornea or conjunctiva. The swabs should be gently wiped away from the surgical site (in the same way as for all routine surgical preparation).
3. Flush the conjunctival sac with a 1:50 dilution of povidone–iodine solution using a 5–10 ml syringe that can be refilled as required (Figure 6.6). If corneal rupture is suspected, povidone–iodine should not be used as it can be toxic to the intraocular structures (e.g. corneal endothelium). The low concentration (1:50 dilution) has enhanced virucidal, bactericidal and fungicidal activity, and causes minimal damage to the ocular surfaces compared with higher concentrations.
4. Remove any mucus or debris from the conjunctival sac using sterile cotton buds or cellulose spears soaked in a 1:50 dilution of povidone–iodine solution. Any residual ophthalmic ointments should also be removed. Carefully flush the conjunctival fornix following the removal of any debris.
5. Flush the conjunctiva with sterile saline solution or lactated Ringer's solution (at least 10 ml) to remove the antiseptic.

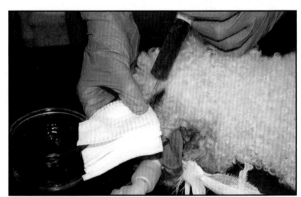

6.6 Surgical preparation includes flushing the conjunctival sac with a 1:50 dilution of povidone–iodine solution using a syringe.

If a bilateral procedure is being performed, the patient can be turned, with the newly cleansed eye protected by a clean, dry, woven (i.e. non-gauze) lint-free swab, whilst the second eye is prepared. When the surgeon is ready to operate on the second eye, a final skin preparation with a 1:10 dilution of povidone–iodine solution is completed in the operating theatre. It is not usually necessary to repeat the entire surgical preparation procedure unless contamination is known to have occurred. It

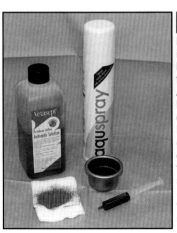

6.5 Dilutions of povidone–iodine solution should be made up fresh from the stock solution. A dilution of 1:10 can be used on soft woven (i.e. non-gauze) lint-free swabs for skin disinfection. A dilution of 1:50 can be used to flush the conjunctival sac (providing there is no corneal rupture), followed by sterile saline.

is recommended that fresh dilutions of stock povidone–iodine solution are decanted into sterile gallipots for each procedure (see Figure 6.5).

Use of magnification

With the exception of the simplest eyelid procedures, all ophthalmic surgery should be performed using appropriate magnification. Lower magnification, such as 2.0–4.0x, may be sufficient for precise eyelid and third eyelid surgery. A minimum of 4.0–5.0x (up to 25.0x) magnification should be used for corneal, conjunctival and intraocular procedures. The main methods of achieving these degrees of magnification involve the magnifying loupe (fixed magnification generally ranging from 2.0–7.0x) and the operating microscope (for a full range of magnification).

Magnifying loupes

Binocular loupes are available in a range of magnifications (in general, the higher the magnification, the smaller the field of view and depth of field), focal lengths and image qualities. The cheapest and most basic, with optics of the poorest quality, are headband magnifiers (Figure 6.7). These do have value but for anyone seriously interested in ophthalmic surgery, higher quality magnifying loupes are recommended (Figure 6.8).

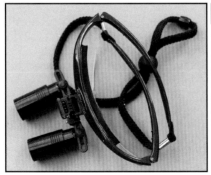

6.7 Headband magnifier for use in ophthalmic surgery. (Courtesy of the University of Wisconsin-Madison, Comparative Ophthalmology Service)

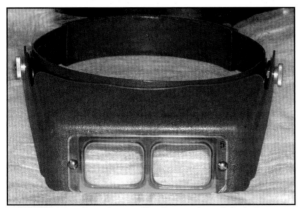

6.8 Surgical loupes provide higher magnification and have better optics compared with headband magnifiers.

When using magnifying loupes, the direction of view can be easily changed, and they are simpler for the general practitioner to master than an operating microscope. Loupes are also much cheaper

than operating microscopes and can be used for other surgical disciplines. For ophthalmic surgery, loupes are most useful for procedures involving the periocular and orbital region (e.g. lid surgery, parotid duct transposition and enucleation) for which the surgeon may wish to see the surgical field from different angles. During corneal surgery this variation in viewing angle is much less important, because manipulation of the globe will suffice if a slightly different viewing angle is required.

The major disadvantages of magnifying loupes are that the focal length is fixed and the depth of field is relatively short, thus at higher magnifications the image 'wobbles' and moves in and out of focus with every small movement of the surgeon's head. This can mimic the feeling of motion sickness and may require practice to overcome. In addition, only moderate magnification can be achieved compared with the far superior magnification attained by even basic operating microscopes. A suggested maximum magnification for loupes is 4.0–5.0x, although higher ranges are available.

When purchasing surgical loupes it is important to remember that they have a fixed focal distance, which should be matched to the preferred operating position of the surgeon. Thus, it is sensible to try out different working distances (34 cm and 42 cm are the most commonly used) to ensure that the surgeon will be comfortable and that they are neither hunched over the patient nor operating at arms' length. Various companies have different styles of spectacle frame and head-mounted versions, and personal preference as well as cost and likely applications will dictate which model to invest in.

Illumination for use with binocular loupes may come from a bright overhead theatre light or from a head-mounted system. Co-axial illumination can be achieved with an appropriately designed headlight, preferably with a fibreoptic light source clipped on to the headband.

Operating microscope

The operating microscope is an essential piece of equipment for the serious veterinary ophthalmologist (Figure 6.9). Both corneal and intraocular surgery can

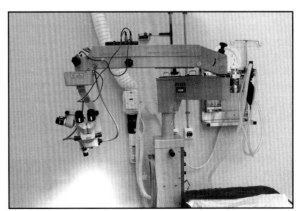

6.9 An operating microscope is essential for the accurate microsurgical techniques required for corneal and intraocular surgery. Operating microscopes are unlikely to be used by general practitioners as they require extensive training and practice to master.

be carried out with much greater accuracy and finesse than with loupes. Use of an operating microscope may also greatly facilitate some eyelid procedures (e.g. removal of ectopic cilia and medial canthoplasty). The operating microscopes used in veterinary practice are most commonly free-standing floor models, although both wall- and ceiling-mounted versions are available. Foot pedal control for focus, zoom and movement of the field of view is desirable.

The obvious advantages of the operating microscope are the enhanced magnification and the fixed image, which does not 'wobble' in and out of focus as can occur with high magnification loupes. It also allows the surgeon to vary the magnification during the procedure (e.g. to 'zoom in' to check the exact depth of a suture) and has a built-in co-axial illumination system, thus ensuring no shadows compromise the field of view. The main disadvantages of operating microscopes are their cost and size. In addition, the viewing position is relatively fixed during the procedure (see above), although this can be overcome by manipulating the position of the globe if necessary. The field of view of an operating microscope is narrow, thus the instruments are introduced 'blind'. The learning curve for using an operating microscope is very steep, requiring extensive training and practice to achieve mastery.

Ophthalmic instrumentation

General considerations

Specific ophthalmic instruments are required for ocular surgery, and those that are most frequently used are discussed. It is not acceptable to use general surgical instruments for ophthalmic surgery, apart from when gross procedures such as enucleation are being performed. A minimum of two types of standard surgical kit are required for ophthalmic procedures: those containing instruments suitable for extraocular and adnexal procedures (e.g. used for eyelid and third eyelid surgery), and those containing instruments suitable for corneal and/or intraocular surgery. A further kit containing larger instruments for enucleation can be prepared if a general surgery kit is not routinely available. A supply of additional instruments packaged individually may also be required. Suggested instruments to be included in pre-prepared packs are listed in Figures 6.10 to 6.12. The selection of specific instruments is very much dictated by personal preference. Instruments for

• Bard–Parker No. 3 scalpel handle
• Adson thumb forceps, 1 x 2 teeth
• Fixation forceps (e.g. Bishop–Harmon), 1 x 2 teeth (heavy)
• Plain dissecting forceps (iris type)
• Cilia forceps (e.g. Bennett)
• Stevens tenotomy scissors, curved
• Ribbon scissors, straight blunt/blunt
• Halsted mosquito artery forceps, curved x 4
• Wells artery forceps, curved x 2
• Castroviejo needle holder, curved without catch
• Foster–Gillies needle holder
• Towel clamp x 4
• Gallipot
• Eyelid speculum (Barraquer or Castroviejo style)
• Chalazion clamp (Desmarres style)
• Lid plate (e.g. Jaeger)
• Callipers

6.11 Suggested instruments to include in an eyelid surgery set.

• Towel clamp x 4
• Beaver handle
• Bishop–Harmon forceps, 1 x 2 teeth (delicate)
• Colibri forceps, corneal
• Harms tying forceps
• Wells artery forceps, curved x 2
• Castroviejo needle holder, curved
• Stevens tenotomy scissors
• Westcott scissors
• Castroviejo spring action scissors, curved
• Barraquer eyelid speculum
• Castroviejo eyelid speculum (for larger patients)

6.12 Suggested instruments to include in a cornea and conjunctiva set.

ophthalmic surgery are designed to be manipulated with minimal movement by the surgeon, because the upper arms and forearms remain still while fine movements of the wrists and hands are used to adjust the position of the instruments.

There are several specific qualities that distinguish ophthalmic instruments from general surgical instruments.

- They are lightweight either by virtue of the material from which they are made (e.g. titanium) or by the presence of holes within their handles to minimize weight. Ophthalmic instruments are shorter (typically 100 mm in length) than general surgical instruments (which are typically 120–140 mm in length), so that they do not touch the bottom of the microscope during the procedure. Although the tips of ophthalmic instruments may be very small, they still need to fit comfortably in the hand.
- Many instruments are designed to be held in a pencil grip and are thus of a similar diameter to a pen or pencil for ease of handling. Since the surgeon is often operating with the assistance of a surgical microscope, there is a need for tactile feedback – the surgeon cannot see the instrument handles, just the tips. Thus, ridging, knurling or flattening of the handles can be useful. These variations also help to prevent slippage and can indicate the correct finger placement for holding and use.

• Adson thumb forceps, 1 x 2 teeth
• Metzenbaum scissors, curved
• Landolt enucleation scissors
• Stevens tenotomy scissors
• Bard–Parker No. 3 scalpel handle
• Towel clamp x 4
• Allis tissue forceps x 2
• Halsted mosquito artery forceps, curved x 3
• Crile artery forceps, curved x 3
• Eyelid speculum (Barraquer or Castroviejo style)
• Needle holder

6.10 Suggested instruments to include in an enucleation set.

- Ophthalmic instruments may have a slightly dulled or dark finish to reduce the scatter of reflected light under the microscope.
- Ophthalmic instruments are often sprung so that the surgeon's hand or wrist position does not need to be altered to re-open the instrument. A pin-stop may be present to prevent excessive pressure on closure, which can lead to damage of the delicate tips.
- Instruments that only operate in one direction (e.g. corneal scissors) often have flat handles whilst those which require rotation during use (e.g. needle holders) may have rounded handles.
- In addition, needle holders may have a lock to allow grasping of the delicate needle without continued digital pressure.

Instrument care

Ophthalmic instruments represent a considerable investment and are easily damaged. It is therefore important that they are well looked after, to maximize their useful life and to ensure their satisfactory function. The instruments should be checked carefully, with magnification, after every few uses. It should be ensured that the tips of forceps and needle holders meet properly, that there are no bends in the tips of the tines on the fixation forceps, and that the catch-lock (if present) opens and closes easily without snagging. Damaged instruments can often be repaired by the manufacturer, or a certified repairer, for a fraction of the cost of replacement instruments.

As previously discussed, ophthalmic instruments fall into two basic categories: those used for eyelid and adnexal manipulations and those used for corneal and intraocular procedures. In general, these categories of instrument should not be used interchangeably, otherwise either tissue or instruments will be damaged. Coloured tape can be applied to the instrument handles to ensure that the instrument kits do not get mixed up. It is often helpful to prepare a list of the instruments that should be included in each kit, together with images of each instrument. The latter can be easily accomplished by laying the instruments out on the glass screen of a photocopier and copying them, or by compiling a set of digital photographs.

Sterilization of most ophthalmic instruments can be achieved by chemical (cold) or heat sterilization. An autoclave using steam under pressure at a temperature of 121°C is routinely used. Ethylene oxide is also efficient and prevents the blunting of delicate surgical blades (such as corneal scissors), which can occur with repeated steam autoclaving. However, ethylene oxide sterilization is not commonly used in general practice owing to health and safety concerns.

The following guidelines will help to prolong the useful life of ophthalmic instruments:

- Learn how to care for the instruments and make designated nursing staff responsible for cleaning and packing them
- Instruments may be wiped on cellulose sponges during surgery to dislodge debris from the tips. Use of the fingers to dislodge debris should be avoided

- Gauze swabs should be avoided in the kit, because these may catch and bend instrument tips
- Care should be taken to ensure that blood and all other contaminants are rinsed off the instruments before they dry
- Spring-handled instruments should be opened for cleaning
- An ultrasonic cleaner or a gentle sponge should be used to wipe the instruments. A scrubbing brush should **never** be used
- The instruments should be rinsed in an appropriate lubricant from time to time.

Another important consideration is to ensure that the instruments are stored appropriately. Given that ophthalmic instruments are particularly delicate, they should be packed in specially designed boxes that prevent them from contacting each other. Both metal and plastic boxes are available and those with silicone rubber 'fingers' to separate the instruments are ideal (Figure 6.13). Individual instruments should have appropriately sized rubber tips or sleeves placed on any sharp or delicate parts. It is usual to include a chemical indicator strip within the box as well as in the outer wrapping, to ensure adequate sterilization. Indicator tape is not a reliable method for checking sterilization (it does not show that the correct time/pressure/temperature has been reached, only that exposure has occurred). Instrument boxes should be wrapped in a paper or fabric drape, placed in a self-seal sterilization bag and labelled and dated prior to sterilization.

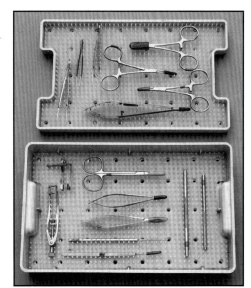

6.13 Ophthalmic instruments are best stored in specialized boxes with silicone 'fingers' to prevent instrument movement and potential damage. Note that the delicate sharp tips are also enclosed in plastic covers to prevent damage.

Eyelid specula

Eyelid specula are essential in veterinary ophthalmic surgery for a wide range of procedures. They are used to retract the lids and enhance exposure of the conjunctiva, cornea and globe. They should be strong enough to retract the lids easily, but sufficiently lightweight to prevent direct pressure on the globe. They should not have large protruding ends around which sutures can become caught. Barraquer wire eyelid specula are very commonly used and are available in paediatric and adult sizes. The former are useful for cats and small dogs. Larger breeds may require the Castroviejo type of eyelid speculum, which has a screw to adjust the opening width of the blades and is a much stronger instrument. Different lengths of blade are available, depending on the eyelid length of the patient. Larger blades are generally only used in dogs and cats if a canthotomy is being performed. The blades of eyelid specula are tucked under the lids in the closed position (or with the Barraquer speculum, held closed) and gently opened to the required position. Figure 6.14 illustrates the two commonly used types of eyelid speculum.

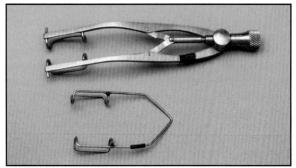

6.14 Eyelid specula: (from the top) Castroviejo and Barraquer.

Tissue forceps

Forceps are used for grasping eyelid skin, conjunctiva and corneal wound edges and for the epilation of cilia. Different designs of instrument are available for each application. Various forceps used for ophthalmic procedures are shown in Figure 6.15. Microsurgical forceps usually have angled tips, such as Colibri forceps, which are used to grasp the cornea. Forceps are usually held in a pencil grip, ensuring that the fingers and thumb are positioned on the handle (approximately one-third from the bottom of the handle and not too close to the tips). Forceps should never be forced tightly closed because damage to the tips could ensue. Forceps should be light enough to limit damage to the tissue being grasped, whilst being strong enough not to be bent or damaged by the tissue. A tying platform can be incorporated close to the tips, to allow suture material to be grasped without being weakened. It is essential that the instrument tips contact each other completely and in perfect alignment on gentle digital pressure. Forceps for conjunctival use usually have 1 x 2 teeth. However, these teeth can cause button-hole tears in the delicate conjunctiva and, as an alternative, Von Graefe fixation forceps, which have 10–14 fine teeth, can be used. These forceps afford greater holding ability but with a reduced risk of tearing the delicate conjunctival tissue. However, Von Graefe forceps are too large for microsurgical procedures. The serrated tips on dressing forceps can be small enough for

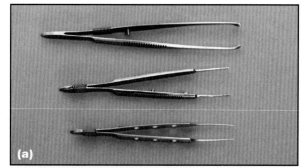

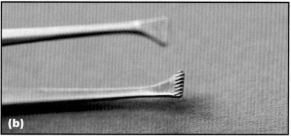

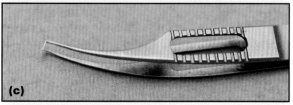

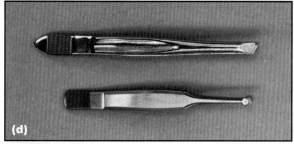

6.15 **(a)** Ophthalmic forceps: (from the top) Von Graefe, St Martins with tying platform and micro rat-toothed. **(b)** Magnified view of the Von Graefe fixation forceps showing the interdigitating fine teeth used to grasp tissue such as the conjunctiva atraumatically. **(c)** Colibri forceps, which are used to grasp the cornea only. **(d)** Cilia forceps: (from the top) Whitfield and Bennett's.

microsurgery, and increase the surface area for grasping without the need to enlarge the instrument tips. Cilia forceps have smooth blunt tips for grasping and removing aberrant lashes. For effective depilation it is essential that the tips meet perfectly to pull out very fine eyelashes and they should never be used for other purposes.

Forceps for grasping the cornea, sclera and limbus require teeth to hold the fibrous tissue. These can be perpendicular (dog-toothed) or splayed. The latter provide a better grasp on smooth surfaces. Mosquito forceps (Halsted haemostatic forceps) are used for haemostasis and to stabilize parts of the globe, such as the limbus or third eyelid. A selection of straight and curved mosquito forceps should be available, along with larger haemostats for general use. Steeply curved forceps are available for enucleation procedures.

Knives

The knives most frequently used in ophthalmic surgery are the standard Bard–Parker handle and blades (No. 11 and 15) and the Beaver handle and blades (No. 64, 65 and 67 plus specialist blades) (Figure 6.16). The latter are used for conjunctival and corneal incisions. Keratomes, either designed to fit the Beaver handles or as separate disposable instruments, are diamond-shaped blades which are mainly used for full thickness corneal incisions (e.g. during cataract surgery). Keratomes provide incisions of accurate width, e.g. the 3.2 mm required for the introduction of most phacoemulsification needles. The diamond knife is a reusable scalpel blade and handle for corneal, limbal and scleral incisions. Although very expensive, with proper care a diamond knife can last for many years. Restricted depth knives are useful for corneal surgery, such as superficial keratectomy for the removal of corneal sequestra. These knives have a sharp blade with a raised button or stop such that the blade can only be inserted a fixed depth into the cornea (e.g. 300 μm, which is approximately half the corneal thickness). Restricted depth knives are much safer for inexperienced surgeons to use, but their cost can be prohibitive.

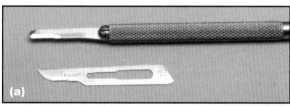

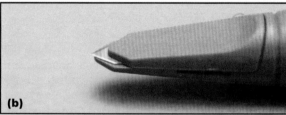

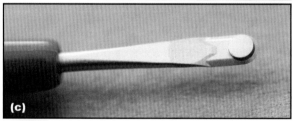

6.16 Ophthalmic knives. **(a)** Beaver handle with No. 64 blade and standard No. 15 Bard–Parker scalpel blade. **(b–c)** Magnified views of the tips of restricted depth knives showing two different styles.

Scissors

A wide variety of ophthalmic scissors are available. They differ in their tips (sharp or rounded; straight or curved) and handles (ringed or spring-handled) (Figure 6.17). For eyelid and conjunctival dissection, Stevens tenotomy scissors are versatile, with either straight or slightly curved tips. A small pair of Metzenbaum scissors are useful for general eyelid skin dissection, while special enucleation scissors are available that have sharply curved blades and

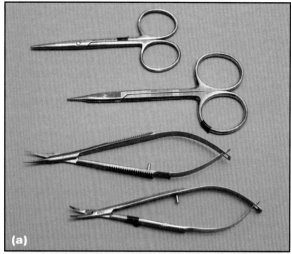

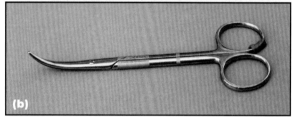

6.17 **(a)** Ophthalmic scissors: (from the top) straight eyelid scissors with blunt tips suited to undermining tissue during blunt dissection, Stevens tenotomy scissors (Straight), Westcott's tenotomy scissors and Castroviejo type corneal scissors. **(b)** Enucleation scissors with acutely angled, curved tips (similarly designed haemostats are also available).

blunt tips. Corneal and corneoscleral scissors tend to have flat spring-handles, allowing more precise control of cutting, and are held in a pencil grip. Universal corneal scissors can cut in either direction, while left- and right-corneal scissors allow the accurate enlargement of a corneal incision in both directions (and are available for both right- and left-handed surgeons). Handles and blades of microsurgical scissors are shorter than those of general ophthalmic scissors. Iris scissors are small and delicate with very sharp, pointed, slightly angled tips.

Needle holders

Needle holders should be chosen according to the size of needle. Ophthalmic needle holders are generally of a similar design to corneal scissors, and are held in a pencil grip. However, the handles are normally rounded, rather than flat, to allow rotation of the instrument, and they incorporate a spring action such that they are open in the resting position. The tips can be straight or curved, with smooth or serrated surfaces. A locking mechanism, which maintains the tips closed when a needle is grasped, may be present but is suitable only for larger sutures because opening of the lock can jar the tips slightly, affecting the precise positioning of the needle required for microsurgical procedures. Microsurgical needle holders without a lock usually possess a pin stop to prevent excessive compression of the handles from damaging the tips, and they are generally suitable for sutures of gauge 8/0 (0.4 metric) and finer. For larger suture material with bigger needles, such as 6/0 (0.7 metric) to 4/0 (1.5 metric), small pairs of Gillies and Hager–Meyer style needle holders are available. These needle holders should never be used with small needles because the blades will bend and snap the delicate needles. Needle holders suitable for ophthalmic procedures are illustrated in Figure 6.18.

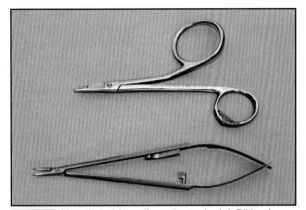

6.18 Needle holders: (from the top) mini-Gillies for large needles such as those swaged-on to 4/0 (1.5 metric) or larger suture material and Castroviejo type with lock.

Needles

By necessity, the diameter of the needle must be considerably larger than that of the suture material to which it is attached (e.g. 8/0 (0.4 metric) suture material, which is typically 40 μm in diameter, is swaged-on to needles that are 200 μm in diameter, creating a needle to suture diameter ratio of 5:1). Although this causes increased tissue damage, it does have the advantage that the knot can be buried within the needle tract, if required.

The variables in needle design are radius, curvature, length and tip configuration. Needles are available with curvatures expressed as fractions of a complete circle (i.e. 1/4, 1/3, 3/8 and 1/2 circle). In general, needles with greater curvature (e.g. 1/2 circle) are used when small but deep bites are required, whereas needles with less curvature (e.g. 1/4 circle) are used to take large but superficial bites of tissue.

Microsurgical suture material can be swaged-on to needles with four different tip designs (Figure 6.19):

- Cutting
- Reverse cutting
- Taper point
- Spatula tipped.

Although taper point needles are the least traumatic, their bluntness limits their use to the conjunctiva. The spatula tipped needle is the most commonly used in corneal surgery because it is designed specifically to accommodate the unique lamellar structure of corneal tissue: the sharpness of the needle allows efficient tissue penetration and the spatulated shaft facilitates atraumatic,

Needle tip design	Features	Use
Cutting	Sharp point and sides; triangular cross-section; traumatic to tissue; difficult to control depth accurately	Skin
Reverse cutting	Sharp point and sides; inverted triangular cross-section; traumatic to tissue; difficult to control depth accurately	Skin
Taper point	Sharp point but smooth sides; little tissue trauma; not sharp enough for skin	Conjunctiva
Spatula tipped	Designed for use in lamellar tissue as remains within same plane, thus accurate placement is possible	Cornea

6.19 Design and use of various ophthalmic needles. (Illustrations redrawn after Eisner (1990) with permission from the publisher)

interlamellar dissection. It is extremely dangerous to attempt to suture corneal tissue with cutting needles of either type, owing to the risks of inadvertent perforation and the sutures being pulled out.

Suture material

The choice of suture material depends upon the site, the procedure and surgeon preference. Factors to bear in mind are:

- Anatomical features of the tissue
- Tensile strength of the tissue
- How long the sutures need to remain in place
- Type of suture pattern to be used
- Whether suture removal will be necessary.

Veterinary ophthalmologists tend to favour 'larger' gauge, absorbable suture materials, in contrast to their medical colleagues. In theory, small-gauge, monofilament, non-absorbable suture materials should be used (e.g. 6/0 (0.7 metric) and finer) because they cause less tissue reaction, are easier to handle, provide longer wound stability and result in less astigmatism. However, in veterinary practice, avoiding the need for suture removal is often a concern that outweighs relatively minor inflammatory and astigmatic effects.

The suture material most commonly used for veterinary ophthalmic procedures is polyglactin 910 (Figure 6.20). This suture material is available in a regular form and also in a form that is associated with faster loss of tensile strength and resorption. The monofilament polyester polydioxanone (PDS) has longer lasting tensile strength and is minimally reactive, but is relatively stiff and difficult to handle. Nylon, monofilament polyester and silk can also be used.

Advantages	Disadvantages
Polyglactin 910	
• Easy to handle – no 'memory' • Less inclined to over-tightening and 'cheese-wiring' than nylon • Absorbable – no need to remove later • Softer and less irritating than nylon	• Promotes a greater tissue reaction than nylon • Knots tend to be relatively large and less secure than with nylon; cannot be rotated into the suture track
Nylon	
• Promotes minimal tissue reaction – particularly important in the axial cornea • Retains its tensile strength for very long periods • Somewhat elastic properties – less likely to break with trauma than polyglactin 910 • Secure knots which can be cut very short and then buried in the suture track, at least for smallest gauge, 10/0 (0.2 metric) and 11/0 (0.1 metric) • Available in small sizes	• Difficult to handle, especially 10/0 (0.2 metric) and 11/0 (0.1 metric) – has 'memory' • Very slippery and tends to cling in any moisture • Easy to over-tighten and 'cheese-wire'; may cause astigmatism (initially at least) • Knots irritating if not buried • May need removal under general anaesthesia

6.20 The advantages and disadvantages of polyglactin 910 *versus* nylon suture material.

Miscellaneous instruments

Lacrimal canaliculus dilator
This is a small pencil-like instrument used to locate and open up the nasolacrimal puncta prior to cannulation. It is an extremely useful instrument, both for diagnostic purposes for nasolacrimal flushing and during surgery for micro- or imperforate nasolacrimal puncta. Several types are available (e.g. Nettleship dilator; Figure 6.21), but they vary little in design.

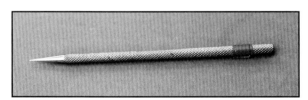

6.21 Nettleship lacrimal dilator.

Chalazion clamp
The chalazion clamp has two plates, one open and one solid, and a screw to tighten and fix the instrument on the eyelid (Figure 6.22). The chalazion clamp has many uses, including facilitating the excision of eyelid masses, ectopic cilia removal and

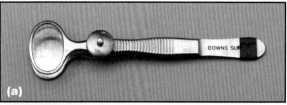

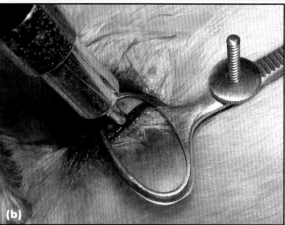

6.22 **(a)** Desmarres chalazion clamp, which is used for eyelid stabilization and haemostasis. **(b)** Chalazion clamp in use during cryoepilation for distichiasis.

cryosurgery for distichiasis. It stabilizes the lid, maintains haemostasis and protects the underlying globe from inadvertent damage, and is available in various sizes.

Chalazion curette
Several sizes of chalazion curettes are available. These are small, sharp curettes that are used to remove inspissated material from the chalazia (and are best employed in conjunction with a chalazion clamp).

Lid plate
This is a smooth plate used to stabilize and put tension on the eyelid tissue for eyelid surgery, so that an incision can be made against the plate. The plate also affords some protection to the underlying globe. Various types are available, with the Jaeger lid plate (Figure 6.23) probably being the most widely used by veterinary surgeons.

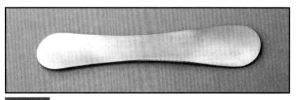

6.23 Jaeger lid plate.

Foreign body spud
A single- or double-ended instrument with sharp pointed tips is sometimes used to remove corneal or intraocular foreign bodies. However, many surgeons simply use two fine gauge (e.g. 25 or 27 gauge) hypodermic needles instead.

Callipers

Callipers (Figure 6.24) are used to obtain the precise measurements that are essential to the success of many ophthalmic procedures, including a number of eyelid and corneal surgical procedures. They are usually sterilized separately from the main ocular kits, because they are not used for every procedure.

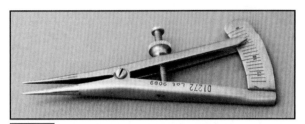

6.24 Ophthalmic callipers (Castroviejo style).

Serrafine clamps

Small cross-action serrafine clamps may be used to help stabilize the globe by anchoring stay sutures.

Disposable items

In addition to the instruments and suture materials described above, several other disposable items are required for routine ophthalmic procedures (Figure 6.25).

Item	Use
Drapes (sticky plastic window is useful for corneal/intraocular surgery)	Assisting with asepsis at surgical site
Microsurgical swabs (soft, woven, lint-free); cellulose spears	Gently removing discharge
Nasolacrimal cannulae (various sizes); 2 ml syringe	Cannulating the nasolacrimal puncta
Balanced salt solution; Hartmanns' solution; lactated Ringer's solution	Flushing the cornea or nasolacrimal duct; intraocular irrigation
Microcautery	Haemostasis

6.25 Disposable items required for ophthalmic surgery.

Drapes

Regular draping materials can be used for routine ophthalmic surgery. Thus, both fabric and disposable drapes can be employed. Fenestrated fabric drapes can be used but because they are not water-resistant they are often reserved for extraocular procedures. Pre-packed sterile disposable drapes are water resistant, and as such are employed for corneal and intraocular surgery where irrigating fluids are used. Some surgeons prefer drapes with a sticky plastic window, which adheres to the skin around the eye. The surgeon carefully cuts into the plastic to expose the cornea. The drape can be folded back under the eyelids and held in place by the eyelid speculum to prevent any stray hairs from entering the surgical site (Figure 6.26). This provides a more reliably aseptic surgical field than fabric or paper drapes alone. Specialized drapes for

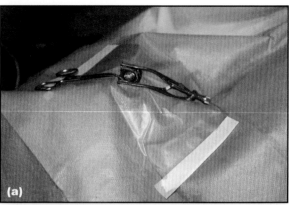

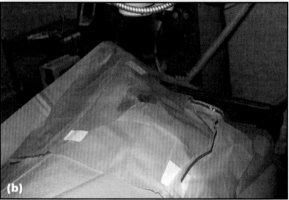

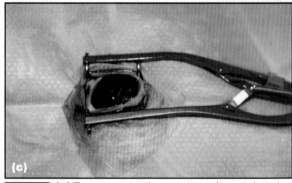

6.26 **(a)** Transparent adherent drape for ophthalmic use, which sticks to the underlying paper drape. Note the placement of fine mosquito forceps at the limbus to aid globe stabilization. **(b)** Drapes with collecting bags are useful when irrigation is used. **(c)** Magnified image showing placement of an eyelid speculum with the cut edges of the sticky drape tucked under the speculum to maintain an aseptic surgical site.

use in intraocular surgery (e.g. phacoemulsification for cataract extraction) include a pouch in the drape or a separate bag to collect excess irrigation fluid.

Swabs

It is essential that the swabs used for ocular surgery are soft and lint-free (Figure 6.27). Routine gauze swabs are not recommended for use in ophthalmic procedures, with the exception of enucleation or adnexal procedures, because fibres left in the ocular area could be irritating. For microsurgery (e.g. keratectomy, conjunctival grafts and any intraocular procedures), cellulose spears are advised. These come in packs of 5, 10 or 20, are safe for swabbing the cornea and can absorb intraocular fluids as necessary.

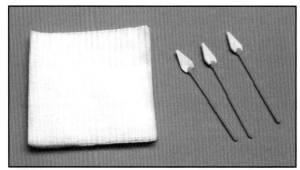

6.27 Swabs for ophthalmic use. For eyelid procedures, woven (i.e. non-gauze), lint-free swabs are ideal. For corneal and conjunctival procedures, cellulose spears are preferred.

Cannulae
Disposable plastic nasolacrimal cannulae should always be available. The two types most frequently used are 0.91 mm and 0.76 mm in diameter. Alternatively, intravenous catheters can be used, if cut short at an angle to provide a bevelled tip. However, if customized intravenous catheters are used they must be introduced to the punctum very gently because the cut edge is sharp and can damage the delicate punctal opening or even cause small lacerations to the canaliculi. In addition to disposable plastic cannulae, metal lacrimal cannulae are available, but these are best reserved for use in anaesthetized patients.

Irrigating fluids
Sterile saline, Hartmann's solution (or lactated Ringer's solution) and balanced salt solution (BSS) can all be used for irrigation in ophthalmic procedures. Saline is usually restricted to cleansing prior to surgery, but can be used to flush the cornea and conjunctival sac or to assess nasolacrimal duct patency. Use of saline as an irrigating solution is not advised if there is a risk of intraocular penetration (e.g. following removal of a perforating corneal foreign body). In such cases, it is more appropriate to use a solution that is similar to aqueous humour (i.e. Hartmann's, lactated Ringer's or BSS). In addition to being balanced with regard to sodium and chloride content, these agents contain buffers such as bicarbonate, which make them physiologically more similar to aqueous humour than saline alone. As such they are non-irritating and cause minimal damage to the delicate intraocular tissues (e.g. corneal endothelium).

Miscellaneous items
Other items which might be used during ophthalmic procedures include contact lenses, collagen shields and tissue adhesives. These items may also be used in the management of corneal disease (see Chapter 12).

Contact lenses (bandage soft contact lenses) are frequently used in dogs and cats. Their most common application is to provide ocular comfort during the healing of a corneal ulcer, whilst protecting the delicate new epithelium from being disturbed by the eyelids during blinking. Several sizes are available and the diameter of the cornea and its radius of curvature should be carefully measured. Most suppliers provide an easy-to-use measuring card for this purpose. In addition to treating corneal ulcers, contact lenses can be used in cases of spastic entropion to relieve the blepharospasm, thus allowing the eyelid to return to its normal position.

Collagen shields can be used as bandages during the healing of a corneal ulcer. They are supplied in individual sterile packets and need to be rehydrated fully before inserting into the eye. They provide only short-term effects and dissolve within a few days.

Tissue adhesives can be used to treat corneal ulcers as well as to improve suture security following temporary everting suture placement in puppies with entropion. Special ophthalmic cyanoacrylate glues are available but sterile general surgical glue is normally sufficient. Tissue adhesives generate heat on polymerization, which occurs as they come into contact with the surface to which they are being applied, and therefore care should be taken to ensure that this reaction does not damage the tissue (e.g. applying too much glue can result in a 'burn' in Descemet's membrane and subsequent corneal rupture). Only a very small amount of tissue glue should be used; if necessary, several thin coats should be applied rather than one larger droplet. This can be achieved using a 25 or 27 gauge needle dipped in the glue, which is then 'painted' over the dried corneal surface.

Principles of ophthalmic surgery

There are four key factors which need to be considered when performing ophthalmic surgery:

- Adequate restraint – this normally requires general anaesthesia, although a few procedures, such as conjunctival biopsy or nasolacrimal flushing, can be performed either under topical anaesthesia alone or in combination with sedation
- Correct surgical instruments for the procedure to be undertaken
- Suitable magnification
- Appropriate, delicate surgical technique, with minimal gross movement on the part of the surgeon. It is essential that tissue trauma is minimized by ensuring fine three-dimensional (3D) control, over both the instruments and the tissues themselves. This can be subdivided into:
  - Techniques for incision (separation of tissue)
  - Tissue stabilization (grasping)
  - Tissue re-alignment (suturing).

Techniques for incision
As with general surgery, the two techniques employed to create incisions in ophthalmic surgery are sharp and blunt dissection.

- Sharp dissection relies on the cutting of tissue fibres using a sharp scalpel blade or scissors. Sharp dissection tends to cause less inflammation than blunt dissection, which is a distinct advantage in ophthalmic surgery, especially when highly vascular structures such as eyelid skin are involved.

- Blunt dissection relies on the overstretching and tearing of tissue fibres, and the scissors used for this must have blunt, not sharp, tips so that they stay within the plane of the tissue being separated. Blunt dissection is most frequently used to undermine skin during eyelid blepharoplastic procedures and to dissect in the correct plane when creating conjunctival grafts.

It is important to appreciate the characteristics and behaviour of different tissues to ensure overall surgical success.

- In general, tissues in which the fibres are readily separated by a cutting motion, rather than those which are displaced by it, are incised with a scalpel. Examples include the cornea, where an accurate depth of cut can be made with minimal displacement.
- Other tissues, such as the loose bulbar conjunctiva, are more likely to be displaced than actually cut into by a scalpel blade. This slippage can be reduced by increasing the tension on the tissue by grasping it with forceps close to the intended incision site and stretching it, or by using scissors to cut the tissue. Failure to recognize these key differences in tissue behaviour could result in the actual incision being several millimetres away from the intended site owing to the tissue sliding away under the blade, which is clearly undesirable.

For eyelid incisions, the eyelid skin should be stabilized (see below) and then incised in one fluid movement using a scalpel blade (e.g. No. 15 Bard–Parker). Multiple short tracks should be avoided because the wound edges will be ragged, resulting in more inflammation and potential scarring, as well as making accurate suturing more difficult. The scalpel handle should be held in a pencil grip with the heel of the hand resting on the patient or the adjacent support cushion. A lid plate or the surgeon's finger should be used to stabilize and exert tension on the tissue, as well as protect the underlying globe from inadvertent damage should the incision be too deep (Figure 6.28). Even sharp scissors will crush the tissue, therefore, although their use has been advocated in the past for eyelid surgery, the author does not recommend them. Such crushing causes swelling and bruising and may compromise surgical success. Once the skin incision has been made, sharp scissors may be used to cut through the rest of the tissue to be excised (e.g. following removal of a lid tumour). Although the eyelids are highly vascular, it is rarely necessary to consider cautery to achieve haemostasis because firm digital pressure and swift, accurate suture placement will generally stem any haemorrhage quickly. If employed, cautery should be used judiciously to limit scarring.

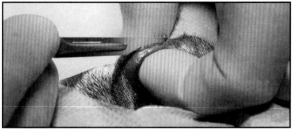

6.28 Stabilization of the eyelid skin can be achieved using the surgeon's finger. A single smooth incision is recommended and the use of a finger not only protects the globe but allows the surgeon to judge the depth of the incision more easily.

Incisions in the conjunctiva are made during the harvesting of conjunctival grafts and during trans-conjunctival enucleation, amongst other procedures, and are best made with a sharp blade to outline the desired area (ensuring that the tissue is properly stabilized to prevent its slippage) and correct depth before continuing with blunt dissection using Stevens or Westcott's tenotomy scissors.

Corneal incisions are required for keratectomy procedures (e.g. to treat corneal sequestra) and stromal corneal ulcers. Full-thickness corneal incisions are not discussed here because these techniques require specialist training. Microblades (such as a No. 64 Beaver blade or a restricted depth knife) are indicated for corneal surgery.

Tissue stabilization

Tissue needs to be grasped in order either to immobilize it (e.g. while making an incision in the third eyelid) or to mobilize it (e.g. while undermining the incised conjunctiva during graft harvesting). All grasping instruments, typically forceps, rely on creating enough friction (grasping pressure) to resist the inherent forces of the tissue and those applied by the surgeon holding the forceps. With too little friction, the tissue will slip through the forceps, causing inflammation and damage, and possibly even tearing of the tissue. Repeated grasping of tissues should be avoided because this results in greater structural damage, as the delicate conjunctiva or eyelid skin is 'chewed up' in the teeth of the forceps, no matter how fine and delicate they might appear to be.

- For eyelid stabilization, the eyelid margins should not be grasped directly. It is better to stretch the lid out to the lateral canthus, using either a finger placed within the conjunctival fornix (see Figure 6.28) or a lid plate.
- Conjunctival stabilization is achieved using forceps with delicate teeth held close to the site of incision to stabilize the globe; fine mosquito forceps may be placed close to the limbus (where the conjunctiva is most closely adherent to the underlying Tenon's capsule). Alternatively, stay sutures may be positioned, very carefully, in the episclera.
- Colibri forceps are specifically designed to grasp the cornea. Only free edges, whether created by an incision, ulcer edge or laceration, should be grasped. Attempts to grasp the intact cornea will

create lacerations or abrasions, and should be avoided. If Colibri forceps are not available, fine 1 x 2-toothed forceps (e.g. with 0.15 mm teeth) with splayed tips can be employed instead.

Tissue re-alignment

The objectives of suturing are to align and compress tissues adequately for wound healing to occur, thus restoring normal function while ensuring good cosmesis. In ocular microsurgery, alignment must be near perfect. The degree of compression required, however, depends on the tissue. For conjunctival surgery, a wide range of degrees of compression may be adequate, from loose apposition to quite tight compression; whereas, for corneal sutures the tension must be exact, to counteract intraocular pressure and prevent wound leakage. Accurate wound alignment is facilitated by:

- Suture placement perpendicular to the wound margin. Inappropriate (e.g. oblique) suture placement can delay healing and contribute to patient discomfort as well as lead to increased scarring. Badly placed corneal sutures are likely to be associated with aqueous leakage and increased infection rates
- Adequate apposition of all tissue layers, not just the superficial layer
- Use of multiple, fine, relatively closely spaced sutures
- Application of the 'rule of bisection' during wound closure (see below).

Wound compression is best achieved by placing sutures sufficiently close together. Although taking larger 'bites' of tissue and tying the sutures more tightly could potentially increase compression, these methods are not recommended for ocular procedures as they may induce tissue distortion and damage the vascular supply.

The choice of suture material and needle type depends on the tissue to be sutured and surgeon preference (Figure 6.29).

Tissue	Suture material	Gauge	Needle
Eyelid skin	Polyglactin 910; nylon; polydioxanone; silk	6/0 to 4/0 (0.7 to 1.5 metric)	Cutting or reverse cutting
Conjunctiva	Polyglactin 910	8/0 to 6/0 (0.4 to 0.7 metric)	Taper point
Cornea	Polyglactin 910; nylon	10/0 to 8/0 (0.2 to 0.4 metric)	Spatula tipped

6.29 Suggested suture materials for use in various ophthalmic tissues.

It is essential that the fine ophthalmic needles are grasped correctly within the needle holders in order to place and direct them accurately without causing damage to the delicate needles. In contrast to general surgical needles, which can be directly picked up and placed in the needle holder, ophthalmic needles require more delicate and precise

handling. The suture material should first be held with the tying platform of the forceps 1–2 cm away from the needle, allowing the needle to dangle and then gently come to rest on the drape close to the surgical site. From here, it is relatively easy to pick up the needle correctly in the needle holders without the need for readjustment (Figure 6.30). The needle should be held in the middle section of its curvature, between one-third and one-half of the distance from the swaged-on end to the needle point (i.e. too close to neither the tip nor the suture). This ensures that the needle does not bend or snap during suture placement, and that the suture material does not break off from the needle.

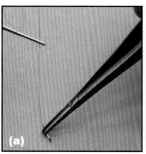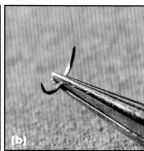

6.30 **(a)** 'Dangle' technique used to pick up delicate ophthalmic suture needles. Tying forceps should grasp the suture material 1–2 cm from the needle, which is dangled and gently brought to rest on the drape. **(b)** Needle holders can then be used to grasp the delicate needle in the correct position (i.e. one-third to one-half of the distance between the swaged end and the needle point).

In addition to ensuring that the needles are not damaged whilst grasping them, it is important to realize that incorrect needle passage through the tissue can also cause bending and thus inaccurate suture placement. Rather than trying to push the needle along, a gentle rolling of the wrist will allow the needle to follow its own angle of curvature (Figures 6.31 and 6.32).

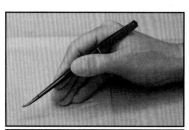
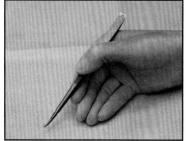

6.31 Accurate placement of sutures is best achieved by gently rolling the wrist and allowing the needle to find its own path, rather than trying to push it through the tissue. The needle should always be re-grasped with needle holders (never with forceps as this may result in damage).

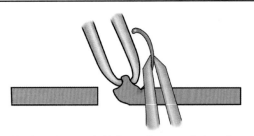

1. The tissue is entered with the needle perpendicular to the tissue surface.

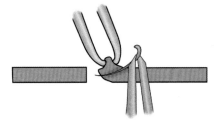

2. The needle is then directed through the tissue using a rolling motion, so that the needle emerges at 90 degrees to the cut tissue surface. The needle may be removed and re-grasped before placement of the next bite, if necessary.

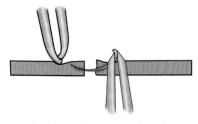

3. The opposite tissue surface is entered exactly opposite the point where the needle emerged, and again at 90 degrees to the cut surface. The needle is rolled up through the tissue to emerge at a point opposite the initial entry point. Forceps can be used to grasp the distal wound edge, or they can be used in a closed position to place gentle pressure at a point just distal to the intended needle emergence site so as to shorten the arc of the needle's tissue path.

6.32 Minimal tissue trauma and maximal wound alignment are achieved by directing the needle along a curvilinear path. This is achieved in a number of steps.

When tying knots, ophthalmic suture material should never be grasped with toothed forceps, which can damage and shred it. A tying platform or plain tying forceps can be used instead, but the latter will need to be exchanged for toothed forceps to stabilize the tissue prior to placement of the next suture. Forceps such as the St Martins (see Figure 6.15a) that combine a tying platform with fine teeth for tissue stabilization are favoured by many ophthalmic surgeons. Generally, standard square knots are used, although an extra throw can be placed on the first suture for eyelid procedures. For corneal incisions three single throws are frequently employed. The suture ends should be cut short to prevent abrasion or ulceration of the ocular surface, although eyelid sutures can be left longer (see below).

There are two important suture patterns that are used frequently for the closure of eyelid wounds.

- **Simple interrupted pattern.** The rule of bisection should be employed following entropion surgery (Hotz–Celsus procedure) where the two crescent-shaped incisions are of unequal length. If suturing is simply begun at one end and sutures placed successively until the opposite end of the wound is reached, a lip of spare tissue often results at the far end. By placing the first suture in the centre of the wound, placing the second and third sutures to bisect the two halves, and continuing with successive bisection of the remaining gaps in the incision as each suture is placed, an even distribution is achieved (Figure 6.33).
- **Figure-of-eight pattern.** Perfect alignment of the lid margin is required to allow proper function – if there is a step along the leading edge it will allow mucus and debris to accumulate, and the smooth even spread of the tear film will be compromised. However, it is equally important that no suture is placed so close to the lid margin that the ends or knot irritate the cornea. For closure of an eyelid margin incision, the figure-of-eight suture pattern achieves these two ideals (Figure 6.34).

With eyelid incisions, particularly those that are parallel to the lid margin, there is not usually much tension on the wound edges, but accurate suture placement is essential to ensure correct anatomical alignment and acceptable cosmesis. A double-layer closure is usually recommended for full-thickness incisions; although in patients with thin eyelid skin, a single layer may be sufficient. If necessary, the subcutaneous layer can be closed with a simple interrupted or continuous pattern, whilst the outer skin layer is generally closed with a simple interrupted pattern. Regardless of whether one or two layers are employed, care must be taken to ensure that the palpebral conjunctiva is not penetrated (which could cause corneal abrasion or ulceration). Normally a cutting or reverse cutting needle is used for the skin, with 6/0 (0.7 metric) to 4/0 (1.5 metric) gauge suture material. The use of absorbable material means that most sutures do not require removal, and therefore the suture ends can be cut short. Alternatively, for incisions perpendicular to the eyelid margin, the

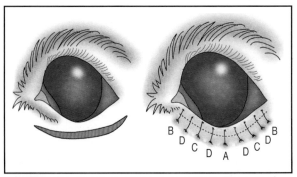

6.33 Simple interrupted suture pattern. The rule of bisection should be used to close entropion incisions where the two incisions are of unequal length. In this example, the order of suture placement would be A – B – C – D.

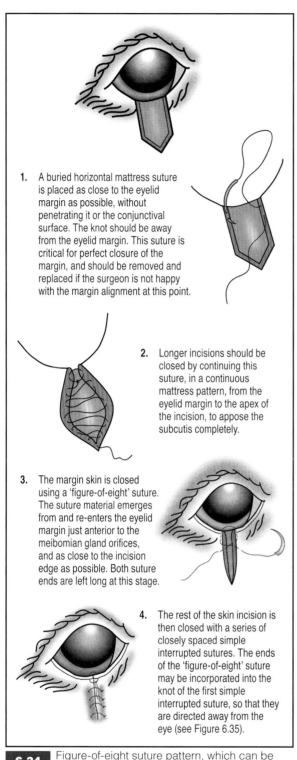

1. A buried horizontal mattress suture is placed as close to the eyelid margin as possible, without penetrating it or the conjunctival surface. The knot should be away from the eyelid margin. This suture is critical for perfect closure of the margin, and should be removed and replaced if the surgeon is not happy with the margin alignment at this point.

2. Longer incisions should be closed by continuing this suture, in a continuous mattress pattern, from the eyelid margin to the apex of the incision, to appose the subcutis completely.

3. The margin skin is closed using a 'figure-of-eight' suture. The suture material emerges from and re-enters the eyelid margin just anterior to the meibomian gland orifices, and as close to the incision edge as possible. Both suture ends are left long at this stage.

4. The rest of the skin incision is then closed with a series of closely spaced simple interrupted sutures. The ends of the 'figure-of-eight' suture may be incorporated into the knot of the first simple interrupted suture, so that they are directed away from the eye (see Figure 6.35).

6.34 Figure-of-eight suture pattern, which can be used for wounds involving the eyelid margin.

suture ends can be left longer and be 'captured' by the next suture to allow easier removal should that prove necessary (Figure 6.35). In some patients, a marked inflammatory reaction develops as the suture material starts to resorb, and removal is advised should this occur.

Conjunctival incisions tend to heal very quickly, and therefore small wounds do not require suturing. Indeed, the placement of sutures could actually cause more irritation than the initial wound. However,

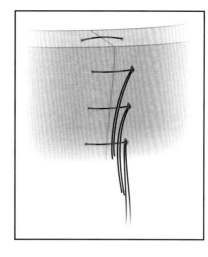

6.35
Closure of wound perpendicular to eyelid margin. Longer suture ends may be 'captured' in successive sutures or suture knots to aid suture removal.

larger defects do require closure with 8/0 (0.4 metric) or 6/0 (0.7 metric) absorbable material, ideally using a simple continuous pattern and buried knots.

To suture the cornea adequate magnification is essential. The most commonly used suture material is 8/0 (0.4 metric) polyglactin 910 with a swaged-on spatula tipped needle. Specialists use even smaller gauges. Sutures must be evenly placed and to the correct depth to ensure a water-tight wound closure with even distribution of tension across the length of the incision (Figure 6.36; see also Chapter 12).

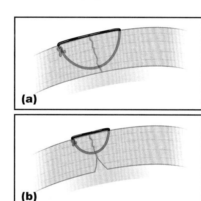
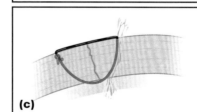
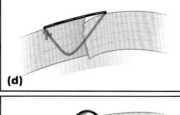
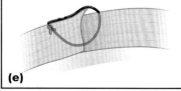

(a)
(b)
(c)
(d)
(e)

6.36
Placement of corneal sutures. **(a)** Correct depth of suture at one-half to two-thirds of the stromal depth. **(b)** Suture placed too shallow, resulting in endothelial gaping. Persistent corneal oedema will result. **(c)** Suture placed too deep, penetrating the anterior chamber and resulting in aqueous leakage. **(d–e)** Uneven suture placement will result in stepping of the cornea and poor apposition.

Postoperative care

In general, there is minimal haemorrhage or contamination during ophthalmic surgery and therefore only gentle cleansing with sterile saline dabbed along the wound using lint-free swabs is required. Postoperative pain relief is obviously essential and is addressed in detail in Chapter 5.

The use of Elizabethan collars is slightly controversial amongst veterinary ophthalmologists, because some feel that they draw the animal's attention to its head, cause the patient to bang into things, and generally distress both patient and owner. However, many resort to the 'safety net' of an Elizabethan collar, for peace of mind. An alternative to the collar is to place soft foot bandages on the front feet (and occasionally also the hind ones) for 12–24 hours, so that if the patient does attempt to rub they are less likely to cause damage. Typically, ophthalmic patients are most likely to rub their eyes during recovery and in the immediate postoperative period, when they must be closely monitored. In addition, they may experience a transient increase in irritation associated with the application of topical medication and the owner should be instructed to prevent them from rubbing.

Patients should be discharged with clear written instructions regarding the type and frequency of medication, when re-examination is required, signs of postoperative complications that the owner should watch for, and other appropriate instructions, such as restricting dogs to lead walks or keeping cats indoors for a number of days.

References and further reading

Eisner G (1990) *Eye Surgery: An introduction to operative technique.* Springer-Verlag, Berlin

Gilger B, Bentley E and Ollivier F (2007). Diseases and surgery of the canine cornea and sclera. In *Veterinary Ophthalmology*, 4th edn, ed. KN Gelatt, pp. 690–752. Blackwell Publishing, Iowa

Macsai S (2007) *Ophthalmic Microsurgical Suturing Techniques.* Springer, Berlin

Miño de Kaspar H, Koss MJ, He L, Blumenkranz MS and Ta CN (2005) Prospective randomized comparison of 2 different methods of 5% povidone–iodine applications for anterior segment intraocular surgery. *Archives of Ophthalmology* **123**(2), 161–165

Troutman RC (1974) *Microsurgery of the Anterior Segment of the Eye. Volume 1 Introduction and Basic Techniques.* CV Mosby, London

Turner SM (2005) *Veterinary Ophthalmology – A Manual for Nurses and Technicians.* Elsevier, London

7

Ophthalmic drugs

James Oliver and Kerry Smith

Drugs may be delivered to the eye by a variety of routes. The route chosen by the clinician depends on several factors, including:

- The intended site of action of the drug
- The frequency of administration required to achieve therapeutic drug concentrations at the intended site
- The ability of the drug to cross the blood–ocular barriers
- Potential side effects
- Owner compliance
- Patient cooperation
- Cost.

The topical route generally reduces the risk of systemic absorption and potential side effects compared with drugs given systemically. Topical drugs are particularly suited for diseases of the ocular surface. However, they do not reach appreciable levels in the posterior segment and systemic drugs are preferred for diseases in this location. For diseases of the anterior segment (e.g. anterior uveitis), a combination of both topical and systemic drugs is usually required. To penetrate the intact cornea, topical drugs need to be both water- and lipid-soluble. This is because the corneal epithelium and endothelium are both lipid-rich and the corneal stroma has a high water content. Most topical antibiotics are water-soluble and do not penetrate the cornea well. Penetration can be enhanced by combining drugs with organic salts (e.g. prednisolone with acetate) and by the use of preservatives that interrupt the corneal epithelium (e.g. benzalkonium chloride). Drug penetration is also increased with corneal ulceration, where the hydrophobic barrier of the corneal epithelium is missing.

Less commonly used routes of administration include subconjunctival, intracameral and intravitreal. Subconjunctival injections are useful for uncooperative patients where application of topical medications is not possible and enhanced penetration of the anterior segment is required. Typically, 0.2–0.5 ml of solution or suspension is injected through a 25 to 27 gauge needle under the dorsal bulbar conjunctiva (Figure 7.1). Absorption can occur directly across the sclera, bypassing the hydrophobic barrier of the corneal epithelium. Some of the drug will also leak through the injection site and may be absorbed across the conjunctival and corneal surfaces or drain away via the nasolacrimal system.

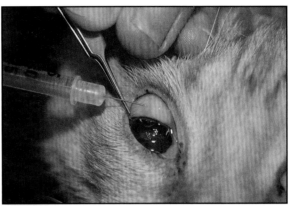

7.1 Subconjunctival injection. The air bubble within the anterior chamber has resulted from a previous intracameral injection.

For the intracameral route, the drug is directly administered into the anterior chamber. This route is most commonly used during intraocular surgery, but is also used in patients with anterior uveitis associated with fibrin accumulation in the anterior chamber. Under sedation and topical anaesthesia, an injection of 25 μg of tissue plasminogen activator is injected intracamerally across the corneoscleral limbus (Figure 7.2).

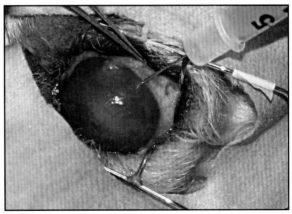

7.2 Intracameral injection.

Intravitreal injections are rarely used in veterinary ophthalmic medicine. The main indications are for the treatment of bacterial endophthalmitis and end-stage glaucoma. In blind and painful glaucomatous eyes, which are not responsive to other therapy, intravitreal gentamicin may be used to destroy the ciliary epithelium pharmacologically. However, the response to treatment is highly variable, and enucleation or evisceration with intrascleral prosthesis is preferable. Furthermore, intravitreal gentamicin injections have been associated with intraocular sarcoma formation in cats.

Topical drug preparations

Eye drops include solutions and suspensions. The ocular surface can only accommodate around 30 µl of fluid and, because the average volume of an eye drop is about 50 µl, a single drop is more than adequate. Any excess will spill over the eyelid margins or will be drained via the nasolacrimal apparatus, from where it may enter the systemic circulation and potentially contribute towards undesirable side effects. Furthermore, simultaneous application of more than one eye drop accelerates drug elimination from the ocular surface, making less available for its intended purpose. When the application of more than one drug is required, it is advisable that 5–10 minutes are allowed to elapse between applications. Eye ointments can be more useful than solutions or suspensions in some instances. Ointments allow prolonged contact time and drainage via the nasolacrimal apparatus is minimal. This results in enhanced drug accumulation at the ocular surface and, thus, may enable a decreased frequency of drug application. However, ointments are contraindicated in the case of corneal or scleral perforation, because the vehicle is toxic to the anterior segment. The relative advantages and disadvantages of solutions, suspensions and ointments are shown in Figure 7.3.

Advantages	Disadvantages
Solutions and suspensions	
• Easy to apply and achieve accurate dosing • Less toxic to anterior segment • Cause minimal visual disturbance	• Short contact time necessitates frequent application • Drainage via nasolacrimal apparatus is significant with potential for systemic absorption • Quickly diluted in irritated eyes by excess tear production • Negligible lubricant effect
Ointments	
• Increased contact time may reduce frequency of application • Lubricate ocular surface • Minimal dilution by excess tear production • Minimal drainage by nasolacrimal apparatus	• Toxic to anterior segment (contraindicated in corneal and scleral perforations) • Blurring of vision • More difficult to apply and achieve accurate dosing

7.3 Advantages and disadvantages of topical ophthalmic solutions, suspensions and ointments.

Antivirals

The main indication for the use of antivirals in small animal ophthalmic medicine is in the treatment of feline herpesvirus type 1 (FHV-1). Treatment for FHV-1 has been recently reviewed (Gould, 2011). Ganciclovir (0.15%) and aciclovir (3%) are the only commercially available topical ophthalmic antiviral medications in the UK. In addition, 1% trifluorothymidine ophthalmic solution can be compounded by some hospital pharmacies. *In vitro* studies have shown that trifluorothymidine has the best activity against FHV-1, ganciclovir has good activity and aciclovir is minimally efficacious (Figure 7.4). One clinical trial, however, demonstrated the benefit of topical 3% aciclovir ointment when applied five times a day (Williams *et al.*, 2005). Topical antivirals usually need to be given frequently, typically five to six times daily, because they are virostatic rather than virocidal. However, cidofovir, in addition to having good *in vitro* activity against FHV-1, has a long half-life, enabling it to reduce viral shedding significantly when applied only twice daily (Fontenelle *et al.*, 2008). Famciclovir is available in an oral tablet formulation and may be of use when topical therapy is not possible or when systemic herpetic disease is present. The active metabolite of famciclovir, penciclovir, has good *in vitro* activity against FHV-1. Oral famciclovir has been shown to reduce the severity of clinical signs in cats experimentally infected with FHV-1 when given at a dose of 90 mg/kg q8h (Thomasy *et al.*, 2011).

Trifluorothymidine > idoxuridine = ganciclovir > cidofovir > penciclovir > vidarabine > aciclovir > foscarnet

7.4 *In vitro* efficacy of antiviral drugs in descending order (Nasisse *et al.*, 1989).

Dietary supplementation with L-lysine has been advocated as a treatment for FHV-1, and some clinicians suggest that it reduces the incidence of recrudescent disease. However, there is very little evidence of the benefits of this treatment and, in fact, the largest studies have shown either no benefit or an increase in severity of the clinical signs and viral shedding in cats supplemented with L-lysine (Maggs *et al.*, 2007; Rees and Lubinski, 2008; Drazenovich *et al.*, 2009).

The use of interferons (IFNs) has also been suggested for FHV-1 infections. Feline IFN-ω and human IFN-α have good *in vitro* activity against FHV-1 (Siebeck *et al.*, 2006). However, pre-treatment with topical feline IFN-ω had no beneficial effect on the course of experimental FHV-1 infection in cats and no controlled clinical trials have been performed (Haid *et al.*, 2007).

Antibacterials

Topical antibiotics are indicated for ocular surface and anterior segment infections and as prophylaxis in cases of ulcerative keratitis and following corneal and intraocular surgery (Figure 7.5). Systemic antibiotics are indicated for infections of the eyelids, orbit, anterior segment and posterior segment.

Penicillins
The penicillins are bactericidal and owe their activity to the presence of a β-lactam ring, which interferes with bacterial cell wall synthesis. Penicillins vary greatly in their spectrum of activity. Penicillin G is effective against Gram-positive bacteria but it is susceptible to bacterial β-lactamases. Ampicillin and amoxicillin have more broad-spectrum activity but are also susceptible to β-lactamases. Combination with a lactamase inhibitor such as clavulanic acid or sulbactam protects them from bacterial inactivation. Amoxicillin/clavulanic acid is perhaps the most commonly used systemic preparation for ophthalmic infections. It has the disadvantage of poor blood–ocular penetration but may reach therapeutic intraocular levels in the inflamed eye. In cats with experimentally induced chlamydial conjunctivitis, treatment with amoxicillin/clavulanic acid was as effective as doxycycline (Sturgess *et al.*, 2001). Cloxacillin is available as an ophthalmic suspension and is indicated for ocular surface infections associated with β-lactamase-producing *Staphylococcus* spp. Carbenicillin, piperacillin and ticarcillin have enhanced Gram-negative activity and are potentially useful for the topical treatment of corneal ulcers caused by *Pseudomonas aeruginosa* and other Gram-negative rod bacteria.

Cephalosporins
Cephalosporins are also bactericidal and have a very similar mode of action to penicillins. First-generation cephalosporins include cefazolin and cefalexin and are mainly effective against Gram-positive bacteria. Cefazolin has good intraocular

Drug	Spectrum of activity	Main indications	Intraocular penetration	Comments
Fusidic acid	Bacteriostatic against Gram-positive bacteria, in particular staphylococci; some Gram-negative bacteria	Prophylaxis and bacterial conjunctivitis	Good	Authorized in cats and dogs
Chloramphenicol	Broad spectrum and bacteriostatic	Prophylaxis and bacterial conjunctivitis	Good	Drug of choice for ocular surface bacterial infections or prophylactic treatment of corneal ulcers
Ofloxacin	Broad spectrum and bactericidal	Conjunctivitis and corneal ulceration associated with Gram-negative bacteria. *Pseudomonas* resistant to aminoglycosides	Good	Not suitable for general prophylaxis – reserve for bacterial keratitis
Ciprofloxacin	Broad spectrum and bactericidal	Conjunctivitis and corneal ulceration associated with Gram-negative bacteria. *Pseudomonas* resistant to aminoglycosides	Fair	Not suitable for general prophylaxis – reserve for bacterial keratitis
Gentamicin	Broad spectrum and bactericidal	Gram-negative ocular surface infections	Poor	Authorized in cats and dogs
Tobramycin	Broad spectrum and bactericidal	Gram-negative ocular surface infections	Poor	May be effective against gentamicin-resistant Gram-negative bacteria
Neomycin	Broad spectrum and bactericidal	Gram-negative ocular surface infections including *Pseudomonas* resistant to gentamicin	Poor	May cause local hypersensitivity
Polymyxin B	Bactericidal against Gram-negative bacteria, including *Pseudomonas* and *Escherichia coli*	Gram-negative ocular surface infections	Poor	Combined with bacitracin ± neomycin
Bacitracin	Bactericidal against Gram-positive bacteria, including streptococci	Gram-positive ocular surface infections	Poor	Combined with polymyxin B ± neomycin
Tetracyclines	Broad spectrum and bacteriostatic against *Chlamydophila* and *Mycoplasma*	Feline chlamydial conjunctivitis. Dogs with refractory corneal ulcers	Poor	Topical formulations not available in UK; *Staphylococcus* and *Pseudomonas* usually resistant

7.5 Commonly used topical ophthalmic antibiotics.

penetration when given intravenously in dogs and has been used prophylactically in dogs undergoing cataract surgery (Whelan *et al.*, 2000; Park *et al.*, 2010). Third-generation cephalosporins, such as ceftriaxone, ceftazidime and cefatoxamine, are used in the treatment of endophthalmitis in humans, but their cost limits their use in veterinary medicine. Cefazolin, ceftriaxone and cefuroxime (a second-generation cephalosporin) have been used intra-camerally in humans as prophylaxis against bacterial endophthalmitis following cataract surgery (Lam *et al.*, 2010) but, to the authors' knowledge, there are no published reports of a similar use in dogs and cats.

Aminoglycosides

Aminoglycosides are bactericidal antibiotics which interfere with bacterial protein synthesis. They are active against both Gram-positive and Gram-negative bacteria. Topical gentamicin and tobramycin are good choices for the treatment of bacterial ulcers associated with susceptible Gram-negative bacteria, especially *Pseudomonas aeruginosa*, although resistance is on the increase. The actions of aminoglycosides are synergistic with those of penicillins, but they should be administered separately because aminoglycosides may be inactivated by penicillins. Topical neomycin is available in combination with other antibiotics and/or corticosteroids and is active against Gram-negative bacteria and staphylococci. However, chronic use has been associated with allergic reactions. Amikacin is effective against *Pseudomonas* spp. that are resistant to tobramycin and gentamicin. When administered by intravitreal injection, amikacin is potentially useful in the treatment of bacterial endophthalmitis because it is less retinotoxic than the other aminoglycosides.

Fluoroquinolones

Fluoroquinolones exert a bactericidal effect by interfering with bacterial DNA gyrase and topoisomerase IV. They have activity against Gram-negative and some Gram-positive bacteria. Enrofloxacin and marbofloxacin are available in injectable and oral formulations and are authorized for use in small animals in most countries. Enrofloxacin has been associated with acute retinal degeneration in cats when used above the manufacturer's current dosing recommendations. Ofloxacin and ciprofloxacin are available as topical ophthalmic solutions and are frequently used in dogs and cats; although in cats ciprofloxacin may be more poorly tolerated than ofloxacin. These drugs are especially useful for the treatment of infected corneal ulcers in the presence of organisms resistant to aminoglycosides. Ofloxacin has better corneal penetration than ciprofloxacin and, for this reason, may be more appropriate for prophylaxis following cataract surgery (Yu-Speight *et al.*, 2005). In humans, topical ofloxacin has been associated with an increased risk of corneal perforation, possibly as a result of increased expression of matrix metalloproteinases in the cornea (Mallari *et al.*, 2001; Reviglio *et al.*, 2003). This complication has not yet been reported in dogs and cats.

Tetracyclines

Tetracyclines are bacteriostatic agents that interfere with bacterial protein synthesis. They are active against Gram-positive and Gram-negative bacteria, mycoplasmas, rickettsiae and *Chlamydophila* spp. *Pseudomonas* and staphylococci are usually resistant. Oral doxycycline has been recommended as the treatment of choice for feline chlamydial conjunctivitis. Possible side effects include enamel discoloration in growing kittens and puppies and oesophagitis in cats. Topical tetracyclines are available in some countries and are beneficial in the treatment of feline chlamydial conjunctivitis. In addition, topical oxytetracycline has been shown to hasten the healing of spontaneous chronic corneal epithelial defects (SCCEDs) in dogs through a supposed immunomodulatory mechanism (Chandler *et al.*, 2010).

Macrolides and lincosamides

Macrolides and lincosamides prevent bacterial protein translocation and are bacteriostatic. Macrolides include erythromycin, azithromycin and clarithromycin. They have efficacy against Gram-positive bacteria, mycoplasmas, rickettsiae and *Chlamydophila* spp. Azithromycin, an erythromycin derivative, has enhanced activity against Gram-negative bacteria, such as *Bartonella henselae* and *Borrelia burgdorferi*. Azithromycin has also been recommended for the treatment of feline chlamydial disease. Clindamycin, a lincosamide, is of particular interest in veterinary medicine owing to its activity against *Toxoplasma gondii*. For feline toxoplasmosis, it is orally administered at a dose of 25 mg/kg daily in divided doses.

Sulphonamides

Sulphonamides prevent bacterial folic acid synthesis and are broad spectrum and bacteriostatic. They are rarely used in veterinary ophthalmic medicine. Orally administered trimethoprim/sulphonamide reaches therapeutic levels in the vitreous and aqueous in dogs, however, which makes it potentially useful in the treatment of bacterial endophthalmitis. A potential side effect of trimethoprim/sulphonamide in dogs is keratoconjunctivitis sicca (KCS), which occurs in approximately 4% of cases.

Chloramphenicol

Chloramphenicol is bacteriostatic and interferes with bacterial protein synthesis. It has efficacy against Gram-positive and Gram-negative bacteria. It is available as a 0.5% ophthalmic solution and 1% ointment and is an excellent choice for the topical treatment of bacterial conjunctivitis and as prophylaxis for corneal ulceration in dogs and cats. Owing to its lipophilic nature, it penetrates the cornea well and achieves therapeutic concentrations in the aqueous, and thus is often used prophylactically following intraocular surgery.

Polypeptide antibiotics

These include bacitracin and polymyxin B, which are both bactericidal. Bacitracin inhibits bacterial cell wall synthesis and polymyxin B interferes with the formation of bacterial cell membranes. Bacitracin is mainly effective against Gram-positive bacteria whilst polymyxin B has mainly Gram-negative activity, including *Pseudomonas aeruginosa*. Bacitracin and polymyxin B are available as a combined topical preparation to provide broad-spectrum activity for mixed ocular surface infections.

Fusidic acid

Fusidic acid is mainly bacteriostatic but may be bactericidal at high concentration. Its main activity is against Gram-positive bacteria, in particular staphylococci. It is available as a 1% gel and is indicated for the treatment of ocular surface infections. It has good corneal penetration, is effective even when given only once daily and is one of the few ophthalmic preparations authorized for use in small animals.

Antifungals

Ocular fungal infections are rare in small animals in the UK, although keratomycosis is occasionally encountered. There are no commercially available topical ophthalmic antifungal preparations in the UK, but clotrimazole, econazole, miconazole, voriconazole and amphotericin can be compounded by some hospital pharmacies. Antiseptic agents such as povidone–iodine and chlorhexidine digluconate also have antifungal properties and can be used topically in aqueous solution if other topical antifungal agents are unavailable, but are not particularly efficacious. Intraocular mycoses warrant the use of systemic antifungals. Itraconazole has been used successfully in dogs with ocular blastomycosis and is authorized for use in dogs and cats. Ketoconazole may be effective against *Aspergillus* spp. but penetrates the vitreous poorly when given systemically. In addition, long-term ketoconazole therapy has been associated with cataractogenesis in dogs. Fluconazole has enhanced intraocular penetration and may be useful for the treatment of intraocular cryptococcosis in dogs and cats. Voriconazole may be a good choice for systemic mycoses. Amphotericin B is available as an injectable formulation and is sometimes used in conjunction with other antifungals for the treatment of intraocular mycotic infections. It should be noted that antifungal agents are generally fungistatic rather than fungicidal, thus requiring protracted therapy and being reliant on a functional host immune system to clear the infection.

Parasiticides

Sarcoptes and *Demodex* may affect the eyelid skin as part of a more generalized skin infection. Amitraz is authorized for the treatment of both demodectic and sarcoptic mange, and selamectin is authorized for sarcoptic mange in dogs in the UK. Current dermatological texts should be consulted for more detailed treatment protocols for these diseases. Pentavalent antimonials, such as sodium stibogluconate, and/or allopurinol are used systemically to treat ocular and systemic leishmaniosis. Oral albendazole and fenbendazole have been used in conjunction with phacoemulsification surgery to treat phacoclastic uveitis associated with *Encephalitozoon cuniculi* in rabbits. Recently, *E. cuniculi* has also been reported as a cause of focal anterior cortical cataracts and uveitis in cats (Benz *et al.*, 2011). Effective treatment was achieved using oral fenbendazole in combination with other medications and phacoemulsification. Moxidectin and milbemycin are authorized in dogs for prevention of heartworm (*Dirofilaria immitis*) and moxidectin is authorized for the treatment of lungworm (*Angiostrongylus vasorum*), both of which may present with ophthalmic signs.

Anti-inflammatory, anti-allergy and immunosuppressive drugs

Anti-inflammatory drugs

Corticosteroids and non-steroidal anti-inflammatory drugs (NSAIDs) inhibit the formation of pro-inflammatory products of the arachidonic acid pathway (Figure 7.6).

Corticosteroids

Corticosteroids inhibit the formation of arachidonic acid from cell membrane phospholipids and thus prevent the induction of both the cyclooxygenase (COX) and lipoxygenase (LOX) pro-inflammatory pathways. In the eye, corticosteroids act to reduce cell and protein exudation, inhibit chemotaxis and neovascularization and stabilize lysosomal membranes and the blood–aqueous barrier. They should be used with extreme caution, or not at all, in the face of infection and, when used topically, are contraindicated in the presence of corneal ulceration.

Several topical ophthalmic corticosteroids are available, which differ in potency and corneal penetration (Figure 7.7). Prednisolone acetate 1% has excellent corneal penetration and is widely used in the treatment of anterior uveitis and in the perioperative treatment of patients undergoing cataract surgery. Dexamethasone 0.1% penetrates the cornea less effectively, and is more suitable for the treatment of immune-mediated diseases of the ocular surface, including chronic superficial keratitis in dogs and eosinophilic keratoconjunctivitis in cats. Less potent topical corticosteroid drops include betamethasone sodium phosphate, prednisolone sodium phosphate, fluorometholone and hydrocortisone (Figure 7.7).

Frequent use of topical corticosteroids may be associated with systemic signs, including polydipsia and polyuria, and diabetic patients may be difficult to stabilize during their use. Chronic use of topical corticosteroids may induce corneal lipidosis, and has been associated with subcapsular cataract formation in cats (Zhan *et al.*, 1992).

Non-steroidal anti-inflammatory drugs

NSAIDs inhibit the COX pathway. COX-1 is constitutively present in normal tissues, whereas COX-2 is

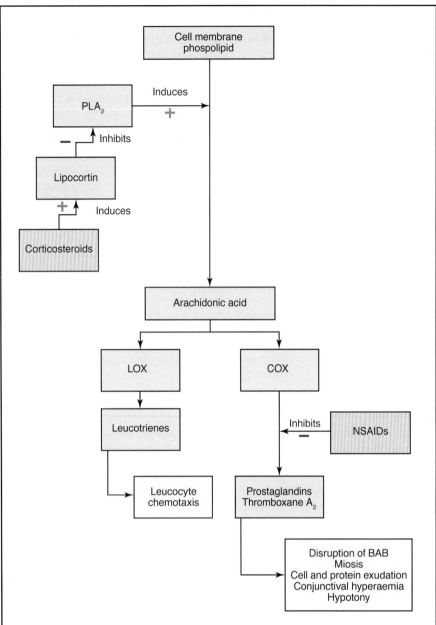

7.6

Inflammation and the eye.
BAB = blood–aqueous barrier;
COX = cyclooxygenase;
LOX = lipoxygenase;
NSAIDs = non-steroidal
anti-inflammatory drugs;
PLA$_2$ = phospholipase A$_2$.

Drug	Main indication
Prednisolone acetate (1%)	Anterior uveitis
Dexamethasone (0.1%)	Ocular surface inflammation and anterior uveitis
Betamethasone sodium phosphate (0.1%)	Ocular surface inflammation
Prednisolone sodium phosphate (0.5%)	Ocular surface inflammation
Fluorometholone (0.1%)	Ocular surface inflammation
Hydrocortisone	Ocular surface inflammation

7.7 Topical ophthalmic corticosteroids, in descending order of potency, and their indications.

induced by inflammation. COX-2 selective drugs are therefore generally preferred and their use should minimize undesirable side effects. NSAIDs authorized for systemic use in dogs include carprofen, meloxicam, tepoxalin, firocoxib, robenacoxib and mavacoxib. Carprofen, meloxicam and robenacoxib are also authorized in cats. In one study, tepoxalin was found to be more effective than carprofen and meloxicam in controlling experimentally induced uveitis in dogs, leading the authors to conclude that it may be a preferred treatment for anterior uveitis in this species (Gilmour and Lehenbauer, 2009). However, tepoxalin is not COX-2 selective and is not authorized for preoperative use in the UK. There are no authorized topical NSAIDs for use in small animals, although ketorolac, flurbiprofen and diclofenac are widely used in the treatment and prevention of intraocular inflammation, especially when corticosteroids are contraindicated. In cats, 0.1% diclofenac was found to be as effective as 1% prednisolone, and more effective than 0.03% flurbiprofen and 0.1% dexamethasone, in controlling experimentally induced intraocular inflammation (Rankin et al., 2011). However, diclofenac and flurbiprofen were found to increase intraocular pressure significantly and should be used with caution in cats with ocular hypertension. In addition, because NSAIDs may inhibit platelet function they should be used with caution in cases in which intraocular haemorrhage is a feature.

Anti-allergy drugs

There is limited knowledge about the treatment of ocular allergies in dogs. Oral antihistamines such as chlorphenamine are commonly used in the treatment of atopic dermatitis in dogs and may be useful in dogs with atopic conjunctivitis. In humans, topical antihistamines used for ocular allergies include levocabastine and emedastine, but there are no reports of their use in small animals. The mast cell stabilizer sodium cromoglicate has been suggested as a topical treatment for allergic conjunctivitis in dogs and cats. It is available as a 2% ophthalmic solution and should be applied every 6 hours.

Immunomodulatory agents

In addition to corticosteroids, several other immunomodulatory agents are of importance in the treatment of ophthalmic diseases in small animals. Ciclosporin, tacrolimus and pimecrolimus are calcineurin inhibitors. They bind to intracytosolic immunophilins in T-helper lymphocytes and block the production of lymphokines necessary for T lymphocyte activation.

Ciclosporin is authorized as a 0.2% ophthalmic ointment for the treatment of canine immune-mediated KCS and chronic superficial keratitis. Topical ciclosporin is also useful in the treatment of

superficial punctate keratitis in dogs and feline eosinophilic keratoconjunctivitis (Spiess et al., 2009).

The most common ophthalmological indication for the use of azathioprine is canine uveodermatological syndrome that is poorly responsive to corticosteroids. It may be used in combination with corticosteroids or as a sole agent. Side effects of this drug include bone marrow suppression, gastrointestinal and pancreatic disorders and hepatotoxicity. For this reason, regular monitoring of haematological and serum biochemical parameters is necessary.

Oral megestrol acetate has been used as a treatment for feline eosinophilic keratoconjunctivitis that is refractory to first-line topical treatments.

Anti-glaucoma drugs

A summary of commonly used anti-glaucoma preparations in dogs and cats is provided in Figure 7.8.

Hyperosmotic agents

Hyperosmotic agents are indicated in the management of acute glaucoma and are administered either orally or intravenously. Following administration, they are distributed to the extracellular fluid compartment. This results in an increased osmotic gradient between the extracellular fluid (plasma) and intraocular fluids (aqueous and vitreous humours). The diffusion of water from the aqueous and vitreous humours into the plasma results in a reduction in intraocular pressure (IOP). The effect of hyperosmotic agents can be increased by withholding water for up to 4 hours following administration. Use of these agents results in osmotic diuresis and consequent dehydration, therefore, close monitoring of hydration and electrolyte status is necessary. It is also prudent to assess cardiac and renal function before administration. Hyperosmotic agents have reduced efficacy when anterior uveitis is present, owing to the breakdown of the blood–aqueous barrier.

Drug	Dosage	Main indications	Side effects	Contraindications
Hyperosmotics: Mannitol (10% and 20%)	Dogs: 1–2 g/kg i.v. over 30 minutes (= 10–20 ml/ kg of a 10% solution)	Acute glaucoma in dogs	Fluid and electrolyte disturbance; acute renal failure	Congestive heart failure; pulmonary oedema; anuric renal failure
Prostaglandin analogues: Latanoprost (0.005%) Travoprost (0.004%)	Dogs: 1 drop in eye q12–24h	Acute primary glaucoma and chronic glaucoma in dogs	Conjunctival hyperaemia; miosis; blood–aqueous barrier disruption	Uveitis; anterior lens luxation; ineffective in most cats
Carbonic anhydrase inhibitors (CAIs): Dorzolamide (2%) Brinzolamide (1%)	Dogs: 1 drop in eye q8–12h Cats: 1 drop in eye q8–12h	All types of glaucoma in dogs and cats; brinzolamide ineffective in normal cats, but effective in glaucomatous cats	Local irritation may be greater with dorzolamide (pH 5.6) than brinzolamide (pH 7.5)	Severe hepatic or renal insufficiency
Beta-blockers: Timolol (0.25% and 0.5%)	Dogs: 1 drop in eye q8–12h Cats: 1 drop in eye q12h	Canine and feline glaucoma	Miosis; conjunctival hyperaemia; local irritation; bradycardia; hypotension	Uveitis; anterior lens luxation; heart failure

7.8 Anti-glaucoma drugs commonly used in cats and dogs.

Mannitol is the most commonly used hyperosmotic agent in veterinary ophthalmology. It is given at a dose of 1–2 g/kg i.v. over 30 minutes. IOP is usually reduced within 1 hour of administration and the effect can last up to 24 hours. Administration can be repeated 2–4 times over the following 48 hours.

Glycerol is given orally at a dose of 1–2 g/kg. IOP reduction occurs within 1 hour and lasts about 10 hours. Administration may be associated with nausea and vomiting and, because it is rapidly metabolized to glucose, glycerol can cause hyperglycaemia and glycosuria. It is contraindicated in diabetic patients.

Prostaglandin analogues

Prostaglandin analogues mediate a reduction in IOP through interaction with prostaglandin F (FP) receptors in the uveal tract and trabecular meshwork. They are thought to work mainly by increasing uveoscleral outflow of aqueous humour and are effective in primates and dogs. They are not effective in normal cats, in which IOP reduction is mediated by EP, not FP, receptors. Latanoprost, travoprost, bimatoprost and tafluprost are available as topical ophthalmic solutions. Latanoprost, travoprost and bimatoprost have been evaluated in dogs and are effective at reducing IOP. Latanoprost is also available in combination with timolol (a beta-blocker). Prostaglandin analogues are indicated in the emergency treatment of acute primary glaucoma and in the treatment of postoperative ocular hypertension and chronic glaucoma. In dogs, they are usually administered twice daily to minimize the occurrence of IOP 'spikes'. They can cause disruption of the blood–aqueous barrier, thus should be used with caution in patients with uveitis. Topical prostaglandin analogues cause marked miosis, which has led some clinicians to advocate their use in the management of posterior lens luxation, to decrease the chance of the lens moving anteriorly. However, caution should be exercised because entrapment of vitreous within the miotic pupil can lead to raised IOP. Owing to the miotic effect of these drugs, they should not be used in cases of anterior lens luxation.

Carbonic anhydrase inhibitors

Carbonic anhydrase inhibitors (CAIs) suppress the formation of aqueous humour by preventing the formation of bicarbonate ions in the ciliary epithelium. CAIs may be given systemically or topically. Systemic CAIs are rarely used, however, because side effects are common and often severe (metabolic acidosis, hypokalaemia, anorexia, vomiting and diarrhoea). Dorzolamide and brinzolamide are both available as topical ophthalmic preparations and are usually applied every 8–12 hours. Combined dorzolamide/timolol appears more effective at reducing IOP in glaucomatous dogs than either drug used alone (Plummer *et al.*, 2006). In normal cats and those with primary congenital glaucoma, dorzolamide significantly reduces IOP (Sigle *et al.*, 2011). Brinzolamide has no effect on IOP in normal cats. CAIs are not as effective at reducing IOP as prostaglandin analogues, but are helpful in the management of chronic glaucoma and postoperative ocular hypertension.

Autonomic agents

Drugs acting at cholinergic receptors

Pilocarpine is a direct-acting parasympathomimetic and may be useful in treating primary open angle glaucoma in dogs. Pilocarpine hydrochloride is available as a 1%, 2% or 4% ophthalmic solution. The 1% solution appears as effective as the more concentrated solutions and is usually applied 2–3 times daily. Pilocarpine is rarely used to treat other forms of glaucoma in dogs and should not be used in patients with anterior uveitis or anterior lens luxation owing to the side effects of blood–aqueous barrier disruption and miosis, respectively. The use of pilocarpine as a lacrimostimulant is discussed later in this chapter.

Carbachol acts as both a direct- and indirect-acting parasympathomimetic. Its main indication in veterinary ophthalmology is the prevention of postoperative ocular hypertension following lens extraction surgery: 0.3–0.5 ml of 0.01% carbachol is administered intracamerally at the conclusion of surgery.

Drugs acting at adrenoreceptors

Adrenaline and its pro-drug dipivefrin are sympathomimetics. They are rarely used to treat glaucoma because they cause mydriasis, which may further compromise aqueous humour outflow. However, topical adrenaline has been shown to reduce IOP in dogs with primary open angle glaucoma.

Brimonidine and apraclonidine are alpha-2 agonists. In humans, topical brimonidine is authorized to treat open angle glaucoma and ocular hypertension in patients where beta-blockers are inappropriate. Topical apraclonidine is used to manage IOP in patients before and after anterior segment laser surgery. Apraclonidine has been evaluated in cats and dogs. However, the severity of the side effects in cats and the relative inefficacy of the drug in dogs mean that its use cannot be recommended. Topical brimonidine does not cause a significant reduction in IOP in glaucomatous dogs.

Topical beta-blockers are commonly used in the management of glaucoma in humans. Beta-blockers may reduce IOP via several mechanisms, although their main effect is from the blockade of beta-adrenergic receptors in the non-pigmented ciliary epithelium. Commercially available topical beta-blockers include timolol, betaxolol, carteolol, levobunolol and metipranolol. Timolol is the most widely used beta-blocker in the dog and cat. It is available as a 0.25% or 0.5% solution and is usually applied every 8–12 hours. Timolol is also available in combination with latanoprost, travoprost, dorzolamide and brinzolamide. Timolol appears to have only a small effect in reducing IOP in dogs with normal eyes, but seems to be more effective in eyes with glaucoma (Plummer *et al.*, 2006). Timolol has not been evaluated in glaucomatous cats, but in normotensive cats it reduces IOP by around 20%. Ocular side effects include local irritation, conjunctival hyperaemia and miosis. Owing to its miotic effect, it should not be used in cases of anterior lens luxation. Adverse systemic side effects include bradycardia and hypotension; thus, it has been suggested that the 0.25% solution may be more appropriate in cats and in dogs weighing <10 kg.

Mydriatic and cycloplegic drugs

Pupil dilation is necessary for both diagnostic and therapeutic purposes, to allow visualization of the posterior segment and to facilitate intraocular surgery. Cycloplegic drugs relax the ciliary body, relieving painful spasm, and help prevent the formation of posterior synechiae in uveitis.

Mydriatic agents have either a sympathomimetic action on the iris dilator muscle (adrenergic agonists) or a parasympatholytic action on the iris sphincter muscle (cholinergic antagonists). Parasympatholytic agents also cause varying degrees of cycloplegia, making them useful in the treatment of uveitis. Speed of onset, duration and completeness of effect vary between species (Figure 7.9) and are affected by the presence of uveitis. Mydriatics should be used with caution in patients with lens instability.

Adrenergic agents

These are generally used in combination with other mydriatics to achieve maximal pupil dilation. Potential side effects include systemic arterial hypertension and bradycardia. Whilst these usually do not cause clinical complications (Herring *et al.*, 2004), caution is advised in animals with preexisting cardiovascular disease and those of low bodyweight (Franci *et al.*, 2011).

Phenylephrine, a direct-acting alpha-1 agonist, is available in a topical 2.5% or 10% solution. Its main ophthalmic use is in the diagnosis of Horner's syndrome (see Chapter 19) but it may also be used as a mydriatic to aid maximal pupil dilation. Its vasoconstrictive effects can also be used to differentiate conjunctival from episcleral blood vessel hyperaemia: application of topical phenylephrine leads to rapid blanching of the conjunctival blood vessels within seconds, whilst the deeper episcleral vessels take longer

(1–2 minutes) to vasoconstrict. In dogs, 10% phenylephrine causes significant increases in systemic arterial blood pressure and bradycardia but without arrhythmias (Herring *et al.*, 2004; Martin-Flores *et al.*, 2010). In cats, 10% phenylephrine is ineffective as a sole mydriatic agent (Stadtbaumer *et al.*, 2006).

Adrenaline, a direct-acting alpha and beta agonist, has minimal mydriatic effect when used topically. It is used intracamerally during intraocular surgery for both mydriasis and haemostasis, and can be directly injected at a dilution of 1:10,000, or added to the irrigating fluids at a 1:1,000,000 dilution. A preservative-free form must be used to avoid corneal endothelial toxicity.

Anticholinergic agents

These cause mydriasis by reversibly blocking cholinergic receptors on the iris sphincter muscle, and cycloplegia by blocking receptors in the ciliary body. Cycloplegia can cause IOP elevation, possibly as a result of the relaxation of tension on the trabecular meshwork, so these agents should not be used in animals with or at risk of glaucoma.

Tropicamide, available as a 0.5% or 1% solution, is most commonly used diagnostically owing to its rapid onset of action and relatively short duration. It is also used prior to phacoemulsification, although multiple doses are required. It is preferred to atropine because the short duration of action means that postoperative IOP spikes are less likely. It results in less cycloplegia and stabilization of the blood–aqueous barrier compared with atropine, making it less useful in the treatment of uveitis. Tropicamide 1% has been shown to cause a small increase in IOP in dogs (Taylor *et al.*, 2007) and, in cats, it increases IOP significantly, in both the treated and the untreated eye (Stadtbaumer *et al.*, 2002, 2006; Gomes, 2011). A single drop of 1% tropicamide does not reduce Schirmer tear test (STT) readings in dogs but does so transiently in cats (Margadant *et al.*, 2003).

Atropine is a potent mydriatic and cycloplegic, making it ideal for the treatment of uveitis. Initially used up to four times daily to effect, it should be withdrawn when maximal dilation is achieved, and then used to effect. Owing to its relatively slow onset and long duration of action, it is not suitable

Topical drug	Time to maximal dilation (h)		Duration of dilation (h)		Extent of dilation	
	Dog	Cat	Dog	Cat	Dog	Cat
Sympathomimetics						
Phenylephrine (10%)	2.0	No effect	12–18	No effect	Maximal	None
Adrenaline (0.1%)	No effect	NDA	No effect	NDA	None	NDA
Parasympatholytics						
Atropine (1%)	1.0	0.5	96–120	60	Maximal	Maximal
Tropicamide (1.0%)	0.5	0.75	12	8–9	Maximal	Maximal

7.9 Mydriatric and mydriatic/cycloplegic drugs used in the dog and cat. NDA = no data available.

for diagnostic purposes. It is available as a 1% solution and potential side effects include salivation (due to the bitter taste), reduced tear production and IOP elevation. Cats, in particular, may dislike the bitter taste of the aqueous solution; therefore, atropine ointment (if available) is preferable in this species. Topical atropine may induce severe systemic side effects, especially when used frequently, so it should be used cautiously in small patients and in young animals.

Tear substitutes and stimulants

Strategies to improve ocular health in qualitative and quantitative KCS include tear substitution and tear stimulation. Tear substitutes/lacrimomimetics should mimic the trilaminar tear film as closely as possible. The ideal lacrimomimetic should restore ocular comfort, improve optical clarity, aid clearance of surface debris and enable the surface epithelium to perform its barrier function. Desired features include:

- A pH close to that of tears
- Sufficient surface tension
- Suitable osmolality and osmolarity
- Adequate corneal adhesion
- Prolonged contact time
- Preservatives if administered from a multidose bottle.

Preservatives are essential to inhibit microbial growth but are epitheliotoxic, disrupt tear film stability and may cause hypersensitivity reactions. Preservative-free medications are available but expensive. Tear substitutes currently available in the UK can be broadly categorized according to the phase of the trilaminar tear film they mimic, although there is some crossover.

Tear substitutes

Aqueous tear substitutes
These include solutions containing cellulose polymers or vinyl derivatives. Commonly used in human dry eye conditions, they are seldom sufficient as sole agents to treat the more severe KCS seen in dogs. Cellulose polymers increase viscosity without altering the refractive index of the cornea or causing ocular toxicity. They include methylcellulose, which provides good viscosity at physiological pH, and hydroxypropylmethylcellulose, which is less viscous but maintains cohesive and emollient properties better than methylcellulose. They are all inert chemicals which stabilize the tear film and mix well with other drugs.

Vinyl derivatives are water-based polymers. Polyvinyl alcohol is the most widely used and, although less viscous than cellulose polymers, it has better retention time and stabilizes the tear film in a similar manner. Caution must be exercised when it is used in combination with other drugs because it has a tendency to coagulate in the presence of some buffers. Polyvinylpyrrolidone increases the viscosity of tear replacement solutions and has adsorptive properties similar to those of naturally occurring mucin, hence also functions as a mucinomimetic.

Autologous serum has been used to treat KCS in humans with documented improvements in tear film break up time, corneal vital staining, pain scores and impression cytology, as well as an increase in mucin expression. To date there have been no clinical trials in animals, and difficulties in obtaining, storing and handling autologous serum may render it unsuitable for long-term use.

Mucinomimetics
These linear polymers mimic the mucin layer of the tear film and have a longer corneal contact time than aqueous tear substitutes, making them more suitable for the treatment of canine KCS. They can be combined with cellulose polymers for a more comprehensive effect. Polyacrylic acid (Carbomer 980) is one of the most effective artificial tear preparations in dogs. Replacing both the aqueous and mucin layers of the tear film, it can be used 4–6 times daily in dogs.

Viscoelastics
Sodium hyaluronate and chondroitin sulphate are naturally occurring mucopolysaccharides frequently used in intraocular surgery. Sodium hyaluronate is involved in wound healing and increases corneal epithelial migration. It has prolonged ocular retention time owing to its high viscosity, and its pseudoplasticity facilitates blinking. Viscoelastics do not stabilize the tear film as well as some other polymers and their cost may be prohibitive. Sodium hyaluronate has been shown to increase tear film break up time and reduce corneal vital staining in humans (Herring, 2007). In dogs, a clinical improvement was seen in 50% of animals with congenital dry eye (Herrera *et al.*, 2007). Chondroitin sulphate has been found to increase the speed of corneal healing in dogs with SCCEDs (Ledbetter *et al.*, 2006).

Hydroxypropyl guar (HP-Guar) is a branched polymer of mannose and galactose which becomes a gel at tear film pH. A matrix forms which promotes adhesion of viscosity-enhancing agents, prolongs contact time and provides mechanical protection to the ocular surface. Its use in dogs has yet to be evaluated.

Lipid-based tear substitutes
Ointments containing lanolin, petrolatum or mineral oil mimic the lipid layer of the tear film and prevent evaporation of existing tears. Excellent corneal retention means that they only require application 3–4 times daily. However, they can be difficult to apply owing to the high viscosity and are likely to cause blurred vision.

Lacrimostimulants
Ciclosporin, a fungal-derived immunosuppressant, improves clinical signs and tear production in dogs with immune-mediated KCS by a variety of mechanisms, including T cell suppression of the

immune-mediated destruction of lacrimal tissue, increased lymphocyte apoptosis and decreased apoptosis of glandular and conjunctival epithelial cells, as well as a postulated direct lacrimostimulant effect. The authorized treatment is a topical 0.2% ointment which should be used twice daily, long-term. Compounded solutions of 1–2% in corn oil can be used if the former is ineffective. Administration for up to 3 months may be needed before improvement is seen, and dogs with an initial STT of 2 mm/min or above are most likely to respond. Ciclosporin reduces corneal vascularization and pigmentation in patients with KCS, even in the absence of increased tear production.

Tacrolimus and pimecrolimus (macrolide antibiotics) are drugs with a similar immunosuppressive mode of action. Topical tacrolimus and pimecrolimus increase tear production and clinical signs in dogs with immune-mediated KCS, including some animals that are non-responsive to ciclosporin (Berdoulay et al., 2005; Nell et al., 2005; Ofri et al., 2009). These agents are currently unavailable in an authorized ophthalmic preparation in the UK and have to be imported under a Special Treatment Certificate (STC). A 0.03% dermatological cream is available in the UK and has anecdotally been used with success and without obvious serious adverse reactions. Topical application of these immunosuppressive drugs has been associated with carcinogenesis in humans and, although rare, this could also be the case in dogs (Dreyfus et al., 2011).

Pilocarpine directly stimulates tear secretion by mimicking acetylcholine at the effector lacrimal cell (cholinergic agonist). It is therefore useful in cases of neurogenic KCS that have functional lacrimal gland tissue but lack parasympathetic innervation. Topical pilocarpine results in no significant or long-term elevation in tear production in normal dogs and causes signs of ocular discomfort (due to the low pH) (Smith et al., 1994). There is much anecdotal support for the use of oral pilocarpine in the treatment of neurogenic KCS, but these claims are unsubstantiated in clinical trials. A starting dose of 1 drop of 2% pilocarpine per 10 kg bodyweight given twice daily in food has been suggested. The dose should be increased by 1 drop every 2–3 days until STT results have improved or signs of systemic toxicity develop ('SLUDGE': salivation, lacrimation, urinary incontinence, diarrhoea, gastrointestinal disturbances and emesis), at which stage the dose should be decreased.

Oral IFN-α and topical nerve growth factor have both been postulated as potential treatments for dogs with KCS, but further investigation is warranted.

Local anaesthetics

All local anaesthetics reversibly block conduction of nerve impulses, preventing depolarization by inhibiting sodium ions from entering the axon. In ophthalmology they may be used topically, intracamerally, regionally by local infiltration or retrobulbar injection, or intravenously.

Topical anaesthesia

Topical anaesthesia facilitates many diagnostic and therapeutic procedures, including tonometry, corneal or conjunctival sampling, removal of surface foreign bodies, flushing of the nasolacrimal duct and intracameral injection. When used intraoperatively they enhance corneal anaesthesia. Given that they have deleterious effects on the corneal epithelium and retard wound healing, topical anaesthetics should never be used therapeutically.

Contraindications include known hypersensitivity and penetrating ocular injury (because the preservatives can damage the corneal endothelium). Swabs for corneal and/or conjunctival culture should be taken prior to their instillation because both the preservatives and the anaesthetic agent itself exhibit antibacterial and antifungal activity. They should not be applied prior to performing a STT-1, which measures reflex, as well as baseline, tear production.

Proxymetacaine (proparacaine), available as a 0.5% solution, is the most commonly used topical anaesthetic. In dogs, a single drop starts to have an effect 1 minute after application, maximal desensitization is achieved after 15 minutes and the duration of effect is 45 minutes, which can be extended to 55 minutes by application of a second drop 1 minute after the first (Herring et al., 2005). In cats, the onset of action also begins after 1 minute and lasts for 25 minutes (Binder and Herring, 2006). Proxymetacaine can be kept at room temperature for up to 2 weeks before losing efficacy (Stiles et al., 2001), but otherwise it should be refrigerated. Vials should be discarded if discoloration develops.

Amethocaine (tetracaine), available as a 0.5% or 1% solution, has a similar onset, intensity and duration of action to proxymetacaine in humans, but the occurrence of allergic reactions and level of discomfort on administration are greater. Signs of ocular sensitivity have been reported in dogs (Koch and Rubin, 1969). The duration of effect in domestic species has not been reported.

Injectable anaesthesia

Intracameral anaesthesia (1% lidocaine, 0.5% bupivacaine) is widely used in humans undergoing cataract surgery, as an adjunctive method of analgesia. In dogs, intracameral administration of 0.1 ml of preservative-free lidocaine caused no adverse effects on the corneal endothelium, corneal thickness or IOP (Gerding et al., 2004). Use of intracameral lidocaine in dogs undergoing phacoemulsification significantly reduces intraoperative isofluorane and postoperative analgesia requirements (Park et al., 2010), and also has a mydriatic effect (Park et al., 2009). Regional and intravenous anaesthesia are covered in Chapter 5.

Ocular irrigation solutions

Surface irrigants may be used to flush debris and discharge, or to prepare the ocular surface for surgery. For the former, normal sterile saline (0.9%) or a balanced salt solution (BSS) are commonly used.

Sterile distilled water is hypotonic and not suitable for use. In order to reduce bacterial load prior to surgery, an antiseptic agent is needed. Dilute aqueous solutions (not alcohol solution or surgical scrub, which damage the corneal epithelium) of povidone–iodine are widely used for ophthalmic surgical preparation. The 10% aqueous solution is diluted 1:50 to 1:20 with normal saline to give a final concentration of 0.2–0.5%. In cases of ocular perforation, povidone–iodine should be avoided because severe endothelial toxicity has been demonstrated; however, solutions of ≤0.1% are deemed to be safe (Naor *et al.*, 2001). Chlorhexidine gluconate is also safe at a concentration of 0.05%, and as effective an antiseptic as 0.2% povidone–iodine (Fowler and Schuh, 1992), but higher concentrations are irritant. It is unstable in saline and should be diluted with sterile water. Chlorhexidine diacetate is toxic to the corneal epithelium.

Intraocular irrigants are used during surgical procedures. Functions include maintenance of the anterior chamber, cooling of the phaco-handpiece, and removal of cataract fragments and viscoelastic agents. The irrigating fluid must be as close as possible to aqueous humour in terms of pH, osmolality and ionic composition in order to avoid corneal endothelial damage. The solutions used include lactated Ringer's solution, BSS and BSS Plus (which contains the antioxidant glutathione, believed to help preserve corneal endothelial cell function; Herring, 2007). The corneal effects of irrigation with 0.9% NaCl, BSS and BSS Plus on dogs and cats are minimal and comparable (Glasser *et al.*, 1985; Nasisse *et al.*, 1986).

Potential irrigant additives which have been used and evaluated include:

- Heparin to decrease intraocular fibrin
- Adrenaline for mydriasis and haemostasis
- Local anaesthetics for analgesia and to augment mydriasis
- Antibiotics to minimize the risk of postoperative endophthalmitis
- Ascorbic acid to protect against free-radical damage.

Any potential additive should be preservative-free and the possible effect on the corneal endothelium considered prior to inclusion. Use of cooled irrigating solutions may have a stabilizing effect on the blood–aqueous barrier but the effect appears to be transient (Herring, 2007).

Anticollagenases

Collagenases (e.g. matrix metalloproteinases (MMPs) and serine protease) released by neutrophils, bacteria (especially *Pseudomonas* spp. and β-haemolytic *Streptococcus* spp.) and keratocytes cause corneal stromal lysis in 'melting' ulcers. Topical corticosteroids are contraindicated in the presence of ulceration because they stimulate the release of collagenases by neutrophils. Several different compounds have

been utilized as anticollagenases and because their modes of action vary (e.g. metal chelating agents only inhibit MMPs, not serine proteases), they can be used in combination for synergistic effects.

Acetylcysteine has been shown to decrease MMP activity *in vitro*, but *in vivo* studies are equivocal. Concentrations of between 1% and 20% have been suggested. Lower concentrations have been shown to increase re-epithelialization in dogs, whilst higher concentrations can cause epithelial necrosis. Sodium or potassium ethylenediamine tetra-acetic acid (EDTA) strongly inhibit MMP activity *in vitro* and are thought to work by chelating zinc and calcium.

Tetracycline antibiotics concentrate in the cornea and lacrimal gland when used topically and systemically and have anticollagenase effects independent of their antimicrobial activity. Mechanisms of action are thought to include chelation of cations, inhibition of gene expression, inhibition of α1-antitrypsin degradation and inhibition of leucotaxis (Herring, 2007).

Autologous serum contains α2-macroglobulin and α1-antitrypsin (serine protease and MMP inhibitors) and is the broad-spectrum anticollagenase of choice for melting ulcers. Epitheliotropic properties mean that it may have indications for treating non-healing indolent corneal ulcers. Serum is preferred to plasma as it contains higher concentrations of epithelial growth factor, platelet-derived growth factor and vitamin A, leading to increased stimulation of epithelial growth, migration and differentiation (Herring, 2007). Serum must be prepared in an aseptic manner with strict attention to handling and storage. A fresh blood sample is collected from the patient, allowed to stand for 30 minutes, centrifuged and the supernatant is harvested. It should be stored in a refrigerator and, owing to the lack of preservatives and the fact that it is an excellent growth medium for bacteria, the sample is best discarded after 48 hours. Serum is initially applied hourly during the acute phase of a corneal melting ulcer.

Fibrinolytic and antifibrotic agents

Fibrinolytic agents

Fibrin, which forms during activation of the clotting cascade to control haemorrhage, can have devastating consequences in the eye, including synechia formation, pupillary seclusion leading to iris bombé, formation of vitreal traction bands and occlusion of glaucoma filtration devices. Tissue plasminogen activator, a serine protease, is the most commonly used fibrinolytic in veterinary ophthalmology. It is used at a dose of 25 μg, with doses of ≥50 μg causing intraocular toxicity in dogs and cats (Gerding *et al.*, 1992ab; Hrach *et al.*, 2000). When frozen at −70°C it retains fibrinolytic activity for over a year. Intracameral injection results in rapid fibrinolysis within 15–30 minutes. The extent of fibrinolysis depends on the duration of the clot. Owing to the potential for re-bleeding in cases of hyphaema, treatment should be delayed until at least 48 hours after the most recent bleed.

Antifibrotic agents

Mitomycin C (MMC) and 5-Fluorouracil (5-FU) are agents that inhibit fibrosis. The main use of MMC is to suppress fibrosis around implants in glaucoma surgery, although it has also been used to treat malignancies and may be useful in the prevention of corneal scarring (Gupta *et al.*, 2011). There are several reports of the use of 5-FU in glaucoma implant surgery, but it is a less favourable option than MMC because repeated subconjunctival injections are required. Prospective studies in canine glaucoma surgery have yet to be performed with either compound.

References and further reading

Benz P, Maaß G, Csokai J, *et al.* (2011) Detection of *Encephalitozoon cuniculi* in the feline cataractous lens. *Veterinary Ophthalmology* **14**(Suppl. 1), 37–47

Berdoulay A, English RV and Nadelstein B (2005) Effect of topical 0.02% tacrolimus aqueous suspension on tear production in dogs with keratoconjunctivitis sicca. *Veterinary Ophthalmology* **8**, 225–232

Binder DR and Herring IP (2006) Duration of corneal anaesthesia following topical administration of 0.5% proparacaine hydrochloride solution in clinically normal cats. *American Journal of Veterinary Research* **67**, 1780–1782

Chandler HL, Gemensky-Metzler AJ, Bras ID, *et al.* (2010) *In vivo* effects of adjunctive tetracycline treatment on refractory corneal ulcers in dogs. *Journal of the American Veterinary Medical Association* **237**, 378–386

Drazenovich TL, Facetti AJ, Westermeyer HD, *et al.* (2009) Effects of dietary lysine supplementation on upper respiratory and ocular disease and detection of infectious organisms in cats within an animal shelter. *American Journal of Veterinary Research* **70**, 1391–1400

Dreyfus J, Schobert CS and Dubielzig RR (2011) Superficial corneal squamous cell carcinoma occurring in dogs with chronic keratitis. *Veterinary Ophthalmology* **14**(3), 161–168

Fontenelle JP, Powell CC, Veir JK, *et al.* (2008) Effect of topical ophthalmic application of cidofovir on experimentally induced primary ocular feline herpesvirus-1 infection in cats. *American Journal of Veterinary Research* **69**, 289–293

Fowler JD and Schuh JCL (1992) Preoperative chemical preparation of the eye: a comparison of chlorhexidine diacetate, chlorhexidine gluconate, and povidone iodine. *Journal of the American Animal Hospital Association* **28**, 451–457

Franci P, Leece EA and McConnell JF (2011) Arrhythmias and transient changes in cardiac function after topical administration of one drop of phenylephrine 10% in an adult cat undergoing conjunctival graft. *Veterinary Anaesthesia and Analgesia* **38**(3), 208–212

Gerding PA, Essex-Sorlie D, Vasaune S and Yack R (1992a) Use of tissue plasminogen activator for intraocular fibrinolysis in dogs. *American Journal of Veterinary Research* **53**, 894–896

Gerding PA, Essex-Sorlie D, Yack R and Vasaune S (1992b) Effects of intracameral injection of tissue plasminogen activator on corneal endothelium and intraocular pressure in dogs. *American Journal of Veterinary Research* **53**, 890–893

Gerding PA, Turner TL, Hamor RE and Schaeffer DJ (2004) Effects of intracameral injection of preservative-free lidocaine on the anterior segment of the eyes in dogs. *American Journal of Veterinary Research* **65**, 1325–1330

Gilmour MA and Lehenbauer TW (2009) Comparison of tepoxalin, carprofen and meloxicam for reducing intraocular inflammation in dogs. *American Journal of Veterinary Research* **70**, 902–907

Glasser DB, Matsuda M, Ellis JG and Edelhauser HF (1985) Effects of intraocular irrigating solutions on the corneal endothelium after *in vivo* anterior chamber irrigation. *American Journal of Ophthalmology* **99**, 321–328

Gomes FE, Bentley E, Lin TL and McLellan GJ (2011) Effects of unilateral topical administration of 0.5% tropicamide on anterior segment morphology and intraocular pressure in normal cats and cats with primary congenital glaucoma. *Veterinary Ophthalmology* **14**(Suppl. 1), 75–83

Gould DJ (2011) Feline herpesvirus 1. Ocular manifestations, diagnosis and treatment options. *Journal of Feline Medicine and Surgery* **13**, 333–346

Gupta R, Yarnall BW, Giuliano EA, Kanwar JR, Buss DG and Mohan RR (2011) Mitomycin C: a promising agent for the treatment of canine corneal scarring. *Veterinary Ophthalmology* **14**(5), 304–312

Haid C, Kaps S, Gönczi E, *et al.* (2007) Pretreatment with feline interferon omega and the course of subsequent infection with feline herpesvirus in cats. *Veterinary Ophthalmology* **10**, 278–284

Herrera HD, Weichsler N, Gomez JR and de Jalon JA (2007) Severe unilateral, unresponsive keratoconjunctivitis sicca in 16 juvenile Yorkshire Terriers. *Veterinary Ophthalmology* **10**(5), 285–288

Herring IP (2007) Clinical pharmacology and therapeutics In: *Veterinary Ophthalmology, 4th edn*, ed. KN Gelatt, pp. 332–354. Blackwell Publishing Professional, Iowa

Herring IP, Bobofchak MA, Landry MP and Ward DL (2005) Duration of effect and effect of multiple doses of topical ophthalmic 0.5% proparacaine hydrochloride in clinically normal dogs. *American Journal of Veterinary Research* **66**, 77–80

Herring IP, Jacobson JD and Pickett JP (2004) Cardiovascular effects of topical ophthalmic 10% phenylephrine in dogs. *Veterinary Ophthalmology* **7**, 41–46

Hrach CJ, Johnson MW, Hassan AS, et al. (2000) Retinal toxicity of commercial intravitreal tissue plasminogen activator solution in cat eyes. *Archives of Ophthalmology* **118**, 659–663

Koch SA and Rubin LF (1969) Ocular sensitivity of dogs to topical tetracaine HCl. *Journal of the American Veterinary Medical Association* **154**, 15–16

Lam PTH, Young AT, Cheng LL, Tam PMK and Lee VYW (2010) Randomised controlled clinical trial on the safety of intracameral cephalosporins in cataract surgery. *Clinical Ophthalmology* **4**, 1499–1504

Ledbetter EC, Munger RJ, Ring RD and Scarlett JM (2006) Efficacy of two chondroitin sulfate ophthalmic solutions in the therapy of spontaneous chronic corneal epithelial defects and ulcerative keratitis associated with bullous keratopathy in dogs. *Veterinary Ophthalmology* **9**, 77–87

Maggs DJ, Sykes JE, Clarke HE, *et al.* (2007) Effects of dietary lysine supplementation in cats with enzootic upper respiratory disease. *Journal of Feline Medicine and Surgery* **9**, 97–108

Mallari P, McCarty D, Daniell M and Taylor H (2001) Increased incidence of corneal perforation after topical fluoroquinolone treatment for microbial keratitis. *American Journal of Ophthalmology* **131**, 131–133

Margadant DL, Kirkby K, Andrew SE and Gelatt KN (2003) Effect of topical tropicamide on tear production as measured by Schirmer's tear test in normal dogs and cats. *Veterinary Ophthalmology* **6**, 315–320

Martin-Flores M, Mercure-McKenzie TM, Campoy L, *et al.* (2010) Controlled retrospective study of the effects of eyedrops containing phenylephrine hydrochloride and scopolamine hydrobromide on mean arterial blood pressure in anaesthetized dogs. *American Journal of Veterinary Research* **71**(12), 1407–1412

Naor J, Savion N, Blumenthal M and Assia EI (2001) Corneal endothelial cytotoxicity of diluted povidone iodine. *Journal of Cataract and Refractive Surgery* **27**, 941–947

Nasisse MP, Cook CS and Harling DE (1986) Response of the canine corneal endothelium to intraocular irrigation with saline solution, balanced salt solution, and balanced salt solution with glutathione. *American Journal of Veterinary Research* **47**, 2261–2265

Nasisse MP, Guy JS, Davidson MG, Sussman W and De Clercq E (1989) *In vitro* susceptibility of feline herpesvirus-1 to vidarabine, idoxuridine, trifluridine, acyclovir, or bromovinyldeoxyuridine. *American Journal of Veterinary Research* **50**, 158–160

Nell B, Walde I, Billich A, Vit P and Meingassner JG (2005) The effect of topical pimecrolimus on keratoconjunctivitis sicca and chronic superficial keratitis in dogs: results from an exploratory study. *Veterinary Ophthalmology* **8**, 39–46

Ofri R, Lambrou GN, Allgoewer I, *et al.* (2009) Clinical evaluation of pimecrolimus eye drops for treatment of canine keratoconjunctivitis sicca: a comparison with cyclosporine A. *The Veterinary Journal* **179**(1), 70–77

Park SA, Kim NR, Park YW, *et al.* (2009) Evaluation of the mydriatic effect of intracameral lidocaine hydrochloride injection in eyes of clinically normal dogs. *American Journal of Veterinary Research* **70**, 1521–1525

Park SA, Park YW, Son WG, *et al.* (2010) Evaluation of the analgesic effect of intracameral lidocaine hydrochloride injection on intraoperative and postoperative pain in healthy dogs undergoing phacoemulsification. *American Journal of Veterinary Research* **71**, 216–222

Plummer CE, MacKay EO and Gelatt KN (2006) Comparison of the effects of topical administration of a fixed combination of dorzolamide-timolol to monotherapy with timolol or dorzolamide on IOP, pupil size, and heart rate in glaucomatous dogs. *Veterinary Ophthalmology* **9**, 245–249

Rankin AJ, Khrone SG and Stiles J (2011) Evaluation of four drugs for inhibition of paracentesis-induced blood–aqueous humor barrier breakdown in cats. *American Journal of Veterinary Research* **72**, 826–832

Rees TM and Lubinski JL (2008) Oral supplementation with L-lysine did not prevent upper respiratory infection in a shelter population of cats. *Journal of Feline Medicine and Surgery* **10**, 510–513

Reviglio VE, Hakim MA, Song JK and O'Brien TP (2003) Effect of topical fluoroquinolones on the expression of matrix metalloproteinases in the cornea. *BMC Ophthalmology* **3**, 10

Siebeck N, Hurley DJ, Garcia M, *et al.* (2006) Effects of human recombinant alpha-2b interferon and feline recombinant omega interferon on *in vitro* replication of feline herpesvirus-1. *American Journal of Veterinary Research* **67**, 1406–1411

Sigle KJ, Camaño-Garcia G, Carriquiry AL, *et al.* (2011) The effect of dorzolamide 2% on circadian intraocular pressure in cats with primary congenital glaucoma. *Veterinary Ophthalmology* **14**(Suppl. 1), 48–53

Smith EM, Buyukmihci NC and Farver TB (1994) Effect of topical pilocarpine on tear production in dogs. *Journal of the American Veterinary Medical Association* **205**, 1286–1289

Spiess AK, Sapienza JS and Mayordomo A (2009) Treatment of proliferative feline eosinophilic keratitis with 1.5% cyclosporine: 35 cases. *Veterinary Ophthalmology* **12**, 132–137

Stadtbaumer K, Frommlet F and Nell B (2006) Effect of mydriatics on intraocular pressure and pupil size in the normal feline eye. *Veterinary Ophthalmology* **9**, 233–237

Stadtbaumer K, Kostlin RG and Zahn KJ (2002) Effects of topical 0.5% tropicamide on intraocular pressure in normal cats. *Veterinary Ophthalmology* **5**, 107–112

Stiles J, Krohne SG, Rankin A and Chang M (2001) The efficacy of 0.5% proparacaine stored at room temperature. *Veterinary Ophthalmology* **4**, 205–207

Sturgess CP, Gruffydd-Jones TJ, Harbour DA, *et al.* (2001) Controlled study of the efficacy of clavulanic acid-potentiated amoxicillin in the treatment of *Chlamydia psittaci* in cats. *Veterinary Record* **149**, 73–76

Taylor NR, Zele AJ, Vingrys AJ and Stanley RG (2007) Variation in intraocular pressure following application of tropicamide in three different dog breeds. *Veterinary Ophthalmology* **10**, 8–11

Thomasy SM, Lim CC, Reilly CM, *et al.* (2011) Evaluation of orally administered famciclovir in cats experimentally infected with feline herpesvirus type-1. *American Journal of Veterinary Research* **72**, 85–95

Whelan NC, Richardson RJ, Kinyon JM, *et al.* (2000) Ocular and serum pharmacokinetics of intravenous cefazolin in dogs. 31st Annual Meeting of the American College of Veterinary Ophthalmology, Montreal, Canada

Williams DL, Robinson JC, Lay E and Field H (2005) Efficacy of topical aciclovir for the treatment of feline herpetic keratitis: results of a prospective clinical trial and data from *in vitro* investigations. *Veterinary Record* **157**, 254–257

Yu-Speight AW, Kern TJ and Erb HN (2005) Ciprofloxacin and ofloxacin aqueous humor concentrations after topical administration in dogs undergoing cataract surgery. *Veterinary Ophthalmology* **8**, 181–187

Zhan G-L, Miranda OC and Bito LZ (1992) Steroid glaucoma: corticosteroid-induced ocular hypertension in cats. *Experimental Eye Research* **54**, 211–218

8

The orbit and globe

David Donaldson

Investigation of orbital disease is challenging and in many emergency situations rapid recognition of signs of orbital disease and instigation of appropriate management are critical to the final outcome for the patient. Familiarity with the anatomy and physiology of the region facilitates an understanding of the basic principles of orbital disease pathogenesis. Furthermore, recognizing the key signs associated with different orbital diseases allows a logical approach to the investigation and management of these patients.

Anatomy and physiology

The bony orbit
The bony orbit of predatory species such as dogs and cats is classified as an open type, being incomplete in the dorsolateral region, thus leaving the orbit continuous with the temporal fossa (Figure 8.1). The orbital ligament bridges the incomplete region of the bony orbital rim, extending from the zygomatic process of the frontal bone to the frontal process of the zygomatic bone. The ligament is a taut band of fibrous tissue that is readily palpable in the conscious animal. The zygomatic and maxillary bones define the lateral limits of the orbit. A projection of frontal bone, which contains the frontal sinus, extends over part of the dorsal roof of the orbit. Most of the medial bony orbital wall is formed by the thin septum of frontal bone, which separates the orbit from the nasal cavity. The optic canal and

orbital fissure pass through the sphenoid bone and define the caudal apex of the orbit.

The soft tissue orbit
Owing to the incomplete nature of the bony canine orbit much of the dorsal, lateral and ventral orbit is bordered by muscle. The temporal muscle confines the dorsal orbit and some of the lateral orbit. The masseter muscle lies medial and ventral to the zygomatic arch and forms part of the lateral border of the orbit. The pterygoid muscles provide the ventral floor of the orbit. The soft tissue structures within the orbit may be separated into the anatomical compartments referred to as the intraconal and extraconal spaces. These compartments are defined by the four rectus muscles and the periorbital fascial sheath which envelops them. This forms an anatomical cone which is widest anteriorly, where it surrounds the globe and lacrimal gland, then tapers towards the orbital apex (caudally, medially and ventrally) and inserts at the orbital apex where it surrounds the optic canal and orbital fissure. The anatomical relationship between the intraconal and extraconal structures is shown in Figure 8.2.

The intraconal structures include:

* Extraocular muscles – four rectus muscles, two oblique muscles and the retractor bulbi muscle
* Cranial nerves – optic nerve (CN II), oculomotor nerve (CN III), trochlear nerve (CN IV), ophthalmic branch of the trigeminal nerve (CN V) and abducens nerve (CN VI)

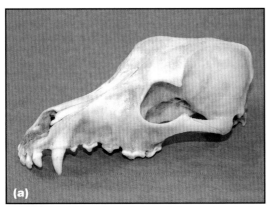

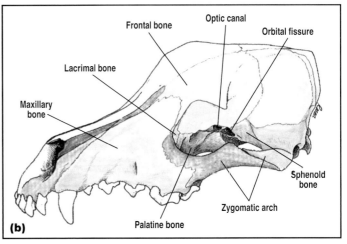

8.1 **(a)** Dorsolateral view of the canine skull. **(b)** The bones of the canine orbit.
(b, Courtesy of Roser Tetas Pont)

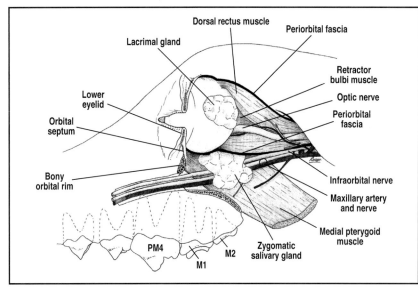

8.2 Soft tissue anatomy of the canine orbit. All structures within the periorbital fascia are termed intraconal, whilst those outside this plane are termed extraconal. The orbital septum is shown in cross-section: the septum extends from the bony orbit to the eyelids and encircles the globe. This structure is a critical barrier separating the more superficial adnexal structures such as the eyelids from the orbit. (Courtesy of Roser Tetas Pont)

- Orbital lacrimal gland (positioned under the orbital ligament)
- Orbital fat within the cone and separating extraocular muscles
- Autonomic nerves, arteries and veins
- Smooth muscle which envelops the periorbita.

The extraconal structures include:

- Zygomatic salivary gland (dogs) – positioned dorsal to the pterygoid muscles and occupying most of the orbital floor
- The base of the nictitating membrane
- Neurovascular structures traversing the orbital floor, including the maxillary artery (largest branch of the external carotid artery), the palatine nerve, the infraorbital nerve, the maxillary branch of the trigeminal nerve and the parasympathetic pterygopalatine nerve and ganglion
- Orbital fat cushion inferior to the orbital cone.

The orbital septum is an important anatomical barrier, which forms the anterior border of the orbit. The orbital septum extends from the bony orbit across the base of the orbit into the eyelids (see Figure 8.2) and is continuous with the periorbital fascial sheath. Functionally, it separates the orbital contents from the more superficial structures. The orbital septum has been referred to as the 'firewall of the orbit' because it represents a critical barrier preventing inflammation of the more superficial adnexal structures (such as the eyelids) from extending into the orbit, which may be associated with much more serious morbidity and potentially mortality.

Surrounding structures

- The nasal cavity and paranasal sinuses are separated from the orbit by only a thin septum of frontal bone and as such extension of disease from these regions to the orbit is not uncommon.
- The caudal roots of the maxillary fourth premolar and first and second molar teeth are in close proximity to the orbital floor. Only a thin layer of alveolar bone separates them from the soft tissues of the orbital floor, so orbital cellulitis/abscessation may be a sequel to tooth root abscessation or related to iatrogenic trauma during dentistry.
- The close proximity of the brain to the orbital apex makes extension of neoplastic and inflammatory diseases via the calvarial bone or foramina in the region possible.
- Disease of the temporal and/or masseter muscles that border a large area of the orbit directly affects the orbital tissues. Orbital disease is a common feature of conditions such as immune-mediated masticatory myositis.
- The zygomatic salivary gland is an extraconal structure which lies on the floor of the canine orbit. Acute inflammation of this gland (sialadenitis) may lead to signs of orbital cellulitis or abscessation. In contrast, zygomatic sialoceles tend to have a more insidious clinical progression.

Clinical signs

The orbital structures lie deep to the surface, thus many of the clinical signs seen with orbital disease reflect the secondary effects on the overlying structures. The classical signs associated with orbital disease are:

- Exophthalmos – anterior displacement of the globe along the orbital axis is a hallmark sign of orbital disease
- Enophthalmos – posterior displacement of the globe
- Strabismus – deviation of the globe away from the normal orbital axis (e.g. exotropia or esotropia).

Important differential considerations for exophthalmos and enophthalmos are given in Figures 8.3 and 8.4 respectively.

Developmental conditions
• Brachycephalic skull conformation • Orbital arteriovenous fistula • Orbital varices • Orbital dermoid cysts • Craniomandibular osteopathy (canine)
Acquired conditions

• Inflammatory disease:
  – Orbital cellulitis/abscess [a]
  – Masticatory myositis (canine) [a]
  – Extraocular muscle myositis (canine) [a]
  – Fibrosing extraocular muscle myositis with restrictive strabismus (canine)
  – Restrictive orbital myofibroblastic sarcoma (previously known as orbital pseudotumour) (feline)
• Orbital neoplasia [a]:
  – Primary
  – Secondary
• Trauma:
  – Traumatic proptosis [a]
  – Fracture of the orbital or periorbital bones [a]
  – Orbital varices
  – Orbital arteriovenous fistula
• Orbital cystic disease:
  – Zygomatic mucocele
  – Dacryops
• Orbital haemorrhage:
  – Trauma
  – Coagulopathy

8.3 Differential diagnoses for exophthalmos. [a] = most common conditions.

Developmental conditions
• Dolichocephalic skull conformation • Microphthalmos
Acquired conditions
• Horner's syndrome • Dehydration • Anterior segment pain with active globe retraction • Loss of orbital fat pads (senile) • Atrophy of temporal muscle (senile) • Chronic masticatory myositis (canine) • Fibrosing extraocular muscle myositis with restrictive strabismus (canine) • Orbital or periorbital fractures • Phthisis bulbi

8.4 Differential diagnoses for enophthalmos.

Other clinical signs associated with orbital disease include:

• Protrusion of the nictitating membrane
• Periocular swelling
• Conjunctival hyperaemia or congestion/chemosis
• Epiphora or mucopurulent ocular discharge
• Lagophthalmos (incomplete eyelid closure) ± exposure keratopathy
• Keratoconjunctivitis sicca (KCS)
• Pain or difficulty in opening the mouth, or reluctance to eat and chew
• Swelling/induration/fistulation of the pterygopalatine fossa (i.e. the oral mucosa caudal to the upper molar teeth)

• Reduced ocular motility
• Afferent or efferent nerve deficits due to disease affecting CN II to CN VI and/or autonomic nerves within the orbit
• Mild elevation in intraocular pressure (IOP)
• Retinal folds or scleral indentation
• Tortuous engorged retinal blood vessels (primarily venules)
• Papilloedema.

Investigation of disease

The investigation of orbital disease requires a comprehensive evaluation of the eye and orbit as well as a general examination of the patient for signs of systemic disease. The initial investigation should include:

• History
• Physical examination:
  – Differentiation of exophthalmos from pseudo-exophthalmos
  – Orbital palpation
  – Oral examination
  – General physical examination
• Ophthalmic examination
• Neurological and neuro-ophthalmic examination
• Differentiation of intraconal and extraconal orbital disease
• Routine haematology and biochemistry
• Orbital imaging.

History

Important information obtained from the history of the patient includes the apparent rate of disease progression and the presence of signs of pain. A sudden onset of clinical signs, often including swelling of the eyelids and conjunctiva as well as pain when opening the mouth, is commonly associated with orbital inflammation or acute masticatory myositis. A more insidious disease progression and relatively little pain suggests neoplasia or other space-occupying lesions. Although this provides a useful clinical guide, these findings should not be over-interpreted. This is particularly the case for aggressive orbital neoplastic disease, which may mimic the clinical presentation of acute orbital inflammatory disease (Hendrix and Gelatt, 2000).

Physical examination

Differentiation of exophthalmos from pseudo-exophthalmos

Exophthalmos is the hallmark sign of orbital disease and must be differentiated from the false impression of exophthalmos (pseudo-exophthalmos) created by certain orbital and ocular asymmetries. The most common cause of pseudo-exophthalmos is globe enlargement secondary to glaucoma (hydrophthalmos or buphthalmos). Careful ophthalmic examination should readily rule out pseudo-exophthalmos in these cases, as other prominent signs of chronic glaucoma should be apparent, including an increase in corneal diameter in the affected eye (see Chapter 15).

It is particularly useful to examine the position of the eyes from above to compare the level of the axial corneas. The upper eyelids may need to be retracted gently to view the corneas clearly. Creating an imaginary line between the two corneas should show them to be at the same level: any difference in their anterior position indicates the presence of either exophthalmos or enophthalmos. Enlargement of a glaucomatous globe may lead to the false impression that the globe is anteriorly displaced when the patient is viewed from the front (Figure 8.5), but examination from above reveals minimal changes in the level of the axial cornea compared with the unaffected eye. Careful globe retropulsion is also particularly sensitive for the detection of orbital space-occupying lesions. In the normal dog and cat, the degree of globe retropulsion possible is surprisingly large, except in brachycephalic breeds which have shallow orbits. In the case of the enlarged glaucomatous globe, there is typically no resistance to globe retropulsion compared with the contralateral eye.

In some situations, a globe may appear enlarged owing to a fixed dilated pupil, contralateral enophthalmos or asymmetry of the eyelid fissures (Figure 8.6), and this may also create the false impression of exophthalmos. Examination from above and careful ophthalmic and neuro-ophthalmic examination should rule out the false impression of exophthalmos in such cases. In addition to exophthalmos, the globe may be abnormally deviated (strabismus). This can occur in any direction. Exotropia refers to a strabismus where the globe is deviated laterally, in contrast to esotropia where the globe is deviated medially. Strabismus may be caused by orbital space-occupying lesions or neuro-ophthalmic disorders (see Chapter 19). When the strabismus is secondary to an orbital space-occupying lesion, the globe is typically displaced away from the mass (Figure 8.7).

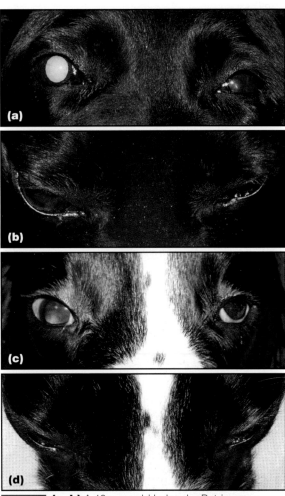

8.5 **(a–b)** A 10-year-old Labrador Retriever presented with an acute history of bilateral blindness and right-sided exophthalmos. (a) The widened palpebral fissure and pronounced pupillary dilatation on the right side give the impression that the globe is enlarged. (b) When viewed from above, the anterior displacement of the right globe is readily appreciated. **(c–d)** A 1-year-old English Springer Spaniel with glaucoma and hydrophthalmos of the right globe. (c) The widened palpebral fissure, pupillary dilatation and slightly increased scleral show could be mistaken for exophthalmos. (d) When viewed from above, the anterior displacement of the right globe is only marginal and is consistent with the degree of hydrophthalmos rather than exophthalmos.

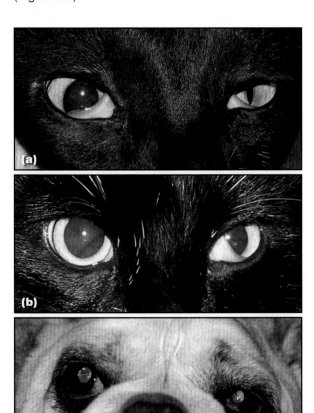

8.6 A false impression of right globe enlargement and/or exophthalmos can be created by differences in pupillary size, contralateral enophthalmos and asymmetry of the eyelid fissures. **(a)** A 6-year-old male neutered Domestic Shorthaired cat with a fixed dilated right pupil due to an efferent pupil defect. **(b)** A 9-year-old female neutered Domestic Shorthaired cat with Horner's syndrome and enophthalmos affecting the left eye. **(c)** An 8-year-old neutered Bulldog bitch with left-sided ptosis due to facial nerve paralysis.

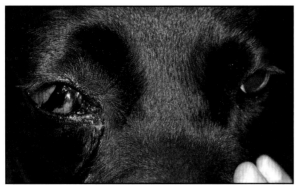

8.7 A 9-year-old entire Labrador Retriever bitch with an orbital tumour causing extreme dorsolateral strabismus of the right globe. The ventral limbus is just visible below the upper eyelid margin. MRI revealed a tumour in the ventromedial orbit.

Orbital palpation
Palpation of the periocular tissues, starting at the bony orbital rim and then progressing away from the eye, to detect areas of pain or swelling can be extremely informative. Mass lesions in the region of the temporal fossa (dorsolateral to the globe) or anterior to the equator of the globe may potentially be palpable. Palpation of the temporal muscles elicits a pain response in cases of acute masticatory myositis. In cases of orbital neoplasia, particularly when the bony orbit is affected, the patient will often resent palpation of the affected or contiguous orbital bones. Palpation may also reveal crepitus due to subcutaneous emphysema or bony fracture. Direct auscultation of the orbit (using the bell of the stethoscope placed on closed eyelids or over the frontal sinus or temporal fossa) may (rarely) reveal a bruit suggestive of an orbital vascular abnormality.

Oral examination
The oral examination in patients with orbital disease may be restricted and painful owing to the pressure exerted by the vertical ramus of the mandible on the soft tissues of the orbit when the mouth is opened. Orbital pain needs to be differentiated from pain arising from other regions, including the mouth, temporomandibular joint, nasopharynx and ears. If the patient is compliant, the buccal mucosa in the pterygopalatine fossa should be examined for swelling, induration and fistulous tracts. Neoplasia involving the nasal cavity or orbit may also extend into the oral cavity. The caudal maxillary teeth should be inspected for disease. Dental fractures exposing the pulp cavity will eventually lead to endodontic disease, which extends to the apical region of the tooth. A periodontal probe should be gently used to examine the gingival sulcus, which is 2–3 mm deep in a normal dog and 1–2 mm deep in the cat. Periodontal probing is an accurate method of detecting and evaluating periodontal tissues for the presence of pockets and/or discharge suggesting periodontal disease. The stoma of the zygomatic salivary gland duct, which opens into the oral cavity on a papilla opposite the first upper molar tooth, may be examined for evidence of erythema, swelling or discharge indicating zygomatic adenitis.

Ophthalmic examination
A thorough ophthalmic examination, including Schirmer tear tests, fluorescein staining and tonometry (when available) should be performed in all cases. The presence of an orbital mass may obstruct venous drainage from the orbit and periorbital tissues, resulting in conjunctival hyperaemia, chemosis and blepharoedema, which may be dramatic. Mild episcleral congestion may occur and the IOP may be elevated above the normal reference range (or relative to the unaffected eye) as a result of an increase in episcleral venous pressure. Epiphora may occur if tear drainage through the nasolacrimal duct is obstructed by orbital or periocular disease. Examination of the posterior segment of the eye may reveal engorgement of the retinal vasculature (primarily venules) when orbital venous drainage is obstructed. Acute compression of the optic nerve may result in papilloedema and, in chronic cases, optic nerve atrophy. If an orbital mass impinges directly on the globe, an area of scleral indentation may manifest as a region of apparent retinal detachment or elevation on funduscopic examination; such mass effects are usually readily visible on B-mode ultrasonography (Figure 8.8).

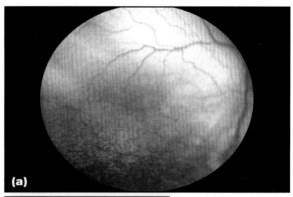
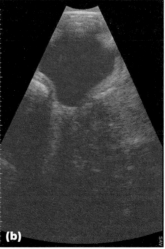

8.8 Pressure from an extraconal mass has led to indentation of the posterior aspect of the globe in a dog with orbital multilobular osteochondrosarcoma. **(a)** Ophthalmoscopic appearance showing indentation of the fundus, deviation of the superficial retinal blood vessels and reduced tapetal reflectivity. **(b)** B-mode ultrasonography confirms gross indentation of the posterior aspect of the globe. (Courtesy of the University of Wisconsin-Madison Comparative Ophthalmology Service)

Neuro-ophthalmic examination

Many neuro-ophthalmic abnormalities may manifest with orbital disease owing to interference with the cranial and autonomic nerves present in the region. Vision, corneal sensation, ocular movements (vestibulo-ocular reflexes), pupillary size and symmetry and pupillomotor function should be assessed. Abnormalities in eyelid position, movement and sensation may also be apparent (see Chapter 19).

Differentiation of intraconal and extraconal orbital disease

The differentiation of intraconal (within the orbital muscle cone) and extraconal (outside the orbital muscle cone but within the soft tissue and bony confines of the orbit) disease is useful because this may influence the differential diagnoses being considered. The most frequently reported intraconal orbital diseases in dogs and cats include neoplasia of the optic nerve and inflammatory myopathies of the extraocular muscles. The clinical characteristics of intraconal orbital disease include:

- Axial exophthalmos (anterior displacement of the globe in the same axis as the normal orbit) (Figure 8.9)
- Minimal or no protrusion of the nictitating membrane (may occur with extensive intraconal masses)
- Absent or minimal strabismus
- Limited ocular motility in some instances.

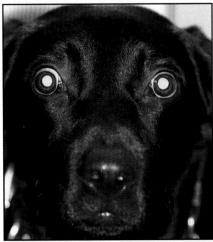

8.9 A 1-year-old Labrador Retriever with bilateral extraocular muscle myositis. The typical presentation is seen in this case, with signs of intraconal disease including bilateral exophthalmos without third eyelid protrusion, 360-degree scleral show and retraction of the upper eyelids.

Neoplasia, orbital inflammatory diseases (including periapical dental abscess and zygomatic adenitis) and masticatory myositis are the most common causes of extraconal orbital disease in dogs. The clinical characteristics of extraconal orbital disease include:

- Non-axial exophthalmos (exophthalmos with strabismus, whereby the globe is anteriorly displaced but also deviated from the normal

orbital axis; Figure 8.10). The direction of the strabismus can provide information regarding the location of the space-occupying lesion
- Protrusion of the nictitating membrane
- Retention of ocular motility.

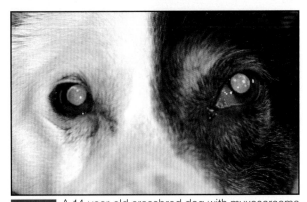

8.10 A 14-year-old crossbred dog with myxosarcoma affecting the left orbit. Signs of extraconal orbital disease include non-axial exophthalmos with the globe displaced dorsolaterally and third eyelid protrusion.

Orbital imaging

A detailed discussion of ocular and orbital imaging is provided in Chapter 2. Useful techniques include:

- Conventional radiography:
  - Optimization of radiographic studies
  - Dental radiography
- Ultrasonography
- Cross-sectional imaging:
  - Computed tomography (CT)
  - Magnetic resonance imaging (MRI).

Conventional radiography

Optimization of radiographic studies: The limitations of conventional orbital radiography include the superimposition of the complex skull anatomy and the poor ability to differentiate orbital soft tissues. The main applications of conventional radiography are:

- To evaluate the bony orbit for evidence of osteolysis, bone remodelling and fractures
- To assess the nasal cavity, frontal sinuses and maxillary dental arcades for pathology
- To assist in the identification of radiodense foreign bodies.

Skull radiographs should be obtained under general anaesthesia. Positioning of the patient is critical because rotation or tilting in any plane will severely compromise the ability of the clinician to accurately interpret the radiographs. A routine radiographic orbital study should include a lateral, dorsoventral (DV) and (sometimes) an intraoral DV radiograph, which provides finer detail of the nasal cavity, maxillary recess and medial orbital wall. Radiographic views that are more topographically specific may be used to assess the orbit, nasal cavity and sinuses, maxillary molar teeth and tympanic bullae. Improvised skyline views may be used to image any region of pathology identified in the skull surface, and may provide information not discernible on a routine orthogonal view. In cases where there is a high index of suspicion of orbital malignancy, survey left and right thoracic radiographs should be obtained prior to taking the skull radiographs. This reduces the pulmonary atelectasis secondary to prolonged patient recumbency, which complicates the interpretation of thoracic radiographs.

Dental radiography: Radiographs to assess the maxillary dental arcades may be obtained using conventional radiography or human non-screen dental film. The use of human non-screen dental film provides exquisite detail of the tooth roots, periodontal ligament and surrounding alveolar bone. These radiographs can be obtained with either a stationary X-ray machine or a dedicated dental X-ray machine.

Dental radiographs may reveal dental caries or regions of periapical lucency at the root apices typical of endodontic disease. Other findings may include sclerosis of the pulp chamber, which occurs secondary to pulpitis, and calcification of the periodontal ligament in older dogs, which increases the chance of tooth fracture during chewing (the periodontal ligament acts as a shock absorber and the associated nerve regulates the force of chewing).

For conventional radiography, the lateral oblique view should be obtained (Figure 8.11). The following technique is recommended:

- The side of interest is positioned closest to the radiographic plate
- The jaw is held open with a mouth gag
- The head is rotated so the opposite maxillary dental arcade is positioned dorsally (i.e. will not be superimposed on the area of interest).

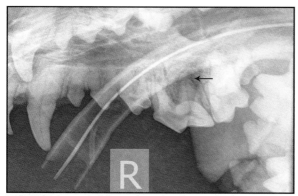

8.11 Lateral oblique dental radiograph of a 10-year-old West Highland White Terrier with a history of recurrent orbital inflammation. There is an area of periapical lucency (arrowed) around the fourth premolar (carnassial) tooth consistent with a periapical tooth root abscess.

Ultrasonography

Two-dimensional (2D) real-time (B-mode) ultra-sonography is an excellent imaging modality for examining the soft tissues of the orbit. The use of a 7.5 or 10 MHz transducer (either linear array or mechanical sector scanner) is recommended for the evaluation of orbital disease in dogs and cats.

Orbital ultrasonography can be performed on conscious patients, either via the eye with direct corneal contact (following the application of topical local anaesthesia) or via a lateral (temporal) approach with the probe placed on the skin directly posterior to the orbital ligament. Direct placement of the transducer on the cornea is the most commonly used technique. It is important to align the transducer with the orbital axis, which is directed in a caudal, medial and ventral direction. With this alignment, the orbital cone should be clearly visible. Being proficient in identifying the orbital cone facilitates categorization of lesions as intraconal or extraconal. The contralateral orbit and eye often provide an ideal 'normal' reference for comparison. A routine study includes both vertical (sagittal) and horizontal (dorsal) scan planes. The horizontal plane provides the best images of the retrobulbar space and the medial bony orbital wall.

In the normal animal, the extraocular muscles, orbital fat and optic nerve can be identified. The more ventrally located zygomatic gland is often seen as a relatively hypoechoic structure. Orbital ultrasonography provides valuable information regarding the presence, location and nature of orbital diseases. The differentiation of soft tissue masses, cystic lesions and abscesses is normally possible owing to their differing ultrasonographic characteristics. In some cases, the characterization of a lesion may be enhanced by advanced techniques, including colour flow Doppler, power Doppler and contrast-enhanced ultrasonography (see Chapter 2). Although ultrasonography may assist in the broader characterization of orbital disease, it is important to remember that the ultrasonographic appearance is not pathognomonic for the tissue of origin or the malignant potential of lesions. Furthermore, orbital ultrasonography is of little value for evaluation of the orbital apex.

Cross-sectional imaging

CT and MRI have greatly improved the diagnosis and management of a diverse range of orbital and neuro-ophthalmic conditions. The advantages and disadvantages of these techniques, as well as their utility in the investigation of orbital disease are discussed in Chapter 2.

Canine and feline conditions

Developmental abnormalities: globe

Anophthalmos

Anophthalmos (a complete absence of the eye) is extremely rare. Almost invariably, primitive ocular tissue (extreme microphthalmos) is seen on histological examination of the orbital contents.

Microphthalmos

Microphthalmos is an abnormally small eye. Some breeds, such as collies and Shetland Sheepdogs normally have small globes. Microphthalmos may occur sporadically in any breed and may involve a small but functional globe (nanophthalmos) or one in which multiple malformations are present. Concurrent malformations can include:

- Anterior segment dysgenesis – persistent pupillary membrane (PPM) being the most common manifestation
- Cataracts
- Persistent hyperplastic primary vitreous/persistent hyaloid artery (patent or non-patent)
- Retinal dysplasia.

In breeds in which microphthalmos has been identified as a hereditary defect, the condition tends to be associated with a specific spectrum of concurrent ocular defects (see Chapter 17 for further information):

- Dobermann – anterior segment dysgenesis and retinal dysplasia
- Miniature Schnauzer – cataracts, microphakia, posterior lenticonus, nystagmus and retinal dysplasia
- Cavalier King Charles Spaniel – cataracts, nystagmus, posterior lenticonus and persistent hyaloid artery
- Australian Shepherd – equatorial staphyloma, persistent pupillary membranes, iris colobomas and retinal dysplasia are features of merle ocular dysgenesis (see below).

Microphthalmos is a prominent feature in merle ocular dysgenesis (MOD). As normal ocular embryogenesis is dependent on the initial development of the pigmented layers of the eye, defects in ocular development may be directly related to ocular pigment dilution. The merle locus in dogs has the alleles m (normal) and M (merle). Homozygous merle dogs (MM) may have severe MOD as well as defective hearing and sterility. Breeds with the merle coat colour include collies, Shetland Sheepdogs, Australian Shepherds, Dachshunds, Old English Sheepdogs and Great Danes (Figure 8.12).

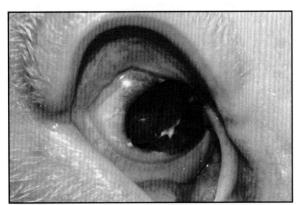

8.12 A 3-month-old Great Dane with the merle coat colour. The ophthalmic abnormalities include microphthalmos, third eyelid protrusion (the third eyelid covered most of the globe and was retracted for ophthalmic examination), iris coloboma (note the localized absence of the iris from the 3–6 o'clock position), dyscoria, microphakia and cataract. Both eyes were similarly affected.

In addition to microphthalmos, the merle gene may be associated with:

- Iris hypoplasia
- Corectopia (eccentric pupil)
- Iris coloboma
- PPM
- Scleral equatorial coloboma or scleral ectasia (thinning) leading to staphyloma (the ocular vascular tunic of the eye bulges beyond the scleral coat)
- Optic nerve coloboma
- Retinal dysplasia.

In some cases of microphthalmos, there may be excessive third eyelid protrusion, which functionally impairs vision (see Figure 8.12). In such cases, shortening of the third eyelid cartilage may be indicated, but the third eyelid should not be removed owing to the significant negative impact on the quantity and spread of the tear film.

Globe enlargement

Congenital glaucoma may be unilateral or bilateral and occurs due to abnormalities in the aqueous outflow pathways. This leads to enlargement of the globe (hydrophthalmos or buphthalmos) which may be dramatic in young animals, especially cats (Figure 8.13).

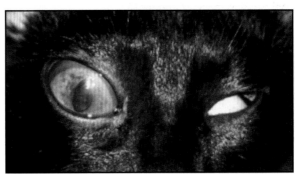

8.13 A 6-month-old Domestic Shorthaired cat with a history of hydrophthalmos affecting the right eye since kittenhood. Globe enlargement can be dramatic in young animals, especially cats, in which the fibrous tunic of the eye is more elastic. Note the dark appearance of the sclera. This is due to advanced scleral thinning exposing the underlying darkly pigmented choroid.

Developmental abnormalities: orbit

Enophthalmos

Enophthalmos is a condition in which the globe has an abnormal posterior position within the orbit. Developmentally this occurs due to a combination of a relatively deep orbit and a small globe. This is commonly seen as a 'normal' trait in dolichocephalic breeds such as the English Bull Terrier, Rough and Smooth Collie, Dobermann and Flat-coated Retriever. Passive third eyelid protrusion is often evident and medial canthal pocket syndrome may be seen as a gap or pocket at the ventromedial canthus in which mucus and debris accumulate. This is usually just an aesthetic issue and, apart from regular cleaning to remove the accumulation of mucus and debris from the region, no specific treatment is prescribed. Topical antibiotic therapy is not indicated and is largely ineffective because the problem is conformational and not infectious.

Exophthalmos
The degree of clinically significant exophthalmos related to shallow orbits in brachycephalic breeds varies considerably. Some dogs present at a very early age with recurrent problems associated with ulcerative keratitis due to the inability to blink over the exophthalmic globes (lagophthalmos). Although complete blinks are often elicited when testing the palpebral reflex, when these patients are observed without stimulation, the majority (and sometimes all) blinks are seen to be incomplete. This deficient spreading of the tear film over the axial cornea predisposes these dogs to axial corneal ulceration, for which they are often presented. The owners should be asked to check whether the eyelids are closed when the dog is asleep; it is not uncommon for severely brachycephalic dogs to sleep with their eyes open. The use of artificial tear supplements is indicated in these dogs (even if tear production is normal) to help protect the axial cornea, with a more viscous paraffin-based ointment being used at night. Surgical reduction of the palpebral fissures (by medial or lateral canthoplasty) may also help to improve the efficiency of the blink and facilitate corneal protection (see Chapter 9).

Orbital arteriovenous fistula
Orbital arteriovenous (AV) fistulas are rare congenital or acquired (spontaneous, post-traumatic or associated with highly vascular neoplasia) defects in which there is an abnormal communication between the orbital arteries and veins. This AV shunting leads to increased venous and orbital pressure. This may result in an exophthalmos which is pulsatile (i.e. in time with the heartbeat) or associated with a bruit that can be auscultated over the temporal region. Diagnosis may be confirmed in some cases with colour-flow Doppler ultrasonography. Successful treatment whilst preserving the globe has not been reported in the veterinary literature. Treatment in humans may involve conservative monitoring or attempted embolization of the AV fistula.

Orbital varices
Varices of the orbital veins are rare defects, which are probably primary in most cases but may be acquired following trauma. They are associated with an intermittent exophthalmos, which worsens with exercise, and eventually becomes persistent. As with AV fistulas, treatment of orbital varices in humans may be conservative or involve attempted embolization of the affected vein. Successful coil embolization of a congenital orbital varix in a dog has been reported (Adkins *et al.*, 2005). In canine patients with orbital varices leading to clinically significant exophthalmos, in which such advanced intervention is not possible, careful exenteration may be indicated. Preoperative planning should consider the risk of significant intraoperative haemorrhage.

Orbital dermoids
Dermoids are developmental choristomas (normal tissue in an abnormal location). Orbital dermoids may contain many tissue types, including skin, hair, bone and cartilage. The imaging characteristics of dermoids on B-mode and Doppler ultrasonography, MRI and CT may all assist in making a diagnosis (see Chapter 2). Confirmation of the diagnosis is based on histopathology of the excised tissue. The growth rate of the dermoid may determine the age of the animal at presentation; slow-growing dermoids may not be associated with clinical signs of disease until adulthood. Leakage of lipid and keratin tends to occur from dermoids, inducing marked inflammation in the dermoid wall and secondary fibrosis. This may complicate surgical dissection and removal without damaging normal neighbouring structures. During the surgical excision of orbital dermoids, avoidance of iatrogenic rupture reduces subsequent inflammation and the risk of recurrence.

Craniomandibular osteopathy
Craniomandibular osteopathy (CMO) is a non-neoplastic, proliferative bony disease most commonly seen in young Scottish, Cairn and West Highland White Terriers. It affects primarily the mandible, tympanic bullae and, occasionally, other bones of the head, including the occipital, temporal, sphenoid and/or parietal bones. This may lead to asymmetry of the bony orbit, although the clinical problems generally relate to mandibular swelling and pain, an inability to open the mouth, or pain on opening the mouth. Radiography is the best method for demonstrating the lesions of CMO. At present, the cause of the disease is not known and there is no curative treatment.

Acquired abnormalities: globe

Globe enlargement
Buphthalmos/hydrophthalmos refers to enlargement of the globe secondary to chronic glaucoma and elevated IOP. The fibrous tunic of the eye becomes stretched and thinned. Other signs of glaucoma will also be evident (see Chapter 15).

Phthisis bulbi
Phthisis bulbi refers to an acquired shrunken blind eye. This is the end-stage response to severe ocular injury or disease. In these cases, the severe intraocular pathology leads to the loss of aqueous humour production and a reduction in IOP, which are needed to maintain normal globe size and physiology. Clinically, the phthisical globe is soft and shrunken and the cornea often has a greyish opacification (Figure 8.14). These eyes often appear to be comfortable, but complications associated with secondary entropion or medial canthal pocket syndrome (see above) may be evident. If chronic clinical problems develop, enucleation is indicated. This is particularly the case for feline globes, which may develop intraocular sarcoma years after the initial insult to the globe.

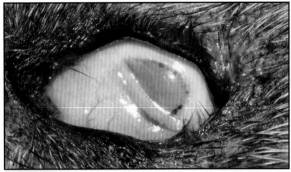

8.14 A 12-year-old neutered Jack Russell Terrier bitch with phthisis bulbi affecting the left eye. The eye is severely shrunken with a small grey cornea. The eyelids have been actively retracted to allow visualization of the globe. Although lower lateral entropion is present, the globe is usually completely covered by the third eyelid and the dog was asymptomatic.

Trauma

The presentation of patients with ocular trauma is highly variable, depending on the force and nature of the injury (penetrating or non-penetrating) and whether or not there are concomitant craniofacial and central nervous system (CNS) injuries or trauma to other parts of the body. Trauma to the globe can affect all anatomical compartments from the fibrous tunic (cornea and sclera) to the uveal tract (iris, ciliary body and choroid) as well as the lens, retina and optic nerve. Assessment of these patients needs to be performed carefully and may be facilitated by the administration of sedatives or general anaesthesia, assuming that this is not contraindicated by the systemic status of the animal. If debris or adherent exudate is present on the ocular surface, this can be gently removed by irrigating the ocular surface with a warmed balanced saline or Hartmann's solution. Topical anaesthesia should not be instilled until it has been established whether or not the globe has ruptured. If the cornea and anterior sclera appear to be intact, a topical anaesthetic solution may be applied, which will facilitate inspection of the conjunctival fornices for foreign material and debris. An intraocular examination may be possible at this stage if the ocular media are clear. If the ocular media are not transparent, B-mode ultrasonography can be used to help determine the integrity of the intraocular structures, in particular the integrity of the lens, the presence of retinal detachment and the integrity of the posterior sclera. Skull radiography or CT may also be useful if orbital or other skull fractures are suspected and to rule out the presence of ballistic lead shot pellets.

Blunt ocular trauma: This is often associated with damage to the uveal tract and intraocular haemorrhage. Contusion of the uvea results in uveitis and typical signs include hypotony, miosis, iridal congestion and the presence of fibrin and debris or frank blood in the anterior chamber. The pressure exerted on the globe during blunt trauma may result in a 'blow-out' scleral rupture. The location of the scleral rupture is variable and may include the posterior pole, optic nerve and limbus. If the fibrous tunic of the eye is disrupted anteriorly, this is normally evident on ophthalmic examination and typically the wound is sealed by uveal tissue that has prolapsed into the defect. Rupture of the posterior sclera, in contrast, is not generally appreciated on direct examination. Detecting posterior scleral rupture on ultrasonography can also be difficult. Ultrasonographic findings suggestive of posterior scleral rupture include a region with an ill defined or irregular echo from the posterior eye wall, with lack of continuity, adjacent to which there may be echogenic/hyperechoic material consistent with vitreal haemorrhage and/or areas of retinal detachment.

The treatment for blunt globe injuries depends on the extent of the pathology and the prognosis for retaining a functional globe. If severe intraocular damage has been sustained (lens rupture/dislocation, vitreal haemorrhage, retinal detachment, posterior scleral rupture), enucleation should be considered owing to the likelihood of chronic intraocular inflammation and eventual phthisis bulbi. More anterior ruptures of the ocular tunics involving the limbus or anterior sclera can be successfully repaired following replacement of the uveal tissue. Cases in which contusion of the globe is not associated with rupture, and the main findings are consistent with intraocular haemorrhage and inflammation, may be treated intensively as for uveitis (see Chapter 14).

Penetrating ocular trauma: Penetrating injuries occurring through the cornea or anterior sclera are normally readily apparent on ophthalmic examination. The resultant tract from the penetrating injury may be visible and in some cases retained foreign material may be present. Small wounds may heal spontaneously; however, larger wounds are normally presented with uveal prolapse into the defect. This appears as darkly pigmented tissue protruding through the corneal or scleral wound. Other signs of uveitis include iris thickening and congestion, fibrinous clots and haemorrhage in the anterior chamber, and miosis or dyscoria due to the iris being drawn towards the rupture site. The anterior chamber is often shallow.

A critical part of the initial assessment of these cases is to ascertain whether or not the lens capsule is intact. Rupture of the lens capsule may lead to phacoclastic lens-induced uveitis (see Chapters 14 and 16). Some small rents in the lens capsule may be managed conservatively with fibrous tissue sealing the ruptured lens capsule, although larger rents with significant prolapse of lens material into the anterior chamber often require lens removal using phacoemulsification (see Chapter 16). Some penetrating injuries may also affect the posterior segment, leading to retinal trauma and detachment. If the ocular media are not clear, the use of ultrasonography may be very important in determining concurrent damage to the intraocular structures. If severe intraocular damage has been sustained (e.g. lens rupture and dislocation, vitreal presentation at the wound, retinal detachment with disruption of the posterior sclera) a severely guarded prognosis should be given and enucleation recommended.

Wounds involving the cornea, limbus or anterior sclera may be repaired by a specialist, usually by direct suturing of the wound following replacement of the uveal tissue into the eye. A topical antibiotic treatment with good ocular penetration (e.g. chloramphenicol or ofloxacin) should be prescribed, along with broad-spectrum systemic antibiotics such as amoxicillin/clavulanate or a cephalosporin. Treatment for uveitis includes systemic corticosteroids, non-steroidal anti-inflammatory drugs (NSAIDs) and topical atropine. Use of topical corticosteroids should be delayed until the corneal epithelium has healed. Topical NSAIDs may be used, although some caution should be exercised because these drugs may potentiate intraocular bleeding and can increase IOP.

It should be noted that not all penetrating injuries are obvious, especially if the wound has occurred through the posterior aspect of the globe. These cases are frequently unilateral and present with a severe panophthalmitis. In such cases, the history may be suggestive (e.g. recent maxillary molar tooth extraction during which iatrogenic damage to the posterior globe was suspected, suspicion of a ballistic injury or a cat or dog fight). The ocular media are likely to be opaque in these situations and initial investigations are usually directed towards ultrasonographic assessment of the globe contents and the posterior aspect of the globe.

Ballistic lead pellets: Ballistic wounds often present with severe unilateral panuveitis. Lead ballistic pellets are occasionally identified within the globe and orbit. Accurate localization relies on obtaining two orthogonal radiographic views of the orbit or CT examination. Given that lead is relatively inert within the body, many cases are best treated conservatively rather than attempting to remove the foreign material surgically. The prognosis for lead shot retained within the globe ultimately depends on the concomitant injuries sustained at the time of the initial insult. Some of these patients do retain functional globes and as such empirical treatment for traumatic uveitis may be justified in appropriate cases.

Acquired abnormalities: orbit

Orbital abscess and cellulitis
Orbital abscess refers to a localized region of purulent material within the soft tissues of the orbit. In contrast, orbital cellulitis refers to a diffuse inflammation of the soft tissues of the orbit. Both conditions are frequently attributed to aerobic or anaerobic bacterial infection. Orbital abscesses tend to become walled off by reactive fibrous tissue, whilst in cellulitis the inflammation spreads through the interstitial tissue planes and tissue spaces. The inflammation often affects the extraconal space initially and then may extend into the intraconal space. The aetiopathogenesis may include:

- Infectious or non-infectious inflammatory disease of contiguous periorbital structures or spaces (periodontal or endodontic disease, sinusitis, dacryoadenitis, sialoadenitis or panophthalmitis)
- Direct inoculation of infection (transconjunctival, transpalpebral or transoral)
- Secondary to orbital foreign bodies or septicaemia.

Clinical signs: Patients with acute orbital cellulitis or abscessation typically present with a history of a relatively acute onset of rapidly progressive signs, which include pain and difficulty on opening the mouth, and swelling and increased sensitivity of the periocular tissues. The clinical presentation of these cases can be highly variable and often the signs of extraconal disease are the most prominent (see Figure 8.15). Clinical findings can include:

- Pain/discomfort during retropulsion of the globe or when the mouth is opened
- Exophthalmos
- Erythema and oedema of the eyelids
- Chemosis and conjunctival hyperaemia (commonly with a mucopurulent discharge)
- Protrusion of the nictitating membrane
- Visual and afferent pupillary deficits
- Decreased ocular movements
- Decreased eyelid and periorbital sensation
- Exposure keratitis
- Modestly increased IOP
- Induration or fistula of the oral mucosa in the pterygopalatine fossa (caudal and medial to the second maxillary molar tooth)
- Pyrexia and neutrophilia with left shift.

Such cases should be treated as emergencies, requiring urgent investigation and instigation of appropriate management and treatment if globe function is to be retained. Furthermore, the direct communication between the orbit and the CNS means that infective processes can potentially lead to meningoencephalitis and as such can be life-threatening.

Diagnosis: The investigation should include orbital ultrasonography and examination of the oral cavity, with particular attention to the pterygopalatine fossa and maxillary molar teeth. An ultrasound examination of both the normal and affected orbit should be performed because the comparison facilitates interpretation of the findings in the pathological orbit. Retrobulbar abscesses often have a well defined hyperechoic wall surrounding a uniformly hypoechoic region. With orbital cellulitis, subtle changes may be recognized in the normal retrobulbar space, including distortion or obliteration of the normal retrobulbar architecture, and decreased definition of the normal retrobulbar structures with an abnormal mixed echogenicity (medium/high amplitudes) (Mason *et al.*, 2001). Where available, advanced cross-sectional imaging (CT and MRI) may further characterize the disease process (see Chapter 2). Examination of the oral cavity may only be possible under general anaesthesia. In a systemically unwell patient (e.g. with pyrexia and dehydration), a period of stabilization may be necessary before this can be performed safely. Induration or fistulation of the pterygopalatine fossa is highly suggestive of orbital abscessation affecting the ventral orbit. Dental radiographs should be obtained to assess for evidence of periodontal or endodontic disease.

Treatment: The treatment depends on the severity of the clinical signs. In cases where a distinct abscess is not identified on orbital imaging and changes are more consistent with diffuse cellulitis, drainage of the extraconal orbital space via the pterygopalatine fossa is not normally indicated. In these cases, intensive medical treatment with broad-spectrum antibiotics and NSAIDs should be instigated, along with appropriate topical treatments if ulceration and/or lagophthalmos are apparent, to manage or prevent exposure keratitis. Close monitoring of the afferent function of the optic nerve (CN II) is essential. If deterioration in afferent CN II function is detected (e.g. reduction in pupillary light reflex (PLR) or menace response), drainage and/or decompression of the extraconal orbital space through the pterygopalatine fossa may be necessary to reduce intraorbital pressure, even if a distinct fluid pocket is not apparent.

If radiographs of the maxillary dental arcade reveal evidence of periapical abscessation, extraction of the affected tooth is indicated. In these cases, a purulent discharge is normally evident at the time of tooth extraction. Gentle probing of the alveolar bone may reveal a direct communication with the orbit and allow drainage of the orbital abscess. If drainage by this route is inadequate, surgical drainage via the pterygopalatine fossa should be performed. In the absence of dental disease, dependent drainage should be facilitated through the pterygopalatine fossa (Figure 8.15). The procedure for draining the orbital space via the pterygopalatine fossa is summarized below.

- The patient should be anaesthetized, intubated with a cuffed endotracheal tube and the pharynx packed with moistened swabs.
- The mucosa in the region should be prepared for aseptic surgery. A 1 cm incision should be made through the mucosa of the swollen pterygopalatine fossa caudal and medial to the maxillary second molar tooth in a rostral to caudal direction. It is essential that this initial incision penetrates no further than the mucosal tissue. Deeper sharp dissection runs the risk of damaging the neurovascular structures on the floor of the orbit, including the maxillary artery. Severing this artery (a major branch of the external carotid artery) can be associated with severe haemorrhage.

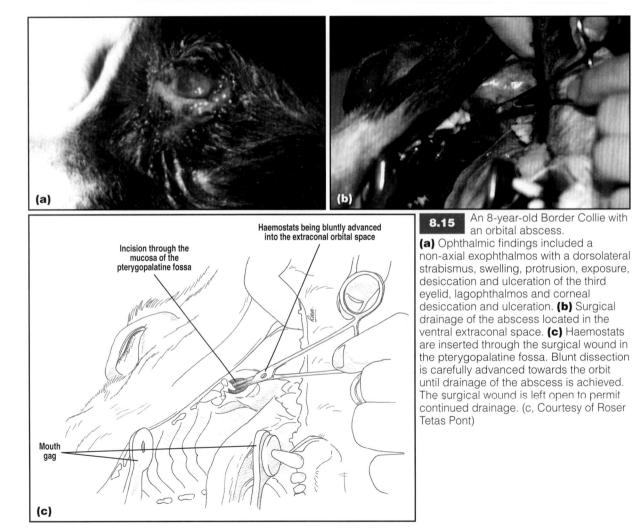

8.15 An 8-year-old Border Collie with an orbital abscess.
(a) Ophthalmic findings included a non-axial exophthalmos with a dorsolateral strabismus, swelling, protrusion, exposure, desiccation and ulceration of the third eyelid, lagophthalmos and corneal desiccation and ulceration. **(b)** Surgical drainage of the abscess located in the ventral extraconal space. **(c)** Haemostats are inserted through the surgical wound in the pterygopalatine fossa. Blunt dissection is carefully advanced towards the orbit until drainage of the abscess is achieved. The surgical wound is left open to permit continued drainage. (c, Courtesy of Roser Tetas Pont)

Incision through the mucosa of the pterygopalatine fossa

Haemostats being bluntly advanced into the extraconal orbital space

Mouth gag

- Following the initial incision through the mucosa, closed haemostats should be placed into the surgical wound, gently opened, and then withdrawn from the orbital space (the forceps should not be re-closed within the orbital space before removal). The process should be repeated as the forceps are gradually advanced into the extraconal orbital space. This blunt dissection allows a communication to be established between the orbit and the oral cavity, which runs through the pterygoid muscles on the floor of the orbit and may also pass through the zygomatic salivary gland. Extreme care is needed when performing surgical drainage of the orbital space to avoid iatrogenic damage to the orbital tissues and posterior aspect of the globe.
- In cases of orbital abscessation, purulent material will start to drain from the surgical wound soon after the haemostats have been advanced into the orbital space; the distance varies depending on the size of the patient and the amount of swelling of the pterygopalatine fossa. Ideally, more precise drainage can be achieved using B-mode ultrasonography with direct corneal contact for guidance. This demonstrates when the haemostats have entered the abscess cavity.
- As soon as purulent material is present, a swab should be taken for microbial culture and sensitivity as well as samples for immediate cytology.
- In some instances, frank purulent material is not evident when lesions are drained and a more serosanguineous fluid may be apparent, but similar sampling should be performed.
- In some cases, temporary tarsorrhaphy sutures may be placed to reduce corneal exposure. The benefits of this must be weighed against the degree of tension necessary to close the eyelids because this may significantly increase intraocular and intraorbital pressure, with resultant damage to sensitive structures such as the retina and optic nerve, as well as pressure necrosis of the eyelid tissue.
- Intensive topical treatment with antibiotics and lubricants needs to be continued until any corneal ulceration and lagophthalmos have resolved.
- Mixed aerobic and anaerobic bacterial infections of the orbit occur commonly in dogs and cats, and initial treatment with a potentiated penicillin (amoxicillin/clavulanate) or cephalosporin is appropriate whilst waiting for the results of culture and sensitivity analysis. The length of treatment is somewhat empirical but should be at least 4 weeks.

Masticatory muscle myositis

Masticatory muscle myositis (MMM) is an immune-mediated disorder that affects muscles derived from the first branchial arch, innervated by the mandibular branch of the trigeminal nerve and containing type 2M myofibres. The condition can affect dogs of any age, sex or breed, although large dogs are more commonly affected. MMM is usually bilaterally symmetrical and leads to inflammation of the temporal, masseter and pterygoid muscles. The immune response involves cellular and humoral components, selectively directed against type 2M myofibres. Although this condition is sometimes referred to as eosinophilic myositis, the predominant cell types in most muscle biopsy samples are lymphocytes and plasma cells, with the finding of eosinophils being variable and inconsistent.

Clinical signs: In the acute stage of the disease, swelling of the temporalis muscle leads to signs of extraconal disease, including exophthalmos and third eyelid protrusion. Complications due to exposure keratitis may be present, as may more generalized signs such as pyrexia and anorexia. Trismus is often evident, as are signs of pain when attempting to open the mouth or on palpation of the temporal or masseter muscles. In the chronic stages of the disease, fibrosis and atrophy of the masticatory muscles may lead to enophthalmos with possible secondary entropion. Interestingly, this seems to occur in some patients without clinically detectable antecedent acute MMM. Trismus may also occur in the chronic stages of the disease, presumably due to fibrosis of the masseter muscle.

Diagnosis: A presumptive diagnosis may be based on the typical clinical signs. Serum creatine kinase levels may be increased and neutrophilia (less commonly eosinophilia) may be present. Definitive diagnosis relies on demonstrating serum autoantibodies against type 2M myofibrils, which are present in the majority of cases. Serological testing for the protozoan parasites *Toxoplasma gondii* and *Neospora caninum* could be considered but, given the location of the myositis, this is usually not performed. Biopsy of the temporalis muscle is diagnostic, showing muscle fibre degeneration and inflammatory cell infiltration.

Treatment: The treatment involves immunosuppressive doses of prednisolone (2 mg/kg orally q24h, may be given in divided doses), which are maintained until resolution of the clinical signs is apparent, followed by a slow tapering of the dose whilst monitoring for clinical evidence of recrudescence. Alternative immunosuppressive drugs such as azathioprine may be included in the treatment regime if the response to treatment is poor or the corticosteroids are not well tolerated. Azathioprine is initially prescribed at a dose of 2 mg/kg orally q24h for 2 weeks followed by a gradual tapering, depending on the clinical response of the patient.

Liquidized food should be provided if trismus prevents the dog from prehending its normal food. The corneas should be protected by the frequent application of ocular lubricants if exposure is a concern. Some patients presenting in the chronic stages of MMM may have severe trismus and enophthalmos associated with fibrosis and loss of masticatory muscles. An ongoing physiotherapy regime may improve jaw opening. In some cases, courses of immunosuppressive therapy improve the situation, suggesting that despite the severe atrophy/fibrosis, an active inflammatory component may be complicating these cases.

Extraocular muscle myositis

Extraocular muscle myositis is a rare immune-mediated inflammatory myopathy of dogs that is restricted to the extraocular muscles (Carpenter *et al.*, 1989). The extraocular muscles have unique myofibres that differ significantly from those of limb and masticatory muscles. The syndrome usually affects young (about 1 year of age) entire bitches, with the Golden Retriever being over-represented (Ramsey *et al.*, 1995). An antecedent 'stressor' such as ovariohysterectomy, the oestrous cycle, or boarding at a kennel was reported in many cases prior to the onset of clinical signs of extraocular muscle myositis.

Clinical signs: The inflammation of the extraocular muscles leads to signs consistent with intraconal disease. The bilateral exophthalmos without pronounced third eyelid protrusion, often with 360-degree scleral show and retraction of the upper eyelid, results in a very characteristic appearance in these patients (see Figure 8.9). Clinical signs of pain during retropulsion or oral examination are usually absent and the dog remains clinically well.

Diagnosis: The diagnosis is usually based on the clinical presentation and ultrasonographic findings revealing thickening of the extraocular muscles (Figure 8.16), which is also readily appreciated on CT and MRI (see Chapter 2). Extraocular muscle myositis is not associated with the antibodies to 2M myofibres seen in masticatory myositis or with elevated serum creatine kinase levels.

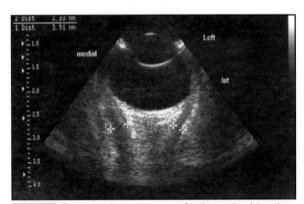

8.16   B-mode ultrasonogram of a 9-month-old entire Labrador Retriever bitch with bilateral extraocular polymyositis. The enlarged hypoechoic lateral and medial rectus muscles are denoted by the callipers.

Treatment: The treatment involves immunosuppression, as outlined for MMM (see above). Given that recurrence appears to be common, especially in association with antecedent stressors, longer term immunosuppressive therapy may be necessary in some cases. In these situations, the use of alternative immunosuppressive drugs such as azathioprine may be preferable to avoid the side effects associated with long-term corticosteroid use.

Fibrosing extraocular muscle myositis with restrictive strabismus

Fibrosing extraocular muscle myositis is a rare condition of young dogs, with the Shar Pei, Irish Wolfhound and Akita being the breeds most commonly reported (Allgoewer *et al.*, 2000). The clinical syndrome leads to enophthalmos and severe unilateral or bilateral, ventral or ventromedial strabismus (esotropia) (Figure 8.17). The globe deviation can be so marked as to cause significant visual deficits. Histologically, the primary pathological change involves fibrosis of the extraocular muscles with lymphocytic/plasmacytic mononuclear cell infiltration. These cases do not respond to immunosuppressive treatment. Surgical correction, in which the fibrotic extraocular muscles leading to the strabismus are resected, may restore the globe to a more normal position. A specialist ophthalmologist should be consulted in such cases.

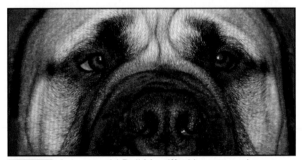

8.17   A 1-year-old Bull Mastiff with progressive bilateral medial strabismus associated with fibrosing extraocular muscle myositis. Note that the medial strabismus is more severe on the right side.

Restrictive orbital myofibroblastic sarcoma

A chronic, non-specific fibrosing process of the orbit has been reported in cats. The condition was originally termed idiopathic sclerosing orbital pseudotumour. The disease is insidiously progressive, poorly responsive to treatment and frequently results in euthanasia. It has been suggested that the condition represents a true neoplastic process, which preferentially affects the orbit and adjacent tissues, and should more appropriately be termed feline restrictive orbital myofibroblastic sarcoma (Bell *et al.*, 2011).

Clinical signs: The condition affects middle-aged to old cats without an apparent sex or breed predisposition. Clinically, most cats present with insidious unilateral ocular involvement, including exophthalmos with progressive restriction of globe and eyelid motility, eyelid retraction, lagophthalmos and thickening of the eyelids. Subsequent progression of the tumour occurs, involving the contralateral eye and/or oral tissues. The lack of eyelid function may lead to severe exposure keratitis with corneal perforation, often necessitating enucleation.

Diagnosis: Biopsy is required to confirm the diagnosis, with the recommended tissue specimens being thickened eyelid or thickened haired skin with subcutis (Bell *et al.*, 2011). If enucleation is performed and there is clinical suspicion of feline restrictive orbital myofibroblastic sarcoma, the globe should be submitted for histological evaluation with the eyelids and orbital tissues in place, contrary to the routine recommendations for dissection and fixation of enucleation specimens.

Treatment: There is no curative treatment for this disease. Some palliation of signs may be seen with anti-inflammatory or immunosuppressive therapy, but euthanasia eventually becomes necessary on humane grounds in most cases.

Orbital neoplasia

Primary orbital neoplasia arises from orbital structures, whilst secondary neoplasia involves local extension from adjacent structures or metastases from distant sites. In dogs and cats, approximately 90% of orbital tumours are malignant. This, combined with the late presentation, means that the prognosis for these patients is usually guarded or grave. The most commonly reported primary and secondary neoplasms of dogs and cats are summarized in Figure 8.18.

Primary neoplasms
• Osteosarcoma
• Fibrosarcoma
• Chondrosarcoma
• Myxosarcoma
• Orbital meningioma
• Neurofibrosarcoma
• Adenoma
• Adenocarcinoma
• Lipoma
• Histiocytoma
• Mast cell tumour
• Rhabdomyosarcoma

Secondary neoplasms
• Lymphoma
• Squamous cell carcinoma
• Melanoma
• Adenocarcinoma
• Cerebral meningioma
• Metastatic disease

8.18 Primary and secondary orbital neoplasms seen in dogs and cats.

Primary orbital tumours may arise from epithelial, glandular, bony, neural, haemolymphatic or connective tissue structures. Secondary tumours include those extending from the nasal and oral cavity (e.g. epithelial and glandular tumours), the brain or the globe (e.g. melanoma). Multicentric and metastatic tumours include lymphosarcoma and adenocarcinoma. In dogs, most orbital tumours are primary neoplasms with osteosarcoma, fibrosarcoma, undifferentiated sarcomas, adenocarcinoma and meningioma being the most commonly reported. In contrast, orbital tumours in cats are mostly secondary neoplasms and include squamous cell carcinoma and undifferentiated carcinomas invading from adjacent tissues (e.g. nasal and oral cavities) and lymphosarcoma associated with multicentric disease.

Clinical signs: Orbital neoplasia generally affects older patients (>8 years of age) and often follows an insidious course, leading to a late presentation when tumours are well advanced. Most cases have a history of slowly progressive unilateral exophthalmos without pain on opening the mouth or palpation of periocular tissues. Despite this classical clinical presentation, some orbital neoplasms (aggressive lymphoma, mast cell tumour, sarcoma) may be misdiagnosed as orbital inflammation because they mimic the clinical signs of acute inflammatory orbital disease (Hendrix and Gelatt, 2000; Attali-Soussay et al., 2001). Furthermore, some tumour types (e.g. lymphoma, rhabdomyosarcoma and mast cell tumours) may also affect younger patients. Common ophthalmic findings are those of extraconal disease and include non-axial exophthalmos, strabismus and protrusion of the third eyelid (see Figure 8.10). Signs of intraconal disease, including axial exophthalmos without strabismus or protrusion of the third eyelid, may be seen in canine orbital meningioma.

Diagnosis: The investigation of suspected orbital neoplastic disease should include:

• Definitive diagnosis of neoplastic disease
• Determining the tumour type
• Determining the tumour grade
• Determining the tumour stage.

Physical examination is important because the identification of lymphadenopathy or organomegaly may increase the index of suspicion for disseminated or locally invasive disease. Initial investigations should ideally include orbital radiography, ultrasonography and MRI, as well as survey radiography of the thorax and abdomen and abdominal ultrasonography for tumour staging. If neoplasia is suspected, survey radiographs of the thorax and abdomen should be obtained prior to imaging the skull. The main aim of the radiographic assessment for orbital disease is to identify bony pathology, including fractures, osteolysis and osteoproliferative lesions. Although bone lysis is highly suggestive of malignancy in dogs and cats, orbital radiography is not highly sensitive in detecting orbital bone pathology (Dennis, 2000).

Determining the type and grade of the tumour relies on obtaining a tissue sample, which in the first instance should be attempted via fine-needle aspiration or Tru-cut biopsy. This is often facilitated by ultrasound or CT guidance. In some cases, sampling of more accessible, non-orbital tissues may be appropriate to determine the nature of the orbital pathology. Exploratory surgery to perform incisional or excisional biopsy is not recommended before information regarding tumour grade and stage has been acquired, owing to the high likelihood of malignant disease. Subjecting the patient to procedures with greater morbidity should be reserved for situations where curative or perceived palliative benefits of orbital surgery have been established.

If financially practical, MRI or CT should be performed because they provide information regarding the local extension of orbital neoplasia, which is superior to that obtained using conventional radiography and ultrasonography (Figure 8.19). This often avoids putting the patient through unnecessary invasive procedures in situations where there is little chance of a positive outcome.

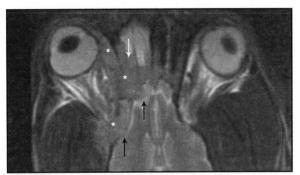

8.19 An 11-year-old Labrador Retriever presented with an acute history of blindness and exophthalmos affecting the right eye. The T2-weighted dorsal MR image revealed an extensive orbital tumour (*) with invasion through the calvarium into the brain (black arrows) and nasal cavity (white arrow).

Treatment: In situations where surgical excision of an orbital tumour is considered for curative or palliative purposes, specialist advice should be sought. Such cases often require a multidisciplinary approach with involvement of specialists in diagnostic imaging, oncology, ophthalmology and general soft tissue and orthopaedic surgery. Curative surgery with partial orbitotomy for solitary, well defined and benign tumours may be indicated in some cases. The surgical approach in such cases should be directed through non-pathologically involved tissue planes. Exenteration is indicated for invasive or infiltrative orbital masses that do not extend beyond the confines of the orbit. When tumours extend beyond the confines of the orbit, subtotal or partial orbitectomy combined with adjuvant radiation or chemotherapy (based on histopathological findings) for palliative or curative purposes may be indicated. On occasion, enucleation or exenteration of an exophthalmic, exposed globe may be considered palliative even if the outcome is not expected to be curative.

Traumatic proptosis
Traumatic proptosis refers to an acute condition in which the globe has been forced anteriorly beyond the rim of the bony orbit and eyelids, where it often becomes entrapped (exacerbated by spasm of the orbicularis oculi muscle at the equator of the globe). Traumatic proptosis is invariably secondary to trauma. Brachycephalic breeds (e.g. Pekingese, Boston Terrier, Pug, Shih Tzu and Lhaso Apso) are predisposed because of their prominent globes, shallow orbits and large palpebral fissures. In contrast, cats with a typical mesaticephalic conformation are less prone to traumatic proptosis. The corollary to this is that traumatic proptosis in non-brachycephalic dogs and cats is usually associated with more severe trauma and concurrent injuries and has a poorer prognosis for recovery of vision (Gilger *et al.*, 1995).

Clinical signs: Patients may present with a proptosed globe that is complicated by the eyelids being 'clamped' posterior to the equator of the globe. Strabismus as a result of torn extraocular muscles is common; the medial rectus muscle is most frequently affected, owing to its more anterior insertion on the globe, resulting in lateral strabismus (Figure 8.20). Chemosis and corneal ulceration are often present and other findings may include uveitis, glaucoma or hypotony and hyphaema. Neuro-ophthalmic examination often reveals visual deficits and pupillary abnormalities. Concurrent craniofacial and CNS trauma is common, particularly in non-brachycephalic breeds.

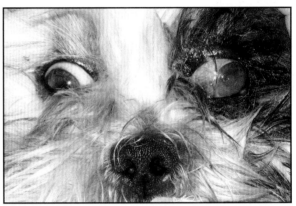

8.20 A 2-year-old male neutered Shih Tzu with lateral strabismus of the left eye following traumatic proptosis. Other ophthalmic findings in the left eye included blindness, loss of direct and consensual pupillary light responses, reduced corneal sensation, lagophthalmos and corneal ulceration.

Treatment and prognosis: The presentation of acute traumatic proptosis invariably involves an extremely distressed patient and client. Initially, it is important not to focus on the proptosis as the most important lesion. In non-brachycephalic patients, the force needed to induce traumatic proptosis may be severe, and identification and assessment of other traumatic injuries may take priority over the obvious ocular trauma. Evaluation of concurrent craniofacial and CNS injury is particularly important. Primary assessments of the airways, breathing and circulation (ABC) are the first priorities. It is essential that interventions for life-threatening injuries are implemented whilst ongoing examination to determine the severity of the ocular injury (assessing vision, PLR, extraocular muscle damage) is being carried out.

Once the patient has been admitted and life-threatening injuries have been ruled out or are being managed, discussions with the client regarding the prognosis for the globe and the possibility that enucleation may be indicated, can be conducted in a less stressful environment. The initial reaction of the client is usually to request replacement and preservation of the globe (whether functional or non-functional), often for cosmetic reasons. Once the potential for long-term complications (see below) has been communicated, the client will be better informed to decide whether attempts to preserve the globe are warranted or enucleation is a better alternative.

The prognosis for vision is poor in affected dogs and very poor in cats, owing to tractional optic nerve damage, which occurs at the time of the traumatic proptosis. In one review, 64% of dogs and 100% of cats were blind following traumatic proptosis (Gilger *et al.*, 1995). Positive prognostic indicators for vision include proptosis in brachycephalic dogs, sight in a globe that is proptosed and positive direct and consensual PLRs (Gilger *et al.*, 1995).

If the damage to the globe, extraocular muscles and/or the optic nerve is severe and the prognosis for salvaging even a non-functional globe is poor, enucleation should be performed. In cases where an attempt at globe replacement to preserve vision and/or salvage the globe is considered appropriate, general anaesthesia is needed. Replacement of a proptosed globe is often difficult because of swelling and haemorrhage of the adnexal and orbital tissues, and can be further complicated by the shallow orbit in brachycephalic breeds.

- The ocular surface should be cleansed with povidone–iodine solution (1:50 dilution with saline) and a lateral canthotomy performed.
- Gentle forward traction is placed on the eyelids to return them to a more normal position. As a result of tissue swelling, it is usually not possible to return the globe to a normal position in which the corneal surface is adequately protected by the eyelids. As such a temporary tarsorrhaphy is invariably needed (Figure 8.21).
- Empirical topical antibiotic treatment should be administered until the temporary tarsorrhaphy is removed and the integrity of the cornea can be evaluated. A broad-spectrum systemic antibiotic should also be prescribed, especially when tearing and exposure of the extraocular muscles is apparent and a direct route for bacterial contamination of the orbit is present. Application of topical atropine twice daily for the first week may help to reduce any secondary uveitis and associated painful ciliary body muscle spasm.
- The initial use of prednisolone (anti-inflammatory doses) tapering over a 1-month period is indicated because of the need to reduce intraocular and orbital inflammation. Although a high dose of methylprednisolone sodium succinate (MPSS) has been previously advocated to reduce optic nerve damage, numerous studies have now refuted the benefits of this treatment.

Complications: The long-term complications associated with this disease can lead to significant patient morbidity. This should be emphasized during the initial decision-making process involving the client to determine whether attempts to preserve a proptosed globe are undertaken. The long-term complications include:

- Permanent blindness
- Lagophthalmos – inability to blink over the entire corneal surface due to persistent exophthalmos and reduced orbicularis oculi muscle function. Management of this may require a long-term (3–6 month) temporary tarsorrhaphy or, in some

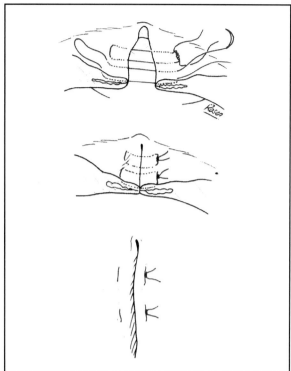

8.21 Temporary tarsorrhaphy technique. Partial thickness horizontal mattress sutures are placed using 4/0–5/0 (1.5–1.0 metric) non-absorbable suture material (e.g. polyamide) on a reverse cutting or micropoint needle. If eyelid swelling is severe, placement of the suture through a stent (see Chapter 12) may help to prevent pressure necrosis. The suture should pass through the anterior eyelid margin (anterior to the meibomian gland openings) to reduce the chance of corneal contact. The medial aspect of the palpebral fissure (over the third eyelid) may be left open to facilitate administration of topical medication. (Courtesy of Roser Tetas Pont)

instances, a permanent partial tarsorrhaphy to reduce the size of the palpebral fissure
- Neurotrophic keratitis (keratitis secondary to trigeminal denervation of the cornea). The loss of corneal sensation is associated with loss of trophic factors supplied by the sensory nerves and may lead to ongoing problems associated with ulcerative keratitis (see Chapter 12)
- KCS due to corneal denervation interfering with the afferent reflex arc responsible for corneal sensation stimulated lacrimation. KCS may also occur due to direct damage to the parasympathetic innervation of the lacrimal gland (see Chapter 10)
- Permanent strabismus, which if the affected eye is sighted can lead to diplopia (double vision)
- Phthisis bulbi, in which the globe shrinks due to severe intraocular damage. This may necessitate enucleation if chronic discomfort ensues.

Fracture of the orbital or periorbital bones
Fractures of the orbital bones are not uncommon following facial trauma. Fractures affecting the more exposed orbital bones, including the frontal and maxillary bones and those forming the zygomatic arch, are the most commonly encountered.

Diagnosis: Physical examination may reveal obvious facial asymmetry associated with orbital fractures. Palpation of the bony orbital rim and adjacent bony structures may reveal instability or crepitation of the affected bones. The full length of the zygomatic arch should be palpated. The mandible should also be palpated, including the symphysis, body, angle and coronoid process in the temporal fossa. Fractures involving the frontal bones may result in communication with the frontal sinus, leading to orbital and/or periorbital emphysema, which may be clinically apparent as a subcutaneous swelling and a 'crackling' crepitus on palpation.

Routine survey imaging demonstrates most traumatic bony injuries, although it is less sensitive in detecting fractures in the region of the orbital apex. In human medicine, CT is replacing plain films for the evaluation of orbital trauma because of higher sensitivity and better definition of the bony pathology; where available, CT also represents the imaging modality of choice for veterinary patients.

Treatment: The majority of orbital fractures are treated conservatively. The principal morbidity associated with orbital fractures is globe injury. If globe function is compromised by bony fractures, then surgical intervention is indicated. On occasion, palpable bony fragments may be manipulated into a more anatomically correct position (closed reduction), whilst larger or unstable fractures may require internal fixation and may necessitate referral.

Orbital cystic disease

Cystic structures may arise from epithelial or glandular tissue within or adjacent to the orbit. Cysts may arise from the orbital lacrimal gland, gland of the nictitating membrane, zygomatic salivary gland or developmentally from retained or buried conjunctival mucosa or other epithelia. Cysts involving the paranasal sinuses may lead to pressure necrosis of the adjacent orbital bony structures and may extend into the orbit. Cysts may also result from incomplete removal of epithelial and/or glandular tissue during enucleation surgery. Certain orbital tumours may also have significant cystic components (e.g. adenocarcinoma).

Radiography, cross-sectional imaging and cytological examination of fine-needle aspirates of cystic fluid (collected using ultrasound or CT guidance) may facilitate characterization of the cyst and inform management strategies. Surgical excision can be complicated and the approach to orbitotomy will be dictated by the location and size of the cystic structure. Thus, referral to a specialist is recommended. Generally, careful blunt dissection to remove the intact cystic mass following limited orbitotomy is indicated. Histopathology is always required to rule out neoplasia with cystic components.

Zygomatic mucoceles: The zygomatic salivary gland lies on the ventral floor of the orbit in the dog (see Figure 8.2). Leakage of saliva from the gland or duct may lead to orbital mucocele formation in the ventral orbit. This may occur in association with

zygomatic sialadenitis (Cannon *et al.*, 2011). This leads to clinical signs consistent with extraconal disease, but signs of pain on opening the mouth or retropulsion are typically minimal.

Diagnosis: Oral examination reveals a fluctuant swelling in the region of the pterygopalatine fossa (Figure 8.22a). Further diagnostic tests include orbital ultrasonography, which may reveal a well delineated hypoechoic or anechoic cavitary lesion in the ventral orbit. Zygomatic sialography may be considered to confirm communication with the zygomatic salivary gland. This involves the retrograde instillation of a non-ionic iodinated contrast

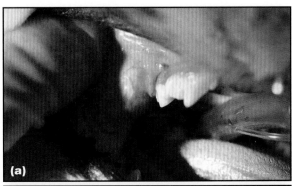

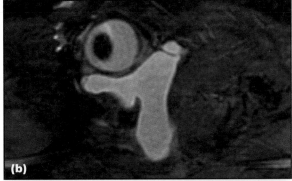

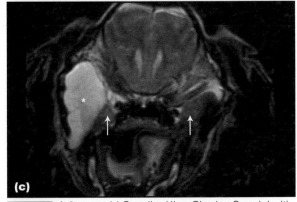

8.22 A 3-year-old Cavalier King Charles Spaniel with a salivary mucocele. **(a)** Oral examination revealed a painless fluctuant swelling in the pterygopalatine fossa. **(b)** T2-weighted sagittal MR image showing a complex fluid-filled cavity in the right orbit. Note the ventral extension of the mucocele towards the oral cavity, which presented as the swelling in the pterygopalatine fossa. **(c)** T2-weighted transverse MR image showing the left and right zygomatic salivary glands (arrowed). Serial transverse MR images demonstrated a direct communication between the right zygomatic salivary gland and the mucocele (∗).

medium into the salivary gland duct: the zygomatic papilla is located lateral and caudal to the last upper molar tooth. The zygomatic papilla should be examined for swelling and redness. Prior to contrast medium instillation, a sample of saliva can be collected for cytology, culture and sensitivity testing. Lateral and DV radiographs should also be obtained prior to contrast medium instillation to ensure correct exposure, or CT may be used if available.

The papilla is cannulated using a 22–25 gauge cannula and the contrast medium is instilled at a rate of 0.5–1 ml per 10 kg bodyweight; instillation may be repeated prior to each exposure. The sialogram reveals the zygomatic salivary gland to be large, single lobed and positioned ventral to the rostral end of the zygomatic arch. On radiographs, the contrast medium will demonstrate a fluid-filled cavity associated with the zygomatic gland, thus helping to distinguish it from cystic lesions associated with other orbital structures. Where available, MRI provides detailed information regarding the location and extent of salivary mucoceles (Figure 8.22bc). Fine-needle aspiration of the mucocele typically reveals a viscous fluid consistent with saliva. Despite this appearance, cytology should be performed to help rule out neoplasia with a cystic component and infectious diseases.

Treatment: Drainage of the mucocele should be attempted by aspiration of the fluid through the pterygopalatine fossa (Figure 8.23). A large-gauge needle facilitates removal of the highly viscous salivary secretion. If drainage of the majority of the saliva is possible, the exophthalmos will resolve immediately. If drainage via needle aspiration is not successful, then the mucocele may be drained by creating a fistula through the pterygopalatine fossa (connecting the mucocele with the oral cavity; see description above for draining an orbital abscess). Drainage, in combination with anti-inflammatory

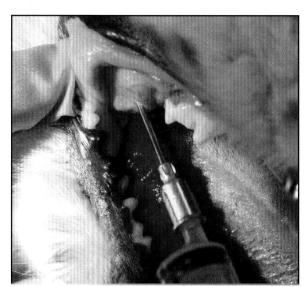

8.23 Drainage of a salivary mucocele (same dog as in Figure 8.22). A large-gauge needle is inserted into the mucocele through the pterygopalatine fossa. Approximately 20 ml of blood-stained saliva was removed from the mucocele.

therapy for any accompanying zygomatic sialadenitis, often leads to resolution of the disease, but in recurrent cases removal of the zygomatic gland via a lateral orbitotomy may be necessary.

Dacryops: This condition relates to cysts of lacrimal gland tissue. These are uncommon and may be developmental or result from trauma. Canine dacryops have been found in the orbit, third eyelid and associated with ectopic lacrimal glandular ductal tissues. Treatment of canine dacryops is surgical excision and complete removal is curative.

Orbit fat pad and temporal muscle atrophy

Loss of orbital fat or temporal muscle mass, leading to enophthalmos, may be a senile process or associated with more generalized conditions that involve cachexia. The loss of masseter muscle volume in chronic masticatory myositis may similarly lead to significant enophthalmos. Complications associated with severe enophthalmos include entropion (usually of the lower eyelid) and visual deficits due to third eyelid protrusion. Only in rare instances is surgical intervention needed to address these problems by augmenting orbital tissue volume with inert implants. A Hotz–Celsus procedure is usually adequate for entropion correction (see Chapter 9), whilst third eyelid shortening may be considered in cases where protrusion leads to significant vision deficits (see Chapter 11).

Enucleation

Owners are often reluctant to consent to enucleation on aesthetic grounds or because of their perception that the eye is not painful or retains some vestige of visual function. Once owners have been counselled regarding the irreversible loss of vision and ongoing discomfort associated with conditions such as chronic glaucoma, removal of the eye is usually seen as the most appropriate option. There is often a significant improvement in the general demeanour of the patient following removal of a chronically painful eye and this reinforces to the owner that the correct decision was made. Retrobulbar anaesthesia may be considered to augment intraoperative and postoperative analgesia.

Transconjunctival enucleation

Transconjunctival enucleation (Figure 8.24) is technically the most straightforward procedure. It should not be performed in situations where there is known infection or a neoplastic process involving the ocular surface.

Transpalpebral enucleation

Transpalpebral enucleation (Figure 8.25) should be performed in situations where there is known infection in the conjunctival sac (e.g. infected stromal ulcer) or where there is the possibility of tumour cells outside the eye. A course of NSAIDs and broad-spectrum antibiotics is normally prescribed for a week following surgery.

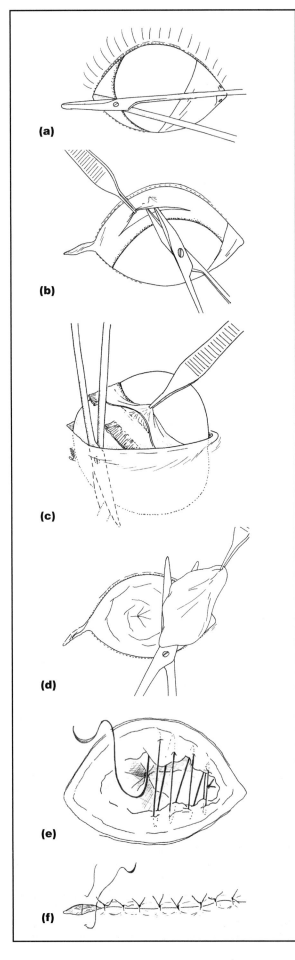

(a)

(b)

(c)

(d)

(e)

(f)

8.24 Transconjunctival enucleation technique. **(a)** A lateral canthotomy is performed to improve exposure of the globe and an eyelid speculum is then inserted. **(b)** Using tenotomy scissors, an incision is made through the bulbar conjunctiva and Tenon's capsule to the level of the sclera, approximately 5 mm posterior to the limbus (this allows haemostats or Allis tissue forceps to be attached to the remaining conjunctiva at the limbus and the globe to be manipulated into the desired position to assist the surgeon). Blunt dissection is continued caudally on this scleral plane to identify the insertion of the superior rectus muscle, which is transected close to the sclera, minimizing haemorrhage. Dissection is continued around the globe through 360 degrees in the scleral plane in order to identify and transect the other rectus and oblique muscles at their insertions on the sclera. **(c)** Once all the rectus muscle and superior and inferior oblique muscle insertions have been sectioned, the globe should be rotated medially in order to identify the retractor bulbi muscles, which surround the optic nerve (direct observation of the optic nerve is usually not possible owing to their presence). Medial rotation of the globe is preferable to placing forward traction on the globe. The optic nerve and retractor bulbi muscles are transected with fine curved Metzenbaum scissors (with or without prior clamping). Exposure and ligation of the optic nerve is not recommended because this may place excessive traction on the optic nerve and chiasm, which could lead to damage of the contralateral optic nerve fibres. This is particularly important in cats, in which the globe occupies most of the orbital space and therefore forward traction on the globe carries a greater risk of a blinding tractional injury to the optic chiasm. **(d)** Once the globe has been removed, the orbit is packed with gauze sponges to control any haemorrhage from the extraocular muscles and orbital vasculature: typically packing the orbit for 5 minutes will control bleeding. The third eyelid, third eyelid gland and associated conjunctiva are excised. The eyelids are removed using large Mayo scissors. The excision should extend approximately 7 mm from the lateral eyelid margins to ensure removal of the meibomian glands. The margin of the excision should taper towards the medial canthus, where only about 3–4 mm of skin should be removed. Dissection of the medial canthal skin and medial caruncle tissue is performed using tenotomy scissors: staying close to the medial canthus reduces the chance of transecting the angularis oculi vein, which can be associated with significant haemorrhage. Any remaining conjunctival tissue is dissected and removed. The lacrimal gland, which lies deep to the orbital ligament, can be identified and dissected from the orbit (although this is not typically performed). After removal of the gauze packing from the orbit, most of the haemorrhage is controlled, but specific bleeding vessels may need to be ligated or cauterized. Haemorrhage from some eyelid vessels can be more significant and require ligation or cautery. **(e)** Closure of the deep surgical wound should be in two layers: closure of the deep fascia over the orbital opening followed by closure of the subcutaneous layer using a continuous 4/0 (1.5 metric) absorbable suture. The dead space caused by removal of the globe will fill with serosanguineous material, and closure of the deeper layer will prevent the extensive subcutaneous haematoma and swelling often seen post enucleation. **(f)** The eyelid skin is closed in a simple interrupted pattern with 4/0 (1.5 metric) non-absorbable monofilament suture material. (Courtesy of Roser Tetas Pont)

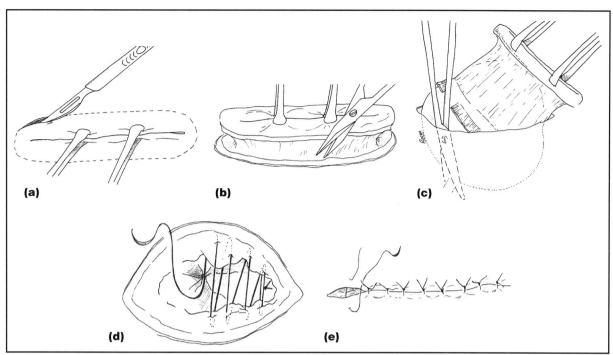

8.25 Transpalpebral enucleation technique. **(a)** The eyelids may be sutured together using a large-gauge non-absorbable monofilament suture such as 2/0 (3 metric) nylon, or they may be held together using Allis tissue forceps to allow an assistant to provide traction on the eyelids in an appropriate direction depending on the area of surgical dissection. Two curved skin incisions are made in the periocular skin of the upper and lower eyelids approximately 7 mm away from the eyelid margin and joined near the medial and lateral canthi. At the medial canthus, the incisions should meet approximately 3–4 mm from the medial canthal margin. **(b)** Blunt dissection is performed towards the globe, taking care not to penetrate the conjunctival sac, until the sclera is identified. Sectioning of the lateral canthal ligament aids exposure, and digital palpation helps guide the blunt dissection and facilitates finding the appropriate plane of dissection. **(c)** Once the sclera is exposed, this plane of dissection should be maintained around the superior, temporal and inferior aspects of the globe. The extraocular muscles should be identified as transected (as described for the transconjunctival enucleation technique). Medially, the dissection continues on the outer surface of the third eyelid. Sectioning the short medial canthal ligament facilitates exposure and freeing of the outer surface of the third eyelid. As with the transconjunctival enucleation technique, rotation of the globe medially to expose and allow transection of the retrobulbar muscles and optic nerve is recommended, rather than direct forward traction on the globe. **(d–e)** Wound closure and aftercare are as described for the transconjunctival enucleation technique. (Courtesy of Roser Tetas Pont)

Orbital prosthesis

To improve the cosmetic appearance post enucleation, implantation of a prosthetic silicone sphere into the orbital space may be performed. The size of the implant is selected in accordance with the size of the orbital space and in dogs the diameter varies from 12–28 mm. They are placed within the orbit after the globe and nictitating membrane have been removed. It has been suggested that flattening the anterior quarter of the sphere using a scalpel blade improves the cosmetic appearance and reduces rotation. Once the prosthesis has been placed, the wound may be closed in a routine manner. This should prevent the sinking of the skin into the orbital space, which often occurs following enucleation. Possible complications include extrusion of the sphere following inadequate wound closure, infection or (rarely) reactions to the foreign material.

Intrascleral prosthesis

Evisceration of the contents of the globe via a perilimbal incision, leaving the corneoscleral shell into which a silicone implant can be placed, has gained popularity in recent years. This may be particularly useful for blind glaucomatous eyes or eyes that have suffered severe injury, but should not be considered if there is any possibility of intraocular infection or neoplasia. Following the procedure, the patient retains a globe with normal motility and adnexa. Most intrascleral prostheses are black, but with the eventual corneal scarring most eyes eventually take on a greyish appearance. Intrascleral prostheses are not without complications, including regrowth of unidentified intraocular neoplasms, scleral wound dehiscence, postoperative infections, corneal mineralization, ulceration and KCS. This procedure involves specialist equipment and, importantly, proper case selection and experience with the surgical technique to minimize unfavourable outcomes and manage the postoperative discomfort adequately. Consultation with a veterinary ophthalmologist is recommended if this procedure is being considered.

Pathological examination

Submission of an enucleated eye for pathological examination is strongly recommended in all cases, and in particular where the underlying aetiology of the disease process leading to the globe being enucleated is not clearly defined. This is often the case in patients with chronic intraocular inflammation, suspected neoplasia, glaucoma and intraocular haemorrhage. Pathological examination of the eye may provide invaluable information, which may influence the management of the contralateral eye or have implications for the overall wellbeing of the patient. Even in situations where the ocular pathology seems more obviously associated with a specific condition (e.g. trauma, corneal perforation due to stromal ulceration), if owners are initially unwilling to pursue histopathological evaluation on the grounds of cost, it is wise to store these eyes for possible future submission, in case there is an unexpected development in the contralateral eye.

The protocol for globe submission for pathological examination is reviewed in Chapter 3. It is generally recommended that the globe be trimmed of all adnexal tissue apart from the optic nerve. Exceptions are cases of suspected restrictive orbital myofibroblastic sarcoma in cats and neoplastic lesions that may extend beyond the globe. Globes are generally fixed in formalin (ratio of 10:1 fixative to globe volume). The clinician should submit as much information as possible regarding the patient, including signalment, history, prior treatments, suspected location of the pathology within the eye and any relevant findings in the contralateral eye.

References and further reading

Adkins EA, Ward DA, Daniel GB *et al.* (2005) Coil embolization of a congenital orbital varix in a dog. *Journal of the American Veterinary Medical Association* **227**(12), 1952–1954

Allgoewer I, Blair M, Basher T *et al.* (2000) Extraocular muscle myositis and restrictive strabismus in 10 dogs. *Veterinary Ophthalmology* **3**(1), 21–26

Attali-Soussay K, Jegou JP and Clerc B (2001) Retrobulbar tumors in dogs and cats: 25 cases. *Veterinary Ophthalmology* **4**(1), 19–27

Bell CM, Schwarz T and Dubielzig RR (2011) Diagnostic features of feline restrictive orbital myofibroblastic sarcoma. *Veterinary Pathology* **48**(3), 742–750

Cannon MS, Paglia D, Zwingenberger AL *et al.* (2011) Clinical and diagnostic imaging findings in dogs with zygomatic sialadenitis: 11 cases (1990–2009). *Journal of the American Veterinary Medical Association* **239**(9), 1211–1218

Carpenter JL, Schmidt GM, Moore FM *et al.* (1989) Canine bilateral extraocular polymyositis. *Veterinary Pathology* **26**(6), 510–512

Dennis R (2000) Use of magnetic resonance imaging for the investigation of orbital disease in small animals. *Journal of Small Animal Practice* **41**(4), 145–155

Donaldson D, Matas Riera M, Holloway A, Beltran E and Barnett KC (2013) Contralateral optic neuropathy and retinopathy associated with visual and afferent pupillomotor dysfunction following enucleation in cats. *Veterinary Ophthalmology* doi: 10.1111/vop.12104

Gilger B, Hamilton H, Wilkie D *et al.* (1995) Traumatic proptosis in dogs and cats: 84 cases (1980–1993). *Journal of the American Veterinary Medical Association* **206**(8), 1186–1190

Hendrix DVH and Gelatt KN (2000) Diagnosis, treatment and outcome of orbital neoplasia in dogs: a retrospective study of 44 cases. *Journal of Small Animal Practice* **41**(3), 105–108

Mason DR, Lamb CR and McLellan GJ (2001) Ultrasonographic findings in 50 dogs with retrobulbar disease. *Journal of the American Animal Hospital Association* **37**(6), 557–562

Miller PE (2008) Orbit. In: *Slatter's Fundamentals of Veterinary Ophthalmology*, 4th edn, ed. DJ Maggs *et al.*, pp. 352–373. Saunders Elsevier, Missouri

Ramsey DT and Fox DB (1997) Surgery of the orbit. *Veterinary Clinics of North America: Small Animal Practice* **27**(5), 1215–1264

Ramsey DT, Hamor RE, Gerding PA *et al.* (1995) Clinical and immunohistochemical characteristics of bilateral extraocular polymyositis of dogs. In: *26th Annual Meeting of the American College of Veterinary Ophthalmologists*, pp. 130–132. Newport, USA

Ramsey DT, Marretta SM, Hamor RE *et al.* (1996) Ophthalmic manifestations and complications of dental disease in dogs and cats. *Journal of the American Animal Hospital Association* **32**(3), 215–224

Smith MM, Smith EM, La Croix N *et al.* (2003) Orbital penetration associated with tooth extraction. *Journal of Veterinary Dentistry* **20**(1), 8–17

Stiles J and Townsend WM (2007) Feline Ophthalmology. In: *Veterinary Ophthalmology*, 4th edn, ed. KN Gelatt, pp. 1095–1164. Blackwell Publishing Ltd, Iowa

9

The eyelids

Sue Manning

Embryology, anatomy and physiology

Embryology
The eyelids develop as folds above and below the eye on about day 25 of gestation. These grow towards each other and elongate to cover the developing eye, meeting and fusing together by day 40. The eyelids separate 10–14 days postnatally in dogs and cats. The eyelid epidermis, cilia, lacrimal gland, nictitans gland, meibomian (tarsal) glands and the sweat and sebaceous glands (glands of Moll and Zeis, respectively) are all derived from the embryonic surface ectoderm. Neural crest-derived mesenchyme contributes to the development of the tarsal plate and dermis, and the eyelid muscles are derived from mesoderm.

Anatomy
The eyelids comprise three layers (Figure 9.1):

- Haired eyelid skin on the outer surface
- Muscle extending to a fibrous tarsal plate containing meibomian glands. The tarsal plate is poorly developed in the dog and better developed in the cat
- Palpebral conjunctiva on the inner surface extending to the conjunctival fornix, where it is reflected to become the bulbar conjunctiva covering the sclera.

The upper eyelid bears two or more rows of cilia (eyelashes) in the dog, whilst in the cat, the first row of skin hairs is often well developed and these act as cilia. Neither cats nor dogs have cilia on the lower lids.

The width of the eyelid opening is controlled by two opposing groups of muscles. The orbicularis oculi muscle closes the palpebral fissure and enables blinking. The upper eyelid is more mobile

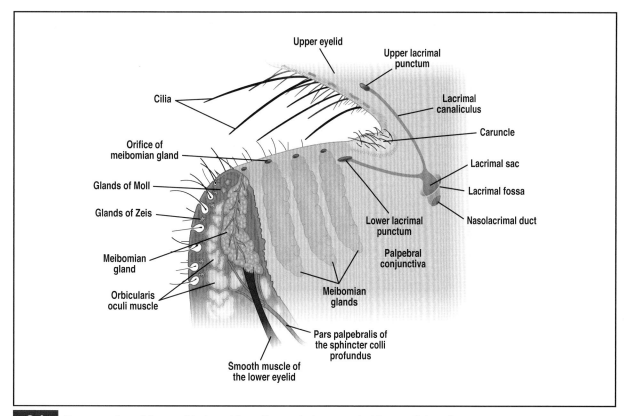

9.1 Cross-section of the eyelid viewed from the posterior aspect of the medial canthus.

than the lower eyelid, resulting in greater coverage of the cornea during each blink. The orbicularis oculi muscle is innervated by the palpebral branch of the auriculopalpebral nerve, which is a branch of the facial nerve (cranial nerve (CN) VII). The levator palpebrae superioris (innervated by the oculomotor nerve (CN III)), the pars palpebralis of the sphincter colli profundus (innervated by the dorsal buccal branch of the facial nerve (CN VII)) and the Müller muscle (smooth muscle with sympathetic innervation also known as the superior tarsal muscle) all widen the palpebral fissure (Figure 9.2). The levator palpebrae superioris and superior rectus extraocular muscles have a common innervation, so that the globe and upper eyelid are elevated together.

The upper and lower eyelids join at the medial and lateral canthi (see Figures 9.1 and 9.2). The medial and lateral canthi are stabilized by the medial and lateral canthal tendons and the retractor anguli oculi muscle. The medial canthal tendon is a distinct fibrous band originating from the periosteum of the frontal bone, whilst the lateral canthal tendon is a musculofibrous band which lies immediately subconjunctivally and connects the muscle at the lateral canthus to the orbital ligament. The alignment of this fibrous band varies with skull shape and can result in involution of the lateral canthus in broad-skulled breeds (see Entropion below).

Sensation is provided to the eyelids by branches of the ophthalmic and maxillary nerves from the trigeminal nerve (CN V). Although the ophthalmic nerve branches are predominantly medial and the maxillary nerve branches are lateral, there is extensive overlap in the areas they innervate.

Sensory deficits in the eyelid skin cause loss of the palpebral reflex. The palpebral reflex should be assessed by touching the periocular skin at both medial and lateral canthi. The observation of spontaneous blinking in the absence of a palpebral reflex helps distinguish a sensory deficit from facial paralysis.

Just posterior to the mucocutaneous junction of the palpebral margin of each eyelid there is a slight groove, sometimes called the margo-intermarginalis or grey line, in which the openings of the meibomian glands can be seen (Figure 9.3). Meibomian glands are modified sebaceous glands. There are 20–40 glands in each eyelid, which are visible through the palpebral conjunctiva when the eyelid is everted (Figure 9.4). They are white or yellow columnar structures that run at right angles to the palpebral margin and are responsible for producing meibum, which forms the lipid fraction of the tear film. Meibum is liquid at body temperature and is expressed from the meibomian gland opening during blinking, forming the superficial layer of the precorneal tear film. Meibum decreases the surface tension of the tear film, drawing water in and increasing the tear film thickness. It also stabilizes the tear film, reducing evaporation, and coats the eyelid margins, minimizing tear overflow over the eyelid margin itself. Additional eyelid glandular structures include the glands of Zeis and Moll. The glands of Zeis are sebaceous glands associated with the eyelid cilia. The glands of Moll are modified sweat glands. Their functional significance in animals is unknown, but they can become infected, resulting in eyelid styes or external hordeola.

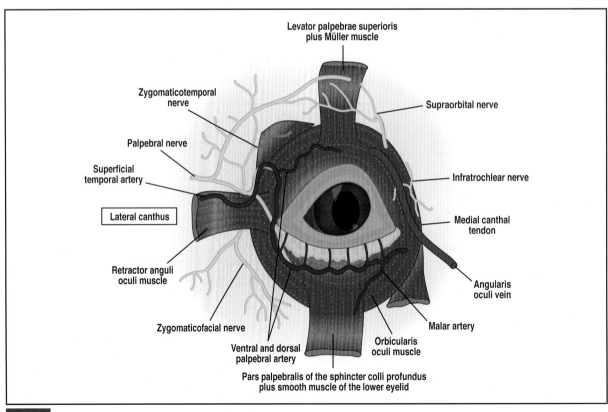

9.2   Gross anatomy of the eyelids of the dog.

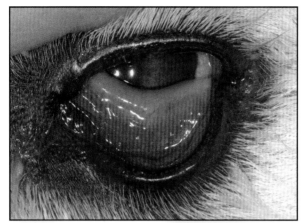

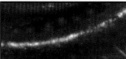

9.3 The meibomian gland orifices can be visualized along the eyelid margins in a shallow groove in this 2-year-old male Samoyed.

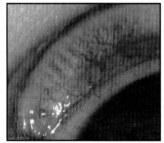

9.4 The vertically aligned meibomian glands in this 5-year-old Shih Tzu bitch can be visualized through the palpebral conjunctiva perpendicular to the eyelid margin.

There is a small protuberance at the medial canthus called the caruncle, from which fine hairs project. The tear film drains to the nasolacrimal duct through lacrimal puncta, which are present in the conjunctival surfaces of both the upper and lower medial eyelid in the dog and cat, approximately 2–5 mm from the eyelid margin (see Figure 9.1).

Function

The eyelids are vital in maintaining ocular surface health:

- Once the menace response has been learnt, it is the resultant eyelid closure that protects the eye from traumatic insult
- Cilia and sensory vibrissae in the eyelid contribute to the protective effect
- The eyelids contribute mucin and lipid to the tear film. Mucin is produced in the goblet cells of the palpebral conjunctiva, whilst lipid is released from the meibomian glands
- The action of blinking is responsible for:
  - Distributing the tear film and therefore providing nutrition and hydration to the ocular surface
  - Draining the tear film to remove toxic waste. Blinking creates pressure changes in the lacrimal sac, which draws tears down the lacrimal canaliculi. As the eyelid opens, pressure is put on the lacrimal sac, pushing the tears down the nasolacrimal duct
  - Physical removal of debris from the ocular surface.

In order to carry out these functions efficiently, the smooth eyelid margin should rest against the ocular surface. Unfortunately, in many breeds of dog and a few breeds of cat, the eyelid conformation is far from optimal. The resulting poor eyelid–globe apposition is a contributory factor in the development of ocular surface disease.

Investigation of disease

Ophthalmic examination

The ophthalmic examination is covered in Chapter 1. However, where there is eyelid disease, particular attention should be paid to:

- The initial examination, which should be performed from a distance, noting any asymmetry in eyelid conformation, signs of discomfort or any periocular skin changes
- The presence, nature and distribution of any ocular discharge. The distribution of discharge can give clues as to the areas of cilia contact with the ocular surface or tear film (Figure 9.5)
- Assessment of the presence of spontaneous and effective blinking and evaluation of the blink rate
- A 'hands-on' focal examination with the naked eye and a light source ± magnification. Any abnormalities should be noted as should the eyelid conformation and eyelid–globe apposition in a variety of head positions (see Entropion below)
- A systematic examination of the eyelids, with particular attention to the periocular skin, upper and lower eyelid margins and (following eyelid eversion) the palpebral conjunctiva. The presence and appearance of the meibomian glands and the nature of the discharge that can be expressed from them can be assessed (see Figure 9.3). The meibomian glands can be visualized through the palpebral conjunctiva (see Figure 9.4). All four lacrimal puncta should be identified and their size assessed, as well as any

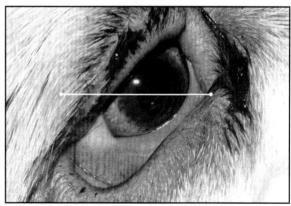

9.5 A 2-year-old male Clumber Spaniel with discharge adherent to the upper eyelashes, which is an indication that these lashes are contacting the cornea or lower conjunctival fornix at times of low head carriage. The white line demonstrates the difference in the horizontal position of the medial and lateral canthi, indicating lateral canthal instability.

discharge within them noted as this may indicate dacryocystitis. Pressure applied over the lacrimal sac whilst observing the puncta may result in the expression of purulent material in such cases
- The presence of entropion. If entropion is diagnosed, topical local anaesthetic should be applied to abolish any spastic component, allowing any residual anatomical or cicatricial contribution to be assessed
- Subsequent findings during the ophthalmic examination following eyelid examination, such as corneal ulceration, which may direct the examiner to look back at the immediately adjacent eyelid to check for an inciting cause for the ulcer (e.g. an ectopic cilium)
- The application of fluorescein. This is usually applied at the end of the ophthalmic examination to check for corneal ulceration, corneal perforations and nasolacrimal duct patency. It is also used to evaluate tear film quality by assessing the tear film break up time (TFBUT), which may indirectly provide the examiner with information about the meibomian gland and conjunctival goblet cell function (see Chapter 10). The fluorescein-stained tear film will be disrupted by any facial hairs or eyelashes contacting the corneal surface, which may make them easier to identify (Figure 9.6). The dye may also pool around and highlight ectopic cilia as they perforate the palpebral conjunctival surface
- A general physical examination, which is mandatory as eyelid disease may be part of a systemic disease or a generalized skin disease.

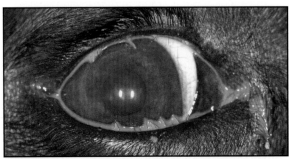

9.6   Distichiasis in a 1-year-old Staffordshire Bull Terrier bitch. The extra lashes are highlighted by fluorescein application.

Laboratory investigation
Laboratory investigation has been covered in Chapter 3. Specific tests that may be indicated for eyelid disease include:

- Cytology using tape strips examined 'in-house' to identify bacteria and yeast colonization of the periocular skin
- Swabs for bacterial culture and sensitivity testing of ulcerated periocular skin lesions or of discharge expressed from abnormal meibomian glands
- Periocular skin scrapes and hair plucks for diagnosis of parasitic disease. These are obtained in the same way as anywhere else on the body, avoiding abrading the eyelid margin

- Microscopic examination of material expressed from the meibomian glands, which may identify bacteria or parasites (particularly *Demodex* spp.)
- Microscopic examination of hair plucks and submission for fungal culture
- Fine-needle aspiration of eyelid masses
- Surgical biopsy:
  - Punch biopsy of the periocular skin
  - Full-thickness eyelid wedge resection may be necessary if the eyelid margin is involved
  - Biopsy of eyelid masses.
- Aspirates and biopsy samples are generally submitted for histopathology and/or immunohistochemistry, but may also be submitted for polymerase chain reaction (PCR; for feline herpesvirus-1 or leishmaniosis) or tissue culture (for mycobacterial disease).

Canine conditions

Congenital abnormalities

Abnormalities of eyelid opening
The eyelids normally open 10–14 days postpartum in dogs and cats. If they open prematurely, when the lacrimal apparatus is still immature, corneal desiccation, conjunctivitis, keratitis and corneal ulceration can develop. If this is left untreated, corneal perforation and endophthalmitis can result. Treatment involves frequent lubrication and possibly also a temporary tarsorrhaphy.

In contrast, delayed opening (ankyloblepharon) is more commonly seen and is caused by the failure of the bridge between the two eyelids to atrophy. Fluid can collect beneath the fused eyelids of neonates and, if infected, results in a build-up of pus and inflammatory debris (ophthalmia neonatorum). The application of warm compresses and gentle digital traction may encourage eyelid opening. If this conservative approach is unsuccessful within about 24 hours, the eyelids should be very carefully prised apart using a blunt-ended instrument such as fine haemostats or blunt-ended scissors. The appropriate instrument should be inserted into the spontaneous first opening, or into the groove of the future fissure, starting at the medial canthus and taking great care not to damage the cornea. The fused eyelid margins should never be incised using a scalpel or scissors because this will cause irreversible damage to the eyelid margins. Once the palpebral fissure has been opened, topical treatment should be commenced with an appropriate antibiotic ointment.

Coloboma
Eyelid colobomas are congenital defects in which a partial or full-thickness length of eyelid is absent (eyelid agenesis). In dogs, it is usually the lower lateral eyelid that is affected and it can be unilateral or bilateral. The effect of this is that there is increased corneal exposure, increased evaporation of tears, poor tear film distribution and trichiasis, as the adjacent skin hairs contact the cornea. The extent of the defect can vary, from a small notch that can be closed directly by creation of a wedge resection, to

complete eyelid agenesis. Where large defects are present, more complicated blepharoplastic techniques are needed. A variety of techniques can be used depending on the position and extent of the defect (see below). Eyelid colobomas are less common in dogs than in cats and, when they do occur, may be associated with other congenital defects such as dermoids.

Dermoid

The term dermoid refers to the presence of aberrant tissue containing skin. Dermoids may occur as a result of abnormal differentiation of an isolated group of cells or inclusion of surface ectoderm during closure of fetal clefts. Dermoids may affect the limbus, cornea, conjunctiva and eyelids (see Chapters 11, 12 and 13). Dermoids are often referred to as choristomas, which are defined as 'histologically normal tissue in an abnormal location'. Blinking is abnormal and trichiasis can result in corneal irritation and damage (Figure 9.7). Treatment comprises removal of the abnormal tissue with repair and realignment of the eyelid margin. The fissure length is usually sufficient to enable direct closure following a simple wedge excision without complicated blepharoplastic techniques.

Macropalpebral fissure

Macropalpebral fissure (euryblepharon) is usually bilateral and describes an enlarged palpebral fissure. It is typically seen in the St Bernard, Neapolitan Mastiff, Clumber Spaniel and Bloodhound, in which the combination of overlong eyelids and weak lateral canthal support leads to ectropion, frequently combined with lateral lower eyelid entropion (see Figures 9.5, 9.8 and 9.9). The resulting eyelid conformation is colloquially referred to as 'diamond eye'. In brachycephalic breeds, the orbits are shallow and the eyelids are taut, so the effect of the eyelid being overlong is the development of varying degrees of exposure keratitis and a tendency to proptosis (Figure 9.10). Surgical shortening of the palpebral fissure is indicated and the appropriate surgical techniques are discussed in the section on Entropion (see below).

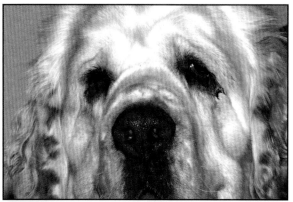

9.8 Macropalpebral fissure in a Clumber Spaniel (same dog as in Figure 9.5).

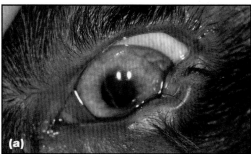

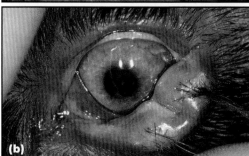

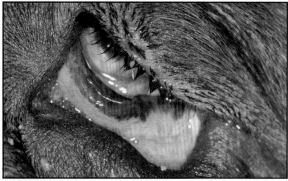

9.9 Macropalpebral fissure in a 1-year-old male Neapolitan Mastiff with lower eyelid ectropion, lateral lower eyelid entropion and upper eyelid ptosis, resulting in the upper eyelid cilia contacting the exposed lower conjunctival fornix.

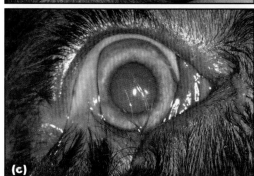

9.7 Bilateral eyelid dermoids in a 5-month-old male Labrador Retriever. **(a)** Left eye. **(b)** Lower left eyelid everted to demonstrate the extent of the dermoid. **(c)** Right eye. (Courtesy of S Monclin)

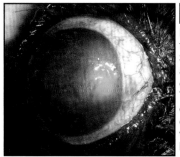

9.10

Macropalpebral fissure in a 9-year-old Shih Tzu with associated axial exposure keratitis. There is also medial canthal entropion and caruncular trichiasis with medial ulcerative keratitis.

Micropalpebral fissure

Abnormally small eyelid fissures are commonly seen in certain breeds of dog, such as the Shetland Sheepdog, Rough Collie and Schipperke. Surgical lengthening of the eyelid fissure is not usually indicated, although the tight eyelid–globe apposition can lead to reduction or loss of the lacrimal lake and resultant epiphora.

Lagophthalmos

Lagophthalmos is the inability to close the eyelids. It may be the result of facial nerve dysfunction preventing eyelid closure, but is most commonly encountered in brachycephalic breeds (such as the Pekingese and Pug) which have prominent globes and/or large palpebral fissures. Incomplete eyelid closure leads to poor tear film distribution, corneal desiccation and exposure keratitis with associated corneal neovascularization and ulceration (Figure 9.11). Owners of dogs with lagophthalmos may have noticed that the eyelids are not completely closed when the dog is asleep. The application of ointment or gel-based tear substitutes may help to halt corneal changes, but if corneal pathology does progress, surgical shortening of the eyelids is required.

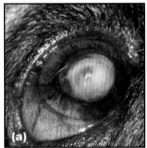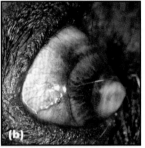

9.11 Axial corneal stromal ulceration in the right eye of a 5-year-old male neutered Pug due to lagophthalmos and exposure. **(a)** Front view. **(b)** Side view.

Cilia abnormalities

Distichiasis

Distichiasis is a condition whereby extra eyelashes arise from or adjacent to the meibomian gland orifices (see Figures 9.6 and 9.12 to 9.16). When more than one hair emerges from a single orifice, it is termed districhiasis. Predisposed breeds include the Miniature Longhaired Dachshund, American and English Cocker Spaniels, Flat-coated Retriever, Miniature Poodle, Shetland Sheepdog, Rough Collie, Cavalier King Charles Spaniel, Pekingese, Welsh Springer Spaniel, Bulldog, Boxer, Weimaraner and Staffordshire Bull Terrier. In many of these breeds, the extra eyelashes are fine and incidental findings that do not require treatment.

If a dog with distichiasis presents with ocular discomfort, it is important to perform a full ophthalmic examination and exclude other potentially inciting causes before concluding that distichiasis is responsible. It should be remembered that distichiasis develops at a young age, so if problems arise in an older dog, or if the discomfort is unilateral when the

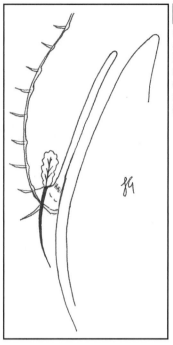

9.12 Cross-section of an eyelid showing the location of an abnormally situated eyelash shaft within the meibomian gland. (Courtesy of J Green)

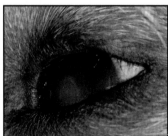

9.13 Distichiasis contributing to corneal ulceration in an 11-month-old Jack Russell Terrier bitch.

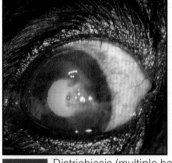

9.14 Distichiasis (multiple hairs emerging from one meibomian gland) contributing to corneal ulceration in a 5-year-old male Pug. Management of corneal disease in this dog should address not only the distichiasis but also the macropalpebral fissure and medial lower eyelid entropion.

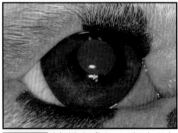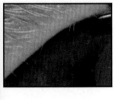

9.15 Multiple fine eyelashes in an 18-month-old Boxer bitch, which are unlikely to be clinically significant.

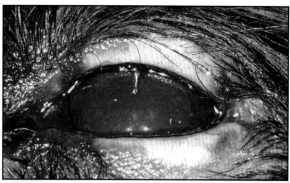

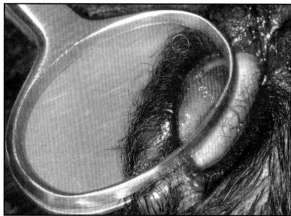

9.16 Eversion of the eyelid using a chalazion clamp prior to cryosurgical treatment for long curly ectopic cilia and distichiasis in an 8-month-old Toy Poodle bitch.

9.17 Eyelid depigmentation 10 days following cryosurgery (same dog as in Figure 9.16).

extra eyelashes appear equally distributed bilaterally, then they are unlikely to be responsible. If there is any doubt, the response to simple epilation of the eyelashes should be assessed before considering permanent removal techniques. Permanent removal techniques include:

- Eyelid wedge resection – for the removal of a solitary eyelash
- Cryotherapy – scarring is minimized and the meibomian gland tissue can recover because the hair follicle is differentially temperature sensitive. Cryotherapy has the benefit of being able to treat more extensive areas of the eyelid, thus addressing any aberrant lashes present in the meibomian glands but unerupted at the time of treatment. A chalazion clamp is used to stabilize and evert the eyelid to allow cryotherapy to be applied transconjunctivally, directly over the meibomian glands, with either a cryoprobe or controlled application of a cryospray. The chalazion clamp also limits the rich blood supply to the area being treated, which allows more rapid freezing and slows thawing, increasing the effectiveness of cryonecrosis. Use of an operating microscope improves the precision of cryoapplication. A double freeze–thaw cycle is usually used. Eyelid swelling occurs postoperatively and should be routinely managed with perioperative analgesics and anti-inflammatory drugs, but resolves within a few days. Eyelid depigmentation often occurs (Figure 9.17) but the eyelids generally re-pigment within 2–6 months. A 20% recurrence rate can be anticipated
- Electrolysis – this is a time-consuming procedure when there are large numbers of eyelashes. Scarring and distortion of the eyelid margins can occur, as well as irreversible

meibomian gland damage in the treated areas. This procedure can only be used to treat those aberrant lashes that are erupted at the time of surgery and, because growth is cyclical, the procedure may need to be repeated as new hairs emerge. Gentle pressure on the eyelids over the meibomian glands can expose some eyelashes that have not yet erupted, reducing the need for additional treatments

- Sharp knife surgery – techniques used include lid splitting or resection of a strip of conjunctiva and tarsal plate containing follicles (Bedford, 1973; Long, 1991). Both techniques can result in incomplete resection and eyelid distortion (Figure 9.18), particularly in breeds with thin eyelids. The complications can worsen the original problem and can be difficult to correct (Pena and Garcia, 1999). A final surgical option is to perform a Hotz–Celsus procedure to evert the eyelid and direct the hairs away from the cornea. However, this option risks altering the all-important relationship between the eyelid margin and ocular surface.

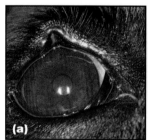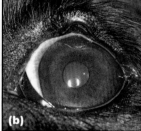

9.18 Eyelid distortion and persistence of distichiasis following attempted subconjunctival surgical resection in a 4-year-old Labrador Retriever bitch. **(a)** Right eye. **(b)** Left eye.

Ectopic cilia

Ectopic cilia are atypical forms of distichiasis that arise from a follicle inside the meibomian gland or from follicles near the meibomian duct. In contrast to distichiasis, ectopic cilia emerge through the conjunctival surface of the eyelid, a few millimetres from the eyelid margin, and are directed towards the cornea (Figure 9.19). They may be solitary or in small clumps, classically occurring in young dogs, and usually (but not always) located in the middle of the

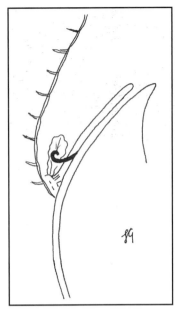

9.19
Cross-section of an eyelid showing an ectopic cilium arising within a meibomian gland and emerging through the palpebral conjunctiva to contact the corneal surface. (Courtesy of J Green)

upper eyelid (see Figures 9.16 and 9.20 to 9.22). Several breeds are predisposed to ectopic cilia, including the Cairn Terrier, Dachshund, Flat-coated Retriever, English Bulldog, Staffordshire Bull Terrier, Lhasa Apso, Maltese, Miniature Poodle, Pekingese, Shetland Sheepdog and Shih Tzu. Ectopic cilia frequently occur in conjunction with distichiasis. They are resected *en bloc* using a chalazion clamp and No. 11 scalpel blade, scleral trephine or 2 mm biopsy punch (Figure 9.23). The surgical site can subsequently be treated with cryotherapy to reduce the potential for recurrence.

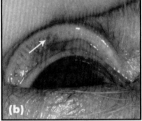

9.20 **(a)** Superior corneal neovascularization and ulceration associated with an ectopic cilium in a 5-year-old Shih Tzu bitch. Note the tendency towards nasal fold trichiasis. **(b)** A non-pigmented ectopic cilium was identified within a raised, slightly discoloured area in the middle of the upper palpebral conjunctiva (arrowed).

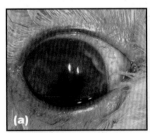
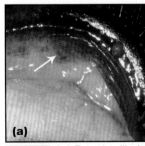

9.21 **(a)** Ectopic cilia (arrowed) in the upper palpebral conjunctiva of a 2-year-old Pug. Note that the meibomian gland openings are also visible. **(b)** Clump of ectopic cilia in the upper palpebral conjunctiva of a 4-year-old Flat-coated Retriever.

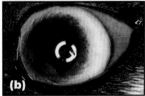
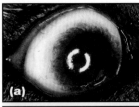
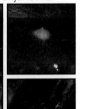

9.22 **(a)** Right and **(b)** left eye in a 2-year-old male Siberian Husky with bilateral distichiasis but only right-sided ocular discomfort and corneal disease (see distorted specular reflection), indicating the likelihood of an ectopic cilium. **(c)** A short stumpy ectopic cilium (solid white arrow) and a long fine ectopic cilium (dashed white arrow) are visible in the lower eyelid conjunctiva.

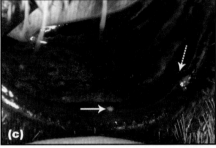

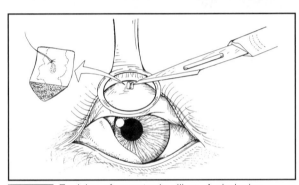

9.23 Excision of an ectopic cilium. A chalazion clamp is applied to the affected eyelid to immobilize and evert it. A biopsy punch or No. 11 scalpel blade is used to excise the cilium and its follicle.

Trichiasis

Trichiasis is the presence of normally located but abnormally directed hairs, which contact and irritate the ocular surface. Misdirected hairs can arise from multiple locations, including:

- Upper eyelid cilia (Figure 9.24)
- Caruncular hair (see Figure 9.10)
- Nasal fold or facial hair (Figures 9.25 to 9.27)
- Hair protruding from other prominent skin protuberances, such as the medial upper eyelid in the Chow Chow (Figure 9.28)
- Hair adjacent to areas of eyelid agenesis
- Misaligned eyelid margin following trauma without surgical repair
- Misaligned eyelid margin following poor surgical repair
- Blepharoplasty techniques involving the transposition of facial skin without creating an eyelid margin (e.g. bucket handle technique, sliding lateral canthoplasty, H-plasty, sliding skin grafts)
- Entropion.

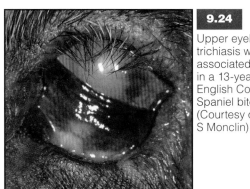

9.24 Upper eyelid trichiasis with associated keratitis in a 13-year-old English Cocker Spaniel bitch. (Courtesy of S Monclin)

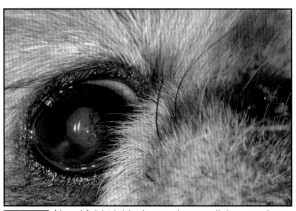

9.25 Nasal fold trichiasis causing medial corneal scarring and pigmentation in a 9-year-old male Pekingese.

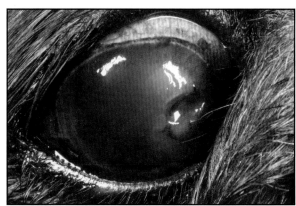

9.26 Nasal fold trichiasis causing deep stromal ulcerative keratitis in an 8-year-old Pekingese. (Courtesy of Willows Referral Service)

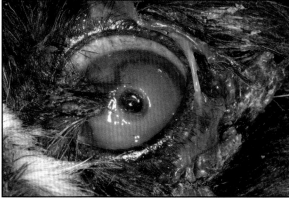

9.27 Descemetocele in a Shih Tzu associated with contact from matted facial hair.

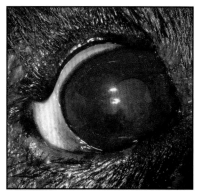

9.28 A 6-year-old male Chow Chow with overlong lower eyelid and lateral lower eyelid entropion (manually everted in this case, but the location can still be seen as a region of depigmentation on the lower eyelid skin), as well as trichiasis from the medial upper eyelid prominence. The distribution of the pathology suggests that corneal irritation has occurred as a result of both areas of trichiasis and both require surgical correction.

Treatment depends on the degree of discomfort and corneal pathology that the trichiasis incites. For example, many Shih Tzus live their whole lives with caruncular hairs that never cause a clinical problem and consequently seldom warrant treatment. Surgical management options for caruncular hairs and nasal fold trichiasis are discussed below.

Eyelid position abnormalities

Entropion
Entropion is the inversion of all or parts of the eyelid margin(s). In this position, the eyelid hairs are in direct contact with the cornea, leading to irritation and corneal pathology. Entropion can be further classified as:

- Breed-related/anatomical entropion
- Spastic entropion
- Atonic/senile entropion
- Cicatricial entropion.

Breed-related/anatomical entropion: Anatomical entropion is common in dogs and is usually bilateral, although it can be unilateral. It occurs as a product of orbital anatomy, skull conformation, eyelid length and the amount of skin around the face. It can develop soon after eye opening, particularly in breeds with heavy periocular skin folds, such as the Shar Pei and Chow Chow, but more usually develops between 4 and 12 months of age as the facial conformation changes. In some cases, it can reduce or completely resolve as the conformation matures. Breed-related entropion may develop in middle-aged animals, especially males. This appears to be associated with increased subcutaneous fat deposits. Most commonly, this results in upper eyelid entropion. The distribution of the entropion, and thus the optimal method for correction, varies with breed and/or predisposing anatomy (see below). Entropion is likely to have a hereditary basis and dogs that require surgical alteration of their facial conformation should not be bred from.

Spastic entropion: Spastic entropion is a secondary entropion that results from spasm of the orbicularis oculi muscle and retraction of the globe due to ocular pain, causing the eyelid to turn inwards. The resultant trichiasis worsens the pain and globe retraction. Most forms of entropion have a spastic component.

Atonic/senile entropion: Atonic entropion occurs as a result of age-related loss of skin elasticity and muscle tone in breeds that already have excessive facial skin, such as the English Cocker Spaniel. As the forehead skin droops, the long upper eyelid cilia are directed inferiorly where they contact the lower conjunctival fornix and/or cornea causing conjunctivitis and keratitis (see Figure 9.24). Lower lid ectropion also develops or worsens.

Cicatricial entropion: Cicatricial entropion is uncommon and results from lid distortion and scarring following injury, chronic dermatitis or inappropriate surgery.

Diagnosis: Successful treatment of entropion requires very careful preoperative assessment of the individual dog. Eyelid conformation should always be evaluated in the non-sedated/conscious patient. Local anaesthetic should always be applied prior to assessment to abolish any spastic contribution to the entropion and to avoid over-correction. It is also important to assess eyelid–globe apposition in a number of different head positions, particularly when the head is held in a downward posture, as most dogs spend a significant amount of time in this position and any entropion/ectropion may be exacerbated by slippage of the facial mask.

This is achieved by examining all but very large-breed dogs on an examination table. The head of the patient is tilted downwards by holding on to the nose and the examiner then crouches at the end of the table and looks up into the eyes of the patient. It is important that the owner/nurse/assistant is not holding the head of the patient either during this process or when the head is in a horizontal position because this will distort the natural orientation of the skin and eyelids.

Observation of the distribution of tearing and ocular discharge also provides clues as to the problematic area; for example, lateral canthal epiphora may indicate lateral canthal entropion, and discharge adherent to the cilia of the upper eyelid suggests that these hairs may be intermittently contacting the inferior conjunctival fornix (see Figure 9.5). Entropion may only be present intermittently and, in these dogs, can usually be provoked by gently inverting the eyelid manually.

Treatment:

Young puppies: Eyelid conformation may change as the puppy ages, so some cases of entropion can self-correct with time. This means that permanent corrective surgery is best delayed until 5–12 months of age (depending on the progression, breed and degree of entropion). Temporary correction is always indicated because the periocular hairs rubbing on the cornea are a source of pain and can cause blepharospasm, globe retraction and worsening of the entropion. This can, in turn, lead to corneal ulceration and scarring or even globe perforation.

Temporary eversion involves placement of non-absorbable interrupted Lembert pattern sutures in the affected region of the eyelid. The sutures should be oriented perpendicular to the eyelid margin. The first bite of the sutures should be placed within 2–3 mm of the eyelid margin to be effective (Figure 9.29). Several rows of stitches may be required in Shar Pei puppies. The sutures can be pre-placed and tissue glue applied to the presumptive skin fold that will be formed before tying the sutures, in order to help prolong the eversion. The sutures should be directed away from the cornea. This procedure may need to be repeated on several occasions if the sutures fail and the entropion recurs before the puppy is old enough for permanent surgical correction.

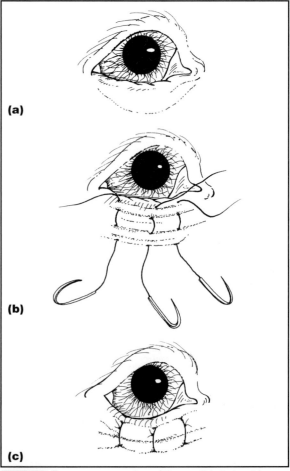

9.29 Temporary eversion of the eyelids to treat lower eyelid entropion. **(a)** The lower eyelid is exhibiting entropion. **(b–c)** Three or four temporary everting sutures of an interrupted Lembert pattern are pre-placed in the eyelid skin before tightening sufficiently to correct the eyelid deformity. This procedure can also be applied to the upper eyelids and multiple rows of sutures can be placed if indicated (e.g. in Shar Pei puppies).

An alternative technique that has been used in puppies with entropion involving only the lateral lower eyelid is temporary partial tarsorrhaphy (Lewin, 2000). This procedure involves placement of a single mattress suture from the lower to upper eyelids (Figure 9.30). The suture enters and leaves the eyelid through the eyelid margin, so that when the mattress suture is gently tightened, the upper and lower eyelid margins become apposed, preventing the lower eyelid from inverting. There is no contact between the suture and the cornea.

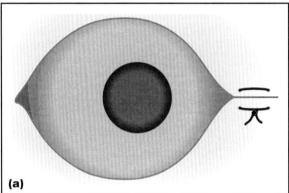

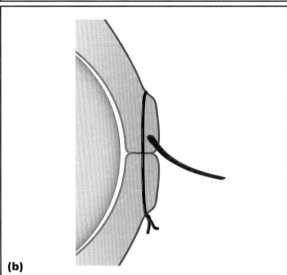

9.30 Temporary partial tarsorrhaphy. **(a)** Sufficient mattress or simple interrupted sutures are placed to close the required length of the eyelid. **(b)** The sutures are placed so that they enter through the haired eyelid and exit through the eyelid margin in the area of the meibomian gland openings. The needle then enters the opposing eyelid through the eyelid margin and exits through the haired eyelid before the suture is tied. When the suture is tied, the eyelid margins abut. Sutures placed in this position should not be able to contact and damage the cornea. This technique may also be useful in the management of proptosis and corneal exposure.

Adults: Entropion in adults requires definitive surgical correction. The basic treatment is a skin or skin–muscle resection (Hotz–Celsus) in which an ellipse of skin and/or underlying muscle is removed corresponding to the degree of in-turning. The eyelid is placed under tension and stabilized using either a finger or lid plate inserted into the conjunctival fornix. The first incision needs to be parallel and close to (2 mm away from) the eyelid margin (Figure 9.31). The wound is closed using simple interrupted sutures of 6/0 (0.7 metric) polyglactin. The use of absorbable sutures in the skin appears to go against the time-honoured doctrines of surgery; however, these dogs are often head shy as a result of prolonged ocular discomfort and the removal of sutures can be challenging without sedation. In addition, braided suture material is softer and less likely to cause problems if it comes into contact with the cornea compared with non-absorbable suture material. The central part of the wound is sutured first. Additional sutures are placed to close the remaining defect. Each subsequent suture is placed such that it bisects the distance still to be sutured in order to prevent unequal traction on the wound edges.

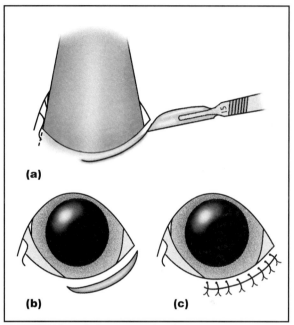

9.31 Hotz–Celsus correction for lower eyelid entropion. **(a)** The degree of correction is assessed in the conscious and non-sedated patient. A lid plate is positioned in the conjunctival sac to support the eyelid and a No. 15 blade is used to incise the strip of skin to be removed. The first incision is parallel to, and 2 mm from, the eyelid margin. **(b)** A piece of skin the required width and length is excised. **(c)** The defect is closed with simple interrupted sutures of 6/0 (0.7 metric) polyglactin, with each suture placed to bisect the wound. The knots are positioned away from the eyelid margin.

In many breeds, the anatomical cause of the entropion is more complex and alternative surgical procedures may be required (Figure 9.32). Corrective eyelid surgery is often described as 'an art, not a science'. There is no 'one-stop surgery' that is effective for all presentations and, occasionally, surgery altering one part of the eyelid conformation can inadvertently and adversely affect another area of the eyelid. The ability to choose the correct technique and estimate the degree of eyelid adjustment required develops with experience. Those patients with more complicated eyelid conformational abnormalities may, therefore, benefit from specialist advice or referral.

Cause of entropion	Treatment	Predisposed breeds
Overlong eyelids (see Figures 9.28, 9.33 and 9.34)	Eyelid shortening by wedge resection (Figure 9.35). In some dogs this alone may be sufficient, or a concurrent (but smaller) Hotz–Celsus skin–muscle resection may be required (Read and Broun, 2007) (see Figure 9.31). Eyelid shortening and support of the lateral canthus can be achieved with a modified Kühnt–Szymanowski technique (Munger and Carter, 1984) (Figure 9.36)	Chow Chow, Labrador Retriever, Shar Pei, setters
Excess facial folds around the eyes (medial brow folds and/or lateral check folds are often seen in conjunction with other eyelid conformational problems; see Figure 9.28)	Local excision of skin folds	Chow Chow, Shar Pei
Inverted lateral canthus due to angled traction on the lateral canthal tendon (affects the lateral lower ± upper eyelid) (Figure 9.37)	Sectioning of the lateral canthal tendon (Robertson and Roberts, 1995ab). The lateral canthus is grasped and reflected laterally to expose the conjunctival surface. A vertical conjunctival incision is made over the fibrous band, which is located by palpation and is situated 10–12 mm beyond the canthus. The fibrous band is then transected with scissors, fanning the blades dorsally and ventrally until the tension on the lateral canthus is released. Lateral canthal tendonectomy is generally performed in combination with a lateral lower eyelid wedge resection, as release of the lateral canthus can result in ectropion. A concurrent lateral lower eyelid Hotz–Celsus skin resection may also be indicated, depending on the preoperative presentation	Broad-skulled breeds with redundant facial skin, including the Chow Chow, Labrador Retriever, Mastiff and Rottweiler
Brachycephalic skull conformation associated with: • Nasal folds and nasal fold trichiasis (see Figures 9.20a, 9.25 and 9.26) • Excessive nasal skin folds causing medial lower ± upper eyelid entropion (see Figures 9.14, 9.39, 9.40 and 9.41) • Medial caruncular trichiasis (see Figures 9.10 and 9.41) • Lagophthalmos and globe exposure (see Figures 9.10, 9.11, 9.39 and 9.40)	• Nasal fold excision (Figure 9.38) • Lower ± upper eyelid modified Hotz–Celsus procedure (Figure 9.42) • Resection of caruncle as part of a medial canthoplasty • Permanent canthoplasty (for treatment of a macropalpebral fissure). Whilst canthoplasties can be performed either medially or laterally, a medial canthoplasty is indicated in breeds with a brachycephalic conformation (Figure 9.43). This will not only reduce the size of the palpebral fissure and remove caruncular hairs (Figure 9.44), but may also protect the medial cornea against nasal fold trichiasis. It can be combined with a modified Hotz–Celsus procedure (Figure 9.45) and/or nasal fold excision	Bulldog, Pekingese, Pug, Shih Tzu (and Persian cats)
Facial droop (Figure 9.46) ± upper eyelid ptosis/trichiasis (see Figure 9.24) in breeds with redundant forehead skin and atonic/senile entropion	Removal of large amounts of skin from the upper eyelids by a Stades procedure (Stades, 1987; Stades and Boevé, 1987) (Figures 9.47 and 9.48) or from the forehead by a face lift (coronal rhytidectomy) (McCallum and Welser, 2004) (Figure 9.49) combined with the appropriate eyelid surgery. Alternative techniques such as brow slings (Willis et al., 1999), stellate (Stuhr et al., 1997) and sagittal rhytidectomies (Bedford, 1990) are also described	Basset Hound, Bloodhound, Chinese Shar Pei, Chow Chow, Clumber Spaniel, English and American Cocker Spaniels, Mastiff
'Diamond eye' conformation: overlong upper and lower eyelids combined with weakness at the lateral canthus (see Figures 9.5, 9.8 and 9.9). (The medial and lateral canthi should be level. In diamond eyes, there is weakness at the lateral canthus which can lead to lateral canthal inversion)	Requires upper and lower eyelid shortening by simple wedge resection, sparing the lateral canthus, combined with a permanent suture to put traction on and anchor the lateral canthus (modified Wyman canthoplasty) (Figure 9.50). More complicated techniques have also been described, but they disrupt the lateral canthus (Bigelbach, 1996; Bedford, 1998)	Basset Hound, Bloodhound, Clumber Spaniel, Great Dane, Neapolitan Mastiff, Newfoundland, St Bernard (the same breeds often need face lifts)

9.32 Causes and treatment options for entropion in dogs.

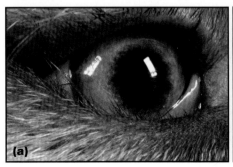

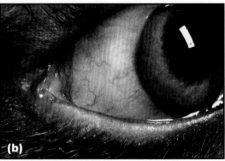

9.33

(a) Lower lateral eyelid entropion in an Italian Spinone. **(b)** Manual eversion reveals that the eyelid is overlong. Deposits and slight depigmentation can be seen on the eyelid margin consistent with it being chronically wet. (Courtesy of Willows Referral Service)

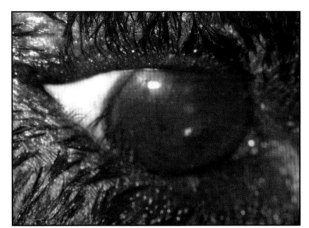

9.34 Lower lateral eyelid entropion in a 6-year-old Chow Chow combined with trichiasis from the medial upper eyelid prominence (same dog as in Figure 9.28). Eversion revealed that the eyelid was overlong.

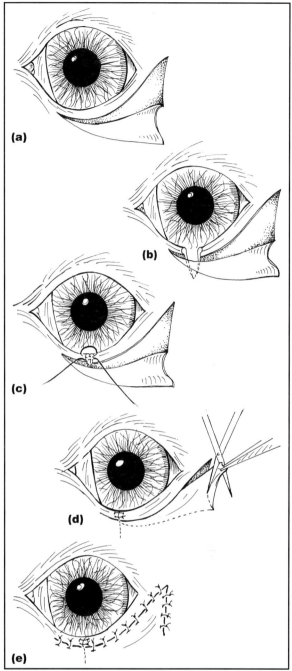

9.36 Munger and Carter's (1984) modification of the Kühnt–Szymanowski procedure for eyelid shortening and correction of lower eyelid ectropion. **(a)** A skin incision is made 3 mm from and parallel to the eyelid margin along the lateral one-half to three-quarters of the lower eyelid. The incision is extended dorsolaterally to 1 cm beyond the lateral canthus. From the lateral end of the incision, a 10–20 mm incision is made vertically in a ventral direction. The resulting skin–cutaneous muscle flap is undermined and mobilized. **(b)** A triangular wedge of tarsoconjunctiva is resected. The width of the triangle base is equal to the length by which the eyelid is to be shortened. **(c)** The defect created in the tarsoconjunctival half of the lower eyelid is sutured using 6/0 (0.7 metric) polyglactin, burying the knots. **(d)** The skin flap is slid laterally and a triangle removed from the lateral end of it. This is a similar size to the triangle removed from the tarsoconjunctiva. **(e)** The skin flap is sutured into its transposed position. The result is eyelid shortening with a double-layered staggered wound. In addition, the lateral eyelid is drawn upwards and laterally.

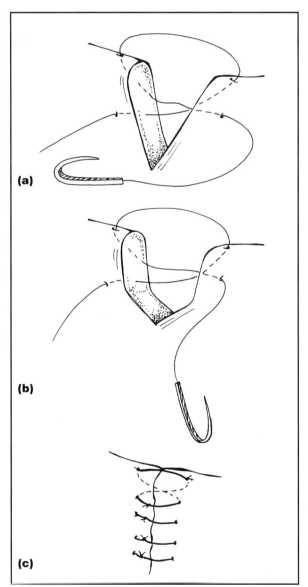

9.35 **(a)** V-shaped and **(b)** four-sided eyelid resection for eyelid shortening or tumour removal. **(c)** The resultant defect is closed in two layers using a figure-of-eight suture to re-appose the eyelid margins (see text).

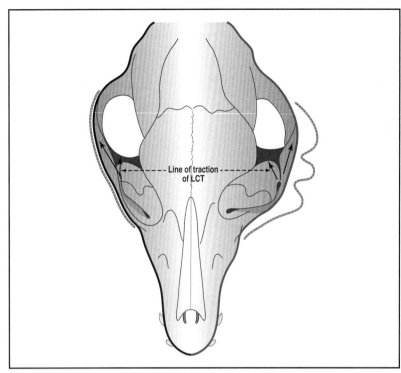

9.37 The lateral canthal tendon (LCT) is a poorly defined musculofibrous band that connects the orbicularis oculi muscle fibres at the lateral commissure to the orbital ligament. It lies immediately adjacent to the palpebral conjunctiva and stabilizes the lateral canthus. In dolichocephalic dog breeds (left-hand side), the line of traction provided by the lateral canthal tendon is parallel to the skin, resulting in normal close eyelid/globe apposition. In certain mesaticephalic breeds with broad skulls and redundant facial skin (right-hand side), traction on the lateral canthal tendon occurs at an angle, resulting in lateral canthal inversion. Associated ocular discomfort results in globe retraction, exacerbating the problem.

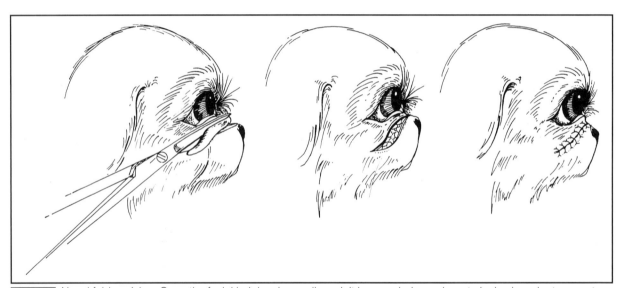

9.38 Nasal fold excision. Once the facial hair has been clipped, it is very obvious where to incise in order to resect the nasal fold. Following a skin incision with a No. 15 blade, the nasal fold is then excised with strong sharp scissors and the skin wound is closed routinely.

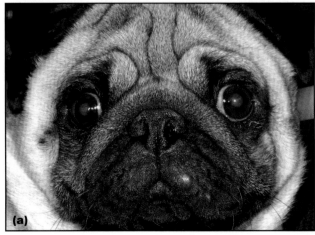

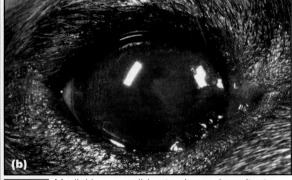

9.39 Medial lower eyelid entropion and resultant medial corneal pathology associated with brachycephalic conformation and prominent nasal folds in a Pug. (Courtesy of Willows Referral Service)

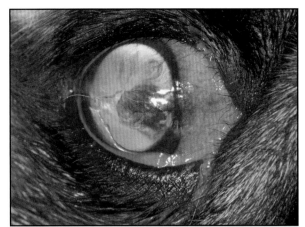

9.40 Medial upper and lower eyelid entropion associated with brachycephalic conformation and prominent nasal folds in an 11-month-old male Pug. The medial corneal neovascularization and pigmentation are made obvious by retro-illumination. The pupil has been pharmacologically dilated as part of the treatment for an unrelated traumatic laceration in the temporal cornea (fluorescein stained).

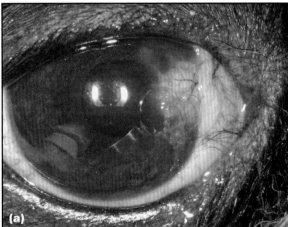

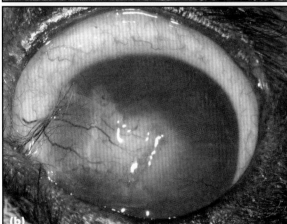

9.41 Bilateral caruncular trichiasis and medial lower eyelid entropion in a Shih Tzu (same dog as in Figure 9.27), which was previously obscured by nasal trichiasis. This dog had bilateral corneal perforations as a result of the trichiasis, which were repaired with **(a)** Biosist™ and a conjunctival pedicle graft in the right eye and **(b)** a corneo-conjunctival transposition in the left eye. This case illustrates the importance of identifying the underlying aetiology in corneal ulceration because eyelid surgery should be recommended in such cases to prevent recurrence or worsening of corneal disease.

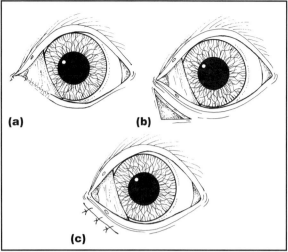

9.42 Modified Hotz–Celsus procedure to address medial lower eyelid entropion/trichiasis in brachycephalic breeds. **(a–b)** A triangular piece of skin (rather than a crescent) is removed. This helps to reduce the potential for recurrence of entropion associated with the excess skin still present in the nasal fold. **(c)** Closure is routine using simple interrupted sutures of 6/0 (0.7 metric) polyglactin.

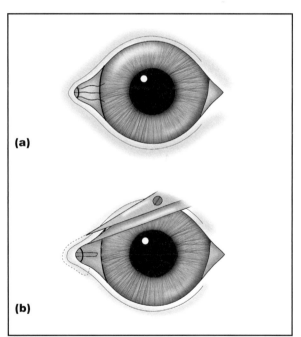

9.43 Medial canthoplasty to shorten the eyelids of brachycephalic dogs. **(a)** The degree of eyelid shortening required should be assessed preoperatively. The length of medial eyelid that can be removed is somewhat limited by the position of the lacrimal puncta and canaliculi, which should ideally be preserved. However, realistically, these patients often have concurrent dry eye or poor tear distribution. It also allows alignment of the eyelid margins with a tougher tarsal plate, which reduces the tendency for postoperative stretching of the eyelid repair. An additional benefit of increased shortening is that the medial canthus is displaced laterally, which may prevent the nasal hairs from coming into contact with the nasal cornea and avoid the need for concurrent nasal fold excision. **(b)** Following a skin incision with a No. 15 blade or Beaver blade, the medial eyelid margins are excised, continuing around the medial canthus to ensure that all the hair-bearing caruncular tissue is included in the excised tissue. (continues) ▶

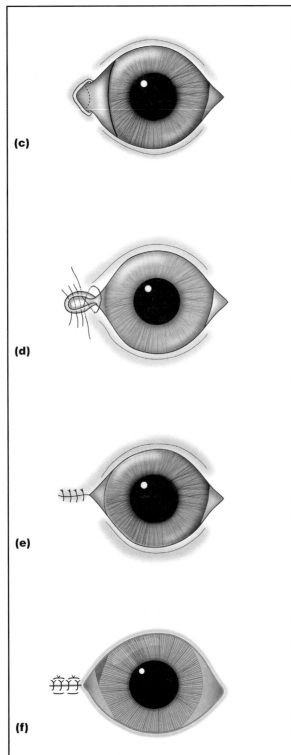

(c)

(d)

(e)

(f)

9.43 (continued) Medial canthoplasty to shorten the eyelids of brachycephalic dogs. **(c)** The tissue has been removed. **(d)** The defect is closed in two layers with a figure-of-eight suture used to realign the eyelid margins. The conjunctival layer is closed with a continuous suture, ensuring that the suture/needle does not penetrate the underlying conjunctiva and that the knots are directed outwards. **(e)** The skin is closed with simple interrupted sutures. The suture closest to the figure-of-eight suture can also catch the ends of the margin suture to ensure that they are directed away from the corneal surface. **(f)** Horizontal mattress sutures are also placed across the wound to relieve tension on the repair. All sutures are of 6/0 (0.7 metric) polyglactin.

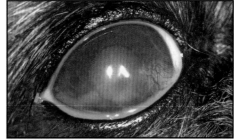

9.44 Postoperative appearance of the eye shown in Figure 9.10 following medial canthoplasty (and conjunctival pedicle grafting). The palpebral fissure is reduced in size, eyelid closure has improved (as indicated by the sharp corneal reflex and lustrous cornea) and the medial caruncular trichiasis has been removed.

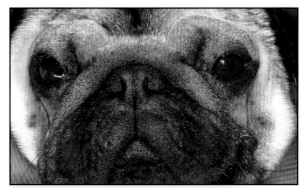

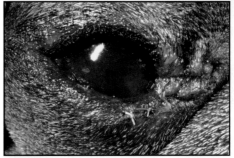

9.45 Postoperative appearance of the eye shown in Figure 9.39 following combined medial canthoplasty and modified lower eyelid Hotz–Celsus skin resection. The palpebral fissure is reduced in size and the medial lower eyelid entropion has been corrected. (Courtesy of Willows Referral Service)

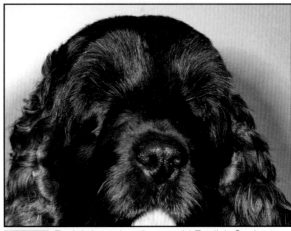

9.46 Facial droop in a 5-year-old English Cocker Spaniel bitch. (Courtesy of Willows Referral Service)

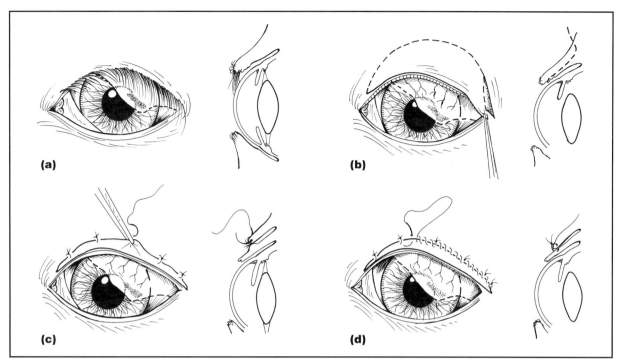

9.47 Correction of upper entropion/trichiasis using a Stades procedure. **(a–b)** A skin incision is made 1 mm superior to the meibomian gland openings so that all cilia can be removed from the upper eyelid. The incision should be made 3–4 mm from the medial canthus and extended 5–10 mm past the lateral canthus. A second incision (arc shaped) should be made with the superior margin at the level of the orbital rim such that a 15–20 mm wide strip of skin is removed. Any hair follicles remaining in this area need to be excised. **(c–d)** The upper skin edge is then mobilized and sutured about half-way across the wound, leaving the lower half to head by secondary intention. It is important to suture the skin to the tarsal plate, just behind the meibomian gland bases. The upper skin edge is sutured with cardinal simple interrupted sutures and, once positioned, secured with continuous sutures using 6/0 (0.7 metric) polyglactin. Healing by secondary intention results in eversion of the upper lid margin and a tough, bald strip remains above the eyelid margin, making recurrence of the entropion/trichiasis unlikely. Incompletely removed follicles with produce hairs following surgery, but they are not usually a problem because the position of the eyelid has been improved.

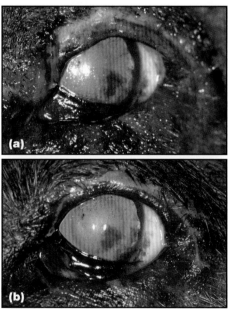

9.48 **(a)** Appearance immediately following a Stades procedure on a 13-year-old English Cocker Spaniel bitch (same case as in Figure 9.24). The upper skin edge is sutured half-way across the wound, leaving the second half to heal by secondary intention. The owners of the dog should be warned in advance of the presence of an open granulating wound following surgery. **(b)** By 13 days following the surgery, the wound has epithelialized, leaving a hairless area above the eyelid. (Courtesy of S Monclin)

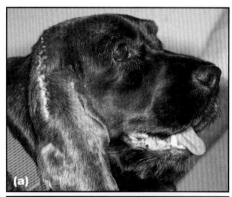
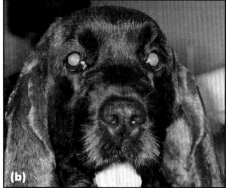

9.49 **(a)** Side view and **(b)** front view of the dog in Figure 9.46 following a coronal rhytidectomy (face lift). Eyelid surgery was not necessary. (Courtesy of Willows Referral Service)

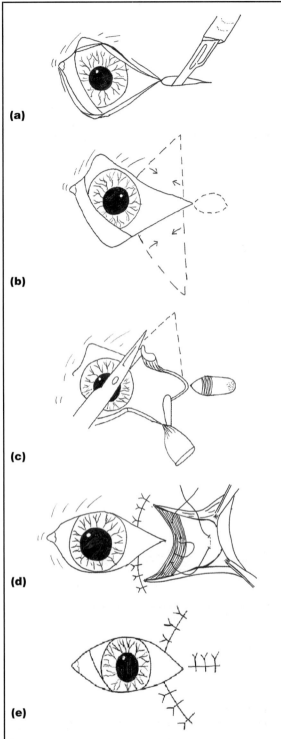

(a)

(b)

(c)

(d)

(e)

9.50 Modified Wyman canthoplasty coupled with eyelid shortening for the treatment of 'diamond eye'. **(a)** A horizontal skin incision is made from the lateral canthus to the zygomatic arch. **(b–c)** Full-thickness wedge resections are performed in both the upper and lower eyelids, which are closed in two layers with a figure-of-eight suture at the eyelid margins. **(d–e)** The zygomatic arch is exposed by blunt dissection. One or two 2/0 (3.0 metric) nylon sutures are used to anchor the lateral canthus permanently to the zygomatic arch. The nylon suture is then tied in such a position that it provides sufficient tension to create a palpebral fissure of reasonably normal size and shape. The lateral canthal skin incision is closed routinely. (Courtesy of J Green)

Figure-of-eight suture: When repairing any eyelid defect, it is important to align the eyelid margins accurately and not to leave any suture material contacting the cornea. This is best achieved using a figure-of-eight suture. When performing this suture, the needle is first placed in the skin away from the eyelid margin and directed obliquely to the other side of the defect to exit the eyelid margin through the meibomian gland orifices. The needle is then directed to the other side of the defect to enter the meibomian gland orifice equidistant from the incision. It then follows the same path in reverse on the other side of the wound. When the suture is tightened, the eyelid margin should be precisely re-aligned with no step and minimal possibility of a suture contacting the cornea (see Figure 9.35). The remainder of the defect is closed in two layers, with a continuous suture used to close the palpebral conjunctiva, ensuring that the suture/needle does not penetrate the underlying conjunctiva. Simple interrupted sutures are then placed to close the rest of the skin defect. The 'ends' of the figure-of-eight suture can be caught in the knots of the adjacent simple interrupted sutures to reduce the risk of corneal contact further.

Ectropion

Ectropion refers to an outward turning or eversion of the eyelid. It is common in dogs and is usually breed-related, occurring in breeds with overlong eyelids and laxity of the lateral canthus. As a result, there is increased conjunctival exposure and collection of debris in the lower conjunctival sac, as well as poor tear film distribution over the corneal surface. This leads to conjunctivitis and increased mucin production. It may be complicated by downwardly directed upper eyelid cilia contacting the exposed conjunctival surface, as commonly seen in the Cocker Spaniel. Ectropion of the central lower eyelid can be combined with entropion of the lateral lower eyelid or trichiasis from the upper eyelid, as occurs with 'diamond eye', and such cases have corneal irritation in addition to the clinical signs described above. Less commonly, ectropion occurs as a result of severe damage, scarring and cicatrix formation. This may be the result of severe skin disease or thermal burns, or may be iatrogenic following inappropriate surgery for distichiasis or over-correction of entropion.

Ectropion correction is indicated when corneal or conjunctival pathology results from the deformity. Simple ectropion may be corrected by wedge resection to shorten the eyelid length. This may be combined with upper eyelid shortening and stabilization of the lateral canthus where indicated (see Figure 9.50). Another eyelid shortening technique is a modification of the Kühnt–Szymanowski procedure (see Figure 9.36), which both shortens the eyelid length and supports the lateral canthus, but requires adequate surgical skill to accurately split the lid thickness. Cicatricial ectropion can be treated with a V-to-Y plasty (Figure 9.51).

Eyelid inflammation

Inflammation of the eyelids (blepharitis) may be localized and associated with infection of one or

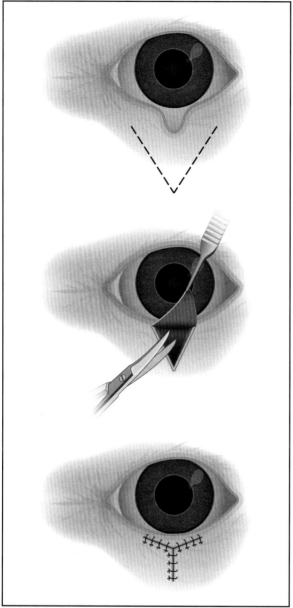

9.51 V-to-Y plasty for the correction of cicatricial ectropion. Converging skin incisions are made commencing 1–2 mm from the eyelid margin. A V-shaped skin flap is separated from the subcutaneous tissues and the cicatricial tissue is excised. The V flap is advanced to correct the eyelid eversion and the resulting Y-shaped wound is closed with simple interrupted sutures of 6/0 (0.7 metric) polyglactin.

more of the glandular structures in the eyelid, or may be part of a generalized skin disease or a systemic disease. All patients presenting with blepharitis or periocular dermatitis should undergo a general dermatological examination because the presence and distribution of concurrent skin disease may assist with making a diagnosis.

Chalazion

A chalazion is a firm, cream, well demarcated, 2–5 mm diameter swelling located in the area of the meibomian glands. It occurs following blockage of the meibomian gland duct and inspissation of the secretory products. It is visible through the palpebral

conjunctiva and, occasionally, through the eyelid skin (Figure 9.52). Chalazia are generally non-painful, unless the gland ruptures, releasing its contents into the surrounding eyelid and inciting a granulomatous inflammatory response. Blockage of the meibomian gland duct can occur following meibomianitis, surgical trauma and neoplasia, particularly meibomian adenoma formation. Chalazia are often incidental findings, only causing a problem by frictional irritation of the eye. Treatment involves lancing and curettage of the individual chalazia via the conjunctival surface, which usually requires general anaesthesia. Where the chalazion is secondary to adenoma formation, surgery to excise both the adenoma and chalazion should be performed.

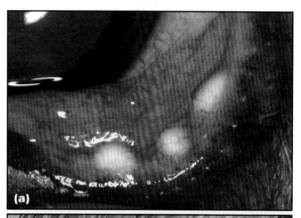

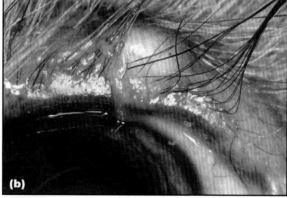

9.52 **(a)** Multiple chalazia visible through the palpebral conjunctiva. **(b)** Solitary chalazion visible through the upper eyelid skin.

Hordeolum

A hordeolum (stye) is a localized infection (usually due to *Staphylococcus* spp.) of one or more of the glands of the eyelid margin. An external hordeolum is an infection of the glands of Moll or Zeis (Figure 9.53); an internal hordeolum is an infection of a meibomian gland. A hordeolum is usually red and painful (Figure 9.54). Management of hordeola may involve lancing the abscess, but this has to be delayed until the abscess is pointing. Pointing can be encouraged by the application of warm compresses. Hordeola should never be opened too early or manually expressed before they have pointed as the infection can be spread to the surrounding tissues. Topical and systemic broad-spectrum antibiotics should be administered for 14–21 days.

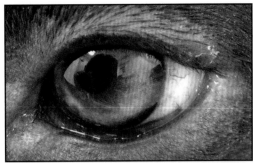

9.53 External hordeolum in the lateral upper eyelid of a 3-year-old male German Shorthaired Pointer.

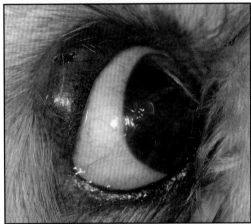

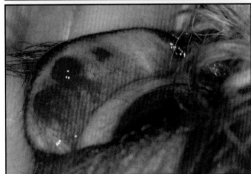

9.54 Granulomatous inflammation erupting through both the eyelid and conjunctival surfaces in a 6-year-old Shih Tzu bitch with presumptive hordeola.

Meibomianitis

This condition affects several meibomian glands simultaneously and often occurs as part of a more generalized dermatological disease. Meibomianitis is most commonly caused by suppurative bacteria such as *Staphylococcus* spp. The pathogenic mechanism is related to the presence of bacteria and the immune-mediated reaction induced by its toxin (Pena and Leiva, 2008). Dogs with acute meibomianitis typically have swollen, painful eyelids with slight pointing of the meibomian gland openings (Figure 9.55). Gentle pressure on the eyelid margins results in the expression of discoloured meibum. Inflammation of the meibomian glands also leads to loss of the meibomian oil layer and thus evaporation of the tear film, resulting in a decreased TFBUT and increased tear osmolarity. Abnormal lipids produced as a result of inflammatory disease can be toxic to the cornea.

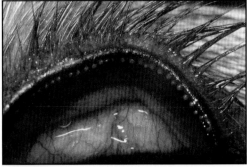

9.55 Prominent meibomian gland orifices in a dog with meibomianitis. (Courtesy of Willows Referral Service)

Treatment includes the application of warm compresses and the use of both topical and systemic antibiotics. In the absence of culture and sensitivity testing, the choice of antibiotic is similar to that for pyoderma elsewhere on the body and includes clavulanate-potentiated amoxicillin or a cephalosporin. Prolonged courses of treatment may be required. Tetracycline may also be beneficial owing to its immunomodulatory as well as antibacterial action. Topical and/or systemic corticosteroids may be necessary in combination with antibiotics in view of the presumed immune-mediated contribution to the pathogenesis and in those cases with significant granulomatous inflammation.

Bacterial blepharitis

Secondary bacterial periocular skin infections can occur with atopy, parasitic disease, fungal disease and self-trauma due to other chronic eyelid diseases such as entropion. Periocular dermatitis can also develop following parotid duct transposition, particularly in longhaired breeds. This occurs as a result of overflow of saliva from the eye, which causes the periocular skin to be constantly moist. The bacterial flora of the conjunctival sac is also markedly different following parotid duct transposition, and there are increased numbers of bacteria. Management comprises hygiene measures such as keeping the facial hair trimmed short, drying the face after feeding and the careful use of wipes and disinfectants.

Idiopathic mucocutaneous pyoderma (Figure 9.56) is a bacterial skin infection of unknown cause. It affects the mucocutaneous junctions (usually the eyelids and/or lips), appearing as erosive lesions that are often bilateral and symmetrical, mimicking an autoimmune disease. German Shepherd Dogs appear to be predisposed. Mucocutaneous pyoderma is responsive to topical and systemic antibiotics.

Bacterial blepharitis may also present as diffuse superficial eyelid inflammation. This is seen initially as hyperaemia, lid swelling and crusting, with ulceration of the eyelid skin and margins (Figure 9.57), alopecia and fibrosis developing over time. Scarring and fibrosis associated with chronic periocular skin disease can lead to cicatricial entropion and/or ectropion. Bacterial infection involving the deeper eyelids presents as single or multiple pyogranulomas (Figure 9.58).

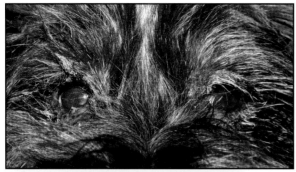

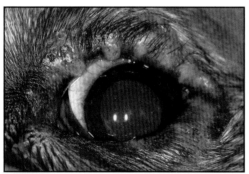

9.56 Mucocutaneous pyoderma.

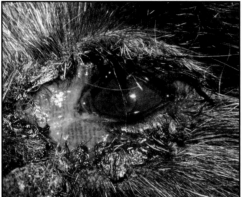

9.57 Diffuse eyelid swelling with ulceration of the eyelid margins and periocular skin in a 4-year-old male Cocker Spaniel. The condition was bilateral and involved only the eyelids. The blepharitis responded to systemic antibiotics alone.

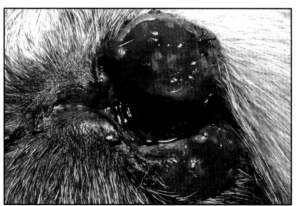

9.58 Granulomatous blepharitis in a 5-year-old German Shepherd Dog bitch. The inflammatory disease process was confirmed on biopsy and complete resolution occurred following systemic corticosteroid and antibiotic administration. (Courtesy of Willows Referral Service)

Parasitic blepharitis

The face, particularly the eyelids, is a predilection site for demodicosis in young dogs. The clinical signs may be localized or more generalized. A non-pruritic, often erythematous, alopecia with comedones and follicular casts is seen (Figure 9.59). Secondary infection leads to pruritus and crusting. Demodicosis and cheyletiellosis are occasionally seen affecting the eyelids of dogs receiving potent ocular corticosteroids. *Sarcoptes scabiei* can also affect the periocular skin, resulting in papules, crusts and scales as well as intense pruritus. Scabies is usually generalized. Less commonly, harvest mite (*Neotrombicula autumnalis*) infestation causes periocular signs (summer and early autumn only). Ticks and *Otodectes cyanotis* are rare causes of periocular disease. Diagnosis is by direct observation, skin scrapings or serology for canine scabies.

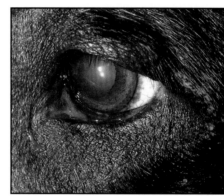

9.59 Periocular alopecia in a dog with demodicosis. (Courtesy of Dr S Shaw)

Leishmaniosis

Systemic leishmaniosis is a chronic and potentially fatal disease, which is endemic in Mediterranean countries as well as India and Central and South America. More than 1000 cases have been diagnosed in the UK since the introduction of the Pet Travel Scheme (PETS) and not all incidences have been in travelled dogs or even in dogs with known contact with travelled dogs. The clinical signs of leishmaniosis are variable, but the eyelids are frequently involved (Pena *et al.*, 2000). The eyelid lesions can vary from periocular alopecia and dry scaly lesions to diffuse eyelid thickening with hyperaemia and ulceration. Focal nodular granulomas may also develop in the eyelids. Diagnosis is by identification of amastigotes in lymph node, bone marrow or skin biopsy specimens, or by PCR testing. Of these options, bone marrow and lymph node aspirates have the highest sensitivity.

Fungal blepharitis

Dermatophytosis commonly affects the face, particularly the area above the eyelids. It may be caused by *Microsporum canis* or *Trichophyton mentagrophytes*. Diagnosis is made by Woods lamp examination in some cases of *Microsporum* infection, by microscopic examination of plucked hairs and by fungal culture. *Malassezia pachydermatis* is a common cause of facial pruritus and erythema and is frequently seen as a secondary infection in a large number of skin diseases, especially atopic dermatitis.

This yeast is common in animals with epiphora and in cases with facial folds. Chlorhexidine- or boric acid-containing wipes can be used for prophylaxis. *Malassezia* can be associated with severe episodic facial pruritus. Systemic mycotic infections (*Cryptococcus*, *Histoplasma*, *Blastomyces* and *Coccidioides*) are rarely seen in the UK at present. Diagnosis is made by identifying the organisms on cytology or histology.

Allergy, atopic blepharitis and hypersensitivity

Acute eyelid inflammation can occur as a result of mast cell degranulation, which may arise due to atopic dermatitis, insect bites and drug reactions.

Atopic blepharitis: Atopic blepharitis is characterized by blepharospasm, erythema and alopecia of the periocular skin, with or without meibomianitis (Figure 9.60). Atopy is an inherited disease with strong breed predispositions and is usually manifest in young dogs. Diagnosis is based on history, physical examination and intradermal allergy testing. The treatment for atopic blepharitis is similar to that described for atopic dermatitis elsewhere on the body and involves avoiding the offending allergen(s),

allergen-specific immunotherapy (ASIT) and pharmacological modification of clinical signs.

Food hypersensitivity: Canine food hypersensitivity is a non-seasonal pruritic skin disorder that can affect the eyelids. Cutaneous signs are not pathognomonic and may include papules, plaques, pustules, wheals, erythema, excoriation, lichenification, alopecia, scales, crusts and moist erosions. Diagnosis is based on exclusion of other likely causes, response to an elimination diet and provocative exposure testing. Treatment comprises allergen detection and elimination with palliative management of the allergic disease until this is achieved.

Contact hypersensitivity: Blepharitis can develop following treatment with certain topical ophthalmic medications. Commonly implicated drugs include gentamicin- and neomycin-containing preparations, ciclosporin preparations and topical carbonic anhydrase inhibitors (dorzolamide and brinzolamide). Brinzolamide has a pH of 7.5, which is more physiological than dorzolamide (pH 5.6) so would be expected to be better tolerated, but both preparations can cause blepharitis and keratitis, which resolve when the drugs are withdrawn.

Immune-mediated blepharoconjunctival diseases

The eyelids are immunologically active structures with an extensive presence of blood vessels, lymphatic vessels and immune cells. Immune-mediated blepharoconjunctival diseases may occur in isolation or in association with systemic diseases, and may be primary autoimmune diseases or occur secondary to exogenous material (e.g. infectious agents and drugs) (Figure 9.61).

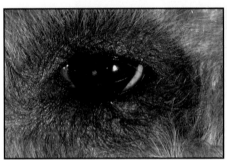

9.60
Periocular atopic blepharitis. (Courtesy of Dr S Shaw)

Clinical signs	Diagnosis	Treatment	Predisposed breeds
Medial canthal ulcerative blepharitis			
Bilateral medial canthal erosions of upper and lower eyelids	Clinical signs and skin biopsy, which reveals lymphocytic and plasmacytic infiltrates	Responsive to topical antibiotics and corticosteroids. Alternative immunomodulatory drugs, including topical tacrolimus and topical or systemic ciclosporin may also be effective	Seen most commonly in German Shepherd Dogs (can be seen in combination with chronic superficial keratitis, pannus and plasmoma; (Figure 9.62), Longhaired Dachshunds (can be concurrent with punctate keratitis), Miniature and Toy Poodles
Uveodermatological syndrome (also known as Vogt–Koyanagi–Harada-like syndrome)			
Dermatological lesions affecting the mucocutaneous junctions, primarily the eyelids, lips and nasal planum. Seen as depigmentation of hair and skin (poliosis and vitiligo), ulceration and crusting (Figure 9.63). Accompanied by panuveitis (anterior uveitis and chorioretinitis) and may lead to retinal detachment and secondary glaucoma	Signalment and clinical signs. Clinical signs are attributed to the effects of immune-mediated destruction of melanocytes. Combination of severe bilateral ocular inflammatory disease with a well defined distribution of skin changes is usually diagnostic (although ocular disease may precede the development of skin lesions and depigmentation). Skin biopsy reveals lichenoid interface dermatitis with infiltration by histiocytes, lymphocytes, plasma cells and multi-nucleated giant cells	Immunosuppression. Historically, treatment comprised immunosuppressive doses of prednisolone in combination with azathioprine plus appropriate topical ophthalmic medication for the uveitis ± glaucoma. The long-term prognosis was very poor and the treatment did not usually prevent bilateral glaucoma and vision loss. Prednisolone combined with systemic ciclosporin may result in a better outcome but can be cost prohibitive, particularly as it is large-breed dogs that are usually affected. Oral ketoconazole has been used to reduce the required dose of oral ciclosporin	Chow Chow, Japanese Akita, Samoyed and Siberian Husky, but has been reported in many other breeds. Seen in adult dogs

9.61 Immune-mediated diseases that affect the eyelids in dogs. (continues) ▶

Clinical signs	Diagnosis	Treatment	Predisposed breeds
Pemphigus complex			
Pemphigus foliaceus and pemphigus erythematosus (common conditions): lesions develop on the face and ears, initially as erythematous macules which progress to pustules that rupture, leaving erosions and ulcers, scaling, crusting and hypopigmentation (Figure 9.64); variably pruritic Pemphigus vulgaris (rare condition): intraepidermal vesicles or bullae develop (rather than pustules as seen with other pemphigus variants)	Histopathology of skin biopsy samples. Immunohistochemistry may be useful	Long-term topical and systemic corticosteroid administration with additional immunosuppression using azathioprine or other immunomodulatory agents in refractory cases. Eyelid surgery may be necessary if chronic eyelid disease has led to cicatricial entropion	
Canine lupus erythematosus (discoid and systemic)			
Facial dermatitis consisting of crusts, depigmentation, erosions and ulcers. Affects the nasal planum, muzzle, eyelids and lip margins. Usually bilaterally symmetrical. With SLE there are clinical signs of other organ involvement	Skin biopsy ± other tests as required for SLE	Topical immunosuppressive drugs (initially). Immunosuppressive doses of systemic prednisolone can be used in refractory cases. Avoidance of exposure to sunlight as photosensitivity may have a role in pathogenesis	
Juvenile cellulitis (puppy strangles)			
Bilateral granulomatous pustular blepharitis with submandibular lymphadenomegaly. Predominantly occurs in dogs <8 months old but occasionally seen in older animals. Can also result in facial swelling, affecting the lips, muzzle and pinnae (Figure 9.65). Presumed to be a hypersensitivity to bacterial toxins	Clinical signs	Early and aggressive systemic therapy with immunosuppressive doses of prednisolone is required to prevent permanent scarring. Treatment is tapered following resolution. Systemic bactericidal antibiotics are only indicated if there is cytological or clinical evidence of secondary infection	Dachshund, Golden Retriever, Gordon Setter, Labrador Retriever, Lhaso Apso

9.61 (continued) Immune-mediated diseases that affect the eyelids in dogs.

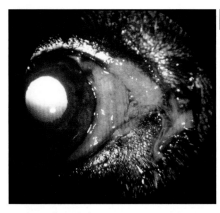

9.62 Medial canthus ulceration and plasma cell infiltration of the third eyelid in a German Shepherd Dog.

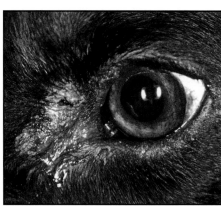

9.64 Pemphigus foliaceus. (Courtesy of Dr S Shaw)

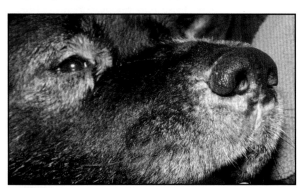

9.63 Poliosis and vitiligo of the periocular skin and muzzle/nasal planum of a Japanese Akita with uveodermatological syndrome. (Courtesy of Willows Referral Service)

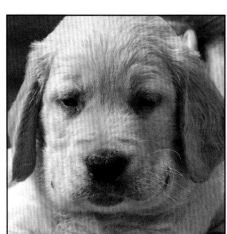

9.65 Juvenile cellulitis. (Courtesy of Dr S Shaw)

Zinc-responsive dermatosis

Periocular alopecia, crusting and erythema can occur as a result of zinc deficiency (Figure 9.66). Northern breeds, such as Siberian Huskies, Alaskan Malamutes and Samoyeds, are predisposed owing to a relative inability to utilize or assimilate zinc. Zinc-responsive dermatosis can also occur in many large-breed dogs if there is reduced zinc in the diet. The diagnosis is made by skin biopsy and response to zinc supplementation therapy.

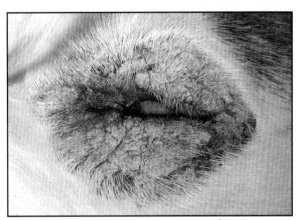

9.66 Zinc-responsive dermatosis in a Siberian Husky. (Courtesy of P Sands)

Eyelid neoplasia

Eyelid neoplasia is common in older dogs, but the majority (at least 75%) of canine eyelid tumours are benign. The most commonly seen tumours include sebaceous adenoma, papilloma, benign melanoma, sebaceous adenocarcinoma and histiocytoma with mast cell tumour, basal cell carcinoma, squamous cell carcinoma and a variety of soft tissue sarcomas, including haemangiopericytoma and fibrosarcoma, also reported (Krehbiel and Langham, 1975; Roberts *et al.*, 1986). The average age for developing eyelid neoplasms is 8 years, although papillomas and histiocytomas typically occur in young dogs. These tumours must be distinguished from conjunctival neoplasms, whose behaviour is generally very different.

Adenoma and adenocarcinoma

Meibomian gland adenomas account for approximately 40% of reported eyelid tumours. They are usually lobulated, pigmented and friable, often bleeding and crusting. The tumour is first noticed erupting through the eyelid margin. The neoplastic tissue often blocks the meibomian duct, leading to chalazion formation, and, if this material is released into the surrounding eyelid tissue by progressive expansion of the neoplasm, it leads to a significant granulomatous response. Occasionally, histology of the excised mass reveals increased mitotic activity, prompting classification as an adenocarcinoma, but these tumours also behave as benign neoplasms in this location. A short course of systemic anti-inflammatory and antibiotic therapy is indicated prior to surgical intervention if a significant granulomatous inflammatory component is suspected. The eyelid margin should be everted to evaluate the full extent of the tumour (Figure 9.67) before planning treatment. A full-thickness four-sided eyelid resection is usually curative, provided all the abnormal tissue is removed. Debulking and cryosurgery may be considered if the tumour is large. Carbon dioxide laser ablation has also been used and may be possible with local infiltration anaesthesia in elderly patients where general anaesthesia is not an option.

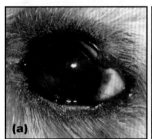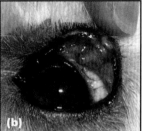

9.67 **(a)** Sebaceous adenoma affecting the upper eyelid. **(b)** Eversion of the eyelid reveals the extent of the tumour. (Courtesy of S Crispin)

Papilloma

Viral papillomas are typically seen in young dogs and may be associated with oral or generalized papillomatosis. They are superficial, pedunculated and have a typical verrucose appearance. They can also occur as solitary eyelid lesions in older dogs. Removal is indicated if they are rapidly growing and associated with corneal irritation. They can be treated by excision, cryosurgery or a combination of both; however, they can spontaneously regress in young dogs.

Melanoma

Canine eyelid melanomas are superficial and may involve the eyelid skin or the eyelid margin. They may develop as single or multiple pigmented masses. Eyelid melanomas exhibit more benign behaviour than melanomas in the mouth or other sites. Surgical excision is usually curative, but they can also be treated by cryosurgery.

Histiocytoma

Histiocytomas develop rapidly, primarily in young dogs. The lesions are raised, pink and hairless, sometimes ulcerate and are usually <1 cm in diameter (Figure 9.68a). They can be diagnosed by fine-needle aspiration. Histiocytomas can spontaneously regress (Figure 9.68b), but this can take anywhere from 6 weeks to 10 months (for multiple lesions or in older dogs). Surgical excision or cryosurgery is usually curative for cutaneous histiocytoma and is recommended for any mass that does not show evidence of spontaneous regression within 3 months. The choice of surgical technique depends on the size of the mass and the position on the eyelid(s).

Epitheliotropic lymphoma

Epitheliotropic lymphoma usually affects the eyelids as part of a generalized disease, but can present with eyelid depigmentation and ulceration as the only signs (Figure 9.69).

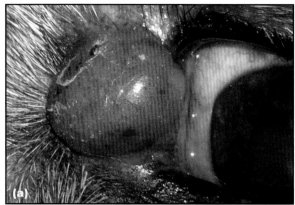

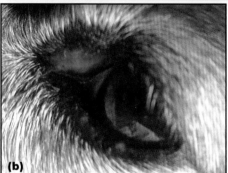

9.68 **(a)** Histiocytoma in a 10-year-old male Jack Russell Terrier. The diagnosis was confirmed by fine-needle aspiration of the mass. **(b)** The same lesion following spontaneous regression.

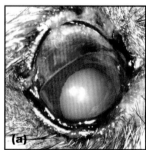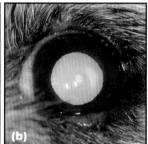

9.69 Bilateral ulceration of the eyelid margins of both the **(a)** right and **(b)** left eye as a result of epitheliotropic lymphoma. Note the subconjunctival haemorrhage in the right eye, indicating possible paraneoplastic disease.

Treatment

Therapy for localized canine eyelid tumours includes surgical excision, cryotherapy or a combination of both. Basic principles of oncological surgery should be observed (comprising complete resection with minimal handling of adjacent healthy tissue). Where surgical management is possible, the technique used will depend on the size, nature and position of the mass. As previously mentioned, the upper eyelid covers a greater area of the cornea during blinking than the lower eyelid, so it is more important for any repairs/reconstruction of the upper eyelid to be anatomically as accurate as possible.

Upper eyelids: Small eyelid masses (up to one-third of the length of the upper eyelid) can be removed by wedge or four-sided full-thickness resection with direct closure of the defect using a figure-of-eight

suture at the eyelid margin (see Figure 9.35). For masses requiring excision of more than one-third of the length of the eyelid margin, specialist consultation or referral is recommended. The resection should be at least one meibomian gland orifice or 1 mm beyond the margins of the tumour. As a general rule, the resulting defect should be closed using the simplest technique possible. Cases that require complex procedures for surgical reconstruction are seldom encountered in general practice. If larger masses are removed, this technique for direct closure can be combined with a sliding lateral canthoplasty to lengthen the upper eyelid (Figure 9.70). The 'new' eyelid margin is produced from haired skin and this may result in trichiasis, although it will be

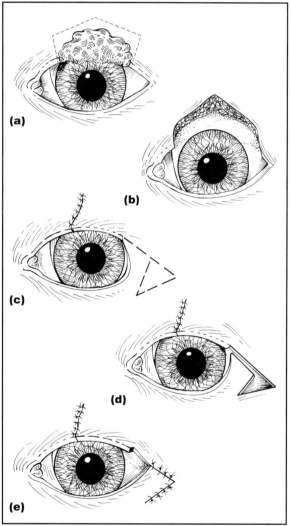

9.70 Sliding lateral canthoplasty. **(a–b)** A large tumour is excised from the eyelid, requiring removal of more than one-third of the eyelid length. **(c–d)** An incision is made at the lateral canthus, extending laterally in a direction that appears as a continuation of the eyelid that is being lengthened (the upper eyelid in this case). The incision is made through the full thickness of the eyelid and continues into the adjacent skin. A triangle of skin is excised at the lateral end of the skin incision, which allows the skin to be slid medially to lengthen the upper eyelid. **(e)** The resulting defect is sutured. The direction of the lateral incision and excised triangle of skin is reversed if elongation of the lower eyelid is required.

restricted to the lateral globe. The direction of the lateral incision and excised triangle of skin in the sliding lateral canthoplasty is reversed if elongation of the lower eyelid is required.

Alternative techniques include the H-blepharoplasty, Z-blepharoplasty (Gelatt, 1994), rhomboid graft flap (Blanchard and Keller, 1976) and the semicircular sliding skin flap (Pellicane *et al.*, 1994). These are partial-thickness grafts and may benefit from being lined by conjunctiva transposed from the adjacent eyelid, from the third eyelid as a rotational graft, or from the oral mucosa. The advantage of these techniques is that they are single procedures involving a single anaesthetic. The disadvantage is that there is a possibility of developing trichiasis, which is more likely when these techniques are performed on the upper eyelid. Contracture and scarring can develop if insufficient care is taken to avoid tension on the conjunctiva and skin, and the reconstructed eyelid can lack strength.

The use of a split eyelid flap (Lewin, 2003) has also been described as a means of repairing defects of up to 50% of the eyelid length, whilst still retaining a smooth margin along the complete eyelid. This is achieved by incising the residual eyelid along its margin through the openings of the meibomian glands from the border of the defect, for a distance equal to the size of the defect. The incision is then deepened beyond the meibomian glands through the tarsal plate by sharp then blunt dissection to elevate a flap of skin, which is mobilized and transposed to fill the defect. The eyelid in the area of the defect contains the outer aspect of the eyelid margin and the tarsal plate. The area from which the flap is transposed retains the conjunctiva and inner eyelid margin. A skin flap is then created from the adjacent eyelid skin and rotated to cover the defect, where it is sutured in place. This is a one-stage technique that avoids trichiasis but damages a significant proportion of the meibomian glands that have not been excised.

A superior technique for the repair of large upper eyelid defects is the Mustardé technique (Munger and Gourley, 1981; Esson, 2001). The advantage of this technique is that it creates a normal smooth eyelid margin but it requires two anaesthetics because it is a two-stage procedure. The original technique involves transposition of part of the lower eyelid to the upper eyelid during the first procedure, leaving it attached by a pedicle. During the second procedure, the pedicle is sectioned and the upper eyelid reconstructed whilst, at the same time, the lower eyelid deficit is repaired using an H-plasty or lip-to-lid flap (see below). This process can be simplified by 'sharing the lid deficit'. For upper eyelid defects that involve 50–60% of the eyelid length, 25–33% of the lower eyelid is transposed. Once the pedicle is incorporated, a further procedure is required to section it, but then both eyelids can be repaired by direct apposition, leaving both eyelids with 66–75% of the original eyelid length and avoiding the need for complicated lower eyelid reconstruction with the potential for trichiasis (Figure 9.71).

Lower eyelids: Wedge resection, wedge resection with sliding lateral canthoplasty, rhomboid graft flap, H-plasty and Z-blepharoplasty can also be used to close defects of the lower eyelid (with the same possible complications as described above). However, because the lower eyelid is less mobile, the incidence of trichiasis and keratitis is lower. The best technique for repairing very large lower eyelid defects is the mucocutaneous subdermal plexus flap from the lip (Pavletic *et al.*, 1982) (Figure 9.72) as it creates a hairless, smooth eyelid margin.

Invasive neoplasms: Despite the generalization that the majority of eyelid neoplasms are benign, inevitably some will be locally invasive or require much larger margins, necessitating wide surgical excision. In these cases, enucleation or orbital exenteration may be indicated, leaving a defect that cannot be closed directly. Surgical planning is imperative to allow closure in these cases using, for example, a caudal auricular axial pattern flap (Stiles *et al.*, 2003). An axial pattern flap based on the cutaneous branch of the superficial temporal artery has also been used, following wide resection of a mast cell tumour involving the medial canthus. Although half the length of the medial upper and lower eyelids was removed, it was possible to repair

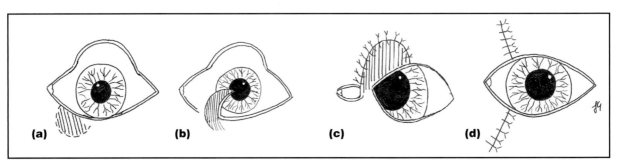

(a)   (b)   (c)   (d)

9.71 Mustardé technique. This is a two-stage procedure in which the upper eyelid is repaired using a pedicle of eyelid transposed from the lower eyelid. There are several variations on this technique, which involve repairing the defect in the lower eyelid using an H-plasty or a lip-to-lid graft. However, it is much simpler to transpose a pedicle of eyelid that is shorter than the defect, leaving a sufficient length of lower eyelid to be closed directly. The result is that both the upper and lower eyelids are slightly shorter, but this procedure avoids the potential for trichiasis associated with H-plasty or the need for another complicated grafting technique. **(a)** A flap of skin and lower eyelid is dissected, leaving a pedicle of attachment at one end. **(b)** The flap is rotated into the defect in the upper eyelid, which has been prepared to accept it. **(c)** The flap is sutured into position and the defect at the donor site is closed. **(d)** Once healed, the donor pedicle is resected and the lid margins are repaired using small wedge resections. (Courtesy of J Green)

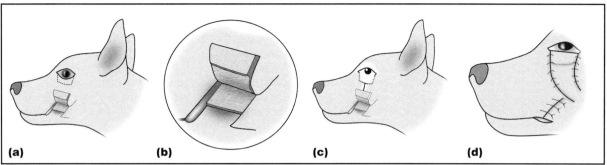

9.72 Lip-to-lid graft (mucocutaneous subdermal plexus flap). Rotation of a graft fashioned from the upper lip can be used to replace the lower eyelid. A portion of oral mucosa is included with the flap to replace the lower palpebral conjunctiva and the oral mucocutaneous junction mimics the eyelid margin. **(a)** There is a large defect in the lower eyelid. A full-thickness dissection of the lip has been started. **(b)** The lip flap only includes oral mucosa to a sufficient depth to mimic the depth of the eyelid itself. The dissection is then continued to separate the skin and subdermal plexus from the deeper structures over a sufficient length to allow the flap to be rotated to reach the eyelid defect. The skin ventral to the eyelid defect is incised and the edges are separated sufficiently to accommodate the rotated flap. **(c–d)** The oral mucosa of the lip flap is sutured to the conjunctiva in the fornix. The lip skin is sutured to the edges of the eyelid defect and the separated edges of the skin incision ventral to the lid defect. The defect in the oral mucosa and lip skin is closed.

this defect with the skin flap, which was lined with the bulbar conjunctiva and leading edge of the third eyelid, after the palpebral conjunctival surface had been removed (Jacobi *et al.*, 2008). Note that this is a complex surgical procedure and specialist advice or referral should be considered when presented with such cases.

Eyelid injuries

Eyelid injuries most commonly occur as a result of bite wounds (Figure 9.73) or road traffic accidents. A thorough physical and ocular examination should be performed to rule out head trauma and damage to the globe or orbit. Reconstructive surgery should be performed as soon as the patient is stable. Following thorough saline irrigation, the wounds and conjunctival sac should be cleaned with dilute povidone–iodine solution (see Chapter 6) not scrub. The eyelid skin has an excellent blood supply, which usually ensures healing of even contaminated wounds. Ischaemia and devitalization are unusual and primary closure should be performed with minimal mechanical debridement. As in the routine management of skin wounds elsewhere, appropriate systemic antibiotics and anti-inflammatory drugs should be administered, along with the provision of adequate analgesia. If the nasolacrimal system is involved, the puncta/canaliculi should be cannulated prior to surgery to maintain patency and an indwelling cannula should be left sutured in place for 7–10 days postoperatively. As with all eyelid surgery, the aim is to accurately restore the eyelid margin and eyelid–globe apposition (using the techniques described above). If eyelid swelling prevents effective blinking, a temporary partial tarsorrhaphy (see Figure 9.30) and/or the application of ocular lubricants is indicated to prevent exposure keratitis.

Neurological diseases affecting the eyelids

Changes in eyelid position and function can occur as a result of neurological disease. Facial nerve paralysis can lead to denervation of the orbicularis oculi muscle, failure to be able to close the eyelid, and an increase in size of the eyelid fissure. With

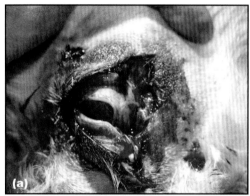

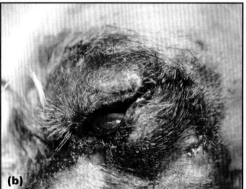

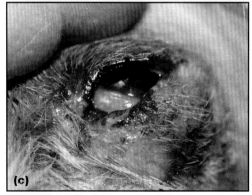

9.73 **(a)** Eyelid laceration following a dog fight. **(b)** Primary repair and temporary tarsorrhaphy. **(c)** Postoperative appearance showing satisfactory eyelid reconstruction, although the dog subsequently developed keratoconjunctivitis sicca. (Courtesy of R Grundon)

chronicity, fibrous contraction of the orbicularis oculi muscle may occur, resulting in a smaller palpebral fissure, which can sometimes be confused with blepharospasm.

Ptosis (drooping of the upper eyelid) can be seen with denervation of the levator palpebrae superioris muscle, which is innervated by the oculomotor nerve (CN III). This is usually seen in association with denervation of the extraocular muscles that are also innervated by CN III (external ophthalmoplegia). Where the oculomotor fibres to the pupil are also affected, a fixed dilated pupil is seen, and this combination is termed total ophthalmoplegia. Denervation of the smooth muscle in the upper and lower eyelids occurs with Horner's syndrome. This leads to ptosis of the upper eyelid and reverse ptosis of the lower eyelid, with a resulting narrow palpebral fissure, which should be differentiated from blepharospasm. Neurological diseases affecting the eyelids are discussed in more detail in Chapter 19.

Feline conditions

Congenital abnormalities

Abnormalities of eyelid opening
The eyelids of a kitten usually open 10–14 days after birth. Delayed opening (ankyloblepharon) has been reported in Persian cats. If the kitten becomes infected with herpesvirus before the eyelids open, the conjunctival and corneal epithelial necrosis and the subsequent neutrophilic response result in the accumulation of large amounts of inflammatory debris in the conjunctival sac, distending the still-fused eyelids (ophthalmia neonatorum) (Figure 9.74). This can then become secondarily infected. A small amount of discharge occasionally escapes at the medial canthus. Treatment involves opening the eyelids along their line of fusion (as described for dogs above). The damage caused by the infection can include:

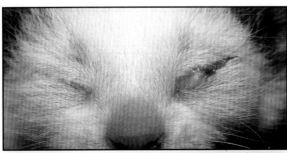
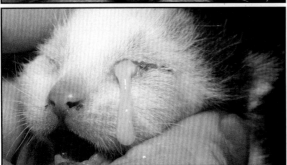

9.74 Ophthalmia neonatorum in a kitten. (Courtesy of Willows Referral Service)

- Symblepharon
- Corneal ulceration and perforation
- Endophthalmitis and panophthalmitis.

Coloboma
Coloboma (or eyelid agenesis) is the most common congenital eyelid abnormality in cats. It can occur sporadically in any breed but has been reported in the Domestic Shorthaired Cat, Persian and Burmese. The extent of the defect can vary from a small notch in the lid margin to complete absence of two-thirds or more of the upper eyelid and its conjunctival lining. The abnormality is usually bilateral and most commonly affects the lateral aspect of the upper eyelid (Figure 9.75), although medial canthal involvement has been reported. Incomplete eyelid closure resulting in corneal exposure and trichiasis from facial hair often occurs. Eyelid colobomas may occur alone or as part of a syndrome of multiple ocular abnormalities. These abnormalities may include colobomas of the iris, choroid and optic nerve, persistent pupillary membranes, choroidal hypoplasia, microphthalmia, absence of the lacrimal gland and cataracts. Affected kittens are often born with the palpebral fissure partly or fully open.

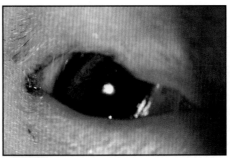

9.75 Agenesis of the lateral portion of the upper eyelid of a cat. The periocular hair has been clipped in preparation for surgical reconstruction. (Courtesy of R Grundon)

Treatment recommendations depend on the severity of the agenesis. Mild cases may require only lubricating ointment. Cryoepilation of the offending hairs can be performed, if the eyelid has sufficient function to protect the cornea. Surgical correction is indicated if impaired eyelid function and trichiasis leads to corneal exposure and irritation, respectively. Small defects can be closed directly following conversion to a simple wedge excision. For larger defects, the most commonly performed surgical procedure involves use of a skin–orbicularis layer from the lower eyelid and conjunctiva from the third eyelid (Dziezyc and Millichamp, 1989). This type of correction can be difficult and sometimes requires more than one procedure, and thus warrants special consultation or referral. Graft contraction can occur and misdirected hairs from the grafted skin may result in corneal irritation, necessitating a further procedure, such as cryoepilation. A modified Mustardé technique may be performed, which uses the full thickness lower eyelid to reconstruct the upper eyelid, avoiding the trichiasis associated with previously described methods (Munger and Gourley, 1981;

Esson, 2001). An H-plasty or lip-to-lid procedure can then be performed to repair the defect in the lower eyelid. A modifed lip-to-lid technique has also been described which involves taking a section from the lip commissure and using it to replace the upper eyelid and lateral canthus (Whittaker *et al.*, 2010), making it a one-stage process that avoids trichiasis and leads to a good cosmetic and functional result.

Dermoid

Dermoids result from faulty differentiation of tissue during ocular development. The anomaly occasionally develops along the eyelid margin and within the palpebral conjunctiva at the lateral canthus, although the temporal perilimbal conjunctiva and cornea are more typical locations. Although rare in cats, dermoids show a familial tendency in the Birman, and their development may be associated with the genetic predisposition to eyelid agenesis in certain lines of Burmese. Treatment is indicated where hairs extending from the dermoid make contact with and irritate the corneal surface. Surgical excision with accurate eyelid repair is usually curative.

Lagophthalmos

Lagophthalmos occurs in cats for similar reasons to those for dogs (see above). It is most commonly seen in Persians owing to the their macropalpebral fissures. Exposure keratitis results with the potential for corneal sequestrum formation (Figure 9.76).

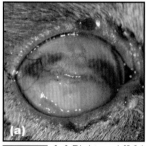
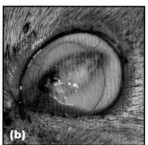

9.76 **(a)** Right and **(b)** left eyes showing lagophthalmos and exposure keratitis with sequestrum formation in a 5-year-old female Persian. The right inferior cornea has developed stromal ulceration. The distribution of corneal pathology, corresponding to the region of the palpebral fissure, is highly suggestive of exposure keratitis, keratitis due to facial paralysis or keratitis due to lack of corneal sensation.

Cilia abnormalities

Distichiasis is uncommon and ectopic cilia are rare in cats. When these abnormalities occur, they may result in increased lacrimation and, occasionally, corneal ulceration and sequestrum formation (Figure 9.77). Burmese and Siamese cats appear to be predisposed, despite the low number of cases reported. Magnification is required to confirm the diagnosis. The treatment options are the same as for the dog and include electrolysis, surgical resection or cryotherapy for distichiasis and surgical excision combined with cryotherapy for ectopic cilia. Although these conditions are rare, they should always be excluded in cases of feline ulcerative keratitis prior to embarking on the investigation and treatment of other suspected causes such as feline herpesvirus-1.

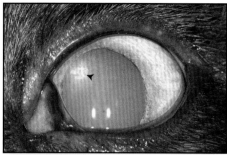
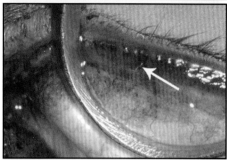

9.77 Superionasal corneal ulceration (arrowhead) secondary to an ectopic cilium (arrowed) in a 3-year-old female Burmese.

Eyelid position abnormalities

Entropion

Entropion is less common in cats than in dogs. It is more usually acquired as a consequence of chronic painful ocular disease, causing spastic entropion that fails to resolve when the initiating painful disease resolves. It is also seen in older cats where loss of orbital volume due to, for example, weight loss, has led to enophthalmos and secondary entropion. Excessive facial 'jowl' tissue in some cats, particularly Maine Coons, can also contribute to in-turning of the lower eyelids. Primary entropion is rare in cats, with only the Persian reported to have a breed predisposition. Treatment involves surgical correction using a Hotz–Celsus procedure, which may be combined with eyelid shortening. Removal of a greater amount of eyelid tissue is generally required for correction in the cat compared with similar procedures in the dog.

Ectropion

Ectropion is much less common in cats than in dogs and is more likely to be cicatricial following periocular injuries (e.g. abscesses and burns). Surgical treatment options include wedge resection of the affected area, V–Y plasty and advancement flaps, depending on the position and extent of the eversion.

Eyelid inflammation

Bacterial blepharitis

Localized abscessation may result from cat fight injuries. Secondary bacterial (and/or yeast) infection can occur as a complication of self-mutilation, which in turn may be the result of allergic skin disease or idiopathic facial dermatitis (especially in Persian cats). Mycobacterial disease is uncommon, but may be responsible for the development of non-healing, discharging cutaneous nodules on the eyelids and other areas. Diagnosis is made by confirmation of acid-fast bacilli on histopathology and culture. It is always advisable to keep a frozen tissue sample so that it is available for culture should this be indicated; however, culture is diagnostic in only approximately 50% of cases of mycobacterial disease. The degree of systemic involvement and zoonotic risk varies with the species of *Mycobacterium* involved (see Chapter 20).

Parasitic blepharitis

Demodicosis is a rare disease in cats. *Demodex cati* mites live in the hair follicle and can be found in clinically healthy cats as part of the normal cutaneous flora. The eyelid, periocular area, head and neck are commonly affected. Variable pruritus, with patchy erythema, crusting, scaling and alopecia results. Generalized demodicosis may be found in Siamese and Burmese breeds associated with diabetes mellitus, feline leukaemia, systemic lupus erythematosus, hyperadrenocorticism or feline immunodeficiency virus. Infestation with *Demodex gatoi* has also been reported; these mites live primarily in the superficial keratin layer of the epidermis. Cats with demodicosis secondary to *D. gatoi* infestation are typically pruritic, and the clinical signs may be indistinguishable from those of cats with allergic or psychogenic dermatological conditions. Dermatitis due to *D. gatoi* is not associated with an underlying disease, but the mites are contagious and can be passed from one cat to another. Feline scabies, which is caused by *Notoedres cati*, is also rare. The associated pruritus is variable, ranging from mild to severe. A diagnosis of parasitic blepharitis can be obtained by microscopic examination of deep skin scrapes.

Fungal blepharitis

Dermatophytosis affecting the feline eyelid is most commonly caused by *Microsporum canis*. Young cats (<1 year of age) and longhaired Persians and Himalayans are predisposed to dermatophytosis. The disease presents as one or more irregular areas of alopecia, with or without scaling. Other lesions occur on the head, pinnae and paws. The diagnosis is made by observation of apple-green fluorescence when viewed with a Woods lamp, microscopic examination of hair plucks and/or fungal culture. Systemic mycotic infections (*Cryptococcus*, *Histoplasma*, *Blastomyces* and *Coccidioides*) are rarely seen in the UK at present. Diagnosis is made by identifying the organisms on cytology or histology.

Viral diseases

Periocular nodules, papules, crusts and ulcerative plaques may be seen as a result of feline poxvirus infection (Figure 9.78). It may also be associated with systemic signs such as pyrexia, conjunctivitis and respiratory disease. A diagnosis is made based on serology, culture of the virus from the crusts, detection of orthopox DNA in the crusts or histopathological examination of skin biopsy samples. There is no specific treatment, but most animals eventually recover unless immunocompromised. Ulcerative facial and nasal dermatitis can also develop as a

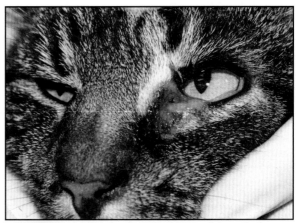

9.78   Poxvirus infection causing medial canthal ulceration in a 2-year-old male neutered Domestic Shorthaired Cat. (Courtesy of P Sands)

dermatological manifestation of feline herpesvirus infection, occurring approximately 10 days following the classic signs of herpesvirus infection. Diagnosis of herpes dermatitis is by histopathological examination and/or PCR testing of skin biopsy samples. Use of systemic antiviral therapy may be indicated in cats with herpes dermatitis (see Chapter 11).

Lipogranulomatous conjunctivitis

Lipogranulomatous conjunctivitis refers to a condition in which multiple smooth, non-ulcerated, cream or white subconjunctival masses can be seen in a typical distribution in the palpebral conjunctiva adjacent to the eyelid margins (Figure 9.79). It is thought to be a reaction to sebaceous secretions from damaged or ruptured meibomian glands and may represent a form of chalazion. It is a condition of older cats (6–16 years) and is typically seen in white or predominantly white cats with poorly pigmented eyelids, which may indicate a role for actinic damage in the pathogenesis of the disease (Read and Lucas, 2001). The nodules can vary in size from 1 mm in diameter to overlapping rows of relatively bulbous lesions up to 5 mm in diameter. Occasionally, these nodules can be seen through the eyelid skin (Figure 9.80). They can affect both the upper and lower eyelids and can be unilateral or bilateral. The masses may be incidental findings or may result in chronic ocular discomfort.

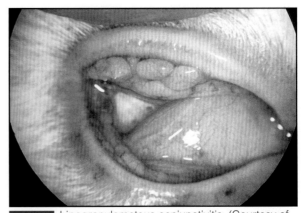

9.79   Lipogranulomatous conjunctivitis. (Courtesy of A Read)

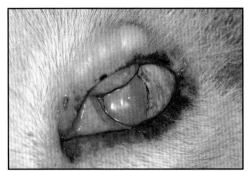

9.80 Unusual presentation of lipogranulomatous conjunctivitis, which was present bilaterally in an elderly cat. The aggregations of creamy inspissated meibomian secretions can be seen through the upper eyelid skin. The adjacent conjunctiva is chemotic and appears to contain small foci of lipid.

Treatment depends on the presence or absence of associated clinical signs. Medical treatment with systemic and topical antibiotic preparations may reduce but not eliminate irritation. In such cases, surgical resection of the lesions is indicated. Two incisions are made in the palpebral conjunctiva, parallel to the eyelid margin and either side of the row(s) of lesions, to a depth equal to the depth of the lesions. A strip of conjunctiva and subconjunctival tissue containing the lesions is then excised in a similar manner to the technique originally described for subconjunctival resection for the removal of distichiasis (Long, 1991). The conjunctival wound is left to heal by secondary intention. Postoperative management consists of topical application of antibiotics.

Immune-mediated eyelid disease

The most common immune-mediated feline eyelid disease is pemphigus foliaceus. This first appears as erythematous macules that rapidly progress to pustules and then become dry brown crusts. The disease starts on the head and ears, progresses to the footpads, and becomes generalized within 6 months.

Idiopathic facial dermatitis

A severe chronic facial dermatitis has been described in young Persian cats (Figure 9.81). Lesions are characterized by a symmetrical distribution of black waxy material adherent to the hair and skin of the chin, perioral and periocular areas. Erythema and exudation are seen in the facial folds and pre-auricular areas, and concurrent ceruminous otitis may be observed. Pruritus is not present initially, but develops as the affected areas become progressively more inflamed and secondarily infected with bacteria and *Malassezia*. The aetiology is unknown and a successful form of therapy has not been identified. Antimicrobial therapy is not curative and the response to glucocorticoids is variable and often poor.

Eyelid neoplasia

Feline eyelid tumours are more likely to be malignant than benign (McLaughlin *et al.*, 1993). Eyelid neoplasms occur most commonly in cats >10 years of age.

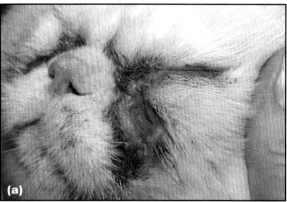

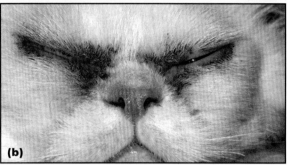

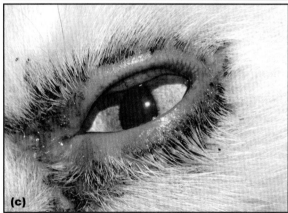

9.81 Idiopathic facial dermatitis in a 2-year-old female Persian. **(a)** Fluorescein application confirmed significant epiphora, which was contributing to the ulceration in the facial fold. **(b)** Modified medial lower eyelid Hotz–Celsus skin resections were performed to correct the entropion and improve the lacrimal lake, in order to reduce the epiphora. This was combined with facial fold resection, which partially improved the dermatitis. **(c)** Characteristic deposits of black waxy material, exudation and ulceration persisted around the eyelids.

Squamous cell carcinoma

Squamous cell carcinoma is the most common eyelid neoplasm in the cat (Figures 9.82 and 9.83). It is seen as a slightly raised or depressed ulcerative lesion either on or adjacent to the eyelid margin, the limits of which can be difficult to identify. Exposure to sunlight is a contributory factor and there is a predilection for white cats. Metastasis does not occur until late in the disease process, but local invasion can be extensive and regional lymph nodes are eventually involved. Treatment options include surgical excision, cryotherapy, radiotherapy (Hardman and Stanley, 2001) and photodynamic therapy (Stell *et al.*, 2001).

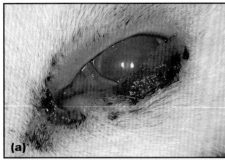

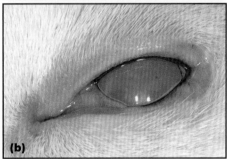

9.82 **(a)** Squamous cell carcinoma in the lateral lower eyelid of a 10-year-old male neutered white Domestic Shorthaired Cat. **(b)** Appearance 3 months following surgical debulking and cryotherapy.

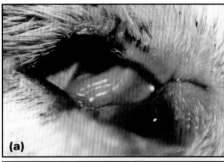

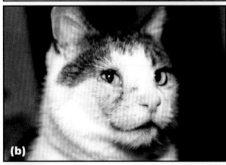

9.83 **(a)** Squamous cell carcinoma in the non-pigmented medial lower eyelid of an 8-year-old male neutered Domestic Shorthaired Cat. **(b)** The patient was initially treated with cryotherapy, but the residual lid defect required reconstructive surgery and a lip-to-lid procedure was performed.

Mast cell tumour

Feline cutaneous mast cell tumours usually occur in older cats and are often located on the head and neck. Of those arising on the head, the most common sites are the temporal area, pinnae, periocular areas and the haired skin of the eyelid. In cats, cutaneous mast cell tumours tend to have a benign clinical course, even when they are histologically pleomorphic. There is a low rate of local recurrence

following surgical excision (<5%), even if the excision is incomplete (Newkirk and Rohrbach, 2009; Montgomery *et al.*, 2010). These results are comparable with those for strontium-90 radiation (recurrence rate of approximately 3%) and combination therapy may be considered where complete surgical margins cannot be achieved.

Peripheral nerve sheath tumour

Peripheral nerve sheath tumours are spindle cell neoplasms arising from the neural sheath of the peripheral, cranial or autonomic nerves. This type of tumour may also be termed a neuroma or neurofibroma. The upper eyelid is more commonly affected and aggressive local recurrence is common following tumour excision. One review of six cases of peripheral nerve sheath tumours, where all cats had undergone surgical excision, reported that tumour regrowth occurred in all cats, necessitating additional surgical procedures on an average of three occasions (range 2–6) (Hoffman *et al.*, 2005). Wide surgical excision combined with enucleation and exenteration may therefore be indicated in the early stages.

Haemangiosarcoma and haemangioma

Despite histopathological features of malignancy, haemangiosarcomas arising from the eyelids of cats appear to have a favourable outcome when excised completely. They more commonly develop in non-pigmented ocular tissues, so may be associated with exposure to ultraviolet radiation.

Adenocarcinoma

Adenocarcinomas in feline eyelids are aggressive tumours and incomplete excision is frequently followed by death or euthanasia.

Lymphoma

Eyelid lymphoma is uncommon but carries a poor prognosis.

Apocrine hidrocystoma

Apocrine hidrocystomas are adenomatous proliferative tumours of the apocrine sweat glands of the eyelids (glands of Moll). They appear as multiple, well circumscribed, tense to fluctuant, smooth nodular structures, 2–10 mm in diameter and are located in the upper and lower eyelid skin (Figure 9.84). They are seen in older cats and there is a breed predisposition in Persians (Cantaloube *et al.*, 2004). Treatment options include monitoring, drainage alone, drainage and subsequent cryotherapy (Sivagurunathan *et al.*, 2010) and surgical excision. The recurrence rate is high following both drainage and surgical excision. Tissue debridement and chemical ablation is the most recent treatment option for this condition in humans; 20% trichloracetic acid has been used following surgical removal of the cyst wall and debridement of the subjacent tissue with a scalpel. The 20% trichloracetic acid was applied to each lesion for approximately 5–10 seconds before suturing the surrounding skin to close the lesion (Yang *et al.*, 2007).

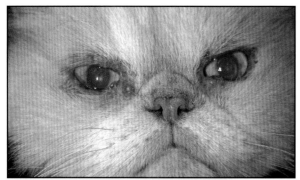

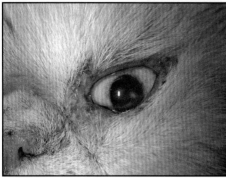

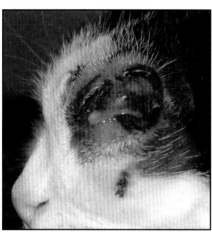

9.84 Apocrine hidrocystomas in a Persian cat.

Other neoplasms

Other feline eyelid tumours that may be encountered include adenomas, basal cell carcinomas, fibrosarcomas (Figure 9.85) and trichoepitheliomas.

9.85

Fibrosarcoma in a Domestic Shorthaired Cat.

Treatment

The surgical treatment options for periocular neoplasia, as in dogs, are determined by the size, nature and position of the tumour. Those procedures described for the dog have also been used in the cat, including split eyelid flaps, lip-to-lid transpositions and cutaneous transposition flaps lined with the bulbar surface of the third eyelid (Hagard, 2005; Schmidt *et al.*, 2005; Hunt, 2006).

Acknowledgements

The author is grateful to those colleagues who contributed photographic material and to Dr Stephen Shaw for advice on the dermatological content.

References and further reading

Bedford PG (1973) Distichiasis and its treatment by the method of partial tarsal plate excision. *Journal of Small Animal Practice* **14**(1), 1–5

Bedford PGC (1990) Surgical correction of facial droop in the English Cocker Spaniel. *Journal of Small Animal Practice* **31**(5), 255–258

Bedford PGC (1998) Technique of lateral canthoplasty for the correction of macropalpebral fissure in the dog. *Journal of Small Animal Practice* **39**(3), 117–120

Bigelbach A (1996) A combined tarsorrhaphy–canthoplasty technique for repair of entropion and ectropion. *Veterinary and Comparative Ophthalmology* **6**(4), 220–224

Blanchard GL and Keller WF (1976) The rhomboid graft flap for the repair of extensive ocular adnexal defects. *Journal of the American Animal Hospital Association* **12**(5), 576–580

Cantaloube B, Raymond-Letron I and Regnier A (2004) Multiple eyelid apocrine hidrocystomas in two Persian cats. *Veterinary Ophthalmology* **7**(2), 121–125

Dziezyc J and Millichamp NJ (1989) Surgical correction of eyelid agenesis in a cat. *Journal of the American Animal Hospital Association* **25**(5), 513–516

Esson D (2001) A modification of the Mustardé technique for the surgical repair of a large feline eyelid coloboma. *Veterinary Ophthalmology* **4**(2), 159–160

Gelatt KNGJP (1994) *Handbook of Small Animal Ophthalmic Surgery.* Oxford, Elsevier Science Ltd

Hagard GM (2005) Eyelid reconstruction using a split eyelid flap after excision of a palpebral tumour in a Persian cat. *Journal of Small Animal Practice* **46**(8), 389–392

Hardman C and Stanley R (2001) Radioactive gold-198 seeds for the treatment of squamous cell carcinoma in the eyelid of a cat. *Australian Veterinary Journal* **79**(9), 604–608

Hoffman A, Blocker T, Dubielzig R *et al.* (2005) Feline periocular peripheral nerve sheath tumor: a case series. *Veterinary Ophthalmology* **8**(3), 153–158

Hunt GB (2006) Use of the lip-to-lid flap for replacement of the lower eyelid in five cats. *Veterinary Surgery* **35**(3), 284–286

Jacobi S, Stanley BJ, Petersen-Jones S *et al.* (2008) Use of an axial pattern flap and nictitans to reconstruct medial eyelids and canthus in a dog. *Veterinary Ophthalmology* **11**(6), 395–400

Krehbiel JD and Langham RF (1975) Eyelid neoplasms of dogs. *American Journal of Veterinary Research* **36**, 115–119

Lewin GA (2000) Temporary lateral tarsorrhaphy for the treatment of lower lateral eyelid entropion in juvenile dogs. *Veterinary Record* **146**(15), 439–440

Lewin GA (2003) Eyelid reconstruction in seven dogs using a split eyelid flap. *Journal of Small Animal Practice* **44**(8), 346–351

Long RD (1991) Treatment of distichiasis by conjunctival resection. *Journal of Small Animal Practice* **32**(3), 146–148

McCallum P and Welser J (2004) Coronal rhytidectomy in conjunction with deep plane walking sutures, modified Hotz–Celsus and lateral canthoplasty procedure in a dog with excessive brow droop. *Veterinary Ophthalmology* **7**(5), 376–379

McLaughlin SA, Whitley RD, Gilger BC *et al.* (1993) Eyelid neoplasms in cats: a review of demographic data (1979 to 1989). *Journal of the American Animal Hospital Association* **29**(1), 63–67

Montgomery KW, van der Woerdt A, Aquino SM *et al.* (2010) Periocular cutaneous mast cell tumors in cats: evaluation of surgical excision (33 cases). *Veterinary Ophthalmology* **13**(1), 26–30

Munger RJ and Carter JD (1984) A further modification of the Kuhnt–Szymanowski procedure for correction of atonic ectropion in dogs. *Journal of the American Animal Hospital Association* **20**(4), 651–656

Munger RJ and Gourley IM (1981) Cross lid flap for repair of large upper eyelid defects. *Journal of the American Veterinary Medical Association* **178**(1), 45–48

Newkirk KM and Rohrbach BW (2009) A retrospective study of eyelid tumors from 43 cats. *Veterinary Pathology* **46**(5), 916–927

Pavletic MM, Nafe LA and Confer AW (1982) Mucocutaneous subdermal plexus flap from the lip for lower eyelid restoration in the dog. *Journal of the American Veterinary Medical Association* **180**(8), 921–926

Pellicane CP, Meek LA, Brooks DE *et al.* (1994) Eyelid reconstruction in five dogs by the semicircular flap technique. *Veterinary and Comparative Ophthalmology* **4**(2), 93–103

Peña MA and Leiva M (2008) Canine conjunctivitis and blepharitis. *Veterinary Clinics of North America: Small Animal Practice* **38**(2), 233–249

Peña MT, Roura X and Davidson MG (2000) Ocular and periocular manifestations of leishmaniasis in dogs: 105 cases (1993–1998). *Veterinary Ophthalmology* **3**(1), 35–41

Peña TM and Garcia FA (1999) Reconstruction of the eyelids of a dog using grafts of oral mucosa. *Veterinary Record* **144**(15), 413–415

Read RA and Broun HC (2007) Entropion correction in dogs and cats using a combination Hotz–Celsus and lateral eyelid wedge resection: results in 311 eyes. *Veterinary Ophthalmology* **10**(1),

6–11

Read RA and Lucas J (2001) Lipogranulomatous conjunctivitis: clinical findings from 21 eyes in 13 cats. *Veterinary Ophthalmology* **4**(2), 93–98

Roberts SM, Severin GA and Lavach JD (1986) Prevalence and treatment of palpebral neoplasms in the dog: 200 cases (1975–1983). *Journal of the American Veterinary Medical Association* **189**, 1355–1359

Robertson BF and Roberts SM (1995a) Lateral canthus entropion in the dog, Part 1: Comparative anatomic studies. *Veterinary and Comparative Ophthalmology* **5**(3), 151–156

Robertson BF and Roberts SM (1995b) Lateral canthus entropion in the dog, Part 2: Surgical correction. Results and follow-up from 21 cases. *Veterinary and Comparative Ophthalmology* **5**(3), 162–169

Schmidt K, Bertani C, Martano M *et al.* (2005) Reconstruction of the lower eyelid by third eyelid lateral advancement and local transposition cutaneous flap after *en bloc* resection of squamous cell carcinoma in 5 cats. *Veterinary Surgery* **34**(1), 78–82

Sivagurunathan A, Goodhead AD and Du Plessis EC (2010) Multiple eyelid apocrine hidrocystoma in a Domestic Shorthaired Cat. *Journal of the South African Veterinary Association* **81**(1), 65–68

Stades FC (1987) A new method for surgical correction of upper eyelid trichiasis–entropion: operation method. *Journal of the American Animal Hospital Association* **23**(6), 603–606

Stades FC and Boeve MH (1987) Surgical correction of upper eyelid trichiasis–entropion: results and follow-up in 55 eyes. *Journal of the American Animal Hospital Association* **23**(6), 607–610

Stell AJ, Dobson JM and Langmack K (2001) Photodynamic therapy of feline superficial squamous cell carcinoma using topical 5-aminolaevulinic acid. *Journal of Small Animal Practice* **42**(4) 164–169

Stiles J, Townsend W, Willis M *et al.* (2003) Use of a caudal auricular axial pattern flap in three cats and one dog following orbital exenteration. *Veterinary Ophthalmology* **6**(2), 121–126

Stuhr CM, Stanz K, Murphy CJ *et al.* (1997) Stellate rhytidectomy: superior entropion repair in a dog with excessive facial skin. *Journal of the American Animal Hospital Association* **33**(4), 342–345

Whittaker CJ, Wilkie DA, Simpson DJ *et al.* (2010) Lip commissure to eyelid transposition for repair of feline eyelid agenesis. *Veterinary Ophthalmology* **13**(3), 173–178

Willis AM, Martin CL, Stiles J *et al.* (1999) Brow suspension for treatment of ptosis and entropion in dogs with redundant facial skin folds. *Journal of the American Veterinary Medical Association* **214**(5), 660–662

Yang SH, Liu CH, Hsu CD *et al.* (2007) Use of chemical ablation with trichloracetic acid to treat eyelid apocrine hidrocystomas in a cat. *Journal of the American Veterinary Medical Association* **230**(8), 1170–1173

10

The lacrimal system

Claudia Hartley

The lacrimal system has two components: the secretory system and the excretory system. The secretory system is composed of the orbital lacrimal gland and the third eyelid gland, as well as the goblet cells of the conjunctiva (see also Chapter 11) and meibomian glands of the eyelids (see also Chapter 9). It is responsible for production of the preocular tear film. The excretory system is composed of upper and lower eyelid nasolacrimal puncta, upper and lower lacrimal canaliculi, the lacrimal sac, the nasolacrimal duct and the nasal punctum. It is responsible for the drainage of tears from the ocular surface (Figure 10.1).

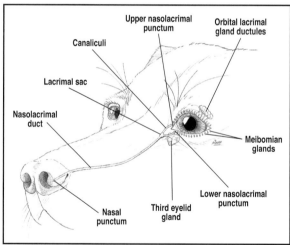

10.1 Lacrimal secretory and excretory systems. (Illustration by Roser Tetas Pont)

Lacrimal secretory system

Embryology, anatomy and physiology

The orbital lacrimal gland, third eyelid gland, conjunctival goblet cells and meibomian glands are derived from surface ectoderm. The lacrimal gland is located in the dorsolateral orbit and comprises 15 to 20 lacrimal ductules, which pass through the dorsolateral conjunctiva to discharge tears on to the ocular surface. The nictitans gland is located at the base of the third eyelid and is attached by connective tissue to the third eyelid cartilage. The numerous nictitans gland ducts discharge tears on to the posterior (bulbar) surface of the third eyelid.

The lacrimal gland acini are largely innervated by parasympathetic nerves, although sympathetic nerves are also sparsely present (predominantly around the gland vasculature). The parasympathetic nerve fibres originate from the parasympathetic nucleus of the facial nerve within the brainstem, and run with the facial nerve via the petrous temporal bone, internal acoustic meatus and facial canal. They subsequently join the greater petrosal nerve, along with the deep petrosal nerve (sympathetic), to form the nerve of the pterygoid canal. From the pterygopalatine fossa, the fibres synapse in the pterygopalatine region. The post-ganglionic parasympathetic fibres then join the zygomatic nerve (a branch of the trigeminal nerve) and finally branch off as the lacrimal nerve to reach the lacrimal gland.

The meibomian glands, which are modified sebaceous glands, are present along the eyelid margins (see also Chapter 9). The glands are located within the tarsal plate of the eyelid and number between 20 and 40 per eyelid. Meibomian glands are holocrine (i.e. the secretory cells rupture and are shed into meibum) and the lipid produced is transported through a ductule to the orifice on the eyelid margin. The openings on the eyelid form a line along the margin, which is sometimes referred to as the 'grey line'. Control of meibomian secretion is not fully understood. Parasympathetic nerves surround the meibomian acini and neurotransmitters can influence lipid synthesis and secretion. Sparse sympathetic innervation is also present, but predominantly found around the vasculature. Androgen sex hormones may also have a role in the regulation of lipid synthesis and secretion; in humans, meibomian gland function has been shown to be regulated by sex hormones, with androgens acting as agonists and oestrogens acting as antagonists.

Tears are distributed across the cornea by eyelid blinking and third eyelid excursions, and are essential for the maintenance of ocular surface health. Not only do they lubricate the surface, flushing away debris and allowing atraumatic eyelid closure, they also provide nutrition to the avascular cornea and contain protective antimicrobial proteins. However, certain breeds are at greater risk of poor tear film distribution. Brachycephalic breeds may have degrees of lagophthalmos, which prevents complete tear coverage, with the central cornea most prone to drying, even when tear production is normal.

The tear film

The tear film is composed of three components: mucus, aqueous and lipid. Previously, these layers were thought to form a trilaminar film; however, more recent studies have shown that the layers are more intricately mingled (Figure 10.2).

The mucus layer

This is secreted by goblet cells present in the conjunctiva, concentrated particularly in the lower conjunctival sac. This layer is believed to allow adherence of the tear film to the corneal surface. Mucins are classified as either secretory or membrane bound. Membrane-bound mucins are found on the edges of the microplicae of the surface epithelial cells, forming a dense glycocalyx at the epithelium–tear film interface. This prevents pathogen penetration and enhances aqueous cohesion. Secretory mucins help to remove debris, hold fluid in place and bind defence molecules. Goblet cell secretion is provoked by stimulation of sensory nerves within the conjunctiva, which subsequently activate the parasympathetic and sympathetic nerves around the goblet cells (i.e. a reflex action).

The aqueous layer

This is produced by the lacrimal and nictitans glands (approximately 70% and 30%, respectively) and makes up the bulk of the tear film. It comprises water, electrolytes, glucose, urea, surface-active polymers, glycoproteins and tear proteins. The tear proteins include secretory immunoglobulin (Ig)A, IgG, IgM, albumin, lysozyme, lactoferrin, lipocalin, epidermal growth factor, transforming growth factors and interleukins.

The lipid layer

The lipid layer (meibum) is thought to stabilize the tear film and reduce evaporative loss and is produced by the meibomian glands. The lipids in meibum include wax monoesters, sterol esters, triglycerides, free sterols, free fatty acids and polar lipids.

Investigation of disease

Quantitative tear film assessment

Tear production is measured by the Schirmer tear test (STT).

Schirmer tear test 1: STT-1 involves the placement of a test strip over the lower eyelid (preferably the lateral third) into the lower conjunctival fornix for 60 seconds, followed by measurement of the length of wetting of the strip (Figure 10.3). Test strips are variable in their absorbency, so use of the same test strip type (by the same manufacturer) is advisable when monitoring tear production over a period of time.

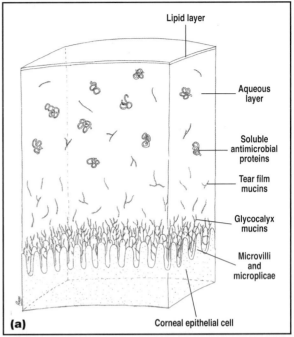

(a)

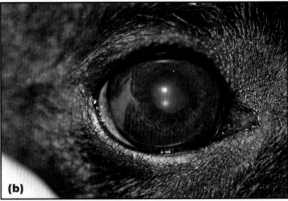

(b)

10.2 **(a)** Normal tear film. The corneal epithelial cells have microplicae and microvilli, which increase the surface area for tear binding. Glycocalyx expressed by the epithelial cells interacts with tear film mucins and promotes retention of tears on the cornea ('wettability'). Secretory mucins are dispersed in the tear film and soluble antimicrobial proteins are also suspended in the aqueous portion of the tear film. A thin lipid layer over the surface of the tear film reduces evaporation. (Illustration by Roser Tetas Pont) **(b)** Normal tear film of an adult Staffordshire Bull Terrier. Note the tear meniscus and crisp corneal reflections (Purkinje image).

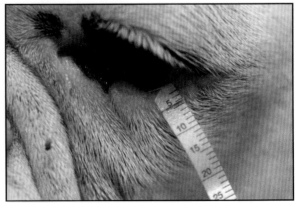

10.3 Schirmer tear testing (22 mm wetting) in an adult Boxer.

The STT-1 is not the most reproducible test, but is widely accepted as the best diagnostic tool available to screen for keratoconjunctivitis sicca (KCS) in veterinary patients. In human medicine, an array of tests and questionnaires are used to diagnose and categorize KCS. The STT-I measures the tear lake, from both basal tear production and reflex tear production (stimulated by the placement of the test strip against the conjunctiva and cornea). Thus, the test should be performed before the application of any drops or manipulation of the eye.

- Dogs:
  - Normal = >15 mm/minute
  - Early/subclinical KCS = 10–15 mm/minute. These readings are equivocal and testing should be repeated at a later date
  - Mild/moderate KCS = 6–9 mm/minute. Values <10 mm/minute are diagnostic for KCS in conjunction with compatible clinical signs
  - Severe KCS = ≤5 mm/minute
- Cats:
  - Normal = 3–32 mm/minute (mean of 17 mm/minute).

All cases presenting with ocular discomfort should have the STT-1 performed, unless there is an obvious contraindication such as globe rupture or descemetocele (where restraint or disturbance of the eye could provoke rupture). West Highland White Terriers, English Cocker Spaniels, English Bulldogs, Lhaso Apsos, English Springer Spaniels and Toy Poodles are predisposed to immunogenic KCS (Sanchez *et al.*, 2007) and should periodically have an STT-1 performed. In addition, all patients with hypothyroidism, diabetes mellitus and hyperadrenocorticism should have their tear production routinely measured because an association with KCS has been reported.

Schirmer tear test 2: STT-2 is undertaken by applying a topical anaesthetic to the eye (e.g. proxymetacaine) followed by gentle drying of the lower conjunctival sac after 1 minute, and then placement of a test strip as for STT-1. The STT-2 measures only basal tear production (the reflex production of tears is abolished by the application of the topical anaesthetic) and the readings obtained are usually approximately half those seen with STT-1.

Qualitative tear film assessment
Tear film quality is assessed by tear film break up time (TFBUT) and Rose Bengal testing.

Tear film break up time: The TFBUT is assessed by applying a single drop of fluorescein to the ocular surface, followed by enforced blinks to ensure that it is distributed evenly. The eyelids are then held open and the corneal surface is observed for the first sign of fluorescein break-up, observed as dark spots, with the aid of a slit-lamp biomicroscope on a blue filter setting. The TFBUT assesses both the ocular mucin component of the tear film (responsible for corneal 'wettability') and the lipid layer (responsible for tear film stability and reduction of evaporation). Normal TFBUT is reported to be 15–25 seconds in the dog and 12–21 seconds in the cat.

Rose Bengal staining: Rose Bengal staining can also identify qualitative tear deficiency because stain uptake is not seen in normal healthy corneas, but is present where the mucin component of the tear film is absent. Rose Bengal stain can be irritant, so the excess should be flushed with saline to minimize discomfort.

Other tests

Meibometry: This is a means of measuring the lipid production from the meibomian glands. It involves the application of a test strip against the eyelid margin surface, followed by placement of the strip into a meibometer, which gives a numerical reading of the lipid level on the strip. Meibometry is currently only used experimentally in veterinary species, but is undertaken in humans with tear film abnormalities.

Tear film osmolarity: This is also assessed in humans with dry eye by taking a minute sample of the tear lake using a specialized piece of equipment, which gives a numerical measure of the tear osmolarity. Tear film osmolarity changes with increasing severity of KCS in humans and can provide an objective grade of the disease. Unfortunately, tear osmolarity readings are not very reproducible in veterinary species. Statistically significant differences in tear osmolarity between cats with and without conjunctivitis could not be demonstrated in one study (Davis and Townsend, 2011).

Canine conditions

Keratoconjunctivitis sicca
Reduction in tear production causes increasing corneal inflammation and, ultimately, permanent damage that may prove blinding. The classic signs of KCS are a tacky mucopurulent ocular discharge that is frequently adherent to the corneal surface in strings, and recurrent conjunctivitis with or without

- Immune-mediated
- Neurogenic (may be associated with middle ear disease)
- Drug-induced (e.g. systemic sulphonamides, systemic and topical atropine, topical and general anaesthetics, opioids and etodolac)
- Congenital alacrima (e.g. Yorkshire Terriers or in conjunction with ichthyosiform dermatosis in Cavalier King Charles Spaniels)
- Irradiation
- In association with metabolic disease (e.g. diabetes mellitus and hypothyroidism; presumed via autonomic neuropathy pathogenesis)
- Trauma/inflammation of lacrimal gland or orbit, or innervation
- Canine distemper virus infection
- Chronic blepharoconjunctivitis
- Iatrogenic (excision of the third eyelid gland)
- Dysautonomia
- Sjögren's syndrome

10.4 Possible causes of canine KCS.

corneal ulceration that is typically slow to heal. However, some cases present with conjunctivitis and only a mild mucoid discharge. Owing to the non-specific, sometimes vague signs, KCS is likely to be under-diagnosed. The possible causes of KCS are given in Figure 10.4. Immune-mediated destruction of lacrimal glandular tissue is believed to represent the largest proportion of KCS cases.

Immunogenic KCS: Histological examination of lacrimal tissue from dogs with idiopathic KCS has revealed lymphoplasmacytic infiltrates associated with acinar fibrosis and atrophy, suggesting an immunological basis for the disease. The predisposition to this immune-mediated disease appears to have a hereditary basis due to the marked breed incidence (see above).

Treatment: Topical treatment with the immunomodulatory drug, ciclosporin (0.2%), is the mainstay of therapy for immune-mediated KCS. Lifelong treatment is required to suppress the immune-mediated attack and allow lacrimal recovery. Early initiation of treatment is more effective because less lacrimal tissue is permanently damaged. There is a lag phase (usually 2–4 weeks, but can be up to 8 weeks) before improvement in tear production is seen, during which time ocular lubricant products should be employed (Figure 10.5) (see Chapter 7). Once the lacrimal tissue recovers, ocular lubricants can often be withdrawn.

In cases where 0.2% ciclosporin is ineffective, a higher concentration can be trialled. However, this is 'off-licence' use and the client should be made aware of this fact. The ciclosporin is made up to 1% or 2% in corn oil and applied twice daily. This topical preparation can be irritant (especially if derived from the intravenous ciclosporin preparation) and some dogs will not tolerate its use.

More recently, tacrolimus (0.03% in oil) has been used to treat refractory KCS with considerable success (Berdoulay *et al.*, 2005). It appears to be better tolerated than ciclosporin in oil, but some patients demonstrate ocular irritation on application. It has been associated with an increased incidence of skin cancer in human medicine, where it is used as a topical ointment in the treatment of atopic dermatitis. Experimentally, it has also been shown to increase lymphoma incidence in mice (Bugelski *et al.*, 2010). It is not authorized for use in any veterinary species and owners need to be made aware of this, as well as the potential side effects encountered in humans.

Patients with KCS are at increased risk of opportunistic secondary bacterial conjunctivitis, and topical antibiotics may be required until tear production is restored to normal levels. Those animals that respond poorly and rely on ocular lubricants are likely to require intermittent antibiotic therapy. The flora found in the conjunctival sac of dogs with KCS is different from that of normal animals; bacterial culture and sensitivity testing should be considered to identify the most appropriate antibacterial therapy. If medical treatment is unsuccessful, then parotid duct transposition surgery should be considered (see below).

Neurogenic KCS: Lacrimal gland secretion is predominantly controlled by parasympathetic innervation (see above). Owing to its intimate connection with the peripheral vestibular system and middle ear, disease processes such as otitis media can affect facial nerve function and therefore tear production (Figure 10.6). In addition, given that the sympathetic innervation to the eye passes in close proximity to the structures of the inner and middle ear, clinical signs of ipsilateral Horner's syndrome may accompany neurogenic KCS. Neurogenic KCS may also be seen in conjunction with an ipsilateral dry nose because the innervation of the lateral nasal gland shares the same preganglionic parasympathetic fibres proximal to the pterygopalatine ganglion (Figure 10.7).

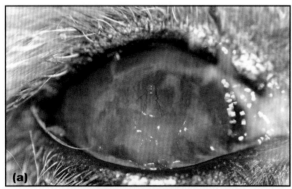

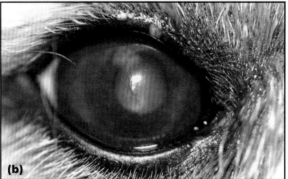

10.5 **(a)** West Highland White Terrier with severe KCS (STT = 0 mm/minute). Note the classic appearance of a tacky mucopurulent discharge adherent to the corneal surface and corneal neovascularization. **(b)** Appearance of the eye 4 weeks after the initiation of topical ciclosporin therapy (STT = 18 mm/minute). Note that a single branching superficial corneal blood vessel remains.

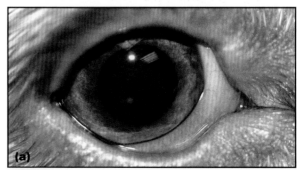

10.6 **(a)** Normal right eye of a dog with unilateral KCS. (continues) ▶

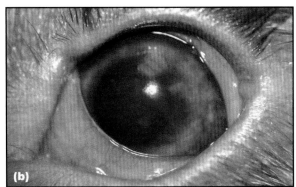

10.6 (continued) **(b)** Neurogenic KCS secondary to otitis media in the left eye. Note the disrupted corneal reflex, conjunctival swelling and third eyelid protrusion.

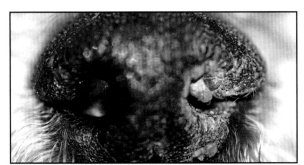

10.7 Dry nares associated with lack of lateral nasal gland function (also under parasympathetic control via the facial nerve) in a Toy Poodle with neurogenic KCS. These cases often present with unilateral dried mucoid material completely occluding the ipsilateral nares.

Treatment: The treatment is aimed at the underlying cause (if identified). Prolonged courses (6–8 weeks) of oral antibiotics may be indicated in cases of otitis media, particularly if it is accompanied by inflammation of the neighbouring petrous temporal bone. Systemic anti-inflammatory drugs may be indicated for treatment of the primary disease, and may be beneficial in reducing the adjacent facial nerve inflammation. Facial trauma can result in facial nerve damage, which may resolve with time. Frequent application of ocular lubricants is indicated. These cases rarely respond to topical ciclosporin or tacrolimus.

In the presence of denervation hypersensitivity, treatment with oral or topical pilocarpine (parasympathomimetic) can prove beneficial. The oral dosage for neurogenic KCS has been reported to be one drop of 2% pilocarpine per 10 kg bodyweight. The dose is increased by one drop increments at each dosing until signs of systemic toxicity (hypersalivation, inappetence, vomiting, diarrhoea, cardiac arrhythmias) appear; the dose is then lowered to the previously highest tolerated dose. Topical pilocarpine is given diluted (0.1–0.25%) in saline and there are anecdotal reports of success in cases of neurogenic KCS. Topical pilocarpine may cause blepharospasm, miosis and conjunctival hyperaemia. A study in normal dogs suggested that topical pilocarpine does not significantly increase tear production; however, the study has not been repeated in the presence of denervation hypersensitivity (Smith *et al.*, 1994).

Drug-induced KCS: Pre-anaesthetic and anaesthetic agents may reduce tear production for up to 24 hours (Herring *et al.*, 2000). In this study, the duration of anaesthesia was shown to affect tear production, with anaesthetics lasting >2 hours having a prolonged effect on tear production. The effect of inhalational anaesthetic agents alone (i.e. mask induction) is less long-lasting, with tear production returning to baseline values at 10 hours post-anaesthesia; the duration of the anaesthetic period had no effect on the time taken to return to baseline in these cases (Shepard *et al.*, 2011). The administration of anticholinergics (e.g. atropine) prior to or during anaesthesia also decreases tear production after the anaesthetic period. Ocular lubrication should be employed for all anaesthetized patients (Figure 10.8) and maintained in susceptible breeds (e.g. brachycephalic breeds with lagophthalmos) for up to 48 hours following the anaesthetic period.

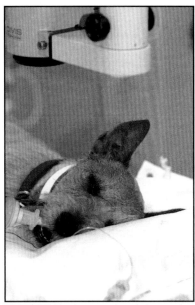

10.8 Terrier crossbred dog under general anaesthesia. All animals should have their eyes lubricated when under general anaesthesia and during the recovery period.

Topical atropine, which is used in the treatment of uveitis, can have a profound and possibly prolonged effect on tear production. In cases of ulcerative keratitis with a reflex uveitis, it is important to measure tear production because treatment of a patient that has undiagnosed KCS with topical atropine may exacerbate the disease.

Systemic sulphonamide therapy (e.g. sulfasalazine, sulfadiazine and trimethoprim/sulphonamide combinations) has been associated with acute onset KCS. The mechanism is not well understood; however, a T-cell mediated response to proteins haptenated by oxidative sulphonamide metabolites may be responsible. Prolonged systemic use of these agents may lead to permanent severe KCS, resulting from complete atrophy of the lacrimal glands. Regular STTs are advised for all patients receiving these drugs.

The non-steroidal anti-inflammatory drug (NSAID), etodolac, has also been associated with KCS in dogs and all patients receiving this drug, particularly for several months, should have their tear production routinely monitored.

Treatment: Withdrawal of the offending medication may result in some recovery of the lacrimal glands when a toxic lacrimal adenitis has occurred. In cases of chronic administration, tear production may never recover. In the case of general anaesthesia and anticholinergic drug administration, tear production returns to normal once the effects of the drug have dissipated (which may be >1 week in the case of topical atropine). Ocular lubricants should be employed in the intervening period, or long-term use may be required when permanent lacrimal gland damage has occurred. If artificial tears cannot be given frequently enough (every 1–2 hours during waking hours if the STT = 0 mm/minute), parotid duct transposition should be considered (see below).

Congenital KCS: Congenital alacrima has been reported in many breeds of dog, although Yorkshire Terriers were over-represented in two studies and bitches were more commonly affected in one of these studies (Herrera *et al.*, 2007; Westermeyer *et al.*, 2009). The mechanism of congenital alacrima is not fully understood, but it has been proposed that these cases have congenital lacrimal gland agenesis or hypoplasia, although a central or peripheral neuropathy could also result in a congenital absence of tear production. In one report, no orbital lacrimal gland was identified on post-mortem examination, consistent with lacrimal gland agenesis. In most dogs, the clinical signs are unilateral but bilateral cases do occur. Most commonly, the STT-1 shows 0 mm/minute in congenital alacrima cases.

Congenital KCS in conjunction with an ichthyosiform dermatosis has also been described in Cavalier King Charles Spaniels (CKCSs) (Barnett, 2006; Hartley *et al.*, 2012). Affected dogs are born with a rough or curly coat, quite distinct from the normal silky coat. After eyelid opening, KCS is apparent with frequent bouts of secondary bacterial conjunctivitis, sometimes in conjunction with corneal ulceration. In the first few months of life, affected puppies demonstrate a scurfy and sparse coat with hyperkeratinisation of the footpads and abnormal nail growth. The mechanism of KCS is not well understood in this syndrome and it is possible that both a quantitative and qualitative tear deficiency may be present. The genetic mutation responsible has been identified and breeding dogs can now be screened prior to mating; the diagnosis can be confirmed in affected puppies, if required.

Treatment: Congenital alacrima requires extremely frequent application of artificial tears to provide comfort to affected dogs. Parotid duct transposition may also be considered.

Congenital KCS and ichthyosiform dermatosis in CKCSs can show a variable response to lacrimostimulants such as ciclosporin; although, subjectively, treated dogs had less severe corneal changes in one long-term study (Hartley *et al.*, 2012). Frequent use of ocular lubricants is also required in affected dogs.

Other causes of KCS: Other causes of KCS include *irradiation* (e.g. when the eye and/or orbit have been included in the field of radiotherapy for a nasal tumour). KCS secondary to irradiation is poorly responsive to lacrimal stimulants and treatment is largely aimed at tear replacement therapy. Given that irradiation may also cause cataracts and retinal degeneration in the long term, some owners may elect to have enucleation performed, rather than committing to prolonged use of intensive medication, if the eye is blind.

Quantitative KCS may also occur in association with *metabolic disease* (e.g. diabetes mellitus or hypothyroidism). In diabetes mellitus, this has been postulated to occur secondary to reduced corneal sensitivity and, therefore, decreased reflex tearing. Qualitative tear deficiency in such cases has also been described and a common aetiopathogenesis may be responsible. Hormonal influence on tear production has been established in humans, although gender and/or neutering have not been shown to affect tear production in normal dogs. However, immune-mediated KCS has been shown to occur more frequently in bitches.

Trauma or inflammation of the lacrimal gland may result in KCS. Orbital trauma (e.g. from road traffic accidents) or cellulitis may involve the lacrimal gland and are typically poorly responsive to lacrimostimulant drugs. Traumatic damage to the parasympathetic nerve supply to the orbital lacrimal gland results in neurogenic KCS (STT-1 = 0 mm/minute). Treatment is aimed at reducing the inflammation associated with the primary disease, with supportive care in the form of artificial tear products. On occasion, the damage is severe and permanent and the prognosis is therefore guarded, with patients requiring long term tear replacement therapy or parotid duct transposition to provide ocular lubrication. Some functional recovery of the gland may occur in a few cases and temporary supportive care with treatment of the secondary bacterial conjunctivitis is sufficient.

Canine distemper virus is capable of inducing lacrimal adenitis as part of the spectrum of clinical signs associated with the infection. Dogs that have recovered from canine distemper virus may demonstrate persistent KCS due to permanent lacrimal gland damage.

Chronic blepharoconjunctivitis may cause damage to the lacrimal ductules from the orbital or third eyelid glands with subsequent KCS. Treatment of the primary disease may result in some recovery of tear production if not all ductules are obstructed.

Iatrogenic KCS can occur as a consequence of excision of the third eyelid gland following gland prolapse. In some dogs, the orbital lacrimal gland is able to compensate for the loss of the third eyelid contribution to tear production. Unfortunately, many breeds susceptible to third eyelid gland prolapse are commonly affected by immune-mediated KCS (e.g. English Bulldog) and are therefore on a lacrimal 'knife-edge' already. In one study of dogs with third eyelid gland prolapse, 48% of those treated by surgical excision of the gland later developed KCS compared with 14% of dogs treated by surgical replacement of the prolapsed gland (Morgan *et al.*, 1993).

Parotid duct transposition: Where KCS is severe and permanent and the patient's comfort cannot be maintained with topical artificial tear preparations, parotid duct transposition should be considered. This involves the relocation of the parotid salivary duct and papilla from the oral cavity to the lower conjunctival sac. There are two techniques described for this procedure and both require magnification and fine surgical instruments. These procedures require a great deal of skill, thus specialist referral is strongly recommended.

Open method: A skin incision over the lateral face allows identification of the parotid duct, which is dissected caudally towards the parotid gland and rostrally to the parotid papilla. The facial nerve and vein should be identified and care taken not to injure either during facial dissection. The parotid duct is usually cannulated with suture material (2/0 (3 metric) nylon) via the papilla to aid its identification during dissection. The papilla should be dissected free from the oral mucosa with enough mucosal margin that suturing into the conjunctival sac will not traumatize the duct. Once the duct has been freed rostrally, a tract is bluntly dissected to the lower conjunctival fornix, and the conjunctiva incised to allow the papilla to be sutured (without tension) into the fornix (using 8/0 (0.4 metric) polyglactin 910 absorbable suture material). Excessive tension or trauma to the duct will result in fibrosis and stricture formation with failure of the procedure.

Closed method: This involves dissection of the parotid duct back to the gland via an oral mucosal incision. This method is more difficult owing to the poor visualization of structures but avoids a facial skin incision. The papilla is sutured into the ventral conjunctival sac as for the open method.

Complications: The possible complications associated with parotid duct transposition include:

- Failure of parotid duct transposition due to excessive traction, twisting, sectioning or trauma to the transposed duct
- Sialolith formation in the duct, which may require surgical removal or massaging from the duct
- Sialadenitis
- Overflow of saliva on to the face with secondary blepharitis and dermatitis
- Deposition of calcium precipitates on the cornea (from saliva), which may be associated with keratitis and discomfort.

Prognosis: With appropriate treatment, the prognosis for immunogenic KCS is very good (those cases diagnosed and treated promptly have the best prognosis). Left untreated, the prognosis is grave for vision because the cornea becomes increasingly vascularized, pigmented and keratinized (Figure 10.9). Ulceration is common in acute cases and can be progressive and/or slow to heal. Perforation of a progressive KCS ulcer is relatively common and is devastating for vision and the globe (Figure 10.10). Neurogenic or drug-induced KCS that does not improve with appropriate treatment has a guarded prognosis, requiring diligent owners who are able to frequently apply artificial tear products. Artificial tears are not a replacement for natural tears as they lack the beneficial immune proteins and epitheliotrophic factors. Parotid duct transposition can improve the comfort of the eye, although side effects are common (see above).

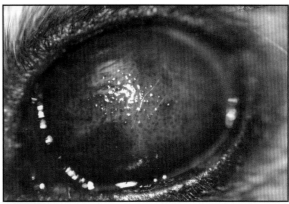

10.9 Severe corneal pigmentation, keratinization and fibrosis in a Cavalier King Charles Spaniel with bilateral KCS that was inadequately treated. The eye was blind.

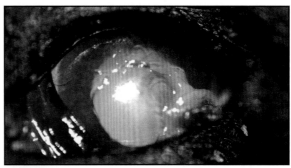

10.10 Descemetocele with mucopurulent adherent discharge in a dog with acute onset KCS.

Meibomianitis
Inflammation causes distension of the meibomian gland (meibomianitis), which may be visible below the palpebral conjunctiva adjacent to the eyelid margin. Inspissated meibum can sometimes be expressed by gently compressing the eyelid margin using thumb forceps. If the meibomian gland ductules are obstructed, meibum cannot escape and this can eventually cause rupture of the gland with release of lipid into the tissue. The lipid stimulates a granulomatous response (e.g. chalazion or lipogranulomatous conjunctivitis; see Figure 10.12). Meibomian gland ducts may be obstructed by eyelid masses or by epithelial metaplasia of the gland opening (e.g. due to actinic damage of the eyelid margin).

Goblet cell dysfunction

Tear film mucins are produced by conjunctival goblet cells (see Chapter 11) and the lacrimal gland. Abnormal tear mucins result in poor tear film stability and qualitative tear deficiency, which may lead to conjunctivitis and/or keratitis. Mucins have both structural and protective functions. Membrane-bound (structural) mucins increase tear film retention on the cornea ('wettability') by binding to the surface glycocalyx of corneal and conjunctival epithelial cells. Soluble mucins within the tear film bind debris and enhance its clearance.

Lacrimal gland neoplasia

Lacrimal gland neoplasia is rare in the dog. The most commonly reported canine primary lacrimal neoplasm is adenocarcinoma, although primary lacrimal pleomorphic adenoma has been reported in an elderly crossbred dog (Hirayama *et al.*, 2000).

Third eyelid gland neoplasia

The reader is referred to Chapter 11 for details on third eyelid gland neoplasia.

Cysts

Dacryops are cysts of the lacrimal gland ductule tissue. They are rare, but have been reported in Basset Hounds and Labrador Retrievers. Ectopic lacrimal tissue with cyst formation most commonly occurs at the medial canthus in these cases. A well defined mass is palpable at the medial canthus. Contrast dacryocystorhinography demonstrates that the swelling is separate from the nasolacrimal system and nasolacrimal flushing is usually possible. Ultrasonography (using a 10 MHz probe) reveals a spherical thin-walled cystic structure. Aspiration of cystic fluid may reveal inflammatory cells, but there is usually an absence of bacteria. Computed tomography (CT) and magnetic resonance imaging (MRI) can assist in surgical planning and confirm the isolation of the cyst from the nasolacrimal system.

As these cysts enlarge, secondary obstruction of the lower canaliculus may result in epiphora. Surgical excision is curative; however, iatrogenic laceration of the lower canaliculus is a fairly common complication of this procedure due to the proximity of the duct. Such lacerations require accurate apposition and catheterization of the canaliculus postoperatively to prevent stricture formation.

Feline conditions

Keratoconjunctivitis sicca

Immune-mediated KCS is not recognized in cats. The most common cause of KCS in cats is secondary to feline herpesvirus-1 (FHV-1) infection (Figure 10.11). FHV-1 has a tropism for conjunctival epithelium and its cytopathic effect can cause conjunctival swelling (obstructing lacrimal ductules from the orbital lacrimal gland and third eyelid gland) and conjunctival ulceration. Conjunctival ulceration may result in adhesions within the conjunctival epithelium or to the cornea (where corneal ulceration is also present), known as symblepharon (see

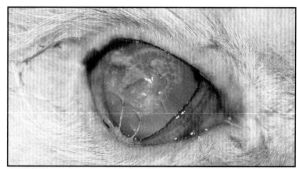

10.11 KCS in an adult Persian can with feline herpesvirus-1. Note the tacky adherent mucoid discharge. The pupil has been dilated for fundus examination.

Chapter 11), which may permanently occlude the lacrimal ductules.

Treatment: Treatment of the underlying FHV-1 infection with topical and/or systemic antivirals and supportive care can result in re-establishment of tear production (when the conjunctival swelling subsides). Prevention of adhesions in young cats and kittens during acute FHV-1 infection by gentle separation of the tissues with a cotton-tipped swab under topical anaesthesia may reduce the risk of long-term KCS. Where permanent occlusion of the lacrimal ductules has occurred, lifelong treatment with frequent application of artificial tear preparations is required. Parotid duct transposition has been described in the cat.

Other conditions

Qualitative tear deficiency in conjunction with ulcerative keratitis has also been reported in cats. Normal aqueous tear production with a reduced TFBUT has been reported in cats with indolent corneal ulcers or sequestra (Grahn *et al.*, 2005). The TFBUT has also been shown to be reduced in cats with conjunctivitis and, in an experimental study, FHV-1 infection was demonstrated to induce qualitative tear deficiency. Meibomianitis and lipogranulomatous conjunctivitis (Figure 10.12) can also result in qualitative tear deficiency in feline patients.

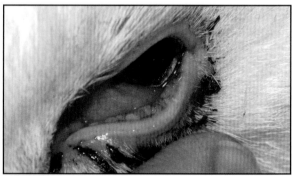

10.12 Lipogranulomatous conjunctivitis in an elderly white Domestic Shorthaired cat. The cat has been treated for pinnal and nasal planum squamous cell carcinoma. It was postulated that actinic damage had occluded the meibomian gland openings, resulting in the condition (which was present bilaterally). The TFBUT was <2 seconds in both eyes.

Lacrimal excretory system

Embryology, anatomy and physiology

The nasolacrimal system develops from surface ectoderm. Ectodermal cells within the nasolacrimal groove (a furrow between the lateral nasal fold and maxillary process) sink into the mesenchyme below, forming a cord. The cord of cells grows towards the eye and nose, with the proximal (ocular) end forming two buds near the medial canthus, which ultimately become the upper and lower canaliculi and puncta. The cord canalizes to become a duct lined by pseudostratified columnar epithelium and is usually present at birth.

The upper and lower eyelid lacrimal puncta are present about 3–7 mm from the medial canthus at the junction between the eyelid margin and palpebral conjunctiva, and approximately where the meibomian glands end. The puncta are oval to slit-like in appearance. The puncta lead to canaliculi, which are 4–7 mm in length and join together at the lacrimal sac (normally very small in the dog). The lacrimal sac lies in a small depression in the lacrimal bone (lacrimal fossa). From the lacrimal sac, the nasolacrimal duct passes through the lacrimal bone, where it is slightly constricted, and this is an important location for foreign body retention. The nasolacrimal duct then runs through a canal in the maxilla (located below the nasal mucosa on the medial aspect of the maxilla) and terminates at the nasal punctum (located on the ventrolateral floor of the nasal vestibule, approximately 1 cm caudal to the external nares) (Figure 10.13). In addition, approximately 50% of dogs have an accessory opening in the oral mucosa of the hard palate at the level of the upper canine teeth.

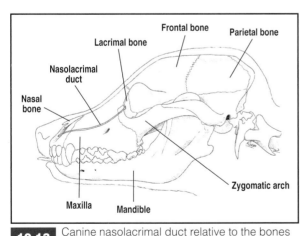

10.13 Canine nasolacrimal duct relative to the bones of the skull. (Illustration by Roser Tetas Pont)

Normal tear drainage occurs via the nasolacrimal system, although evaporation also plays a part in tear loss. Tears collect in a shallow tear meniscus (tear lake). The height of the tear lake in dogs varies with breed; brachycephalic breeds tend to have very shallow lakes as a consequence of their shallow orbits and tight eyelid apposition. From the tear meniscus, the tears largely drain medially to the lower lacrimal punctum, encouraged by eyelid blinking. Tears are drawn into the punctum and canaliculus by capillary action and a siphon effect. Eyelid blinking compresses the lacrimal sac, pushing tears into the nasolacrimal duct, creating a negative pressure as the sac reopens, which consequently draws tears into the canaliculus and lacrimal sac. Pseudoperistalsis within the nasolacrimal duct moves tears toward the nasal punctum.

Investigation of disease

Clinical signs associated with nasolacrimal drainage system obstruction include ocular discharge, which varies from simple epiphora (overflow of normal tears) to a profuse mucopurulent discharge, and conjunctivitis with hyperaemia. Pressure at the medial canthus may cause purulent material to be expelled from the lower lacrimal punctum.

Jones test

Patency of the nasolacrimal system can be assessed with the Jones test. Fluorescein is applied to the tear film, and the ipsilateral external nares should be observed for the appearance of fluorescein up to 10 minutes later (Binder and Herring, 2010) (Figure 10.14). Unfortunately, because 50% of brachycephalic dogs and most cats have accessory nasolacrimal openings, false-negative results can occur with this test. It is worthwhile observing the nasopharynx for signs of fluorescein passage. The use of a cobalt blue light can improve detection of fluorescein.

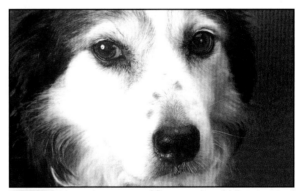

10.14 Normal passage of fluorescein, which appeared at the ipsilateral nostril within 30 seconds of application to the conjunctival sac.

Catheterization and flushing

The patency of the nasolacrimal system can also be tested by catheterization and flushing with saline. Under topical anaesthesia (e.g. proxymetacaine), the upper lacrimal punctum and canaliculus can be catheterized using a nasolacrimal cannula (22–24 gauge) or an intravenous catheter (22–24 gauge; without stylet) and flushed with saline (Figure 10.15). This should result in fluid passing out through the lower lacrimal punctum (via the lacrimal sac and lower canaliculus). Occlusion of the lower punctum with a fingertip should result in fluid passing through the nasolacrimal duct to the distal nasal punctum. Tipping the nose of the patient downwards will encourage the fluid to flow out through the nares, rather than posteriorly into the nasal cavity. Those patients with accessory openings may be observed

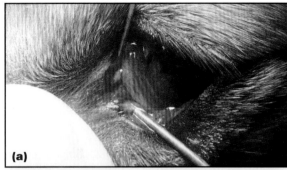

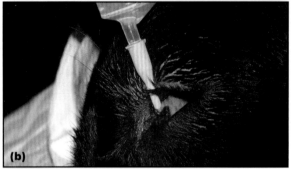

10.15 **(a)** Lacrimal probes placed in the upper and lower lacrimal puncta to demonstrate their location. **(b)** Upper lacrimal punctum cannulated with a 22 gauge cannula attached to a 10 ml syringe filled with sterile saline in a 3-year-old Labrador Retriever. Initially, the lower punctum should be observed for the exit of saline and then occluded by digital pressure and the nostril observed for the flow of saline from the nasal punctum.

to swallow when fluid passes into the mouth or naso-pharynx. If flushing is performed under general anaesthesia, the nasopharynx should be packed to avoid aspiration of the saline.

Cytology

Cytology with microbial culture and sensitivity testing of ocular discharges or fluid flushed from the naso-lacrimal system is recommended. Cytology provides a rapid assessment of any bacterial population and allows a more focused initial choice of antibacterial drug. Culture and sensitivity testing may take a few days (aerobic and anaerobic bacterial culture) to a few weeks (fungal culture) but can determine whether resistant microbial strains are present.

Radiography

Radiography can also be used to assess the naso-lacrimal system. Plain skull radiographs (lateral, intraoral and dorsoventral) should be obtained ini-tially, under general anaesthesia, and assessed for abnormalities within the surrounding tissues (e.g. paranasal sinuses, maxillary dental arcades and nasal cavity). Following plain radiography, the phar-ynx should be packed, the lower lacrimal punctum catheterized and iodinated contrast medium injected into the nasolacrimal system in order to perform con-trast dacryocystorhinography (Figure 10.16).

Placement of a swab in the nasal opening is advisable in order to collect any contrast material that exits from the nasal punctum (rather than allow-ing it to run back into the nasal cavity, or on to the X-ray plate, and obscure detail on the radiograph).

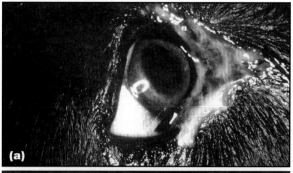

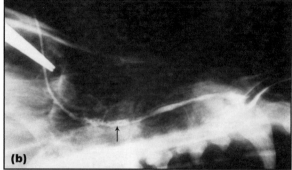

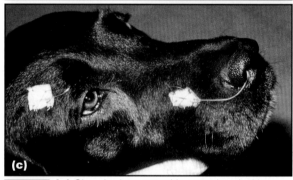

10.16 **(a)** Chronic dacryocystitis associated with disintegration of a foreign body in a Labrador Retriever. The foreign body was inadvertently flushed down the nasolacrimal duct. Repeated irrigation failed to restore patency of the duct and the dog was referred to a specialist. **(b)** Dacryocystorhinography demonstrated the abnormal region in the narrowest part of the intraosseous portion of the nasolacrimal duct (arrowed). **(c)** Patency was restored and maintained by cannulating the entire nasolacrimal system using a feline urinary catheter; the restriction in the nasolacrimal duct was appreciable as the catheter was passed. The catheter (6 gauge) was sutured in place to maintain patency. The condition resolved completely within 2 weeks and the catheter was removed.

In dogs and cats with accessory openings in the mouth or nasopharynx, radiographs may reveal con-trast material in these areas. Ideally, only sufficient contrast medium to fill the nasolacrimal system should be used, in order to avoid pooling in the nasal cavity or pharynx.

Retrograde flushing or injection of contrast medium can also be attempted via the nasal punc-tum, but this approach can be challenging. Magnification and good lighting are required, and grasping the alar cartilage may assist in visualiza-tion of the nasal punctum. A nasolacrimal cannula or intravenous catheter can be used, but the metal stylet on the intravenous catheter should be removed to avoid traumatizing the duct.

Obstructions prevent the contrast material from passing normally through the nasolacrimal system and this can be identified on the radiographs.

- Cysts associated with the nasolacrimal system are outlined by pooled contrast material. The percutaneous injection of contrast medium into cysts that are isolated from the nasolacrimal system but are causing secondary obstruction (e.g. canaliculops or dacryops) has been described in order to identify the lack of continuity with the nasolacrimal system.
- Dilatation of the lacrimal sac secondary to obstruction of the nasolacrimal duct is outlined by pooled contrast material.
- Bony lysis can be identified radiographically and may suggest osteomyelitis or neoplastic erosion of the maxilla or lacrimal bones (neoplasms most commonly originate from the nasal cavity and secondarily involve the nasolacrimal system).

Computed tomography

CT is being increasingly used to assess the naso-lacrimal system (CT-dacryocystorhinography) in veterinary patients, as it is in humans. Iodinated contrast material can be utilized to outline the nasolacrimal system more clearly. In humans, an axial scan (equivalent to the dorsal plane in dogs) is usually chosen to assess the whole nasolacrimal system in one plane. Unfortunately, this is not possible in veterinary patients without continuous contrast medium injection; however, three-dimensional (3D) reconstructions can be achieved using serial transverse images. CT is generally more useful than MRI because of the enhanced bony resolution (MRI is superior for soft tissue resolution). Technical difficulties are associated with overfilling of the nasolacrimal system with contrast material and subsequent leakage into the nasal cavity, resulting in reduced quality images. Dilatation of the lacrimal sac or cystic dilatations confluent with the nasolacrimal system lead to pooling of contrast medium. Obstructions or other abnormalities of the nasolacrimal system cause the flow of contrast material to be impeded (partially or completely) in the distal system. Osteolysis adjacent to the nasolacrimal system may suggest neoplasia or infection.

Canine conditions

Disease conditions involving the nasolacrimal drainage system may lead epiphora or dacryocystitis and include:

- Congenital atresia or agenesis of all or part of the nasolacrimal system
- Obstruction by foreign or inflammatory material
- Cystic expansion adjacent to or within the nasolacrimal system
- Traumatic injury (e.g. road traffic accident, cat fight injury or surgical incision)
- Extension of neoplasia or inflammation (e.g. due to tooth root abscess) in adjacent tissues.

Dacryocystitis

Inflammation of the nasolacrimal drainage system is referred to as dacryocystitis. Clinical signs of dacryo-

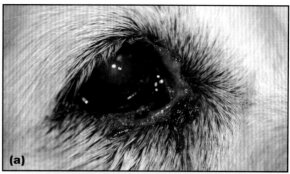
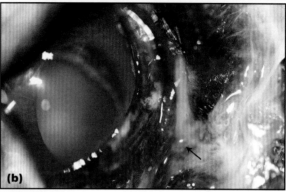

10.17 **(a)** Dacryocystitis in a young Golden Retriever secondary to a foreign body in the lacrimal sac (subsequently removed surgically). **(b)** Mucopurulent discharge emanating from the lower lacrimal punctum (arrowed).

cystitis are characterized by a mucoid to mucopurulent ocular discharge, emanating from the lacrimal puncta (Figure 10.17). Discharge can sometimes be massaged from the lacrimal sac out of the lower lacrimal puncta with gentle digital pressure, and this is pathognomonic for dacryocystitis. Hyperaemia of the inferior conjunctival sac is commonly associated with dacryocystitis. Blepharitis can also occur secondary to dacryocystitis and is associated with eyelid swelling and erythema. Chronic dacryocystitis may result in formation of a draining fistula inferior to the medial canthus.

Atresia

Failure of the nasolacrimal system to canalize fully results in obstruction of tear drainage and ocular discharge within the first few months of life. The most common congenital abnormality in the dog is punctal atresia. Absence of the upper punctum is usually asymptomatic, whereas absence of the lower punctum usually results in epiphora. Flushing of saline from the upper punctum may result in bulging of the conjunctiva overlying the lower canaliculus, which can subsequently be incised and a punctum reformed (Figure 10.18). The mucosal site of the punctum is usually thin walled and devoid of blood vessels, making any surgery relatively free from haemorrhage and the region is less prone to secondary stricture formation. A topical antibiotic/corticosteroid preparation is usually employed for 7 days postoperatively.

The absence of a canaliculus or part of the nasolacrimal duct is less common and more difficult to correct. Creation of a communication between the

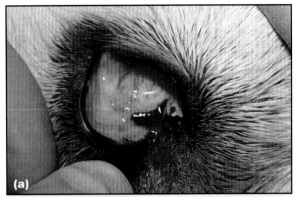

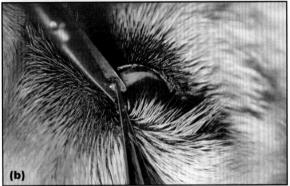

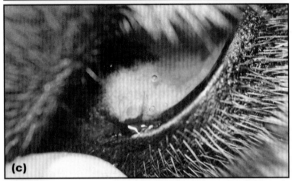

10.18 A 9-month-old Labrador Retriever with bilateral lower lacrimal punctal atresia. **(a)** The upper punctum has been cannulated and flushed with saline. Patency was re-established using a snip technique to open the conjunctiva overlying the lower canaliculus. **(b)** A snip of conjunctival tissue overlying the punctum was excised. **(c)** Following snipping the conjunctiva, the lower canaliculus is exposed. A small amount of haemorrhage is present.

nasolacrimal system and the nasal cavity (conjunctival rhinostomy), maxillary sinus (conjunctival maxillary sinusotomy) or oral cavity (conjunctival buccostomy) has been described. Placement of an indwelling silastic catheter is recommended for 3–6 weeks to promote continued patency and reduce postoperative stricture formation. Topical antibiotic and corticosteroid treatment is recommended until after the silastic tubing has been removed.

Micropunctum

Abnormally small lacrimal puncta may occur as part of the spectrum of congenital nasolacrimal defects, causing epiphora or a mucopurulent ocular discharge. Enlargement of small puncta can be easily achieved using the 1–2–3 snip technique. The lower blade of fine, pointed scissors is introduced into the

punctum and canaliculus to make snip '1'. Small triangles of conjunctiva immediately adjacent to this first linear incision are then excised (snips '2' and '3'). In the absence of surgical haemorrhage, placement of an indwelling catheter in the canaliculus can often be avoided; topical antibiotic and corticosteroid medication should be administered 3–4 times daily for 2–3 weeks postoperatively.

Malpositioned lower lacrimal punctum

The lower lacrimal punctum can be malpositioned within the conjunctiva, resulting in epiphora. Malpositioning of the upper punctum is usually asymptomatic. Malpositioning is a congenital abnormality, but may also occur as a result of conformational problems, particularly in brachycephalic breeds. Lower medial canthal entropion can rotate the lower punctum inwards, occluding it with the lower conjunctival fornix or against the globe and limiting normal tear drainage. Caruncular trichiasis is also often encountered in brachycephalic breeds and promotes wicking of tears on to the medial canthus, compounding the epiphora. In addition, concurrent tight medial canthal ligaments can compress the punctum and canaliculus, further limiting tear drainage. Surgical treatment of the medial entropion (modified Hotz–Celsus procedure) and caruncular trichiasis (excision) can help reduce or eliminate the epiphora. Medial canthoplasty as a treatment for medial entropion and caruncular trichiasis may also address the tight medial canthal ligaments and can be combined with punctal enlargement (see Chapter 9).

Cysts

Canaliculops: These are cysts of the canaliculi, which can become separated from the canaliculus or retain communication with the nasolacrimal system. Both forms can cause secondary obstruction of tear drainage. Cystic expansions may cause distinct palpable swellings over the facial bones. Surgical excision is curative but requires careful reconstruction of the canaliculus with catheterization for a period of 3–4 weeks (with topical antibiotic/corticosteroid treatment) to prevent stricture formation. In addition, dacryops may cause secondary obstruction of the nasolacrimal system, although these cysts originate from lacrimal secretory ductal tissue (see above).

Nasolacrimal duct cysts: These are rare, but may cause recurrent inflammation of the nasolacrimal system characterized by epiphora or a mucoid to mucopurulent discharge emanating from the nasolacrimal puncta and conjunctival hyperaemia. Advanced imaging techniques (CT or MRI) aid in their diagnosis (Figure 10.19). Surgical excision usually requires removal of a section of maxillary bone in order to reach the duct, although endoscopic surgery via the nasal cavity or maxillary sinus has also been described. Cysts should be removed in their entirety or marsupialized to the nasal cavity (dacryocystorhinostomy) or the maxillary sinus (dacryocystomaxillosinusotomy).

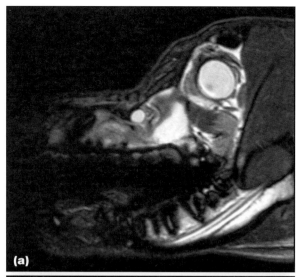

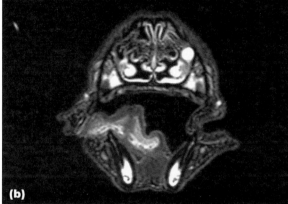

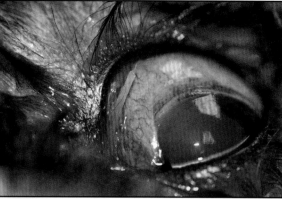

10.20 A young Tibetan Terrier with a grass seed awn lodged in the upper lacrimal punctum. The foreign body was removed under topical anaesthesia and the superficial corneal ulcer (located at approximately 11 o'clock in the superionasal cornea) healed uneventfully with the application of a topical antibiotic solution for 1 week.

10.19 A 2-year-old Labrador Retriever bitch with chronic epiphora due to a nasolacrimal cyst. **(a)** Sagittal T2-weighted MR image showing a hyperintense signal from the fluid-filled cyst. **(b)** Transverse T2-weighted MR image. The cyst is lying within the maxillary bone at the level of the upper right fourth premolar, immediately rostral to the maxillary recess and lateral to the nasal turbinates. The nasolacrimal duct is visible proximal and distal to the cyst. Rhinoscopy was performed but the cyst was not identified. A maxillary bone flap was created to expose the nasolacrimal duct cyst and the medial and rostral walls were resected. The nasolacrimal duct was then cannulated and flushed directly into the nasal cavity. Cannulation with nylon suture material resulted in the suture material entering the nasal cavity.

Maxillary bone epithelial cysts: Secondary obstruction of the nasolacrimal duct has been reported in a Labrador Retriever with a maxillary bone epithelial cyst. These cysts are a rare cause of epiphora as a result of obstruction of the nasolacrimal apparatus.

Obstruction

Obstruction secondary to a foreign body within the nasolacrimal system is relatively common in dogs. Plant material is the most commonly identified cause of the obstruction. Grass seed awns can migrate into the lacrimal puncta, with barbs preventing backward movement (Figure 10.20). These may become lodged within the canaliculus with the tip visible at the punctum, but they are more commonly retained within the lacrimal sac. Another site of foreign body retention is at the entrance of the nasolacrimal bony canal, where the duct is at its narrowest.

Simple flushing may dislodge a foreign body into the punctum, allowing it to be removed, but incision into the lacrimal sac or nasolacrimal duct may be required. Once a foreign body has reached the bony nasolacrimal canal, extraction becomes more technically difficult and requires a section of the maxillary bone to be removed. Postoperative stent placement is necessary to allow healing of the incised canaliculus or nasolacrimal duct without stricture formation. The stent is usually removed after 3–4 weeks and topical antibiotic/corticosteroid treatment is maintained until this occurs.

Obstruction of the nasolacrimal system may also occur secondary to granuloma formation within the lacrimal sac or canaliculi. Stricture formation following healing of a nasolacrimal laceration with granulation tissue (in the canaliculi, lacrimal sac or nasolacrimal duct) may occur if close apposition of tissues is not achieved, or if the sutures are placed into the mucosa of the nasolacrimal system. Closure of a nasolacrimal duct defect (after the surgical removal of a foreign body) has been described using an overlay of porcine small intestinal material to promote re-epithelialization.

Laceration

Laceration or trauma to the nasolacrimal system (e.g. damage sustained in road traffic accidents) requires careful attention to prevent long-term obstruction and epiphora. Lacerations of the upper punctum or canaliculus often heal without long-term clinical implications, whereas lower canaliculi or punctal damage usually results in epiphora. Lacerations of the canaliculi should be repaired meticulously by apposing the surrounding tissues accurately, avoiding direct suturing of the canaliculus, to prevent postoperative stricture formation (Figure 10.21). This procedure should be performed using an operating microscope to provide adequate

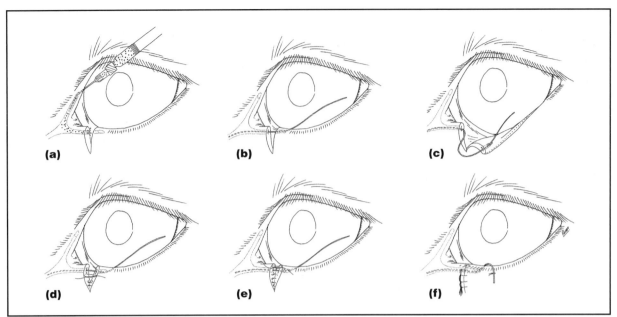

10.21 Lower canaliculus repair. **(a)** The upper punctum is cannulated and viscoelastic containing air bubbles is injected to facilitate identification of the incised canaliculus margin. **(b)** The lower punctum is then cannulated with silastic tubing. **(c)** The silastic tubing is advanced into the lacerated canaliculus. **(d)** The canaliculus is meticulously aligned and figure-of-eight sutures placed in the eyelid margin. **(e)** The subconjunctival tissues are closed. **(f)** The skin laceration is closed routinely and the end of the silastic tubing is sutured to the lower eyelid skin to improve retention. (Illustration by Roser Tetas Pont)

magnification. Flushing of the opposite punctum and canaliculus with saline or air bubbles can help to identify the lacerated margin of the canaliculus. Damage to the nasolacrimal duct within the lacrimal or maxillary bones requires apposition of bony fragments and removal of small fragments that might form sequestra. Placement of an indwelling catheter for 4–6 weeks is recommended to encourage re-epithelialization of the duct and maintain of patency.

Feline conditions

Dacryocystitis
Dacryocystitis is rare in the cat but has been described in conjunction with rhinitis and dental disease. Destructive bony changes associated with rhinitis, dental disease or neoplastic processes may result in a profuse ocular discharge via the nasolacrimal system.

Malpositioned lower lacrimal punctum
The conformation of some cat breeds (e.g. Persian, Burmese) can predispose the animal to epiphora (in a similar manner to brachycephalic dogs) as a result of malpositioning of the lower lacrimal punctum due to medial canthal entropion, caruncular trichiasis causing wicking of tears on to the lower eyelid, and tight medial canthal ligaments compressing the lower canaliculus (Figure 10.22).

Obstruction
Symblepharon (due to FHV-1 infection) can cause obstruction of the lacrimal puncta and/or canaliculi, resulting in epiphora (Figure 10.23). This probably represents the most common cause of nasolacrimal obstruction in cats.

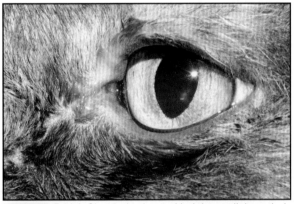

10.22 British Shorthaired cat with tight medial canthal ligaments, medial entropion and epiphora.

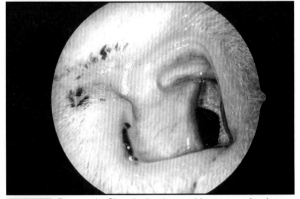

10.23 Domestic Shorthaired cat with an acquired blockage of the upper and lower puncta as a result of extensive symblepharon formation (due to FHV-1 infection). The ventral fornix has been obliterated by the extensive adhesions and the dorsal fornix was also compromised.

Atresia

Atresia of the nasolacrimal system is uncommon in the cat with an imperforate lacrimal punctum being the most commonly reported defect. In cats, the upper punctum is more commonly absent (in contrast to dogs in which the lower punctum is more commonly affected). Treatment, if indicated by the clinical signs, is as described for dogs (see above).

Laceration

Laceration of the medial canthus (e.g. sustained during a cat fight) may involve the nasolacrimal system (lacrimal sac, canaliculi or puncta) and accurate repair is required to avoid long-term epiphora.

References and further reading

Barnett KC (2006) Congenital keratoconjunctivitis sicca and ichyosiform dermatosis in the Cavalier King Charles Spaniel. *Journal of Small Animal Practice* 47(9), 524–528

Berdoulay A, English RV and Nadelstein B (2005) Effect of topical 0.02% tacrolimus aqueous suspension on tear production in dogs with keratoconjunctivitis sicca. *Veterinary Ophthalmology* 8, 225–232

Binder DR and Herring IP (2010) Evaluation of nasolacrimal fluorescein transit time in ophthalmically normal dogs and nonbrachycephalic cats. *American Journal of Veterinary Research* 71, 570–574

Bugelski PJ, Volk A, Walker MR *et al.* (2010) Critical review of preclinical approaches to evaluate the potential of immuno-suppressive drugs to influence human neoplasia. *International Journal of Toxicology* 29, 435–466

Covitz D, Hunziker J and Koch SA (1977) Conjunctivorhinostomy: a surgical method for the control of epiphora in the dog and cat. *Journal of the American Veterinary Medical Association* 171(3), 251–255

Davis K and Townsend W (2011) Tear-film osmolarity in normal cats and cats with conjunctivitis. *Veterinary Ophthalmology* 14(Suppl. 1), 54–59

Featherstone H and Llabres Diaz F (2003) Maxillary bone epithelial cyst in a dog. *Journal of Small Animal Practice* 44(12), 541–545

Gelatt KN, Guffy MM and Boggess TS 3rd (1970) Radiographic contrast techniques for detecting orbital and nasolacrimal tumors in dogs. *Journal of the American Veterinary Medical Association* 156(6), 741–746

Giuliano EA and Moore CP (2007) Diseases and surgery of the lacrimal secretory system. In: *Veterinary Ophthalmology, 4th edn*, ed. Gelatt KN, pp. 633–661. Blackwell Publishing, Iowa

Giuliano EA, Pope ER, Champagne ES and Moore CP (2006) Dacryocystomaxillorhinostomy for chronic dacryocystitis in a dog. *Veterinary Ophthalmology* 9(2), 89–94

Grahn BH and Mason RA (1995) Epiphora associated with dacryops in a dog. *Journal of the American Animal Hospital Association* 31(1), 15–19

Grahn BH and Sandmeyer LS (2007) Diseases and surgery of the canine nasolacrimal system. In: *Veterinary Ophthalmology, 4th edn*, ed. Gelatt KN, pp. 618–632. Blackwell Publishing, Iowa

Grahn BH, Sisler S and Storey E (2005) Qualitative tear film and conjunctival goblet cell assessment of cats with corneal sequestra. *Veterinary Ophthalmology* 8(3), 167–170

Hartley C, Donaldson D, Smith KC *et al.* (2012) Congenital keratoconjunctivitis sicca and ichthyosiform dermatosis in 25 Cavalier King Charles Spaniel dogs – part I: clinical signs, histopathology, and inheritance. *Veterinary Ophthalmology* 15(5), 315–326

Hendrix DV, Adkins EA, Ward DA, Stuffle J and Skorobohach B (2011) An investigation comparing the efficacy of topical application of tacrolimus and cyclosporine in dogs. *Veterinary Medicine International* doi: 10.4061/2011/487592

Herrera HD, Weichsler N, Gomez JR and de Jalon JA (2007) Severe, unilateral unresponsive keratoconjunctivitis sicca in 16 juvenile Yorkshire Terriers. *Veterinary Ophthalmology* 10(5), 285–288

Herring IP, Pickett JP, Champagne ES and Marini M (2000) Evaluation of aqueous tear production in dogs following general anesthesia. *Journal of the American Animal Hospital Association* 36(5), 427–430

Hirayama K, Kagawa Y, Tsuzuki K *et al.* (2000) A pleomorphic adenoma of the lacrimal gland in a dog. *Veterinary Pathology* 37(4), 353–356

Izci C, Celik I, Alkan F *et al.* (2002) Histologic characteristics and local cellular immunity of the gland of the third eyelid after topical ophthalmic administration of 2% cyclosporine for treatment of dogs with keratoconjunctivitis sicca. *American Journal of Veterinary Research* 63(5), 688–694

Kaswan RL, Martin CL and Chapman WL Jr. (1985) Keratoconjunctivitis sicca: histopathologic study of nictitating membrane and lacrimal glands from 28 dogs. *American Journal of Veterinary Research* 45(1), 112–118

Kaswan RL, Martin CL and Dawe DL (1985) Keratoconjunctivitis sicca: immunological evaluation of 62 canine cases. *American Journal of Veterinary Research* 46(2), 376–383

Lussier B and Carrier M (2004) Surgical treatment of recurrent dacryocystitis secondary to cystic dilatation of the nasolacrimal duct in a dog. *Journal of the American Animal Hospital Association* 40(3), 216–219

Morgan RV and Abrams KL (1998) Topical administration of cyclosporine for treatment of keratoconjunctivitis sicca in dogs. *Journal of the American Veterinary Medical Association* 199(8), 1043–1046

Morgan RV, Duddy JM and McClurg K (1993) Prolapse of the gland of the third eyelid in dogs: a retrospective study of 89 cases (1980 to 1990). *Journal of the American Animal Hospital Association* 29, 56–60

Nell B, Walde I, Billich A, Vit P and Meingassner JG (2005) The effect of topical pimecrolimus on keratoconjunctivitis sicca and chronic superficial keratitis in dogs: results from an exploratory study. *Veterinary Ophthalmology* 8(1), 39–46

Nykamp SG, Scrivani PV and Pease AP (2004) Computed tomography dacryocystography evaluation of the nasolacrimal apparatus. *Veterinary Radiology & Ultrasound* 45(1), 23–28

Ofri R, Lambrou GN, Allgoewer I *et al.* (2009) Clinical evaluation of pimecrolimus eye drops for treatment of canine keratoconjunctivitis sicca: a comparison with cyclosporine A. *Veterinary Journal* 179(1), 70–77

Ota J, Pearce JW, Finn MJ, Johnson GC and Giuliano EA (2009) Dacryops (lacrimal cyst) in three young Labrador Retrievers. *Journal of the American Animal Hospital Association* 45(4), 191–196

Rhodes M, Heinrich C, Featherstone H *et al.* (2012) Parotid duct transposition in dogs: a retrospective review of 92 eyes from 1999 to 2009. *Veterinary Ophthalmology* 15, 213–222

Sanchez RF, Innocent G, Mould J and Billson FM (2007) Canine keratoconjunctivitis sicca: disease trends in a review of 229 cases. *Journal of Small Animal Practice* 48(4), 211–217

Sansom J, Barnett KC, Neumann W *et al.* (1995) Treatment of keratoconjunctivitis sicca in dogs with cyclosporine ophthalmic ointment: a European clinical field trial. *Veterinary Record* 137(20), 504–507

Shepard MK, Accola PJ, Lopez LA, Shaughnessy MR and Hofmeister EH (2011) Effect of duration and type of anesthetic on tear production in dogs. *American Journal of Veterinary Research* 72, 608–612

Smith EM, Buyukmihci NC and Farver TB (1994) Effect of topical pilocarpine treatment on tear production in dogs. *Journal of the American Veterinary Medical Association* 205, 1286–1289

van der Woerdt A, Wilkie DA, Gilger BC, Smeak DD and Kerpsack SJ (1997) Surgical treatment of dacryocystitis caused by cystic dilatation of the nasolacrimal system in three dogs. *Journal of the American Veterinary Medical Association* 211(4), 445–447

Wang FI, Ting CT and Liu YS (2001) Orbital adenocarcinoma of lacrimal gland origin in a dog. *Journal of Veterinary Diagnostic Investigation* 13(2), 159–161

Westermeyer HD, Ward DA and Abrams K (2009) Breed predisposition to congenital alacrima in dogs. *Veterinary Ophthalmology* 12(1), 1–5

11

The conjunctiva and third eyelid

Claudia Hartley

Conjunctiva

Embryology, anatomy and physiology

The conjunctival epithelium (along with the eyelids) is derived from surface ectoderm. The conjunctival stroma is derived from mesenchyme, which originates from neural crest cells. From the mucocutaneous junction of the eyelid margin, the palpebral conjunctiva lines the posterior surface of the eyelid (closely adherent to the weak tarsal plate in dogs) and reflects at the inferior and superior conjunctival fornices to become the bulbar conjunctiva overlying the globe (Figure 11.1). The bulbar conjunctiva is more loosely attached to the underlying tissues, except at the limbus, where it is firmly attached to the underlying Tenon's capsule. The looser attachment of the conjunctival fornices and bulbar conjunctiva allow free movement of the globe beneath the eyelids. The conjunctival sac refers to the space between the eyelids and globe that is lined by the conjunctiva.

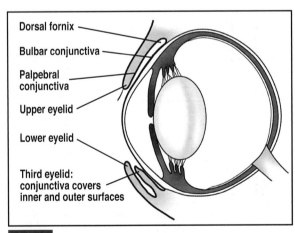

11.1 Anatomy of the conjunctiva.

The normal conjunctival epithelium is non-keratinizing squamous (palpebral and bulbar conjunctiva) to cuboidal (fornices) stratified epithelium, six or more layers thick, with surface microvilli. These microscopic projections act as attachment points for the preocular tear film, most notably the mucoid component. Tear film mucus also interacts with glycoprotein projections (the glycocalyx) expressed on the surface of the conjunctival and corneal epithelium. Within the epithelium and concentrated towards the fornices, especially inferiomedially, are uniformly spaced conjunctival goblet cells, which are responsible for the production of mucin, an important component of the tear film. Underlying the conjunctival epithelium is a superficial stroma containing lymphoid tissue (conjunctival-associated lymphoid tissue; CALT), which is arranged in both a diffuse layer and as multifocal dense aggregates. The superficial and deep stroma are also served by lymphatic vessels, nerves and blood vessels. Sensory innervation of the conjunctiva is via the ophthalmic branch of the trigeminal nerve.

Conjunctival vessels can be identified by their branching, bright red appearance and by their mobility with conjunctival movements (Figure 11.2). These can be differentiated from the deeper, generally straighter and darker, episcleral and scleral vessels (see also Chapter 13). Conjunctival arterioles are derived from the anterior ciliary arteries (bulbar conjunctiva) or from eyelid arteries (palpebral conjunctiva). There is communication between conjunctival vessels and the pericorneal limbal plexus in the episclera and sclera. Endothelial budding from bulbar conjunctival vessels at the limbus results in superficial corneal vascularization. Deep corneal neovascularization originates from deeper limbal (episcleral) vessels.

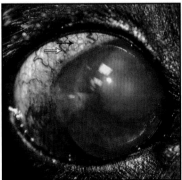

11.2 Conjunctival (white arrow) and episcleral (black arrow) blood vessels. Conjunctival blood vessels are longer, have more branches and are located more superficially than episcleral blood vessels.

Investigation of disease

Cytological analysis can provide rapid and helpful information for diagnosis and for determination of the appropriate antimicrobial therapy in many conjunctival diseases where culture results are pending or culture was not performed. Microbial culture results may be more sensitive than cytology, but the immediacy of cytology allows prompt and focused therapy. Conjunctival biopsy, where indicated, can be undertaken using topical anaesthesia in most cases. Details of techniques to optimize cytology, microbial culture and conjunctival biopsy results are discussed in Chapter 3.

Canine conditions

Epibulbar dermoid

Dermoids are masses that arise during development and consist of well differentiated, non-neoplastic tissue in an abnormal location (choristomas). They commonly occur at the lateral limbus and may involve the cornea (see Chapter 12) or the eyelids (Figure 11.3). They have the appearance of haired skin, frequently sprouting long hairs, which may lie in the tear film. Although congenital, they may be less noticeable in young puppies, but with growth they may become more obvious and associated with clinical signs (ocular discharge, epiphora). Inheritance of epibular dermoids has been postulated in the St Bernard but epibulbar dermoids have also been encountered in other breeds, including German Shepherd Dogs, Basset Hounds, Bulldogs, Labrador Retrievers and Shih Tzus.

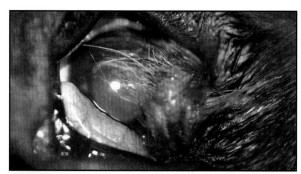

11.3 Epibulbar dermoid in a 4-month-old German Shepherd Dog, involving the conjunctiva and the lateral lower eyelid.

The treatment is surgical excision, which is curative if complete. A superficial conjunctivectomy, with keratectomy if there is corneal involvement, is sufficient but should be performed with the benefit of magnification (using surgical loupes or an operating microscope) to ensure complete excision with minimal damage to the adjacent normal tissue. Where there is corneal involvement, the site of corneal resection will often heal with conjunctivalization.

Conjunctivitis

Conjunctivitis is one of the most commonly encountered ocular diseases in clinical practice and may be either primary or, more often, secondary to other ocular or systemic diseases. It is important to differentiate conjunctivitis from more serious disorders with similar clinical presentations (see Chapter 21) that are caused by orbital, scleral/episcleral, intraocular or systemic diseases. Clinical signs of conjunctivitis include conjunctival hyperaemia, chemosis (oedema of the conjunctiva; Figure 11.4), conjunctival swelling or thickening, blepharospasm, lacrimation and/or ocular discharge (which may be mucoid, mucopurulent, purulent or haemorrhagic). Some

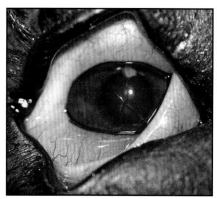

11.4 A 3-year-old St Bernard with chemosis of unknown cause.

forms of conjunctivitis, most notably allergic conjunctivitis, may be associated with ocular pruritus. Doliocephalic breeds of dog may have an accumulation of mucus at the medial canthi as a normal feature, known as 'medial canthal pocket syndrome', due to their relatively enophthalmic conformation (deep-set eyes) and deep conjunctival fornices.

Follicular hyperplasia of conjunctival lymphoid tissue: This is a non-specific reaction to chronic conjunctivitis and is easily recognized by the appearance of nodule-like structures outlined by conjunctival capillaries on the conjunctival surface. Although they may resemble vesicles, they are not fluid-filled but consist of lymphoid tissue. They are commonly encountered in the conjunctival fornices and on the posterior surface of the third eyelid (Figure 11.5). Follicular conjunctivitis may be encountered in young dogs in the absence of clinical signs or underlying disease, and it can often resolve spontaneously without specific treatment.

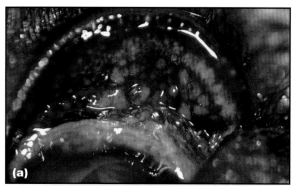

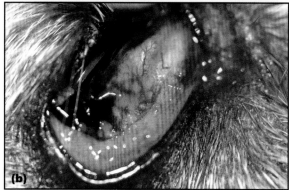

11.5 Follicular conjunctivitis in **(a)** a 5-year-old Leonberger and **(b)** a 10-year-old Jack Russell Terrier.

Thickening of the conjunctiva: This can occur as a result of squamous metaplasia of the epithelium, and may become irreversible if the inciting cause (e.g. keratoconjunctivitis sicca, KCS) is not addressed promptly. Thickening due to cellular infiltration may be accompanied, or incited, by conjunctival inflammation (conjunctivitis), for example with neoplastic disease (see below).

Infectious conjunctivitis:

Viral conjunctivitis: Primary infectious conjunctivitis in dogs is uncommon but has been reported with canine distemper virus (along with other systemic signs), canine herpesvirus-1 and canine adenovirus-2 (Ledbetter *et al.*, 2009) (see Chapter 20). Neonatal conjunctivitis (ophthalmia neonatorum) is seen in young puppies prior to eyelid opening and is described in more detail in Chapter 9. Canine herpesvirus-1 infection from the dam's genital tract is considered the most likely cause, complicated by secondary bacterial infection.

Bacterial conjunctivitis: In the dog this usually occurs secondary to a precipitating event or an underlying disorder, such as conjunctival trauma or KCS, which results in an opportunistic infection (see below). Identification of the predisposing factor is vital to achieve treatment success. Predisposing factors such as entropion, ectropion, eyelid agenesis, distichiasis, trichiasis or KCS should be investigated and treated where present, or recurrence of the conjunctivitis is likely. The most frequently cultured bacteria in canine conjunctivitis represent secondary infection with commensal organisms, including *Staphylococcus* and *Streptococcus* spp. and, less commonly, *Escherichia coli*, *Bacillus* spp., *Proteus* spp. and *Pseudomonas* spp.

Fungal conjunctivitis: This has not been reported in the UK, but conjunctival nodules associated with *Blastomyces dermatitidis* have been reported in the USA (Hendrix, 2007). Yeast infections (*Malassezia* and *Candida* spp.) may be encountered, usually in conjunction with skin or ear disease.

Parasitic conjunctivitis:

- *Thelazia* spp. – these parasites have not been reported in the UK, but *T. callipaeda* is a potential cause of conjunctivitis in dogs as well as cats, foxes and humans in continental Europe. The nematode larvae are transmitted by flies into the host's conjunctival sac and nasolacrimal system, where they moult to adulthood. The cuticle of the nematode can provoke mechanical conjunctival inflammation and epiphora. Treatment is by manual removal or flushing of the nematodes, in conjunction with anthelmintic drugs such as ivermectin and moxidectin.
- *Leishmania* spp. – these are protozoan parasites that are transmitted by the sandfly. Given that the sandfly vector is absent from the UK, the disease is rarely encountered in this country. However, with the advent of pet passports, dogs (and very rarely cats) can demonstrate clinical signs of leishmaniosis on their return from trips abroad. *Leishmania* spp. can cause conjunctivitis, keratitis, blepharitis, uveitis, retinitis, cutaneous signs, cachexia and other systemic signs. Diagnosis can be made on blood tests using quantitative polymerase chain reaction (qPCR) for the parasite and serology for antibody titres.

Non-infectious conjunctivitis:

Irritants: Dust, smoke or grit, as well as several commonly used topical medications (e.g. neomycin, tetracycline) may incite conjunctival inflammation. Removal of the irritant is usually sufficient to resolve the clinical signs. Animals living in a dusty environment or that have accumulated foreign material in the conjunctival sacs (e.g. sand after walking/digging on a beach) may benefit from flushing of the conjunctival fornices with saline to reduce irritation.

Allergic conjunctivitis: This can be associated with immediate or delayed type hypersensitivity reactions. Most cases are bilateral and may be seen in conjunction with atopic dermatitis. Hyposensitization vaccinations for atopic dermatitis may improve the signs of allergic conjunctivitis in these cases. Some animals may demonstrate seasonality of clinical signs, whilst others may respond to an elimination diet.

Autoimmune diseases: Extension of inflammation of the mucocutaneous junctions to involve the conjunctival tissues in autoimmune conditions such as pemphigoid is an uncommon cause of conjunctivitis.

Ligneous conjunctivitis: This is a rare disease characterized by a membranous or pseudomembranous conjunctivitis, which is part of a multi-systemic condition that also involves the oral, upper respiratory tract and urinary tract epithelia. In dogs, ligneous conjunctivitis has most commonly been reported in the Dobermann (Ramsey *et al.*, 1996) (Figure 11.6). Ligneous conjunctivitis in humans has been described in conjunction with mutations of the plasminogen gene, and plasminogen deficiency has been demonstrated in canine cases of ligneous conjunctivitis. Treatment has been reported to be successful in only one case (Torres *et al.*, 2009), but it

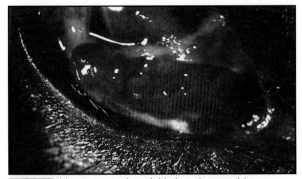

11.6 Ligneous conjunctivitis in a 4-year-old Dobermann. Note the greyish veil of pseudomembrane over the leading edge of the third eyelid.

may involve a combination of topical and systemic immunosuppressive/modulatory and anti-inflammatory therapy, together with topical heparin.

Radiation-induced conjunctivitis: This can occur when the eye(s) have been included in the radiation field (e.g. for sinus neoplasia; Figure 11.7). The condition is poorly responsive to treatment owing to the effect of radiation on the basal stem cell layer of the conjunctival epithelium. KCS can also been seen as an early or late complication of radiation treatment.

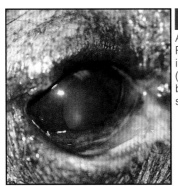

11.7

A 10-year-old Labrador Retriever with radiation-induced conjunctivitis (following external beam radiation for sinus neoplasia).

Extension from local disease: Blepharitis, sinusitis and orbital and lacrimal disease (Figures 11.8 and 11.9) may all secondarily affect the conjunctiva by local extension. A thorough ophthalmic examination, including the adnexa, combined with examination of facial symmetry, the oral cavity and palpation of the orbital and facial bones should identify disease in adjacent structures. Skull radiography and ocular ultrasonography are useful diagnostic modalities for the investigation of sinus and orbital disease, respectively; however, advanced imaging such as magnetic resonance imaging (MRI) or computed

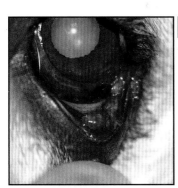

11.8

An 11-year-old Labrador Retriever with pyogranulomatous blepharoconjunctivitis diagnosed on conjunctival biopsy.

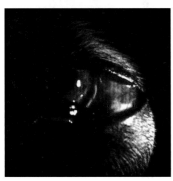

11.9

An 11-year-old German Shepherd Dog with zygomatic gland adenocarcinoma causing increased conjunctival exposure and secondary conjunctival hyperaemia.

tomography (CT) will usually yield better diagnostic information and may be the preferred approach where circumstances allow (see Chapter 2).

Secondary to another ocular disease: Clinical signs associated with conjunctivitis, such as conjunctival hyperaemia, may be observed in conjunction with other ocular signs (e.g. episcleral hyperaemia, corneal oedema) in other ocular conditions. If the underlying ocular disease is diagnosed correctly, and appropriately and successfully managed, the conjunctival hyperaemia will recede without specific treatment. In particular, it is important to examine closely for evidence of:

* Uveitis
* Glaucoma
* Episcleritis/scleritis.

Readers are referred to the relevant chapters for detailed discussion of the above conditions.

Secondary to systemic disease: Conjunctival involvement may be encountered secondary to a broad spectrum of systemic diseases (Figure 11.10; see also Chapter 20). Anaemia may result in conjunctival pallor, although generally the anaemia must be moderate or severe to be obvious. Icterus (due to jaundice) can be noticeable in the conjunctiva and sclera, as well as the oral and urogenital mucosae. Coagulopathies may cause conjunctival haemorrhage (ranging from petechiae to ecchymoses), and polycythaemia or hyperviscosity syndrome may cause conjunctival vessel congestion.

* Anaemia
* Jaundice
* Thrombocytopenia
* Coagulopathy
* Polycythaemia
* Hyperviscosity syndrome
* Systemic hypertension
* Vasculitis
* Systemic histiocytosis
* Multicentric lymphoma
* Idiopathic granulomatous disease
* Autoimmune disease (mucocutaneous junctions)
* Ligneous conjunctivitis

11.10 Systemic diseases that may be associated with conjunctival pathology or signs.

Conjunctival masses

Non-neoplastic masses: Subconjunctival fat prolapse is an important differential diagnosis for a conjunctival mass and is characterized by a soft, non-painful, swelling, usually of acute onset (Figure 11.11). Orbital fat that has prolapsed through the periorbital fascia can be resected, although where large-scale prolapse has occurred, a relative enophthalmos may remain on the affected side. Conjunctival epithelial inclusion cysts may occur following conjunctival surgery or trauma, and surgical excision is curative.

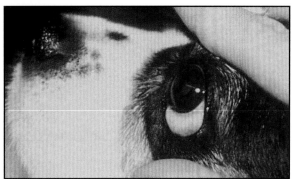

11.11 Subconjunctival fat prolapse. (Courtesy of G McLellan)

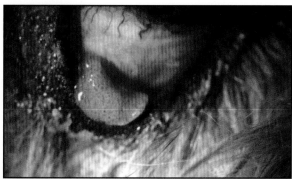

11.14 Conjunctival papilloma in an 8-year-old Lhasa Apso.

Conjunctival neoplasia: Primary conjunctival neoplasia in the dog is rare, although a number of neoplasms have been reported (Figures 11.12 to 11.14). Conjunctival biopsy is diagnostic. Histopathological examination is essential because the behaviour of each of these tumour types is very different. With the exception of conjunctival melanoma, which is often locally invasive and metastatic, primary canine conjunctival neoplasms are usually benign, although they can be locally invasive (e.g. squamous cell carcinoma), necessitating careful resection and adjunctive therapy.

Primary neoplasms
• Mast cell tumour • Squamous cell carcinoma • Papilloma • Haemangioma/sarcoma • Melanoma • Fibroma/sarcoma • Adenoma/carcinoma • Unicentric extranodal lymphoma • Lobular orbital adenoma
Secondary neoplasms
• Lymphoma • Systemic histiocytosis • Haemangioma/sarcoma • Adenoma/carcinoma • Mast cell tumour • Transmissible venereal tumour

11.12 Primary and secondary canine conjunctival neoplasia.

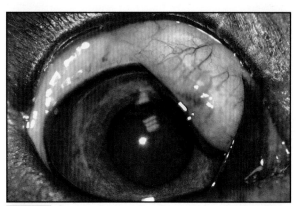

11.13 Conjunctival mast cell tumour in a 9-year-old Labrador Retriever.

Conjunctival thickening due to cellular infiltration may occur with multicentric lymphoma. Conjunctival malignant melanoma, with a predilection for the conjunctiva of the third eyelid, has been reported in dogs. Conjunctival mast cell tumours, in contrast with their cutaneous counterparts, are largely benign, and surgical excision, even with incomplete margins, is frequently reported to be curative (Fife *et al.,* 2011). Conjunctival haemangioma and haemangiosarcoma have been reported in dogs and a link to ultraviolet (UV) light exposure has been proposed (Pirie *et al.,* 2006). A propensity for involvement of the superior temporal bulbar conjunctiva and the leading edge of the third eyelid has been reported. Surgical excision can be curative, although recurrence has been reported and is more common with haemangiosarcomas. Adjunctive treatment with cryotherapy, CO_2 laser and strontium plesiotherapy has been reported.

Conjunctival trauma

The conjunctiva heals very quickly with little scarring, so minimal treatment (topical broad-spectrum antibiotics) and systemic analgesia (e.g. with non-steroidal anti-inflammatory drugs) only is likely to be necessary in cases of sharp conjunctival trauma. However, a conjunctival wound may be deceptively minor in cases of high-velocity foreign body penetration (e.g. air-rifle or shotgun pellets), and careful evaluation of the globe, orbit and periocular structures for further injuries or retained foreign bodies is mandatory.

Where more extensive areas of conjunctiva are lost (or surgically excised) closure with absorbable 6/0–8/0 (0.7 to 0.4 metric) suture material is warranted, taking care to ensure that the knots are buried to minimize irritation and avoid abrasion of the corneal surface. Ulcerated or incised conjunctiva may form adhesions with the adjacent conjunctiva or cornea; this is known as symblepharon formation.

Subconjunctival haemorrhage: Owing to the rich vascular supply of the conjunctiva and the episcleral/scleral tissues, blunt trauma can often result in extensive subconjunctival haemorrhage (Figure 11.15). Blunt force trauma can be very destructive to the intraocular structures; therefore, the presence of subconjunctival haemorrhage should always prompt a thorough ophthalmic examination. The presence of subconjunctival haemorrhage, especially when bilateral and in the absence of witnessed trauma, should provoke a differential diagnosis list that includes coagulopathy (Figure 11.16), systemic hypertension, increased local venous pressure sustained in crush injuries or asphyxia, and vasculitides.

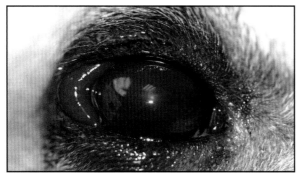

11.15 Subconjunctival haemorrhage and hyphaema in a 12-month-old Whippet following head trauma.

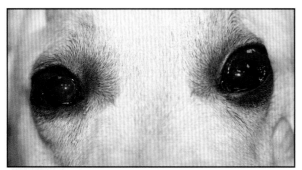

11.16 Bilateral subconjunctival haemorrhage in a 5-year-old Labrador Retriever with a coagulopathy.

Chemical injury: Chemical injury is often extremely serious, especially in the case of alkaline splashes because intraocular penetration is common (in contrast, acidic agents tend to denature tissues on contact, which limits their intraocular penetration) (Figures 11.17 to 11.19). Both acid and alkali burns can lead to destruction of the conjunctival and corneal stem cell populations. Loss of stem cell populations and extensive conjunctival damage frequently results in symblepharon formation. Known or suspected chemical burns should be treated with copious flushing with sterile saline for a minimum of 30 minutes.

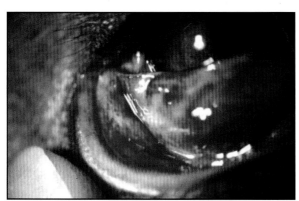

11.17 Conjunctival haemorrhage following a suspected chemical injury in a Labrador Retriever.

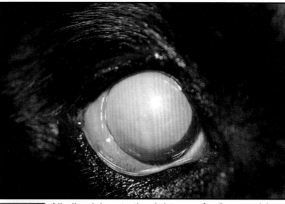

11.18 Alkaline injury to the right eye of a 6-year-old Rottweiler that occurred 24 hours previously.

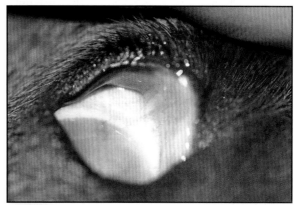

11.19 An 18-month-old Whippet, 2 months following an alkaline injury (caustic soda) to the right eye. Note the conjunctival adhesion and fornix shortening.

Foreign body trauma: Foreign bodies can become lodged in the conjunctival sac or behind the third eyelid. Acute discomfort with chemosis, conjunctival hyperaemia and lacrimation are followed by a mucopurulent discharge in most cases. Organic foreign bodies (Figure 11.20) are the most commonly encountered. Careful examination of the conjunctival fornices and behind the third eyelid, under topical anaesthesia, should reveal and allow removal of the offending material in all but the most aggressive dogs. Foreign material can erode through intact conjunctiva and may migrate into the retrobulbar tissues, or even penetrate the globe,

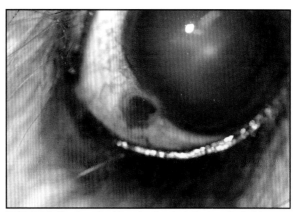

11.20 Conjunctival foreign body (plant material) in a 10-year-old Yorkshire Terrier.

often with discharging sinus tracts. Diagnostic imaging may prove invaluable in many cases. In these instances, where surgical exploration is required to locate and remove the foreign body, general anaesthesia is needed.

Feline conditions

Epibulbar dermoid

Dermoids represent foci of epidermal and dermal tissue (choristomas) in an abnormal location. They occur infrequently in cats, and are usually restricted to the Burmese (Figure 11.21) and Birman breeds, but reports in Domestic Shorthaired cats do exist (Hendy-Ibbs, 1985). The hairs on the dermoids are typically fine and long, so those that contact the cornea tend to float on the tear film.

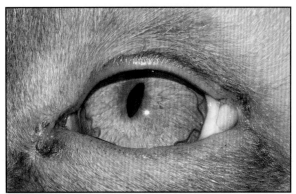

11.21 An 8-week-old Burmese kitten with an epibulbar dermoid (no eyelid involvement).

Conjunctivitis

Primary conjunctivitis: Infectious conjunctivitis is common in the cat and the pathogens implicated include feline herpesvirus-1 (FHV-1), *Chlamydophila felis*, feline calicivirus (FCV) and *Mycoplasma* spp. *Staphylococcus epidermidis*, β-haemolytic *Streptococcus* spp. and non-haemolytic *Streptococcus* spp. have also been cultured from cats with conjunctivitis, usually in combination with other pathogens, and may be considered opportunistic invaders (Hartmann *et al.*, 2010).

Feline herpesvirus-1: This is a DNA alpha-herpesvirus and is widespread amongst cat populations worldwide. Primary infection is common in kittens, typically occurring at 8–12 weeks of age as protection from maternally derived antibodies is waning. The virus has a tropism for the conjunctival, nasal and pharyngeal epithelium and is therefore commonly associated with upper respiratory disease signs and conjunctivitis, as well as general malaise and pyrexia. Neutrophilic infiltrates are marked on histopathological assessment, even in the absence of secondary bacterial involvement. Thus, the presence of a purulent discharge cannot be assumed to represent bacterial involvement in such cases. FHV-1 is also responsible for ophthalmia neonatorum in young kittens (see Chapter 9). Transmission is through close contact and aerosolized respiratory secretions; therefore,

overcrowded conditions promote the spread of infection. FHV-1 is not long-lived in the environment and is killed by most disinfectants.

Replication of FHV-1 within conjunctival and respiratory epithelial cells results in epithelial erosion and inflammation (Figure 11.22). Conjunctival ulceration may result in symblepharon formation (where ulcerated conjunctiva adheres to the cornea, if it is also ulcerated, or other areas of conjunctiva) (Figure 11.23). These conjunctival adhesions may obliterate the lacrimal ductules (resulting in secondary KCS), conjunctival fornices or nasolacrimal puncta, resulting in chronic epiphora. FHV-1 conjunctivitis may also be accompanied by corneal ulceration, which is typically dendritic in its early stages, progressing rapidly to geographical superficial ulceration in most cases. However, in chronic cases, stromal keratitis may be observed (for further details, see Chapter 12).

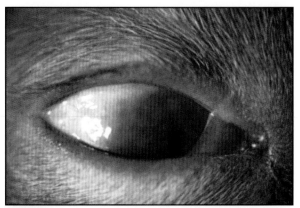

11.22 Conjunctivalization of the limbus in a Siamese kitten with FHV-1 infection. Note also the third eyelid hyperaemia and clear ocular discharge.

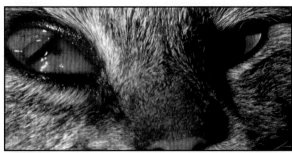

11.23 FHV-1 conjunctivitis in a Domestic Shorthaired kitten.

FHV-1 conjunctivitis may be complicated by secondary opportunistic bacterial infection. Treatment for primary FHV-1 infections is largely supportive, with gentle bathing of ocular secretions, ocular lubrication and prevention of conjunctival adhesions, as well as treatment of any secondary bacterial invasion with topical antibiotics. Topical (e.g. trifluorothymidine) and oral (e.g. famciclovir) antiviral treatments are available, but these are generally reserved for severe primary infections with lower respiratory tract involvement (systemic therapy) or severe, chronic and recurrent disease. Figure 11.24 lists the treatment options for FHV-1 conjunctivitis and keratitis.

Antiviral therapy	Effect	Efficacy *in vitro* against FHV-1 (ED$_{50}$ μM)	Dosage	Comments
Interferon (IFN) omega/alfa	Cytokine mediating innate (non-specific) immunity, including antiviral functions		According to an *in vitro* study, IFN-omega may be the most appropriate of the interferons at high doses (500 000 IU/ml) (Siebeck *et al.*, 2006)	An *in vivo* study showed no benefit of oral or topical IFN-omega pretreatment on subsequent experimental FHV-1 infection (Haid *et al.*, 2007)
L-lysine	L-lysine competitively inhibits arginine (an amino acid essential for viral replication)		250 mg/cat orally q24h to 500 mg/cat orally q12h In feed: 11 g lysine/kg diet to 51 g lysine/kg diet	Conflicting reports on *in vivo* benefit of oral L-lysine. More recent studies show no benefit or even increased severity of disease in treated cats (Drazenovich *et al.*, 2009). Higher in feed concentrations have been shown to reduce diet intake
Trifluorothymidine (trifluridine)	Acyclic nucleoside analogue (analogue of thymidine)	0.67	1% solution q2–6h	No controlled *in vivo* studies
Idoxuridine	Acyclic nucleoside analogue (analogue of thymidine)	4.3–6.8	0.1% ointment q1–6h	No controlled *in vivo* studies. May be irritating to some cats. Difficult to obtain (compounding pharmacists only)
Ganciclovir	Acyclic nucleoside analogue (analogue of guanosine)	5.2	0.15% gel q4–6h for 21 days	No *in vivo* reports exist. Available from UK pharmacies
Cidofovir	Acyclic nucleoside analogue (analogue of cytosine)	11.0	0.5% solution q12h for 21 days	An *in vivo* study reported that twice daily application significantly decreased viral shedding and clinical disease in experimentally induced ocular FHV-1 infection (Fontenelle *et al.*, 2008)
Famciclovir (prodrug of penciclovir)	Acyclic nucleoside analogue	13.9	Recommended dosages vary from 15 mg/kg orally q12–24h to 90 mg/kg orally q12h	Efficacy demonstrated *in vivo*. An *in vivo* study suggested no advantage to dosage >40 mg/kg (Thomasy *et al.*, 2012). Metabolized by the liver and excreted by the kidneys, therefore care required in hepatic and renal disease. *In vivo* efficacy of 1% ointment reported in humans suffering from herpes simplex virus keratitis. Commercial eye preparation not yet available (compounding pharmacies only)
Vidarabine	Acyclic nucleoside analogue (adenosine analogue)	21.4	3% ointment q3–6h for 21 days	No longer available commercially (compounding pharmacies only). No controlled *in vivo* studies
Aciclovir	Acyclic nucleoside analogue	57.9–85.6	3% ointment q4–6h for 21 days	No controlled *in vivo* studies. Not recommended systemically in cats as associated with bone marrow suppression (neutropenia and anaemia)

11.24 Treatment options for FHV-1 conjunctivitis and keratitis. ED$_{50}$ = effective dose 50. The concentration of drug required to reduce plaque numbers by 50% in comparison with controls.

An estimated 80% of primary infections establish latent infection within the trigeminal ganglia. Approximately half of cats with latent FHV-1 infection experience spontaneous reactivation of the virus later in life, with anterograde axonal transport of the virus. Periods of stress and the administration of corticosteroids are associated with reactivation of the latent virus. Ocular signs may be unilateral or bilateral; reactivated cases usually remain limited to the eye originally affected with the contralateral eye remaining clinically normal. Treatment of reactivated FHV-1 conjunctivitis is generally supportive and specific antiviral therapy is usually not required unless corneal involvement is present.

Diagnosis of FHV-1 infection can be confirmed by PCR testing, which has now superseded virus isolation as the gold standard diagnostic test and has a much higher sensitivity. However, reactivation of FHV-1 may occur secondary to trigeminal stimulation. Therefore, the presence of FHV-1 DNA may be coincidental to FHV-1 reactivation or secondary to another ocular disease process, rather than being the cause of the ocular disease under investigation. For this reason, many ophthalmologists rely on a consistent history and ocular findings to make the diagnosis of FHV-1 associated disease (Stiles, 2000; Gould, 2011).

Vaccination does not prevent FHV-1 infection;

however, vaccinated cats tend to have lower clinical scores of disease when challenged with field virus. Cell-mediated immunity, particularly at mucosal surfaces, appears to confer the greatest protection against FHV-1 infection. Vaccination does not reduce the risk of establishment of a latent infection. Live attenuated parenteral vaccines are capable of inducing disease in cats exposed via the oronasal route, so care should be taken to avoid creating an aerosol of the vaccine and ensure that the cat does not lick the injection site.

Chlamydophila felis: This is an obligate Gram-negative bacterium with a primary tropism for the conjunctiva. The human pathogen *Chlamydophila pneumoniae* has also been identified in cats with conjunctivitis (Sibitz *et al.*, 2011). The gastrointestinal, genital and respiratory tracts may also be infected, although clinical signs associated with these systems are usually mild or absent. Infection is typically encountered in cats <1 year old and transmission is by close contact between cats and contact with ocular secretions (via aerosolization or contaminated fomites). *Chlamydophila* elementary bodies can survive a few days at room temperature, but are readily inactivated by solvents and detergents (Ramsey, 2000; Gruffydd-Jones *et al.*, 2009).

Although most infected cats remain systemically well, some may demonstrate inappetence and weight loss with transient pyrexia. Generally, unilateral infections rapidly become bilateral with conjunctival hyperaemia, chemosis, blepharospasm and initially serous and later mucopurulent ocular discharge (Figure 11.25). *C. felis* does not cause corneal lesions and ocular disease is limited to the conjunctiva. In chronic disease, follicular conjunctivitis may be a feature, but it is not pathognomonic for *Chlamydophila* infection in cats. Mild rhinitis with sneezing and/or a serous/mucopurulent nasal discharge may accompany the predominantly ocular signs. Asymptomatic carrier states can occur, complicating control programmes in multi-cat situations. Persistence of the organism in the gastrointestinal and genital systems has also been reported. Concurrent infection with feline immunodeficiency virus (FIV) may prolong the duration of clinical signs and shedding of the organism.

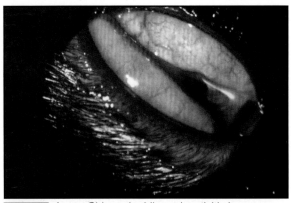

11.25 Acute *Chlamydophila* conjunctivitis in a Domestic Shorthaired kitten. Note the marked chemosis and lacrimation.

The diagnosis of *Chlamydophila* infection by identification of the characteristic cytoplasmic inclusion bodies in conjunctival cell smears has been reported, although these can be easily missed and reduce in number 2 weeks after infection. Rates of detection of inclusion bodies in chronic infections are low. Smears from conjunctival scrapings should be stained with Giemsa or modified Wright–Giemsa (Diff Quik®) stains to identify the basophilic inclusion bodies. Topical ointments may result in cytoplasmic inclusions within conjunctival epithelial cells, known as 'blue bodies', which should be differentiated from *Chlamydophila* inclusion bodies.

Molecular diagnosis by PCR is now the mainstay for confirmation of *Chlamydophila* infection and is sensitive enough to identify chronically infected cats. *Chlamydophila* culture can be undertaken but requires cell samples because of the obligate intracellular nature of the pathogen. Indirect fluorescent antibody testing can be used to diagnose *C. felis* infection, although it is important to remember not to apply fluorescein before collecting samples because false-positive results are likely. Antibody titres obtained by serology can identify exposure to *Chlamydophila* organisms (only to genus level), but cannot distinguish vaccination-associated antibodies from field exposure, or active infection from previous exposure.

Chlamydophila is sensitive to tetracyclines, erythromycin, azithromycin, fluoroquinolones and amoxicillin/clavulanate. Topical treatment alone will not clear gastrointestinal organisms, thus is not recommended for elimination of the infection. Treatment with doxycycline at a dose of 10 mg/kg orally q24h for 28 days is the most efficacious for elimination of the infection compared with amoxicillin/clavulanate, azithromycin and shorter courses of doxycycline. To avoid potential oesophagitis and stricture formation, doxycycline should be given as a suspension or a tablet followed by a water/food bolus to ensure that the drug does not remain in the oesophagus for an extended period of time. To avoid the side effects of tetracyclines in young kittens, a 28-day course of amoxicillin/clavulanate is considered the best option. Treatment of all in-contact cats is also recommended.

Chlamydophila vaccines are available and should be considered for cats at high risk of exposure, such as those in multi-cat households or shelters with a history of *C. felis* infection. *Chlamydophila* is a zoonotic pathogen, but verified transmission from infected cats to humans is rare. Routine hygiene should be encouraged in owners of affected cats, particularly those that are immunosuppressed. Follicular conjunctivitis in humans is considered a strong indicator of chlamydial infection.

The novel chlamydial organism *Neochlamydia hartmannellae* is an endosymbiont of the amoeba *Hartmannella vermiformis,* and has been identified in cats with conjunctivitis (von Bomhard *et al.*, 2003). It has been postulated to be transmitted by amoeba-contaminated water and has been detected in conjunction with FHV-1 and *C. felis*. *N. hartmannellae* has also been associated with eosinophilic conjunctivitis and keratoconjunctivitis.

Feline calicivirus: This is a single-stranded RNA virus capable of causing conjunctivitis in cats. Infection with FCV causes upper respiratory tract disease, as well as oral ulcers and polyarthritis, in addition to conjunctivitis. Whilst most cats eliminate the infection, some animals remain persistently infected and may chronically shed the virus. Topical and systemic antiviral medications are ineffective against FCV because these drugs disrupt DNA (not RNA) replication. Symptomatic treatment, with bathing of ocular discharges and treatment of secondary bacterial infections, is recommended.

More virulent strains of FCV have been identified, which cause systemic disease with significant mortality. Widespread lesions have been described, including subcutaneous oedema and ulceration of the oral mucosa, nares, pinnae and footpads. Liver, spleen, pancreas and lung lesions associated with the viral antigen have also been described on postmortem examination. FCV vaccination, similar to FHV-1 vaccination, does not prevent infection or development of a carrier state, but reduces the severity of clinical disease.

Mycoplasma *spp.: Mycoplasma felis*, *M. gatae* and *M. arginini* have been implicated as a cause of feline conjunctivitis, although *Mycoplasma* spp. have also been isolated from the conjunctival sacs of normal cats. Some investigations have demonstrated *Mycoplasma* spp. to be the most commonly isolated organisms in feline conjunctivitis, and significantly more prevalent in cats with conjunctivitis compared with healthy animals (Low *et al.*, 2007). However, studies involving experimental infection have provided conflicting results on the provocation of conjunctivitis.

Four new species of *Mycoplasma* have been identified in clinical cases of feline conjunctivitis in Germany, namely *M. canadense*, *M. cynos*, *M. lipophilum* and *M. hyopharyngis*, but these have yet to be reported in the UK. *Mycoplasma* spp. are capable of causing severe lower respiratory tract disease in immunocompromised cats, and ocular disease in cats concurrently infected with FHV-1 or *C. felis*. *Mycoplasma* spp. have also been implicated in feline polyarthritis and as opportunistic invaders in ulcerative keratitis.

Diagnosis of feline ocular *Mycoplasma* infection is usually via PCR testing. *Mycoplasma* culture is possible, but requires specialist media (it is advisable to discuss requirements with the diagnostic laboratory prior to sample submission) and is less sensitive than PCR.

Mycoplasma spp. conjunctivitis is sensitive to most topical antibiotics. Treatment with topical tetracyclines is often recommended owing to their efficacy against *Chlamydophila* spp. Oral doxycycline has been reported in the treatment of *M. felis* infections causing systemic disease (respiratory disease or polyarthritis).

Bordetella bronchiseptica: This is a Gram-negative bacterium, which affects the respiratory tract of cats (and dogs) and is capable of causing conjunctivitis.

It is rarely a zoonotic pathogen; therefore, owners of infected cats should be advised to observe general hygiene. Infected dogs can also transmit the organism to cats. *B. bronchiseptica* has been documented in cases of naturally occurring conjunctivitis in cats alone and in association with other respiratory viruses, as well as in experimental infections (Egberink *et al.*, 2009). The bacterium is destroyed by most disinfectants.

B. bronchiseptica may be associated with colonization of the ciliated epithelium of the respiratory tract and chronic respiratory infection. It is shed in the nasal and oral discharges of affected cats. Diagnosis can be confirmed by culture or PCR testing of conjunctival, nasal or oropharyngeal swabs or bronchoalveolar washes. Antibacterial therapy is indicated and doxycycline is reported as the drug of choice (in the absence of specific antibiotic sensitivity results). Vaccination against *B. bronchispetica* is not currently recommended as a core vaccine, although an intranasal modified-live vaccine is available in some European countries and may be beneficial in high-risk situations (catteries or shelters with a high prevalence of respiratory infection).

Other bacterial agents: Conjunctivitis associated with *Salmonella enterica* serovar. *typhimurium* has been described in a cat, and an experimental study has demonstrated that *S. typhimurium* is capable of inducing primary conjunctivitis following conjunctival inoculation (Fox *et al.*, 1984). This study also demonstrated that cats infected by this route may shed bacteria in their faeces.

Secondary conjunctivitis: Secondary bacterial involvement is not uncommon with FHV-1, *C. felis* and FCV infections. Qualitative tear deficiency has been demonstrated in cases of feline conjunctivitis, with a more rapid tear film break up time (TFBUT) compared with healthy cats. It is unclear whether a pre-existing tear film abnormality predisposes to infectious conjunctivitis in cats, or whether it develops secondary to conjunctivitis. Systemic disease, intraocular diseases and extension from local diseases may also involve the conjunctiva as with dogs (see above).

Eosinophilic conjunctivitis: This is an immune-mediated condition in which eosinophils infiltrate the conjunctiva. This condition may progress to involve the cornea with corneal infiltration, ulceration and/or vascularization. Eosinophilic conjunctivitis typically presents with a creamy white, mucopurulent to caseous exudate (resembling cottage cheese) overlying the conjunctiva, associated with erosive or depigmented eyelid lesions, blepharospasm and conjunctival swelling (Figure 11.26). Diagnosis is confirmed by cytological analysis of a smear of the infiltrate. The presence of eosinophils on a smear is diagnostic, although free eosinophilic granules, plasma cells and neutrophils are also often present.

The pathophysiology of the condition is not fully understood, but some authors have postulated a link to FHV-1 infection. This follows the observation that

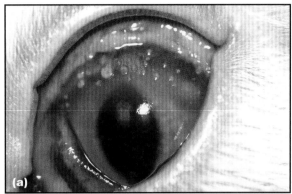

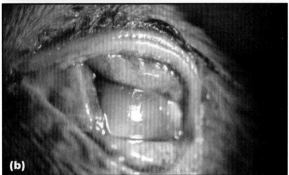

11.26 Eosinophilic keratoconjunctivitis. **(a)** An 18-month-old Maine Coon cat. Note the cream coloured cellular deposits on the cornea and bulbar conjunctiva. **(b)** A 3-year-old Domestic Shorthaired cat with severe disease.

FHV-1 DNA was identified in corneoconjunctival scrapings from 76.3% of cases with eosinophilic keratitis in one study (Nasisse *et al.*, 1998) and in 85.7% of cases in another study (Volopich *et al.*, 2005). Given that recrudescence of FHV-1 to the cornea from latent infection in the trigeminal ganglia can occur following a corneal injury or condition, this finding is not proof of causation. The documentation of viral particles using electron microscopy or FHV-1 DNA by PCR testing was not possible in one retrospective study of 12 cats with eosinophilic conjunctivitis (Allgoewer *et al.*, 2001). A novel chlamydial organism (*Neochlamydia hartmannellae*) has been described in association with eosinophilic keratoconjunctivitis, although direct causation has yet to be demonstrated.

Treatment of eosinophilic conjunctivitis is with topical corticosteroids and/or ciclosporin. In most cases, topical treatment is sufficient to resolve the condition; however, treatment with systemic steroids, including megestrol has been reported to be successful in recalcitrant cases. Owing to the side effects of megestrol (increased risk of mammary hyperplasia, diabetes mellitus, adrenal gland suppression, endometrial hyperplasia and pyometra), this is not recommended as a first-line treatment.

Parasitic conjunctivitis: *Thelazia callipaeda* is a parasite that infects the conjunctival sacs of dogs and cats, causing irritation and conjunctivitis. Transmission is via flies feeding on lacrimal secretions. The parasite has not yet been recorded in the UK; however, cases have been reported in Italy,

Switzerland and France in recent years (the disease was originally reported in Asia). *Thelazia californiensis* has not been reported in Europe and is confined to the western USA.

Symblepharon
Conjunctival adhesions to the eyelids, conjunctiva and cornea may result from neonatal or severe FHV-1 infections or chemical trauma. These adhesions may restrict vision, globe movement, tear flow and/or tear drainage (Figure 11.27). Treatment after they have formed is difficult because surgical resection of symblepharon leads to rapid reformation of the adhesions in most cases. Use of complex surgical procedures to reconstruct the conjunctival fornices, therapeutic contact lenses or conjunctival conformers has been attempted to try and reduce recurrence rates, but with limited success. Recent success in the treatment of affected humans using amnionic membrane transplantation may provide hope for these cases. Prevention of adhesion formation by intensive nursing of affected patients (e.g. bathing of ocular discharges in primary FHV-1 cases and gentle repeated separation of the conjunctival tissues under topical anaesthesia with ocular lubrication) is recommended.

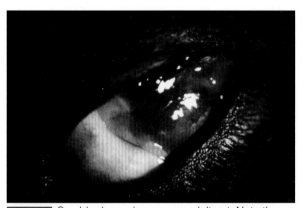

11.27 Symblepharon in a young adult cat. Note the conjunctivalization of the dorsolateral cornea and third eyelid protrusion due to the adhesions.

Conjunctival masses

Non-neoplastic masses: Lipogranulomatous conjunctivitis is a cause of ocular discomfort in cats and is characterized by nodules on the palpebral conjunctiva, adjacent to the eyelid margins (Read and Lucas, 2001) (see Chapter 9). Most cases of lipogranulomatous conjunctivitis are bilateral with the upper eyelid most frequently affected. It has been speculated that actinic damage to the meibomian ductules, with subsequent sequestration of meibum and rupture of the meibomian glands, is responsible for these lesions. Lack of eyelid pigmentation has also been suggested as a risk factor for developing the condition. Surgical curettage of the inspissated material via conjunctival incisions is recommended to resolve the condition. Topical antibiotic ointments have been reported to be soothing, although this is likely to be due to lubrication affording relief of the mechanical irritation associated with the nodules.

Conjunctival neoplasia: Primary conjunctival neoplasia is rare in cats (Figure 11.28). The most common primary neoplasm is squamous cell carcinoma (Figure 11.29). Conjunctival involvement may result from extension of an eyelid squamous cell carcinoma or may involve the conjunctiva on the third eyelid. Feline conjunctival melanoma appears to have a predilection for the bulbar conjunctiva, although palpebral and third eyelid conjunctival melanomas have been reported. Some melanomas may be amelanotic, but most are pigmented. Both local recurrence and metastasis have been reported with a mean survival time of 11 months (Schobert *et al.*, 2010). Other tumours reported include haemangiomas and haemangiosarcomas (Pirie and Dubielzig, 2006).

Primary neoplasms
• Squamous cell carcinoma • Haemangioma/sarcoma • Melanoma • Peripheral nerve sheath tumour • Hodgkin's-like lymphoma • Adenoma/carcinoma
Secondary neoplasms
• Lymphoma • Haemangioma/sarcoma • Adenoma/carcinoma

11.28 Primary and secondary feline conjunctival neoplasia.

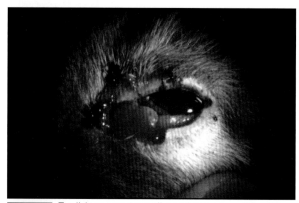

11.29 Eyelid squamous cell carcinoma in a 10-year-old Domestic Shorthaired cat. Note the involvement of the conjunctiva and third eyelid.

Peripheral nerve sheath tumours have also been reported in cats with early recurrence following excision a common feature (Hoffman *et al.*, 2005). Metastasis of this type of tumour has not been reported. Bilateral conjunctival B-cell lymphoma (Figure 11.30) has also been reported in a cat, in which no grossly evident metastasis was observed on imaging at the time of surgery (Radi *et al.*, 2004); however, follow-up information was not available. Extranodal conjunctival Hodgkin's-like lymphoma has also been described in a cat and radiotherapy was reported to be successful in achieving remission (the tumour was not responsive to chemotherapy; Holt *et al.*, 2006).

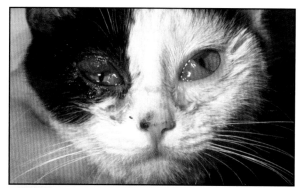

11.30 Lymphoma infiltration of the conjunctiva in a 4-month-old cat with feline leukaemia virus. (Courtesy of D Gould)

Conjunctival trauma

Conjunctival trauma may result from a cat fight, air-gun pellets or as part of the spectrum of injuries sustained in a road traffic accident. Chemical and foreign body trauma may also be encountered in feline patients, although perhaps less frequently than in dogs. The principles of investigation and management of conjunctival trauma are the same as for dogs (see above).

The third eyelid

Embryology, anatomy and physiology

The third eyelid is derived from surface ectoderm. The third eyelid (nictitans or nictitating membrane) comprises a central T-shaped hyaline cartilage surrounded by fibrous connective tissue and covered by conjunctival epithelium (Figure 11.31). The posterior, bulbar surface of the third eyelid also has numerous aggregates of lymphoid tissue beneath the conjunctival epithelium, together with intraepithelial goblet cells. Conjunctival goblet cells are also located, in greater number, on the anterior, palpebral surface of the third eyelid. The third eyelid gland (nictitans gland) is located at the inferior (proximal) end of the cartilage.

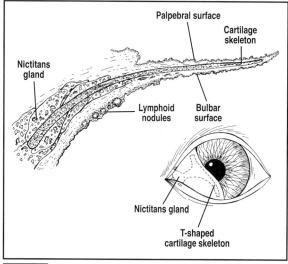

11.31 Anatomy of the third eyelid and nictitans gland.

The third eyelid gland contributes to the preocular tear film. Immunoglobulin (Ig) A secreting plasma cells have been identified adjacent to the conjunctival epithelium on both surfaces of the third eyelid, as well as within the connective tissue of the third eyelid gland, suggesting a role in defence of the ocular surface. The third eyelid gland is considered to contribute approximately one-third of aqueous tear production in normal animals, although some authors have reported that as much as 60% of basal tear production is derived from the third eyelid gland (Saito *et al.*, 2001).

The leading edge of the third eyelid is approximately 4–5 mm in width and is supported by cartilage. The functions of this membrane-like margin are to distribute the tear film evenly across the cornea and to sweep away debris. The margin is usually pigmented; however, in some dogs a non-pigmented margin is present and, if unilateral, this can give the optical illusion of third eyelid protrusion on the unpigmented side. The base of the third eyelid is intimately associated with the fascia of the orbital musculature, and the inferior extent of the cartilage shaft is aligned with the inferionasal peribulbar connective tissue. The canine third eyelid itself lacks musculature; protrusion is achieved passively when the globe is retracted and the retrobulbar tissues push the base of the third eyelid anteriorly. Unlike the dog, the feline third eyelid contains smooth muscle, which serves to retract the third eyelid (Nuyttens and Simoens, 1995). Loss of retrobulbar tissue or reduced globe size may also result in third eyelid protrusion.

Canine and feline conditions

Developmental conditions

Scrolled cartilage: Deformation of the third eyelid (nictitans) cartilage is reported most commonly in large and giant dog breeds. It has also been described in a British Blue cat. Abnormal growth results in a scrolled section of cartilage (Figure 11.32) and subsequent eversion or inversion of the third eyelid. In some cases, the degree of scrolling is minor and not clinically significant; however, where the degree of eversion is moderate or severe,

correction is indicated. Dust, debris and foreign material may collect in or on the everted portion and cause ocular irritation. The scrolled cartilage may also alter third eyelid movement and, thereby, tear film distribution.

Treatment is by careful excision of the scrolled portion of the third eyelid via a conjunctival incision, using surgical loupes for magnification. In addition, some ophthalmologists recommend placement of a third eyelid flap in the affected eye, in order to 'splint' the third eyelid against the contour of the globe postoperatively. In some cases, shortening of the third eyelid is also necessary and this is achieved by performing wedge resections at the temporal and nasal aspects of the third eyelid, which are closed with 6/0–8/0 (0.7 to 0.4 metric) polyglactin suture material. A simpler method of correction has been described that avoids the need for surgical excision of cartilage. The technique utilizes very light application of thermal cautery directly to the bulbar surface of the third eyelid overlying the scrolled region of cartilage to contract and straighten it (Allbaugh and Stuhr, 2013). Whilst this technique appears promising, consultation with a veterinary ophthalmologist is advised and extreme caution must be exercised to avoid excessive thermal damage to tissues and to ensure that abrasion of the corneal surface by charred conjunctiva does not occur.

Prolapsed third eyelid gland: Third eyelid gland prolapse has been described in many dog breeds, including English and French Bulldogs, Lhasa Apso, Shih Tzu, Pekingese, Shar Pei, Beagle, American Cocker Spaniel, Great Dane and Mastiff breeds (Mazzucchelli *et al.*, 2012). It has also been described in Burmese, Persian and Domestic Shorthaired cats (Chahory *et al.*, 2004). The gland is normally located at the base of the third eyelid cartilage and it is believed that laxity of attachment to the cartilage and periorbita, as well as crowding of the inferior orbital space in some brachycephalic breeds, is responsible for prolapse of the gland (Figure 11.33). Gland prolapse occurs most frequently before 1 year of age and may be unilateral or bilateral.

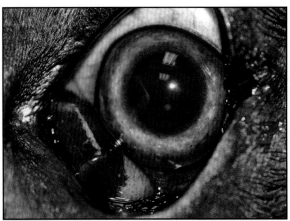

11.32 A 16-month-old Great Dane with scrolled cartilage of the left third eyelid.

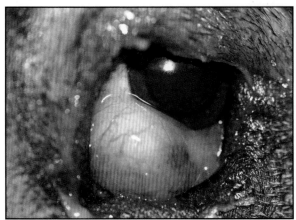

11.33 Third eyelid gland prolapse in a 9-month-old Bulldog.

Removal of the gland is not recommended because approximately one-third of the tear volume originates from the third eyelid gland. In addition, many of the breeds at increased risk of gland prolapse are also at risk of KCS and, therefore, potentially have less functional reserve. In cats, removal of the third eyelid is associated with KCS and changes in tear protein expression. Replacement of the gland is the gold standard of therapy and a number of techniques have been reported, including mucosal pocketing of the gland (Figure 11.34), tacking to the third eyelid cartilage, tacking to the episcleral/scleral tissues, and tacking to the orbital rim periosteum (Figure 11.35) (Kaswan and Martin, 1985; Stanley and Kaswan, 1994; Hendrix, 2007; Plummer *et al.*, 2008).

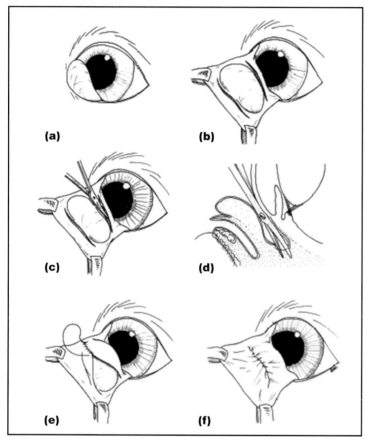

11.34 Mucosal pocket technique for prolapsed third eyelid gland replacement. **(a)** Appearance of prolapsed third eyelid gland. **(b)** A pocket is created inferior to the globe, through the conjunctiva, into which the gland is placed. Conjunctival incisions are made superior and inferior to the gland prolapse on the posterior surface of the third eyelid. **(c–d)** A subconjunctival pocket is bluntly dissected inferiomedial to the globe via the inferior incision in the conjunctiva. **(e–f)** The two incisions are then partially closed using buried absorbable sutures (6/0 (0.7 metric) polyglactin) with the gland 'pocketed'. Care should be taken not to close the ends of the pocket to allow glandular secretion to escape and avoid the possible complication of cyst formation. It is important that the suture material is fully buried and does not contact the cornea, because this usually results in ulceration. The use of surgical loupes is strongly recommended for this technique. (Illustration by Roser Tetas Pont)

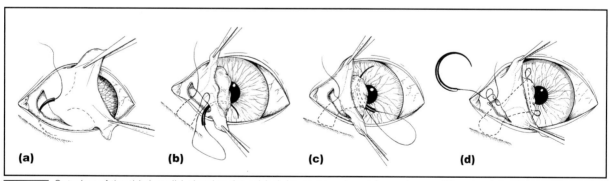

11.35 Suturing of the third eyelid gland to the orbital rim as a treatment for prolapse of the gland. **(a)** Forceps grasp the periphery of the free margin of the third eyelid and pull it across the eye (stay sutures may be used). An incision is made in the inferiomedial conjunctival fornix (at the base of the third eyelid) using scissors. Blunt dissection allows access to the periosteum of the medioventral orbital rim. A firm bite of periosteum along the orbital rim is taken using 3/0 (2 metric) polydioxanone or monofilament nylon: the suture material (with a swaged-on needle) is introduced through the previously made incision. It can be a little difficult to obtain a bite of periosteum and bring the needle out through the original incision, because access to the area is limited. **(b)** After taking a bite of orbital periosteum, the needle is passed through the original incision dorsally to the prolapsed gland to emerge from the gland at its most prominent point of prolapse. **(c)** With the third eyelid everted, the needle is passed back through the exit hole in the gland to take a horizontal bite through the most prominent part of the gland. **(d)** Finally, the needle is passed back through the last exit hole to emerge through the original incision in the conjunctival fornix, thus encircling a large portion of the gland. The suture ends are then tied. This creates a loop of suture through the gland which anchors it to the periosteum of the orbital rim, preventing it from re-prolapsing. The conjunctival incision can now be repaired using 6/0 (0.7 metric) polyglactin or may be left unsutured. Topical antibiotic cover is provided postoperatively.

Protrusion of the third eyelid: Microphthalmos may result in passive protrusion of the third eyelid over the smaller globe. This may have only cosmetic consequences, but in severe cases the protrusion can be sufficient to obscure the pupil, resulting in visual compromise. Shortening of the third eyelid is indicated in such cases. This is achieved by resection of a portion of the third eyelid cartilage via a conjunctival incision on the anterior surface of the third eyelid.

Acquired conditions

Cysts: Conjunctival cysts or cysts of the third eyelid gland may be encountered and are best treated by careful surgical resection (Figure 11.36). Cysts of the third eyelid gland are most frequently seen following third eyelid gland pocketing procedures and entrapment of glandular secretions.

Protrusion of the third eyelid: The causes of protrusion of the third eyelid are listed in Figure 11.37.

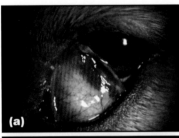
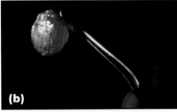

11.36 **(a)** Cyst originating from the third eyelid gland in a Golden Retriever following mucosal pocketing surgery. **(b)** Excised cyst for gland prolapse.

• Enophthalmos (e.g. secondary to cachexia and/or dehydration)
• Microphthalmos
• Retrobulbar (extraconal/non-axial) mass (Figures 11.38 and 11.39)
• Horner's syndrome (Figure 11.40)
• Sedation/anaesthesia
• Dysautonomia
• Cannabis intoxication
• Tetanus (may be associated with 'flicking' protrusion of third eyelid) (Figure 11.41)
• Rabies
• Torovirus in cats (often associated with relapsing diarrhoea)

11.37 Causes of third eyelid protrusion.

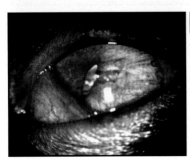

11.38 A 6-year-old Domestic Shorthaired cat with a retrobulbar abscess causing third eyelid protrusion and hyperaemia.

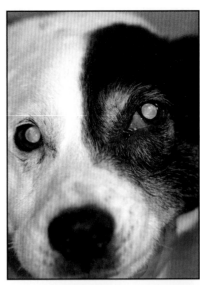

11.39 A 10-year-old Collie cross with orbital neoplasia (myxosarcoma) causing third eyelid protrusion.

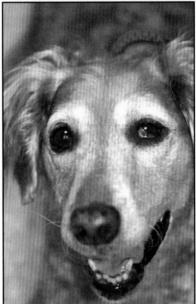

11.40 A 6-year-old Golden Retriever with idiopathic Horner's syndrome, showing third eyelid protrusion with miosis and ptosis affecting the left eye.

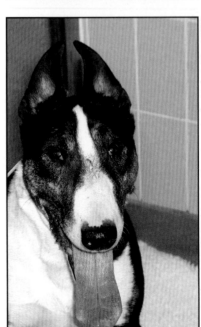

11.41 Tetanus in a 4-year-old English Bull Terrier. Note the pricked ears and bilateral third eyelid protrusion.

Neoplasia of the third eyelid: This is uncommon in canine and feline patients. Third eyelid neoplasia is the only indication for third eyelid resection (including the third eyelid gland). The neoplasms reported to affect the third eyelid conjunctiva and/or gland are listed in Figure 11.42.

Primary neoplasms
• Adenocarcinoma • Squamous cell carcinoma (Figure 11.43) • Melanoma (Figure 11.44) • Histiocytoma (Figure 11.45) • Mast cell tumour • Papilloma • Haemangioma/sarcoma • Angiokeratoma • Plasmacytoma • Mucosa-associated lymphoid tissue (MALT) lymphoma (Figure 11.46) • Fibrosarcoma
Secondary neoplasms
• Lymphosarcoma (Figure 11.47)

11.42 Primary and secondary neoplasms of the third eyelid.

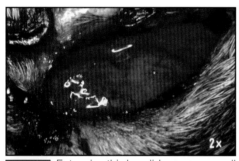

11.43 Extensive third eyelid squamous cell carcinoma in a 12-year-old Domestic Shorthaired cat.

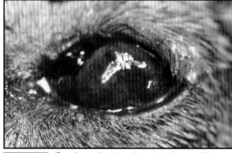

11.44 Conjunctival melanoma in an 8-year-old Great Dane cross.

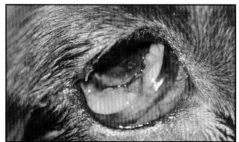

11.45 Third eyelid histiocytoma in a 13-month-old English Springer Spaniel.

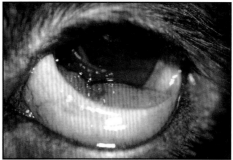

11.46 Multicentric lymphoma presenting as third eyelid thickening in a 5-year-old English Cocker Spaniel.

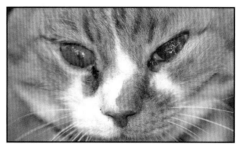

11.47 Conjunctival and third eyelid lymphosarcoma as part of multicentric disease in a 12-year-old Domestic Shorthaired cat.

Inflammatory disease of the third eyelid: The conjunctival surfaces of the third eyelid are usually affected in cases of conjunctivitis. Follicular conjunctivitis involving the posterior surface of the third eyelid is common in patients with chronic conjunctivitis.

Plasma cell infiltration of the third eyelid conjunctiva: This condition, also known as plasmoma and plasmacytic conjunctivitis, is an immune-mediated disease of unclear pathogenesis. German Shepherd Dogs (Figure 11.48), Belgian Shepherd Dogs and collie breeds are over-represented and the condition is often associated with chronic superficial keratoconjunctivitis (CSK) or pannus (see Chapter 12). The disease is recognized as an apparently painless, generally bilateral thickening of the third eyelid (often most pronounced at the leading edge), with depigmentation of the usually pigmented margin and nodular pink–tan cellular infiltrates (predominantly plasma

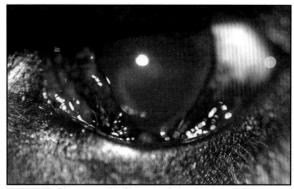

11.48 Plasma cell infiltrates of the third eyelid in a 4-year-old German Shepherd Dog. Note the smooth pink–tan nodules along the third eyelid margin and on the anterior surface of the third eyelid.

cells with some lymphocytes). Clinical presentation alone is often sufficient to allow a diagnosis. However, cytological evaluation of smears obtained from conjunctival scrapings reveals a mixed population of inflammatory cells (predominantly lymphocytes and plasma cells). Initial treatment with 0.2% ciclosporin ointment twice daily is recommended, although topical corticosteroids at a gradually reducing dose may be required as an adjunctive treatment to achieve remission (Read, 1995). Maintenance therapy with long-term topical 0.2% ciclosporin ointment oncde or twice daily is successful at controlling the condition in most cases.

Immune-mediated granulomatous disease: Nodular granulomatous episclerokeratitis (NGE), idiopathic granulomatous disease and nodular fasciitis are thought to represent different forms on a spectrum of related immune-mediated diseases that share clinical and histopathological features.

Inflammatory diseases such as NGE do not usually involve the conjunctiva (the granulomas are subconjunctival); however, they may involve the third eyelid. Collie breeds are over-represented and histopathology reveals a chronic granulomatous infiltrate. Surgical excision alone often results in recurrence, but has been reported to be successful with adjunctive treatment such as cryotherapy. Azathioprine with or without topical corticosteroids has also been reported to be a useful treatment.

Idiopathic granulomatous disease has been reported to involve the conjunctiva, third eyelid, eyelids, skin and nasal mucosa. American Cocker Spaniels, collies and Shetland Sheepdogs appear to be predisposed. The condition has also been described in an Australian Kelpie. Successful treatment with immunosuppressive or immunomodulatory drugs (including azathioprine, L-asparaginase, prednisolone, tetracyclines and niacinamide) has been described. Surgical excision or debulking in combination with medical treatment has also been reported.

Ocular nodular fasciitis has been reported to affect the third eyelid, but is more commonly associated with the sclera, episcleral tissues and cornea (see Chapters 12 and 13).

Third eyelid trauma: This generally heals with minimal intervention; however, trauma involving the free margin or disrupting a large part of the third eyelid should be repaired surgically, taking care to prevent the sutures from rubbing the cornea. Foreign bodies may lodge behind the third eyelid without being visible externally. Application of a topical anaesthetic and a thorough inspection behind the third eyelid is recommended in all cases of conjunctivitis (with the exception of fragile or ruptured eyes where handling may provoke aqueous leakage). Removal of the third eyelid is contraindicated, except in cases of malignancy, since its removal has deleterious effects on the tear film and corneal surface health.

Third eyelid flap surgery: This has very few indications because it provides no nutrition to a compromised cornea (unlike conjunctival grafting procedures) and may obscure visualization of a corneal ulcer or lesion. Third eyelid flap placement may be of limited benefit following grafting procedures, including those utilizing porcine small intestinal submucosa grafts, in providing a moistened environment for the newly placed graft. This needs to be balanced against the risk of trapping neutrophils and other white blood cells against the cornea and promoting keratomalacia (corneal melting).

If placed, it is advisable to suture the third eyelid flap to the bulbar conjunctiva (ensuring that the suture material is not in contact with the cornea). This allows the flap to move with the globe, thereby reducing abrasion of the delicate cornea against the posterior surface of the flap. Although, this technique has been described in conscious animals using topical anaesthesia, local anaesthesia and auriculopalpebral nerve blockade, heavy sedation or general anaesthesia are strongly recommended. Suturing the third eyelid flap through a stent on the upper eyelid (ensuring that the suture material does not contact the underlying cornea by placing sutures through the superior conjunctival fornix) may also allow the opportunity to release the flap temporarily, observe the cornea and then re-tie the sutures as necessary. This approach may be of value in animals that are too elderly or infirm to tolerate prolonged or repeated episodes of general anaesthesia.

References and further reading

Allbaugh RA and Stuhr CM (2013) Thermal cautery of the canine third eyelid for treatment of cartilage eversion. *Veterinary Ophthalmology* **16**, 392–395

Allgoewer I, Schäffer EH, Stockhaus C *et al.* (2001) Feline eosinophilic conjunctivitis. *Veterinary Ophthalmology* **4(1)**, 69–74

Chahory S, Crasta M, Trio S *et al.* (2004) Three cases of prolapse of the nictitans gland in cats. *Veterinary Ophthalmology* **7(6)**, 417–419

Drazenovich TL, Fascetti AJ, Westermeyer HD *et al.* (2009) Effects of dietary lysine supplementation on upper respiratory and ocular disease and detection of infectious organisms in cats within an animal shelter. *American Journal of Veterinary Research* **70**, 1391–1400

Dubielzig R, Ketring K, McLellan GJ *et al.* (2010) Diseases of the eyelids and conjunctiva. In: *Veterinary Ocular Pathology – A Comparative Review*, ed. RD Dubielzig *et al.*, pp. 143–199. Saunders, Philadelphia

Egberink H, Addie D, Belák S *et al.* (2009) *Bordetella bronchiseptica* infection in cats ABCD guidelines on prevention and management. *Journal of Feline Medicine and Surgery* **11**, 610–614

Fife M, Blocker T, Fife T *et al.* (2011) Canine conjunctival mast cell tumors: a retrospective study. *Veterinary Ophthalmology* **14(3)**, 153–160

Fontenelle JP, Powell CC, Veir JK *et al.* (2008) Effect of topical ophthalmic application of cidofovir on experimentally induced primary ocular feline herpesvirus-1 infection in cats. *American Journal of Veterinary Research* **69**, 289–293

Fox JG, Beaucage CM, Murphy JC *et al.* (1984) Experimental *Salmonella*-associated conjunctivitis in cats. *Canadian Journal of Comparative Medicine* **48(1)**, 87–91

Gilger BC (2008) Immunology of the ocular surface. In: *Ophthalmic Immunology and Immune-mediated Disease. Veterinary Clinics of North America: Small Animal Practice*, ed. DL Williams, pp. 223–231. WB Saunders, Philadelphia

Gould DJ (2011) Feline herpesvirus-1: ocular manifestations, diagnosis and treatment options. *Journal of Feline Medicine and Surgery* **13**, 333–346

Gruffydd-Jones T, Addie D, Belák S *et al.* (2009) *Chlamydophila felis* infection ABCD guidelines on prevention and management. *Journal of Feline Medicine and Surgery* **11**, 605–609

Haid C, Kaps S, Gonczi E *et al.* (2007). Pretreatment with feline interferon omega and the course of subsequent infection with feline herpesvirus in cats. *Veterinary Ophthalmology* **10**, 278–284

Hartmann AD, Hawley J, Werckenthin C *et al.* (2010) Detection of bacterial and viral organisms from the conjunctiva of cats with conjunctivitis and upper respiratory tract disease. *Journal of Feline Medicine and Surgery* **12**, 775–782

Hendrix DVH (2007) Canine conjunctiva and nictating membrane. In: *Veterinary Ophthalmology*, 4th edn, ed. KN Gelatt, pp. 662–689. Blackwell Publishing, Oxford

Hendy-Ibbs PM (1985) Familial feline epibulbar dermoids. *Veterinary Record* **116(1)**, 13–14

Hoffman A, Blocker T, Dubielzig R *et al.* (2005) Feline periocular peripheral nerve sheath tumor: a case series. *Veterinary Ophthalmology* **8(3)**, 153–158

Holt E, Goldschmidt MH and Skorupski K (2006) Extranodal conjunctival Hodgkin's-like lymphoma in a cat. *Veterinary Ophthalmology* **9(3)**, 141–144

Ledbetter EC, Hornbuckle WE and Dubovi EJ (2009) Virologic survey of dogs with naturally acquired idiopathic conjunctivitis. *Journal of the American Veterinary Medicine Association* **235(8)**, 954–959

Low HC, Powell CC, Veir JK *et al.* (2007) Prevalence of feline herpesvirus 1, *Chlamydophila felis* and *Mycoplasma* spp. DNA in conjunctival cells collected from cats with and without conjunctivitis. *American Journal of Veterinary Research* **68(6)**, 643–648

Kaswan R and Martin C (1985) Surgical correction of third eyelid prolapse in dogs. *Journal of the American Veterinary Medical Association* **186**, 83

Maggs DJ (2008a) Conjunctiva. In: *Slatter's Fundamentals of Veterinary Ophthalmology*, 4th edn, ed. DJ Maggs *et al.*, pp. 135–150. Saunders, Missouri

Maggs DJ (2008b) Third eyelid. In: *Slatter's Fundamentals of Veterinary Ophthalmology*, 4th edn, ed. DJ Maggs *et al.*, pp. 151–156. Saunders, Missouri

Mazzucchelli S, Vaillant MD, Wéverberg F *et al.* (2012) Retrospective study of 155 cases of prolapse of the nictitating membrane gland in dogs. *Veterinary Record* **170(17)**, 443

Nasisse MP, Glover TL, Moore CP *et al.* (1998) Detection of feline herpesvirus 1 DNA in corneas of cats with eosinophilic keratitis or corneal sequestration. *American Journal of Veterinary Research* **59(7)**, 856–858

Nuyttens JJ and Simoens PJ (1995) Morphologic study of the musculature of the third eyelid in the cat (*Felis catus*). *Laboratory Animal Science* **45(5)**, 561–563

Peña MT and Leiva M (2008) Canine conjunctivitis and blepharitis. In: *Ophthalmic Immunology and Immune-mediated Disease. Veterinary Clinics of North America: Small Animal Practice*, ed. DL Williams, pp. 233–249. WB Saunders, Philadelphia

Petznick A, Evans MD, Madigan MC *et al.* (2012) A preliminary study of changes in tear film proteins in the feline eye following nictitating membrane removal. *Veterinary Ophthalmology* **15(3)**, 164–171

Pirie CG and Dubielzig RR (2006) Feline conjunctival hemangioma and hemangiosarcoma: a retrospective evaluation of eight cases (1993–2004). *Veterinary Ophthalmology* **9(4)**, 227–231

Pirie CG, Knollinger AM, Thomas CB *et al.* (2006) Canine conjunctival hemangioma and hemangiosarcoma: a retrospective evaluation of 108 cases (1989–2004). *Veterinary Ophthalmology* **9(4)**, 215–226

Plummer CE, Källberg ME, Gelatt KN *et al.* (2008) Intranictitans tacking for replacement of prolapsed gland of the third eyelid in dogs. *Veterinary Ophthalmology* **11(4)**, 228–233

Radi ZA, Miller DL and Hines ME (2004) B-cell conjunctival lymphoma in a cat. *Veterinary Ophthalmology* **7(6)**, 413–415

Ramsey DT (2000) Feline chlamydia and calicivirus infections. In: *Infectious Disease and the Eye. Veterinary Clinics of North America Small Animal Practice*, ed. J Stiles, pp. 1015–1028. WB Saunders, Philadelphia

Ramsey DT, Ketring KL, Glaze MB *et al.* (1996) Ligneous conjunctivitis in four Doberman Pinschers. *Journal of the American Animal Hospital Association* **32(5)**, 4339–4447

Read RA (1995) Treatment of canine nictitans plasmacytic conjunctivitis with 0.2% cyclosporin ointment. *Journal of Small Animal Practice* **36(2)**, 50–56

Read RA and Lucas J (2001) Lipogranulomatous conjunctivitis: clinical findings from 21 eyes in 13 cats. *Veterinary Ophthalmology* **4(2)**, 93–98

Saito A, Izumisawa Y, Yamashita K *et al.* (2001) The effect of third eyelid gland removal on the ocular surface of dogs. *Veterinary Ophthalmology* **4(10)**, 13–18

Saito A, Watanabe Y and Kotani T (2004) Morphological changes of the anterior corneal epithelium caused by third eyelid removal in dogs. *Veterinary Ophthalmology* **7(2)**, 113–119

Sansom J, Barnett KC, Blunden AS *et al.* (1996) Canine conjunctival papilloma: a review of five cases. *Journal of Small Animal Practice* **37(6)**, 84–86

Schlegel T, Brehm H and Amselgruber WM (2003) IgA and secretory component (SC) in the third eyelid of domestic animals: a comparative study. *Veterinary Ophthalmology* **6(2)**, 157–161

Schobert CS, Labelle P and Dubielzig RR (2010) Feline conjunctival melanoma: histopathological characteristics and clinical outcomes. *Veterinary Ophthalmology* **13(1)**, 43–46

Sibitz C, Rudnay EC, Wabnegger L *et al.* (2011) Detection of *Chlamydophila pneumoniae* in cats with conjunctivitis. *Veterinary Ophthalmology* **14**, 67–74

Siebeck N, Hurley DJ, Garcia M *et al.* (2006) Effects of human recombinant alpha-2b interferon and feline recombinant omega interferon on in vitro replication of feline herpesvirus-1. *American Journal of Veterinary Research* **67**, 1406–1411

Stanley RG and Kaswan RL (1994) Modification of the orbital rim anchorage method for surgical replacement of the gland of the third eyelid in dogs. *Journal of the American Veterinary Medicine Association* **205(10)**, 1412–1414

Stiles J (2000) Feline herpesvirus. In: *Infectious Disease and the Eye. Veterinary Clinics of North America: Small Animal Practice*, ed. J Stiles, pp. 1001–1014. WB Saunders, Philadelphia

Stiles J and Townsend WM (2007) Feline ophthalmology. In: *Veterinary Ophthalmology*, 4th edn, ed. KN Gelatt, pp. 1095–1164. Blackwell Publishing, Oxford

Thomasy SM, Whittem T, Bales JL *et al.* (2012). Pharmacokinetics of penciclovir in healthy cats following oral administration of famciclovir or intravenous infusion of penciclovir. *American Journal of Veterinary Research* **73**, 1092–1099

Torres MD, Leiva M, Tabar MD *et al.* (2009) Ligneous conjunctivitis in a plasminogen-deficient dog: clinical management and 2-year follow-up. *Veterinary Ophthalmology* **12(4)**, 248–253

Volopich S, Benetka V, Schwendenwein I *et al.* (2005) Cytologic findings, and feline herpesvirus DNA and *Chlamydophila felis* antigen detection rates in normal cats and cats with conjunctival and corneal lesions. *Veterinary Ophthalmology* **8(1)**, 25–32

von Bomhard W, Polkinghorne A, Lu ZH *et al.* (2003) Detection of novel chlamydiae in cats with ocular disease. *American Journal of Veterinary Research* **64(11)**, 1421–1428

Whitley RD (2000) Canine and feline primary ocular bacterial infections. In: *Infectious Disease and the Eye. Veterinary Clinics of North America: Small Animal Practice*, ed. J Stiles, pp. 1151–1167. WB Saunders, Philadelphia

12

The cornea

Rick F. Sanchez

Embryology, anatomy and physiology

The cornea is part of the external tunic of the eye and, peripherally, it is continuous with the sclera through a transition zone known as the corneoscleral limbus. The corneal surface is more curved than that of the sclera. Its outline is somewhat oval and elongated in the horizontal axis (Figure 12.1). Corneal thickness varies slightly with species, breed, age and sex, but it is approximately 0.6 mm centrally in dogs and 0.56 mm in cats and slightly thinner peripherally. Larger animals tend to have slightly thicker corneas than smaller animals, as do males compared with females.

Four layers make up the cornea (Figure 12.2); from superficial to deep they are:

* Epithelium
* Stroma
* Descemet's membrane
* Endothelium.

Each of the corneal layers has a unique set of physical and biochemical properties that affect the overall corneal function and its homeostasis, as well as its response to injury. The most relevant to understanding corneal pathology are detailed below.

Corneal epithelium

Surface ectoderm gives rise to the corneal epithelium, an embryological origin shared with eyelid and conjunctival epithelia (Cook, 2007). The corneal epithelium accounts for approximately one-ninth of the corneal thickness and consists of a single deep layer of columnar basal cells that produce the basement membrane, an intermediate layer of polyhedral or wing cells and an outer layer of squamous cells (Figure 12.3). Squamous cells, which arise from the deeper layers, are ultimately shed from the corneal surface and the entire turnaround time from basal cell to desquamation of the squamous cell takes approximately 7–10 days. The surfaces of the squamous cells contain microplicae and microvillae and secrete the glycocalyx, a complex layer of membrane-bound mucin that interacts with the mucins of the tear film and is secreted by the conjunctival goblet cells. This interaction ensures the adhesion of the tear film to the corneal epithelium and helps maintain the integrity of the tear film, which acts as

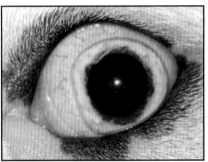

12.1 Normal cornea in a young English Bulldog. The corneal outline is somewhat oval in shape, squared off nasally and temporally.

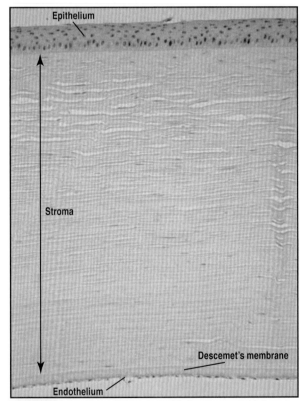

12.2 Histology of the normal feline cornea. Note the relative thickness of the corneal structures. The wide and largely acellular corneal stroma contains scattered quiescent keratocytes (corneal fibrocytes) between its regularly arranged collagen lamellae. It is bordered superficially by the non-keratinizing, stratified squamous corneal surface epithelium (top layer) and at the deep or inner aspect by Descemet's membrane and the corneal endothelium (bottom layers). (©Karen Dunn, FOCUS-EyePathLab)

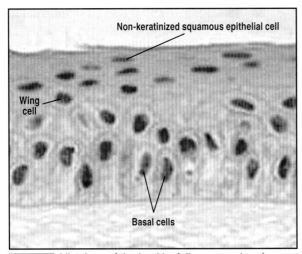

Non-keratinized squamous epithelial cell

Wing cell

Basal cells

12.3 Histology of the healthy feline corneal surface epithelium. Note the normal maturation process, from the larger generative basal epithelial cells at the deep margin of the epithelium, to the smaller 'wing' cells in the intermediate zone, and the superficial squamous cells near the surface. The basal epithelial cells are oriented perpendicular to the underlying basement membrane zone and the deeper, regularly arranged corneal stromal lamellae. (©Karen Dunn, FOCUS-EyePathLab)

a physical barrier against microorganisms and lubricates the corneal surface (see Chapter 10).

The corneal epithelium provides a natural barrier to tears and external contaminants. Healthy epithelium is firmly adherent to the underlying stroma through the basal lamina of the basement membrane by means of fibronectin, anchoring fibrils and hemidesmosomes. Stem cells of the corneal limbus serve as a cellular reservoir for the corneal epithelial basal cells and play a pivotal role in epithelial healing (Secker and Daniels, 2009). Thus, movement of corneal epithelial cells occurs in two directions, one that drives the cells anteriorly towards the corneal surface and another that is centripetal and moves cells from the corneal periphery to its centre. The limbal cornea also contains a variable number of melanocytes. The centripetal migration of corneal cells during corneal healing is also responsible for the undesirable migration of pigment from a peripheral to a more central location over time in some patients.

Corneal stroma

The corneal stroma arises from the mesenchymal neural crest cells, which share an embryological origin with the corneal endothelium, anterior chamber, anterior iris stroma, ciliary muscle and most of the iridocorneal angle (Cook, 2007). The stroma makes up the bulk of the cornea. It is arranged in parallel sheets or lamellae that comprise collagen fibrils and extracellular matrix. There is elastin as well as five different types of collagen, predominantly collagen type I, within the corneal stroma. The extracellular matrix contains several glycosaminoglycans, with two of the most important being keratan and dermatan sulphate. Alteration in the delicately balanced ratio of collagen and glycosaminoglycan types affects corneal transparency because it has a direct effect on factors that alter light transmission (e.g.

collagen fibril arrangement and the water-absorptive capabilities of the stroma). Stromal over-hydration results in corneal oedema, which is associated with an increase in corneal thickness and loss of transparency. In addition, the stroma also contains a sparse population of special fibrocytes, known as keratocytes, which produce and maintain the stromal extracellular matrix.

Descemet's membrane

Descemet's membrane is the hyaline basement membrane of the endothelium. It is produced over the lifetime of an animal and therefore its thickness increases with age. Although clinically Descemet's membrane has elastic properties, it actually comprises collagen fibrils. In cases of chronic glaucoma or buphthalmos, linear breaks in Descemet's membrane may develop and are clinically visible as Haab's striae (Figure 12.4).

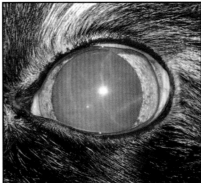

12.4 Haab's striae in a cat with glaucoma.

Corneal endothelium

The corneal endothelium shares its embryological origin with the corneal stroma and several of the structures found in the anterior chamber. It is a monolayer of hexagonal cells with an approximate density of 3000 cells/mm² which have very limited to no regenerative capabilities in adult animals. Due to the inability of the endothelium to replace cells once they have died, endothelial cell density tends to reduce over the lifetime of an animal.

Compared with the external epithelial barrier, the endothelium plays an even more important role in preventing the cornea from becoming oedematous. Hydrostatic forces within the eye push aqueous humour from the anterior chamber into the cornea. The endothelium actively removes this fluid via the action of sodium (Na^+)/potassium (K^+) adenosine triphosphatase (ATPase) pumps contained in the lateral membranes of adjoining cells. These pump Na^+ and chloride (Cl^-) back into the aqueous humour, and water passively follows the ions. In addition, tight junctions between the cells allow the endothelium to act as a barrier between the aqueous humour and the rest of the cornea.

Endothelial cell density reduces over the lifetime of an individual. The loss of endothelial cells is compensated for by the addition of further pumps and the stretching and enlarging of the remaining cells. However, this is not a sustainable process and, if a point is reached at which the collective pump mechanism returns less fluid to the anterior chamber than hydrostatic forces push into the stroma, corneal oedema develops in a process called endothelial cell decompensation. This is thought to occur when endothelial cell density has decreased to approximately <500–800 cells/mm^2 and it may develop to some degree with age, with primary endothelial disease or secondary to intraocular diseases such as anterior uveitis, lens luxation or glaucoma.

Maintaining transparency

Corneal transparency is achieved and maintained by a combination of anatomical and physiological adaptations, including its relative acellularity, a non-keratinized surface epithelium, non-myelinated corneal nerves and a lack of pigment, lymphatic vessels and blood vessels. In addition, the parallel arrangement, precise fibrillar spacing and limited cross-linking of the collagen fibrils that make up the bulk of the corneal stroma permits the almost uninterrupted passage of light through it. In addition, corneal transparency relies critically on the relatively dehydrated state of the stroma (termed corneal deturgescence), the mechanism of which is discussed above.

Corneal refraction

The cornea and tear film account for almost three-quarters of the refractive power of the canine and feline eye. Refraction refers to the amount of bending a beam of light is subjected to, which serves to focus this light as an image on the retina. Refraction is dependent on both the curvature and the change in refractive index of the media the beam of light travels through. The refraction that occurs when light passes from a gaseous medium (such as air) into the tear film and cornea is much greater than that which occurs subsequently when the light travels from the cornea to the aqueous humour to the lens to the vitreous humour. In fact, when taking into account the curvature of the cornea, the sum of the positive refraction of the anterior cornea and tear film and the negative refraction of the posterior cornea, this results in a total refraction of approximately +43 dioptres (D), making the tear film and corneal interface the most refractive site in the eye. Thus, any disease process that results in the loss of corneal transparency through the disruption of any of the special qualities of the cornea, or that affects corneal curvature or any of its refractive properties, will adversely affect vision.

Corneal innervation

The cornea is richly innervated by sensory nerve trunks from the ophthalmic branch of the trigeminal nerve. There are approximately 10 corneal nerve trunks in the dog and 13 in the cat, making the feline cornea more sensitive. However, this is in part dependent on skull shape because brachycephalic dogs and cats have fewer corneal nerve trunks and, thus, lower corneal sensitivity than mesaticephalic and dolichocephalic breeds. The epithelium is particularly richly innervated, with pronounced arborizations at the level of the basal epithelial layer, as well as a prominent anterior stromal network that

becomes less prominent or absent as it reaches the deepest layers of the cornea. This distribution partly explains the clinical observation that some deep ulcers appear to be less painful than more superficial ones.

Corneal sensation is vital to corneal health. Tear production and blink rates are lower in animals with reduced corneal sensation, and corneal dryness develops rapidly in these cases. The corneal surface adopts a pitted appearance and this can progress to epithelial desquamation and even full thickness corneal epithelial loss if dryness persists. In addition, sensory innervation of the cornea plays an important role in corneal epithelial homeostasis and corneal epithelial healing, with the latter being slower in corneas with sensory deficits. However, corneal pain can lead to changes that worsen the ocular pathology; for example, by leading to spastic entropion or reflex uveitis. The latter develops when corneal nerves release pro-inflammatory mediators that cause iridal and ciliary body spasm and disrupt the blood–ocular barrier.

Immunology of the cornea

The corneal surface is an immunologically privileged site, which means that it enjoys a state of relative immune quiescence despite constant exposure to antigenic stimuli. This is of vital importance to corneal health and vision, because immune reactions can lead to the loss of corneal integrity and transparency. In order to achieve quiescence, the cornea makes use of a unique set of innate and adaptive immune systems. The intricate aspects of corneal immunology that allow these two systems to interact with the environment and each other, yet remain as non-reactive as possible for most of the life of the cornea, have been reviewed elsewhere (Gilger, 2008). Corneal immunology is too complex a subject to be comprehensively covered in this chapter, but it may be summarized as the following points.

- The collective action of the eyelids, third eyelid, tears and corneal epithelium comprises the first barrier of the ocular surface. The blink response, the constant renewal of tears and the effects of mucus, lysozyme and lactoferrin, as well as numerous other substances contained within the tear film, maintain a low microorganism and environmental allergen load with relative ease. This first barrier effect makes up the cornea's innate immunity, which is fairly effective despite not being antigen specific.
- The adaptive system, on the other hand, is antigen specific and is mediated by the associated lymphoid tissue of the eye. This comprises lymphocytes located within the conjunctival follicles and a diffuse population of lymphocytes and plasma cells found in the conjunctiva and lacrimal glands. These cells are responsible for the production of immunoglobulins and modulating substances that influence the behaviour of other cells. This process requires antigen-presenting cells, such as macrophages and Langerhan's cells, and the cornea has a

naturally low number of these cells residing in it, which helps to minimize its reactivity. If more of these cells are required the cornea can recruit them via the tear film and conjunctiva.

In addition, toll-like receptors (TLRs) play an important role in the adaptive immune response. There are several types of TLR and each helps recognize a set of specific microorganism-related antigens. Antigen recognition then leads to an immune response directed against the specific pathogen. The strategic absence of TLRs from the corneal surface and their internalization within the epithelial layers boosts the cornea's privileged immune status by creating a relative state of 'immune ignorance' on its surface, where the microorganisms reside. However, once an immune response has been mounted against a microorganism, the immune tolerant state of the cornea is lost and antigen-presenting cells induce an adaptive immune response. This leads to corneal changes that involve events such as the attraction of inflammatory cells, liberation of collagenolytic agents, corneal vascularization and loss of corneal transparency.

Adaptive immunity is further complicated by the cross-reactivity of pathogen-related antigens with potential corneal targets that might act as autoantigens, a situation that can give rise to prolonged autoimmune disease.

Corneal homeostasis

As discussed above, the cornea depends on a number of anatomical and physiological factors that are protective and help maintain homeostasis. The periocular environment and general health of the patient are additional factors that should also be considered when creating a list of differential diagnoses for corneal disease. Figure 12.5 offers an overview of how each individual factor might affect corneal health. Further information on ophthalmic manifestations of systemic disease can be found in Chapter 20.

Ocular and non-ocular factors	Protective effects	Results of factor alteration
Tear film	• Lubrication • Nutrients • Immunity • Cleansing action on corneal surface	• Desiccation and decreased tear film break up time (TFBUT) • Impaired immunity • Accumulation of mucus and other surface debris • Overall conjunctival and corneal irritation ± pigmentation and vascularization • Ulcerative disease of the cornea
Eyelids (including blink as well as structural integrity)	• Mechanical protection • Contribution of lipid layer to tear film • Spreading of tear film • Cleansing action on corneal surface	• Lack of protection leading to trauma • Desiccation by evaporation and more rapid TFBUT, which is worsened by ectropion • Accumulation of mucus and other surface debris • Overall conjunctival and corneal irritation ± pigmentation and vascularization • Persistent trauma in cases of entropion • Ulcerative disease of the cornea
Third eyelid (including tear gland)	• Mechanical protection • Contribution to the aqueous portion of the tear film	• Lack of protection leading to trauma • Desiccation and decreased TFBUT • Reduced tear production • Overall conjunctival and corneal irritation
Epithelium	• Stromal protection: mechanical protection against environment and microorganisms and against overhydration from the tear film • Contribution of glycocalyx to the tear film • Role in immunity	• Exposed corneal stroma, development of oedema and increased sensation of pain • Collagenolysis due to imbalanced stromal repair process
Endothelium and the intraocular environment	• Stromal protection against overhydration • Homeostasis of endothelial cells	• Corneal oedema from endothelial cell failure: – Diffuse: increased intraocular pressure (IOP), uveitis or primary degeneration – Localized: associated with anterior synechiae, persistent pupillary membrane, anterior lens luxation and localized trauma • Subepithelial bulla formation • Loss of vision
Afferent sensory innervation	• Assist the blink and lacrimal tear response • Assist the healing process	• Decreased blinking and/or tearing • Delayed healing response
Periocular environment [a]		• Trichiasis or periocular skin disease causing generalized conjunctival and corneal irritation ± corneal pigmentation and vascularization
General health [a]		• Effects of diabetes mellitus on the tear film and corneal sensitvity • Effects of hypothyroidism on subepithelial corneal lipid deposition and peripheral nerve function • Effects of certain storage diseases on the corneal stroma • Effects of systemic diseases that may lead to uveitis ± secondary glaucoma

12.5 Ocular and non-ocular factors that should be considered when creating a list of differential diagnoses for corneal disease. [a] Non-ocular factors do not necessarily have a direct protective role.

The regeneration of ocular tissues is limited and is age and tissue dependent. Generally, the deeper the corneal layer, the less capacity for regeneration it shows. The greatest regenerative capabilities are seen in the epithelium; the stroma has intermediate regenerative capabilities and the endothelium has limited or no regenerative capabilities (these are reported to be good in young puppies, but are effectively absent in adult dogs).

The following are important aspects of the cornea's response to injury:

- Corneal epithelial healing
- Stromal healing
- Descemetocele development
- Corneal vascularization
- Corneal pigmentation
- Subepithelial bulla formation.

Corneal epithelial healing

Rapid corneal epithelial healing limits exposure of the stroma, stromal overhydration, activation of stromal keratocytes and the release of chemotaxins that attract inflammatory cells; events that are associated with corneal pain, loss of corneal transparency and may lead to further stromal damage. Corneal epithelial defects heal in three phases:

- First phase – epithelial cell elongation followed by migration
- Second phase – marked cell proliferation
- Third phase – cellular differentiation.

Epithelial cells use fibronectin as scaffolding on which they can attach, migrate and grow over the previously denuded stroma. Once a continuous layer of cells has been established and the wound is closed, cellular proliferation and differentiation thicken the epithelial layer and give rise to the cellular subtypes that normally make up the corneal epithelium.

Certain cells in the epithelium play a pivotal role during the healing process. Basal cells located at the limbus are the main progenitor cells (stem cells) of the epithelium. Transient amplifying epithelial cells are located elsewhere in the basal cell layer. They depend on the stem cells and are responsible for the bulk of cell proliferation seen during the healing process. If limbal stem cell depletion occurs as a result of chemical injury or disease, 'conjunctivalization' of the cornea and loss of corneal transparency is likely to ensue.

Healing of the epithelium under normal circumstances occurs rather quickly, with superficial linear scratches expected to heal within 24–48 hours and more extensive superficial ulcers taking from a few days to just over a week. It is worth noting that the anchoring fibrils and hemidesmosomal attachments of the epithelium to the basal lamina of the basement membrane will take longer to form, even after the epithelium has grown over the defect. This process takes even longer (weeks to months) in cases where the basal lamina has been damaged by disease or is missing. Until permanent attachments develop, the epithelium can be easily denuded.

There are many factors that regulate and control epithelial cell migration in mammalian species, including epidermal growth factor, transforming factor growth-β, keratinocyte growth factor and substance P (Haber *et al.*, 2003; Yamada *et al.*, 2005). These factors act to enhance or inhibit epithelial growth and are produced by the tear glands, keratocytes and corneal nerves. Neurosensory deficits of the human cornea are associated with delayed corneal healing and the development or persistence of ulcerative disease, and similar deficits are also likely to play an important negative role in the healing response in animals.

Stromal healing

In general, stromal healing takes longer than epithelial healing and, depending on the severity of the insult, it can lead to various degrees of scar formation. In the early stages of stromal healing, keratocytes closest to the wound undergo apoptosis whereas those around it become activated fibroblasts and lay down glycosaminoglycans and collagen to fill in the corneal defect. The glycosaminoglycan and collagen ratios of the freshly laid matrix are different from the ratios found in the healthy, transparent cornea. This is associated with visible scarring, which is generally worse for deeper defects and in corneas that have recovered from severe disease. However, the cornea has the ability to transform these ratios over time through remodelling of the matrix components. A surprising amount of clarity may be restored in some cases.

It is worth noting that other cells, such as neutrophils, play an active role in stromal repair. Neutrophils are recruited via the tear film, conjunctiva or newly developed corneal blood vessels early in the repair process and produce collagenolytic enzymes such as serine proteases and matrix metalloproteases (MMPs). These proteases join the MMPs produced by keratocytes and epithelial cells to break down small areas of the stromal wound in preparation for reconstruction. It is important that stromal destruction and reconstruction are balanced, as excessive destruction will lead to corneal breakdown in a process known as collagenolysis ('corneal melting'; Figure 12.6).

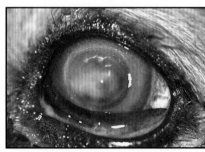

12.6
Large, deep central ulcer with melting stroma.

Descemetocele development

Descemet's membrane is exposed when an ulcerative process erodes through all the overlying corneal epithelium and stroma. This is known as a descemetocele. Descemetoceles may lie flat, deep within the bed of the ulcer, or may bulge anteriorly, but they do not take up fluorescein. They may have the appearance of a deep ulcer surrounded by a 'wall' of oedematous cornea, which is usually fluorescein-positive. The ulcer bed appears to be darker than the oedematous stroma around it (Figure 12.7). This is the descemetocele, which may be extensive enough to allow visualization of the anterior chamber, pupil and iris (Figure 12.8). Descemetoceles should be considered a surgical emergency, with referral strongly advised, because they can easily rupture, leading to corneal perforation.

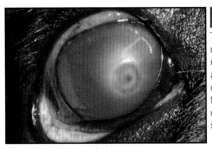

12.7 The small central descemetocele appears dark compared with the surrounding oedematous stroma.

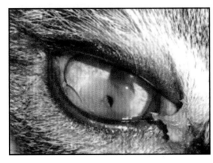

12.8 The transparent descemetocele in this cat's eye, which is at risk of imminent perforation, allows visualization of the intraocular structures.

Corneal vascularization

The healthy cornea of companion animals is naturally avascular (see above). Vascularization originates from the limbus and is a consistent part of the healing response that accompanies a pathological process. It is triggered by inflammatory cytokines and other vasogenic factors released by keratocytes and infiltrating white blood cells. Blood vessels generally arise from the section of limbus closest to the disease process. The early budding of vessels may take up to 4 days. After this, vessels typically grow no more than 1 mm every 2 days in the direction of the corneal lesion, although this can be quite variable.

Vascularization may be superficial or deep. Superficial vascularization is associated with surface ocular disease and appears as an extension of blood vessels from the conjunctiva, with the same dichotomous branching. Deep vascularization is associated with deep stromal and intraocular disease and extends from the limbus in a straight, non-branching pattern. Vessels can coalesce and adopt the appearance of a cluster of bristles, which is sometimes referred to as a 'brush border' pattern. They can also develop into a bed of granulation tissue. Occasionally, vascularization is associated with intracorneal haemorrhage (Figure 12.9). This may result from a variety of corneal conditions and is more frequently observed in older dogs (Matas and Donaldson, 2011).

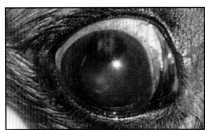

12.9 Intracorneal haemorrhage visible in the superior cornea associated with vascularization.

Vascularization aids the healing process by bringing naturally occurring anti-collagenolytic agents effective against MMPs and serine proteases, oxygen and nutrients to the injured site. However, ulcerative disease and stromal melting can progress much more rapidly than a vascular response, so this response cannot be relied upon to prevent progressive collagenolysis or corneal perforation.

Vascularization can intensify corneal oedema associated with the loss of the epithelial barrier in corneal ulcerative disease, as developing blood vessels leak small amounts of fluid into the stroma. An overhydrated, oedematous cornea is not only opaque but also thicker and softer, and therefore weaker. Once the cornea has healed, the vascular response becomes less obvious as the blood vessels are no longer perfused and form 'ghost' blood vessels. Re-establishment of the epithelial barrier and attenuation of the new blood vessels allow the corneal endothelium to remove excess fluid from the stroma and the cornea to regain its normal thickness and clarity (Figure 12.10). Stromal loss or endothelial damage will naturally affect this process.

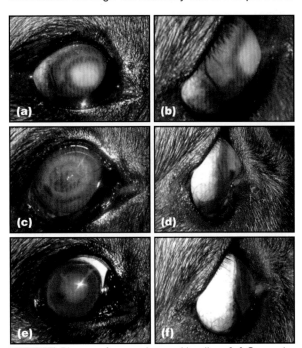

12.10 Phases of corneal wound healing. **(a)** Corneal ulcer highlighted by fluorescein and surrounded by a diffuse stromal infiltrate of inflammatory cells, a ring of vascularization and secondary oedema. **(b)** When viewed from the side, the cornea is obviously thickened and has an exaggerated curvature. **(c–f)** As it heals, transparency and more normal corneal thickness are slowly restored, whilst some scarring with pigment deposition and residual vascularization remain.

Corneal pigmentation

Melanin deposits affect the epithelium and anterior stroma and arise from the limbus and conjunctiva. Surface ocular irritation commonly leads to superficial pigment proliferation and deposition, which is progressive in cases where the source of irritation is not identified and removed (see Pigmentary keratitis). Endothelial pigment deposits are less commonly seen, but may be associated with intraocular diseases, such as rupture of anterior uveal cysts, anterior synechiae and extension of anterior uveal or limbal melanocytomas, and diseases that lead to anterior uveal pigment accumulation or dispersion.

Subepithelial bulla formation

The accumulation of subepithelial and intraepithelial fluid secondary to corneal oedema may lead to the formation of bullae, which can be transient or may rupture into a small ulcer (Figure 12.11). These ulcers tend to heal quickly, but will reform if the oedema persists. If the corneal oedema is successfully treated then the bullae will resolve.

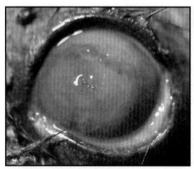

12.11

Subepithelial bullae secondary to marked stromal oedema caused by the ulcerative process. One large bulla is seen in the superior cornea and a cluster of smaller bullae are visible centrally.

Investigation of disease

The interactions between the cornea and the eyelids, third eyelid, preocular tear film, aqueous humour, iris, lens and intraocular pressure (IOP) are all important determinants of corneal health and disease. Thus, a thorough examination of the anterior structures of the eye, adnexa and preocular tear film is vital to understanding the pathogenesis of corneal disease (as described in Chapters 1, 9, 10 and 11).

Equipment

Basic diagnostic equipment for examination of the eyelid, cornea and intraocular structures includes Schirmer tear test (STT) strips, fluorescein dye and a source of bright light (Figure 12.12). The clinician should also have a cobalt blue filtered light for examination of corneal surfaces that have been stained with fluorescein. A detailed examination should be performed in a darkened room. The hand-held slit-lamp is considered the gold standard for corneal examination in veterinary ophthalmology (see Chapter 1). Hand-held ophthalmoscopes do not provide such an exquisitely sharp and detailed image, but are less costly and easier to use. They have a bright light, a set of lenses that allow for examination of the fundus and other intraocular structures and many have a blue filter for use with fluorescein and a

• Source of bright light (with blue filter and magnification if possible)
• Schirmer tear test-1 (STT-1) strips
• Fluorescein stain
• Proxymetacaine 1%
• Tonometers
• Cytology brush and cytology stains
• Von Graeffe forceps (for eyelid and third eyelid manipulation)

12.12 Equipment required for examination of the cornea.

relatively wide slit beam for assessment of corneal contour. Magnifying loupes may also be used to obtain a magnified view of the cornea.

Examination

A complete eye examination protocol is detailed in Chapter 1. Points of particular relevance to corneal disease are listed below:

1. Initially perform a 'hands-off' examination to assess for signs of asymmetry, eyelid or adnexal conformational defects, ocular pain and ocular discharge.
2. Assess blink rate and palpebral blink reflex.
3. Perform an STT-1 prior to the application of any eye drops, excessive eyelid manipulation or the use of a bright light.
4. Inspect the outer and inner aspects of the eyelids to assess for the presence of hair and cilia abnormalities, eyelid margin defects and disease, meibomian gland disease or foreign bodies, using a bright light source and magnification (ideally a slit-lamp).
5. Examine the bulbar conjunctiva, conjunctival fornices and outer aspects of the third eyelid.
6. Perform a thorough examination of the cornea and all its layers using magnification (ideally a slit-lamp).
7. Perform an intraocular examination to check for intraocular disease.
8. Apply fluorescein stain and examine using a cobalt blue light (NB prior use of STT strips or a contact tonometer (e.g. Schiøtz or Tono-pen) commonly causes a faint retention of stain at the point of corneal contact; this should not be confused with corneal ulceration).
9. Perform tonometry if available.
10. If indicated, apply topical anaesthetic and examine the inner aspect of the third eyelid (with the aid of a cotton bud or von Graeffe forceps).
11. If indicated, take swabs for cytology, microbial culture or polymerase chain reaction (PCR) testing (see Chapter 3).

Corneal pain

Signs of corneal pain may be clinically indistinguishable from those of intraocular pain. Application of a topical anaesthetic results in a transient resolution of signs associated with corneal pain, except in those patients with very severe blepharospasm and photophobia. However, repeated applications of topical anaesthetic should **not** be used for the management of surface ocular pain. Persistent blepharospasm is associated with prolonged, marked orbicularis oculi muscle stimulation, which can be difficult to manage. Photophobia is a result of reflex uveitis with secondary iris and ciliary body spasm, all of which are triggered by painful corneal diseases and may be relieved with the use of a mydriatic–cycloplegic preparation such as atropine drops (see Chapter 5).

Lesion recognition

The cornea can suffer from developmental and acquired problems and the latter may include conformational, immune-mediated, traumatic, toxic, infectious, degenerative, neurological and neoplastic processes, all of which should be kept in mind when formulating a list of differential diagnoses. In order to select the appropriate differential diagnoses, the clinician must be familiar with a variety of corneal pathological processes that are common in small animals, as well as the different disease patterns associated with corneal conditions, including lesion progression over time. Some elements of lesion recognition can be simplified by grouping certain problems according to their colour (Figure 12.13).

Canine conditions

Developmental abnormalities

Corneal size and absence

Microcornea is uncommon in dogs and may be seen in an otherwise healthy eye or may be accompanied by other developmental anomalies such as microphthalmos, persistent pupillary membrane, cataract, or

Causes	Comments
White	
Scar	May also contain blood vessels and pigment
Lipid	Covers a range of conditions, including corneal stromal dystrophy, lipid keratopathy and arcus lipoides corneae
Corneal melting	May be yellow depending on the stromal cellular infiltrate
Cellular infiltrate	May be seen with stromal abscess, corneal melting and corneal inflammatory conditions
Eosinophilic keratitis	White deposits on epithelial surface of cornea, often raised (may appear pink due to vascularization)
Corneal oedema	Often appears blue (see below)
Keratic precipitates (KPs) or hypopyon	Sequel to anterior uveitis. KPs located on endothelial (inner) surface of cornea; hypopyon located within anterior chamber. KPs may also be dark; hypopyon may be yellow
Haab's striae	Linear breaks in the Descemet's membrane due to glaucoma
Calcium	Causes include local corneal degeneration, systemic calcium abnormalities and surface deposits secondary to parotid duct transposition surgery
Epithelial inclusion cyst	Rare; presumed due to previous corneal trauma
Lysosomal storage disease	Rare; bilateral corneal clouding associated with systemic signs in young animals; cats more commonly affected
Yellow	
Corneal melting	May be white depending on stromal cellular infiltrate
Cellular infiltrate	May be seen with stromal abscess, corneal melting or stromal inflammatory conditions
Fluorescein	Residue from recent use. May also stain mucus and aqueous humour in the anterior chamber by diffusion through the stroma if not washed off the surface of the eye in cases with an ulcerative lesion
Red/pink	
Vascularization	May be superficial (branching) or deep (brush border effect)
Conjunctivalization	Associated with symblepharon; secondary to severe superficial inflammation (e.g. feline herpesvirus-1 keratitis in kittens, acid or alkali burns)
Extravasated blood	Intracorneal haemorrhage (rare) or hyphaema (intraocular)
Cellular infiltrate	Chronic superficial keratitis/pannus (lymphocytic–plasmacytic infiltrate), eosinophilic keratitis, other corneal inflammatory conditions or neoplastic processes (rare)
Blue	
Corneal oedema	Light blue but to some observers it may appear to be a white haze. Causes include corneal ulceration, anterior uveitis, glaucoma, lens luxation and endothelial disease. Anterior stromal oedema suggests an epithelial lesion (i.e. corneal ulceration). Posterior stromal oedema suggests a localized endothelial lesion or generalized endothelial decompensation. May be vascular in origin: fluid escape from immature blood vessels associated with corneal vascularization
Black	
Pigment	Causes include pigmentary keratitis, corneal scarring, melanoma (especially limbal melanoma) or associated with KPs
Feline corneal sequestrum	Colour ranges from light tan/amber to brown/black when advanced

12.13 A colour guide to lesions of the cornea.

more severe problems such as anterior segment dysgenesis, in which a differentiated cornea may be absent. Congenital or developmental macrocornea is a rare condition and an increase in corneal diameter is more often associated with globe enlargement secondary to glaucoma.

Corneal opacities

Transient corneal oedema may be seen in puppies, particularly those in which the eyelids open prematurely, because maturation of endothelial function does not occur until several days postnatally. Subepithelial corneal opacities within the interpalpebral fissure have been termed infantile corneal dystrophy and are also transient. Permanent, congenital, localized corneal opacification may be observed in patients where persistent pupillary membrane strands contact the posterior surface of the cornea (Figure 12.14). It should be noted that some non-congenital conditions, such as symblepharon in cats or pigmentary keratitis in brachycephalic dogs, may lead to corneal opacification in young animals and should not be confused with congenital problems.

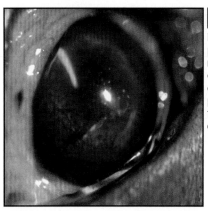

12.14

Persistent pupillary membrane in contact with the cornea, causing permanent, focal, corneal opacities.

Dermoid

This is a choristoma or normally differentiated tissue in an abnormal location. In this case, a patch of skin with a variable number of hair follicles is typically located over the temporal bulbar conjunctiva, limbus and cornea. The hairs that arise from these lesions may wick tears away from the ocular surface and can cause direct irritation of the cornea and conjunctiva, leading to epiphora. In some cases, dermoids are also associated with malformation or absence of the lateral canthus.

Embryologically, dermoids originate from surface ectoderm, as does the corneal epithelium. However, it is not fully understood why the cells at this particular site do not differentiate into corneal and conjunctival epithelia as they should. The area of corneal and conjunctival surface occupied by a dermoid varies: very small dermoids may not affect the limbus and paralimbal cornea, whereas large dermoids can extend a variable distance into the paraxial cornea (Figure 12.15). Dermoids are also variable in depth, from being superficially located in the conjunctiva and limbus to being located as deep as the anterior to mid-corneal stroma.

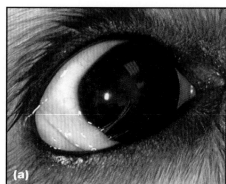

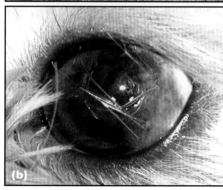

12.15

(a) A small conjunctival dermoid. **(b)** Dermoid affecting the bulbar conjunctiva, limbus and cornea.

Treatment: Lamellar keratectomy with conjunctivectomy is the treatment of choice. The entire lesion must be excised, including the thin, white halo that is often present within the cornea at the margins of the lesion. It is important that the incision reaches the appropriate depth in order to remove the entire lesion and all the hair follicles associated with it. Following keratectomy, depending on its depth, the resulting defect may be closed with an advancement conjunctival graft. Keratectomy and grafting require specialized instrumentation and training in corneal microsurgery and referral is strongly advised. There is a risk of inadvertent corneal perforation during the procedure and postoperative conjunctivilization or recurrence of hair growth at the keratectomy site.

Acquired abnormalities

The term keratitis covers a variety of inflammatory conditions of the cornea. These are among the most common ocular problems that affect companion animals. Keratitis may be further divided into ulcerative and non-ulcerative forms.

Ulcerative keratitis

Corneal ulcerative disease has the potential to pose a significant threat to vision and requires immediate attention. There is a wide range of causes of corneal ulceration (Figure 12.16); therefore, a thorough history and detailed ophthalmic examination are necessary to determine the aetiology, as this is not always immediately obvious and can be a source of frustration to the clinician and owner. It should be remembered that ulcers always have a cause, whether it is an acute, traumatic, single event or a more complex chronic or persistent one.

Superficial epithelial defects of traumatic origin should heal within hours to a few days in the absence of other complicating factors. **Persistent**

Primary corneal disease
• Spontaneous chronic corneal epithelial defect • Corneal degeneration • Punctate keratitis
Trauma (penetrating or non-penetrating and irritants)
• Abrasions, lacerations • Foreign body (corneal, conjunctival, posterior third eyelid) • Heat, smoke, acid or alkali burns
Tear film defects
• Keratoconjunctivitis sicca • Qualitative tear film disease
Eyelid or periorbital disease
• Entropion or trichiasis (e.g. nasal folds) • Ectropion (exposure keratitis) • Ectopic cilium • Distichiasis • Blepharitis • Eyelid margin masses • Loss or distortion of eyelid margin (e.g. traumatic laceration, iatrogenic) • Lagophthalmos due to shallow orbit/incomplete blink in predisposed breeds (e.g. Pug, Pekingese)
Infection
• Bacterial or fungal keratitis (e.g. *Pseudomonas*; NB probably requires corneal traumatic injury to allow bacterial or fungal colonization) • Canine herpesvirus-1
Neurological disease
• Reduced corneal sensation (neurotrophic keratopathy) • Eyelid akinesis (facial nerve paralysis/neuroparalytic keratitis)

12.16 Causes of canine ulcerative keratitis.

superficial ulcers or ulcers that become deeper and/or wider should immediately raise concern. Simply increasing the frequency of topical medication or switching topical antibiotics is rarely the answer in such cases; more commonly, either an underlying cause has been missed or secondary complications have arisen. In these instances a repeat, detailed ophthalmic examination should be performed and specialist advice sought if necessary.

Generic treatment of corneal ulceration is detailed below. Following this, the diagnosis and management of some of the more common types of canine ulcerative keratitis are discussed. These include corneal ulcers due to:

- Eyelid and adnexal disease
- Tear film disorders (primarily keratoconjunctivitis sicca; KCS)
- Spontaneous chronic corneal epithelial defects (SCCEDs; superficial, non-healing, under-run 'indolent' corneal ulcers)
- Acute stromal collagenolysis ('melting' corneal ulcers)
- Corneal trauma (blunt, non-penetrating and penetrating sharp trauma)
- Corneal foreign bodies
- Chemical or thermal burns
- Corneal degeneration
- Neurological disease.

In addition, less common corneal diseases associated with corneal ulceration in dogs such as punctate keratitis, corneal sequestrum, infectious keratitis and symblepharon are briefly reviewed later.

Generic treatment: Treatment of corneal ulcers is based on identifying and treating the cause, supporting the healing process and increasing patient comfort. This may involve medical treatment alone or a combination of surgical and medical treatment. Taking appropriate measures to ensure that the patient does not cause further harm by preventing self-trauma is also very important.

Medical treatment: Uncomplicated, superficial ulcers that are not subject to persistent corneal irritation or trauma should heal quickly and require only supportive medical therapy consisting of prophylactic topical antibiotics and pain relief.

- A broad-spectrum topical antibiotic is indicated in order to prevent secondary infection (see Chapter 7):
  - Chloramphenicol antibiotic drops are a good first choice because the drug is broad-spectrum and displays minimal toxicity towards corneal epithelial cells
  - Fusidic acid is also a reasonable first choice, although it has limited efficacy against Gram-negative organisms
  - Gentamicin drops may be used, although they have been associated with delayed epithelial wound healing (Alfonso *et al.*, 1988)
  - Fluoroquinolones such as ciprofloxacin or ofloxacin drops may be associated with delayed epithelial and stromal wound healing (Mallari *et al.*, 2001) and their reduced efficacy against some streptococci makes them perhaps more suitable as a second-line treatment for infected or collagenolytic corneal ulcers
  - Fortified corneal antibiotics may be compounded for topical use. However, they might also have a negative impact on corneal wound healing and should only be chosen if strictly necessary (Lin and Boehnke, 2000).
- Control of ocular pain is challenging. Ulcerative disease of the cornea is associated with anterior uveal spasm and stimulation of sensory corneal nerves, both of which cause pain. Oral non-steroidal anti-inflammatory drugs (NSAIDs) and mydriatic–cycloplegic drugs are the mainstays of topical medical management of ocular pain:
  - Oral NSAIDs are suitable analgesics in cases of ulcerative keratitis. There is no evidence that they significantly delay corneal epithelialization
  - Topical atropine (0.5–1%) is a mydriatic–cycloplegic drug and as such it reduces ciliary body and iridal spasm:
    - Atropine should be used to effect, aiming to maintain a mid-to-dilated pupil size. Generally, topical atropine should be used no more than four times daily and with

caution in very small patients due to the potential for systemic absorption and serious adverse effects. Patients with significant intraocular inflammation may require more frequent application

- Although it may be necessary to control painful reflex uveitis, atropine should be used with caution in patients with KCS as it temporarily reduces tear production.
  - Oral opioids may be indicated; topical opioids seem to be relatively ineffective as analgesics for corneal pain in dogs (Clark *et al.*, 2011) (see also Chapter 5)
  - **Topical anaesthetics can be used as diagnostic aids, but should never be used for treatment.** They are not only epitheliotoxic but may also cause neurotrophic keratopathy (pathological corneal desensitization) (Heigle and Pflugfelder, 1996)
  - The use of preservative-free tear gels can help reduce corneal pain
  - The use of a contact bandage lens or third eyelid flap, when appropriate, may improve patient comfort
  - If indicated, an Elizabethan collar to prevent self-trauma may be required.
- **Debridement and/or grid keratotomy are NOT indicated for the generic treatment of corneal ulcers and should be reserved *only* for the treatment of superficial, non-healing, under-run 'indolent' ulcers (SCCEDs; see below). The use of these techniques in the routine treatment of corneal ulceration is a common mistake in general practice. When used inappropriately (especially in deep or infected ulcers) they can lead to disastrous consequences, including globe rupture.**
- Topical corticosteroids have been associated with delayed healing of corneal ulcers and corneal melting. Thus, their use is generally contraindicated in ulcerative keratitis.
- Preservatives contained within multi-dose eye drops may be associated with corneal irritation and, possibly, delayed healing. Preservative-free products should be considered in cases in which these complications are suspected.
- Patients with corneal perforation should also receive a broad-spectrum oral antibiotic with good ocular penetration (see Chapter 7).

If an ulcer persists or deepens, despite seemingly appropriate treatment, it is likely that a complicating factor has been missed and a repeat ophthalmic examination should be performed and/or specialist advice sought in order to identify and address any underlying causes (see Figure 12.16).

Bandage contact lenses and third eyelid flaps: These options may be considered in cases of superficial, non-infected corneal ulcers. Both techniques improve patient comfort by protecting the cornea from eyelid movement over exposed corneal stromal nerve endings. They may also protect against adnexal causes of irritation such as distichiasis or entropion, which may delay healing; although, addressing any such problems directly is usually preferable. Both techniques have their advantages and disadvantages, which are summarized in Figure 12.17.

Surgical treatment: Surgery should be considered in cases of significant corneal stromal loss and progressive corneal melting. Corneal ulcers that widen and/or deepen, despite medical therapy, due to progressive collagenolysis are likely to benefit from early surgical debridement of the melting stroma and corneal supportive and/or reconstructive surgery. In addition to the presence of collagenolysis and the response to medical treatment, ulcer depth and diameter are also very important factors to consider when assessing the need for surgery. Ulcers that reach 50% of corneal depth have a significant risk of perforation and should be considered for surgery even if they are of a small diameter and are surrounded by healthy stroma.

Bandage contact lens	Third eyelid flap
Advantages	
• Provides pain relief • May be applied to conscious patient (unless used in combination with partial tarsorrhaphy) • Allows visualization of the cornea following placement • Preserves patient vision during placement period • Allows tears to reach the puncta without being entrapped behind the third eyelid • Allows access of drops to ocular surface	• Provides pain relief • Technically easy to place • Should not dislodge when correctly placed • Physically protects cornea and reduces risk of self-trauma
Disadvantages	
• May dislodge following placement • Contraindicated in cases of ocular surface infection, deep ulcers and keratoconjunctivitis sicca • Use of ointments is contraindicated with soft bandage contact lenses as this limits oxygen access to the cornea • Risk of 'tight lens syndrome' which can lead to corneal oedema	• Requires general anaesthesia • Does not allow visualization of cornea following placement • Temporarily causes blindness during period of placement • Improper placement may lead to corneal trauma due to knot or suture irritation • Limits direct access of eye drops to the corneal surface • Contraindicated in cases of ocular surface infection and progressive deep ulcers

12.17 Advantages and disadvantages of bandage contact lenses and third eyelid flaps.

Commonly used reconstructive techniques include conjunctival pedicle grafting, corneoscleral transposition (CST) and corneoconjunctival transposition (CCT). These techniques utilize the patient's own tissues and do not lead to rejection. They also offer sufficient tectonic support for a variety of corneal reconstruction scenarios.

- Conjunctival pedicle grafting (Figure 12.18) has the advantage of providing a continuous supply of collagen-stabilizing serum through the blood vessels in the graft and has the ability to absorb fluid from the oedematous corneal stroma. However, this technique will interfere with corneal transparency and may occlude the visual axis.
- In CST and CCT grafts (Figure 12.19) the corneal section of the graft is positioned directly over the lesion, thus replacing lost corneal

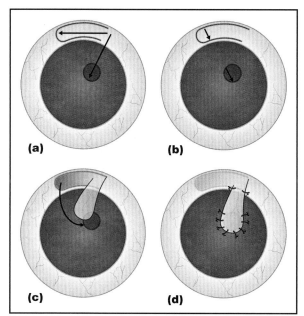

12.18 Conjunctival pedicle grafting. The pedicle must be long and wide enough to cover the corneal defect without having any tension in any direction. The edge of the corneal ulcer must be strong enough to hold the suture material. It is necessary to remove the corneal epithelium at the margins of the lesion, to promote adhesion of the graft to the corneal stroma, and to decide whether devitalized cornea needs to be removed, which invariably will make the defect larger and/or deeper. **(a–b)** The surgeon should measure the distance from the base of the pedicle (the point at which the pedicle will pivot on to the corneal surface) to the distal edge of the ulcer, as well as the width of the ulcer. These measurements are used to prepare the pedicle from bulbar conjunctiva. The use of bulbar conjunctiva that arises from the inferionasal aspect is generally discouraged because the location of the third eyelid fold complicates graft preparation. **(c)** Once prepared, the pedicle should be able to rest on top of the ulcer and cover it completely without retraction caused by excessive tension. **(d)** The base of the pedicle is then sutured on to the limbus and at least four additional single interrupted sutures (cardinal sutures) are used to secure the pedicle to the edge of the ulcer. Once secured, further sutures are used around the edge of the ulcer to fill in the gaps. Excessive manipulation of the pedicle graft during surgery, failure of vascularization of the pedicle and/or progressive collagenolysis postoperatively may contribute to graft dehiscence.

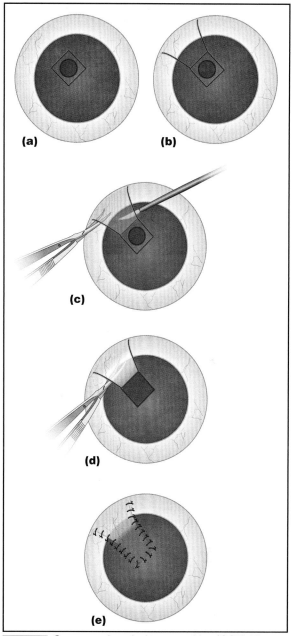

12.19 Corneoconjunctival transposition (CCT). The peripheral cornea and conjunctiva are transposed centrally to the ulcer site. **(a)** The edge of the ulcer is squared off. **(b)** Without removing the outlined 'cut out' around the edge of the ulcer, the rest the graft is outlined on the corneal surface. The path of the graft must be such that the graft is approximately 1 mm wider than the ulcer bed. The graft path is slightly diverging and crosses over the limbus on to the conjunctiva. A diamond knife, beaver blade or a restricted depth blade may be used. **(c)** The corneal and conjunctival sections of the graft are then undermined using a lamellar dissector. The ideal thickness of the corneal portion of the graft is approximately 50% of the corneal depth. Extreme care must be taken not to damage the graft or enter the anterior chamber at any point. **(d–e)** Once the graft is freed from the eye, except at its conjunctival base, it is transposed centrally over the ulcer bed. The outlined tissue at the site of the corneal ulcer is removed and the graft is sutured in place. As with conjunctival pedicle grafting, the surgeon must ensure that there is no graft tension and that the graft is not damaged during surgery. Oedematous corneal tissue is difficult to handle and easy to harm.

stroma with autologous corneal tissue rather than conjunctiva. This has the advantage of providing a relatively clear cornea and, therefore, may be more suitable for ulcers affecting the visual axis.

· A number of other techniques have been described, including the use of cyanoacrylate tissue glue (Watté *et al.*, 2004), fresh or frozen lamellar corneal transplants, porcine small intestinal submucosa and a variety of other graft materials.

Surgical reconstruction of the cornea requires surgical magnification, specialized instrumentation and an in-depth knowledge of a variety of micro-surgical techniques. As such, it should only be performed by surgeons trained and experienced in these techniques.

Eyelid and adnexal disease: This is a common cause of ulcerative keratitis, especially in certain breeds of dog. Entropion may lead to ulcerative disease if the hairs that contact the cornea abrade the epithelial layer. The location of the ulcer normally coincides with the location of the entropion (Figure 12.20), and it may deepen if the insult persists and eyelid spasm worsens due to corneal pain. If diagnosed early, these patients are not likely to require reconstructive surgery as the ulcers tend to remain superficial and are expected to resolve with simple medical therapy once the entropion is corrected. However, deep ulcers may require corneal reconstructive surgery at the time of entropion correction.

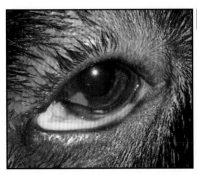

12.20 Lower lateral eyelid entropion in an English Bulldog. The lid margin has been manually everted to expose the associated corneal ulcer, which has been stained with fluorescein.

The presence of an ectopic cilium is often associated with corneal ulcerative disease. As with entropion, the ulcer coincides with the location of the hair, which is commonly under the central upper eyelid, so ulcers usually develop in the superior paracentral cornea. The ulcer is likely to develop soon after the short, stiff hair contacts the cornea. At this early stage of hair growth, the hair is often very small and may be difficult to visualize without slit-lamp magnification. If the hair is removed early and the ulcer is superficial, epithelial healing should be relatively fast and amenable to supportive medical therapy.

Distichiasis typically causes only minor corneal irritation rather than ulceration, but the latter can develop in some cases, especially where the extra eyelashes are short and stubby. This seems to be more common in breeds with shorter hair coats. Trichiasis describes the condition in which normal eyelid or facial hairs contact the corneal surface. It is seen with entropion, but may also occur in breeds with long or curly periocular hairs (e.g. poodles) or excessive nasal folds (e.g. Pugs). Eyelid and adnexal disease is discussed in more detail in Chapter 9.

Tear film disorders: KCS is a common cause of corneal ulcerative disease in dogs. Brachycephalic breeds in particular are likely to develop central to paracentral deep ulcers that are at risk of rapid progression and perforation (Sanchez *et al.*, 2007) (Figure 12.21). If diagnosed early, these rapidly developing ulcers are good candidates for corneal grafting. The use of topical ciclosporin does not delay epithelial or stromal wound healing and it is indicated in cases of KCS, even if the cornea has undergone reconstructive surgery. Qualitative tear film disease is less commonly diagnosed than KCS, but can also contribute to corneal ulceration. It is discussed in more detail in Chapter 10.

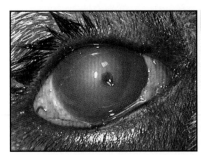

12.21 Paracentral, deep corneal ulcer associated with KCS in a 1-year-old English Bulldog. Distichiasis is also present affecting the lateral upper eyelid.

Spontaneous chronic corneal epithelial defects: SCCEDs ('indolent' corneal ulcers) are superficial ulcers that are characterized by a lip of loose epithelium surrounding a denuded superficial stroma. They persist for 1–2 weeks or longer and are common in middle-aged to older dogs. A breed predisposition in the Boxer and Corgi has been reported, but the condition may occur in any breed. The loose epithelium often folds on to itself around the edge of the ulcer and easily unfolds with each blink. Fluorescein aids the diagnosis as it highlights the exposed stroma and usually travels underneath the loose epithelium (Figure 12.22). The ulcers typically occur spontaneously and are usually unilateral, but have the potential to be bilateral.

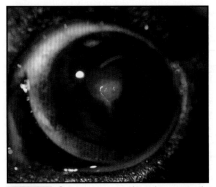

12.22 Spontaneous chronic corneal epithelial defect (SCCED). Fluorescein stains the stroma past the apparent edge of the ulcer. Loose epithelium is seen folding on to itself around the ulcer edge.

Before the diagnosis of SCCED can be made, all other possible causes of corneal ulceration should be ruled out and the clinical criteria outlined above should be met. Bentley *et al.* (2001) showed that SCCEDs exhibit two consistent changes: an absent or discontinuous basement membrane in the ulcerated region; and the presence of a thin, acellular, hyaline zone in the superficial stroma, which have been hypothesized to prevent new epithelial adhesions from forming. As the SCCED persists, stromal neovascularization may develop but this is often unsuccessful at resolving the ulceration. Instead, a granulation tissue response may develop which can further complicate epithelisation and can lead to significant scarring and visual deficits.

Treatment: Medical treatment alone is seldom successful at resolving SCCEDs, as the underlying basement membrane and superficial stromal abnormalities inhibit epithelial attachment. Thus, treatment options are aimed at disrupting this layer to allow epithelial attachment to the stroma. Reported treatments include (Stanley *et al.*, 1998):

- Debridement alone (Figure 12.23a), which has a 63% success rate at the first attempt
- Debridement followed by grid keratotomy (Figure 12.23b), which has an 85% success rate at the first attempt
- Superficial keratectomy, which has a near 100% success rate but requires appropriate general anaesthesia and surgical magnification and microsurgical skills
- Other reported treatments include the use of isobutyl cyanoacrylate tissue adhesive, punctate keratotomy (anterior stromal puncture) or diamond burr debridement; the latter has a success rate of approximately 90% after the first attempt (Gosling *et al.*, 2013).

Grid keratotomy should be performed as a pattern of superficial scratches in the shape of a grid that extends up to 1 mm into the surrounding, apparently healthy cornea and should not be readily visible to the naked eye once completed. To ensure that keratotomy is restricted to the most superficial anterior stroma, the tip of the needle may be bent or grasped with mosquito haemostats, so that just a fraction of a millimetre protrudes, perpendicular to the corneal surface. Repeated grid or punctate keratotomy can lead to significant corneal scarring and, if performed incorrectly, may lead to iatrogenic corneal laceration. If debridement and keratotomy are unsuccessful at the first attempt, they can be repeated at 2–3 week intervals.

Should an SCCED fail to heal, referral for further evaluation and possible superficial keratectomy should be considered. This procedure, which requires an operating microscope and microsurgical equipment, involves removing the superficial layer of the affected corneal stroma to a depth of approximately 100 μm. When performed early in the disease process, this procedure can lead to rapid healing with minimal scarring; however, if stromal neovascularization is present then a granulation tissue response may develop following any surgical intervention, including diamond burring, keratotomy or keratectomy. Following surgical treatment of SCCEDs, patient comfort may be improved with the use of a soft bandage contact lens, with or without a tarsorrhaphy (see Figure 8.21) or third eyelid flap (Figure 12.24). These techniques may aid pain relief, but their effect on healing and the success rate following diamond burring, grid keratotomy or keratectomy have proven difficult to assess; although, early reports support the use of bandage contact lenses (Grinninger *et al.*, 2012; Gosling *et al.*, 2013).

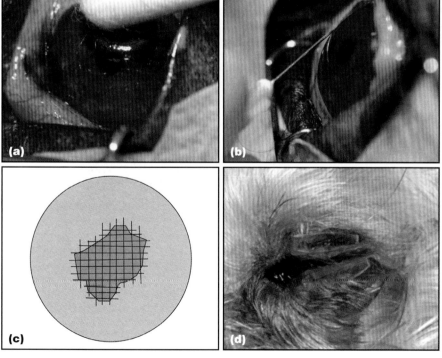

12.23 **(a)** After flushing the ocular surface with a 1:50 saline:povidone–iodine solution, debridement may be performed with a dry cotton tipped applicator. **(b–c)** This may be followed by superficial grid keratotomy with a 27 gauge needle and bandage contact lens fitting. **(d)** A temporary lateral tarsorrhaphy in the shape of a horizontal mattress suture can be used to help secure the lens.

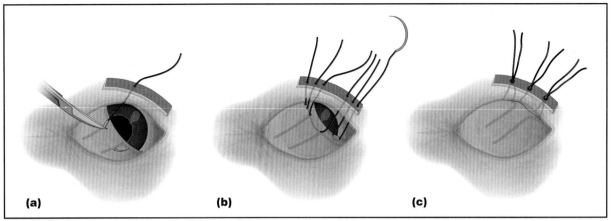

12.24 Placement of a third eyelid flap for palliative management of corneal ulceration if more direct surgical support procedures are contraindicated (e.g. due to systemic health concerns). **(a)** A needle with 2 metric (3/0 USP) non-absorbable suture is inserted through an appropriate stent (thick rubber band, Penrose drain or soft intravenous tubing) and then through the upper eyelid into the superior conjunctival fornix. The needle is then inserted though the anterior surface of the third eyelid, with the aim of encircling the vertical cartilage 'stem' of the third eyelid, taking care to avoid penetrating the conjunctiva on the posterior bulbar surface. Following suture placement, the third eyelid should be everted to confirm that the conjunctiva has not been penetrated on its posterior surface, as this could lead to corneal irritation and abrasion. The needle is then redirected through the superior conjunctival fornix, penetrating both the upper eyelid skin and stent. **(b)** If possible, two further horizontal mattress sutures should be placed in a similar fashion, taking small bites through the horizontal cartilage on either side of the initial suture. **(c)** The sutures are then tightened to pull the third eyelid across the globe, taking care to ensure that the third eyelid is anchored in the superior conjunctival fornix, without undue tension or distortion of the third eyelid. After tying, the suture ends should be left long, to facilitate their temporary untying at subsequent recheck visits (the suture knots should be carefully 'unpicked' and loosened with a hypodermic needle if necessary), releasing the third eyelid flap to permit observation of the eye. If necessary, the third eyelid flap sutures can be retied without the need for repeated surgical procedures.

Acute stromal collagenolysis: Acute stromal collagenolysis ('melting' corneal ulcer, keratomalacia) develops as a complication of an existing corneal ulcer rather than as a primary corneal condition. It may occur at any time during the healing process of an ulcer and can progress to corneal perforation within hours. It is not always possible to determine why it develops, but there are some common factors that may enhance collagenolysis:

- Normal corneal stromal healing represents a balance between collagen synthesis and lysis. Excessive collagenolysis develops when this delicate balance is disrupted
- MMPs and serine proteases are collagenolytic enzymes naturally produced by host cells in the cornea during the tissue response to insult. Chronic corneal irritation can recruit inflammatory cells, which may increase this collagenolytic response
- Microbial invasion of the ulcer (in particular, but not exclusively, *Pseudomonas* and *Streptococcus* infection) may also lead to the release of bacterial collagenolytic enzymes, as well as recruitment of inflammatory cells that are another potential source of collagenolytic enzymes. A stromal abscess (even if sterile) may be another source of collagenolytic enzymes
- The use of topical corticosteroids on a pre-existing corneal ulcer may induce the release of host cell collagenolytic enzymes, which is why their use is contraindicated for most types of corneal ulcer. The relevance of systemic corticosteroids in the aetiology of collagenolysis

is controversial, but it would seem sensible to consider these a potential risk factor
- The association of topical NSAIDs with corneal melting is less clear cut. A number of anecdotal reports have suggested a causative link, but a larger review showed no evidence for a link (Flach, 2001)
- Brachycephalic dog breeds (e.g. Pugs) seem to be at an increased risk of developing stromal collagenolysis; therefore, treatment of any type of corneal ulceration in these breeds must be undertaken with particular caution, involving frequent monitoring and taking care to address any underlying conformational cause. Specialist advice should be sought if the ulcer fails to heal within a few days or becomes progressive despite treatment.

Collagenolysis usually develops quickly, with the affected cornea adopting an opaque and gelatinous appearance. It may first appear as a grey or white dot, which can deepen rapidly or expand to occupy a large area of the corneal surface.

Treatment: Acute stromal collagenolysis should be treated as an ophthalmic emergency because it may lead to corneal rupture within hours. Management aims are:

- To stop progression of the collagenolysis
- To identify and treat ocular surface conditions that might affect healing
- To treat any causal infection
- To provide tectonic support if indicated (i.e. if the ulcer threatens to cause corneal rupture).

If the ulcer is recognized early and treated appropriately, medical treatment may be sufficient to stop the collagenolysis and allow the normal healing process to resume. If possible, the patient should be hospitalized and maintained under very close observation, especially in the early stages of treatment. Medical treatment involves a combination of anti-collagenases, antibiotics and analgesia.

- Anti-collagenases:
  - Serum is the anti-collagenase agent of choice because it is easily obtained and effective against both serine proteases and MMPs. Autologous serum is most commonly used, but donor serum may also be used. A protocol for the collection and use of serum eye drops is detailed in Figure 12.25
  - Ethylenediamine tetra-acetic acid (EDTA) drops, *N*-acetyl cysteine and tetracycline are alternatives, but are only effective against MMPs.
- Topical antibiotics:
  - *Pseudomonas* and *Streptococcus* spp. are the bacteria most commonly associated with stromal collagenolysis. As they have markedly different antibiotic sensitivities, in-house cytology is a simple and quick means of providing the clinician with an indication of the most appropriate type of antibiotic to use. A smear is prepared from a swab or scraping taken from the edge of the area of corneal melting and stained with Diff-Quik (see Chapter 3). The presence of rods or cocci allow a presumptive diagnosis of *Pseudomonas* or *Streptococcus* infection, respectively.
    - Topical fluoroquinolones, gentamicin, tobramycin, neomycin and polymyxin B are appropriate antibiotics for *Pseudomonas* infection.
    - Topical bacitracin, gramicidin, cephalosporins and penicillins are appropriate for streptococcal infections (see Chapter 7).
- Systemic antibiotics with good ocular penetration (e.g. cefalexin) should be administered if there is a risk of globe rupture.
- Analgesia in the form of systemic NSAIDs,

1. Collect 5–10 ml of blood.
2. Place it in one or several small plain or serum gel tubes.
3. Allow the blood to clot.
4. Spin the tube(s).
5. Separate the serum from the supernatant by gently decanting it into several vials, each of which should contain a daily dose of serum (e.g. 6–8 drops).
6. Dispense tubes and small disposable plastic pipettes, if available, one for each day of the treatment. Instructions should clearly state that:
   - The tubes are to be kept frozen until the day of use
   - The tube being used is to be kept in the fridge between doses
   - The unused daily dose of serum and used pipette should be discarded after 24 hours.

12.25 Collection and use of serum eye drops.

topical atropine and, if indicated, oral opioids should be used.

Patients should be medicated once every 30–60 minutes initially and reassessed about every 3 hours, without the repeated use of fluorescein. Improvement of the collagenolytic process, with reduction in the gelatinous appearance of the corneal tissue and arrested ulcer deepening, should be noted within the first 12–24 hours, before the frequency of application of medication is reduced to once every 4–6 hours. If the melting process responds favourably, the patient can be kept on intensive medical therapy under close observation for another 24 hours before reducing the frequency to once every 4–6 hours.

Surgical intervention should be performed if:

- The area of collagenolysis or melting is deep and threatens to cause globe rupture
- Despite intensive medical treatment, the area of cornea melting enlarges, deepens or fails to stabilize over a few hours.

Appropriate surgical treatment includes:

- Conjunctival pedicle or CCT grafting if the area of melting is small
- Conjunctival hood or 360-degree grafts if large areas of the cornea are affected.

Third eyelid flaps or bandage contact lenses are contraindicated in cases of collagenolysis.

Corneal trauma: Corneal trauma may be blunt, sharp or chemically induced and may be penetrating or lead to corneal foreign body entrapment. The term may also be applied to eyelid and adnexal causes of corneal ulceration (see above).

Blunt trauma: In addition to causing corneal ulceration, blunt trauma may also affect other parts of the globe and the consequences can be severe. Additional pathologies may include corneal oedema, scleral rupture, lens luxation, intraocular haemorrhage, retinal detachment and/or orbital fractures. Animals with suspected blunt trauma to the eye should undergo a thorough ocular examination, including assessment of the eyelids, cornea, intraocular structures, bony orbit and periocular structures, as well as an ocular ultrasound examination to identify damage to the posterior segment structures, such as retinal detachment or globe rupture. Scleral rupture (see Chapter 13) may be difficult to identify and carries a poor prognosis (Rampazzo *et al.*, 2006).

Non-penetrating sharp trauma: This is a common ocular emergency and can involve any sharp object such as a cat claw, thorn or nail. In most instances, it results in a partial thickness puncture, a relatively straight cut or a cut at a 90-degree angle, leading to the formation of a corneal flap. In addition, corneal lacerations that are near the limbus may also reach the sclera, causing a scleral laceration or rupture, which may be difficult to identify as the conjunctiva may readily heal over it. The majority of fresh punctures, lacerations and flaps are amenable to direct suturing, although some may require corneal grafting. Some very small non-penetrating punctures do not require suturing, if there is little to no stromal exposure. These lesions may be treated medically but should be re-examined frequently. If corneal oedema develops or worsens, or there is wound edge separation, suturing is necessary to avoid further wound breakdown. Some wounds might contain foreign material, such as hairs or other particulate matter. This is common in lacerations that result in corneal flaps (Figure 12.26). All debris should be removed before suturing or grafting. The identification of particulate matter and its removal, as well as suturing or grafting, requires examination with adequate illumination and magnification and specialized knowledge of corneal microsurgical techniques. Adjunctive medical treatment is as described for corneal ulcers.

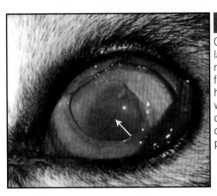

12.26 Corneal laceration resulting in a flap. Note the hair trapped within the corneal stroma, overlying the pupil (arrowed).

Penetrating trauma: It is sometimes difficult to determine whether penetrating corneal injury has occurred in association with sharp ocular trauma. However, there are tell-tale signs of penetrating trauma that the clinician should be aware of (Figures 12.27 and 12.28). Corneal penetrating injuries must be carefully assessed because surgical reduction of

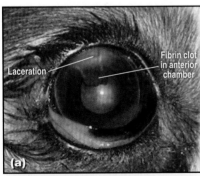

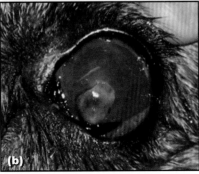

12.27 (a) Cat claw injury through the cornea, resulting in a penetrating horizontal corneal laceration and a clot of fibrin in the anterior chamber. (b) Traumatic perforation of the cornea, resulting in a prominent fibrin plug.

(a) labels: Laceration; Fibrin clot in anterior chamber

Clinical feature	Comments
Cornea	
Fibrin plug	Sudden decompression of the anterior chamber leads to extravasation of protein, including fibrinogen from the vasculature of the iris and ciliary body (plasmoid aqueous). Fibrinogen is converted into fibrin which may reach the cornea and coagulate, forming a protruding plug of a tan to reddish colour that covers the corneal defect
Iris prolapse	Prolapsed iris tissue may not be directly visible within the corneal defect under the coagulated fibrin
Anterior chamber	
Shallow chamber	Sudden decompression of the anterior chamber is also associated with a rapid loss of aqueous humour, a shallow anterior chamber and a marked inflammatory response. The anterior chamber remains shallow if leakage of aqueous through the wound is not stopped by the formation of a fibrin or iridal plug. The accompanying uveitis leads to a low intraocular pressure.
Blood or fibrin	Blood or fibrin may accumulate and coagulate in the anterior chamber forming a clot
Pigment	Strands or segments of pigmented epithelium may break loose from the posterior iris and make their way into the anterior chamber or may be deposited on the lens capsule or corneal endothelium
Lens material	Lens material may protrude into the anterior chamber if the anterior lens capsule is ruptured during the injury
Iris	
Dyscoria	Dyscoria (abnormal pupil shape) results from direct iris trauma or synechiae
Anterior synechia	Anterior synechiae may cause the appearance of a locally shallow anterior chamber as the iris is displaced anteriorly and adheres to the cornea or protrudes from the corneal wound. Anterior synechiae are most readily appreciated by viewing the anterior chamber from the side
Posterior synechia	Posterior synechiae develop when the inflamed iris adheres to the anterior lens capsule
Lens	
Lens rupture	Rupture of the anterior lens capsule may lead to protrusion of varying quantities of cortical or nuclear lens material through the capsular defect, altering the lens contour. Features of lens rupture are described in Chapters 2 and 16

12.28 Clinical features that may be associated with corneal trauma.

iris prolapse may be required and lens surgery may be necessary to prevent the development of phacoclastic uveitis (see Chapters 14 and 16). These very technically demanding procedures require specialist skills and such cases should be referred promptly if possible. Adjunctive medical treatment includes systemic NSAIDs and oral antibiotics, in addition to that described for corneal ulcers.

Corneal foreign bodies: These most frequently comprise organic matter, typically plant material. However, almost anything small and sharp can penetrate the corneal epithelium and become lodged underneath it, or reach various depths within the corneal stroma and remain there. A foreign body may reach the endothelial side of the cornea and penetrate into the anterior chamber, or it may fully enter the anterior chamber where it may become enveloped in fibrin, which might mask its presence. In some cases, the foreign body may enter the irido-corneal drainage angle, where it may remain hidden from view, and elicit a severe anterior uveitis. Certainly, most corneal foreign bodies elicit a significant inflammatory response, especially if made of organic matter.

Penetrating corneal injuries or perforating corneal disease may lead to the stromal entrapment of small amounts of blood, fibrin or iris. These conditions are also associated with an inflammatory response and could be confused with a corneal foreign body response. Entrapment of part of the iris is always associated with a shallow anterior chamber, either focally at the site of anterior synechiae or more generally if there is persistent leakage of aqueous humour, and anterior displacement of the part of the iris that is in contact with the cornea. Viewing the anterior segment structures from a side view with a focal light source (and preferably magnification) should allow identification of such complications.

Treatment: Corneal foreign body removal must be performed with great caution so as not to embed the object further in the cornea or cause more damage than already present. A small needle (23 or 25 gauge) or foreign body spud may be used to engage foreign bodies that are very superficial or partially outside the corneal surface, so that they may be gently retrieved by exerting outward force in the opposite direction from which they are thought to have entered. However, foreign bodies can easily fragment during extraction and the stroma might engage them in a way that makes needle extraction rather difficult. Surgical removal via a carefully planned incision in the corneal surface in the vicinity of the foreign body, retrieval through a full thickness surgical incision into the anterior chamber and the use of needles or forceps may therefore be necessary to avoid causing further corneal or lens damage, leakage of aqueous, intraocular haemorrhage or inadvertent displacement of the foreign body into the anterior chamber. Patients with subepithelial corneal foreign bodies that are easily removed should be treated with supportive medical therapy as for ulcerative keratitis and these lesions would be expected to heal quickly in the absence of other factors that might limit re-epithelialization. Foreign bodies that are more difficult to retrieve require in-depth knowledge of corneal and intraocular microsurgical techniques and necessitate specialist referral.

Chemical or thermal burns: Chemical burns may involve alkaline or acidic substances. Acidic chemicals are found amongst common household cleaning products such as bleach and toilet cleaners containing sulphuric and hydrochloric acids. Alkaline chemicals such as ammonium hydroxide and sodium hydroxide are caustic agents contained in oven and drain cleaners. Calcium hydroxide, which is found in some building materials, is another common caustic agent. Most alkaline chemicals are able to penetrate tissues better than acids because of their lipid solubility. Acidic burns with mild to moderate acids, on the other hand, tend to be somewhat self-limiting because they coagulate the corneal collagen. Coagulated tissue acts as a barrier that stops these acids from penetrating the injured tissue further. Thus, alkali burns usually lead to more serious damage than acid burns and may cause severe and sight-threatening corneal melting, limbal ischaemia/necrosis and severe uveitis. In early injury, pH indicator paper, readily available on urinalysis strips, may be placed in the tear film to help identify the type of burn.

Treatment: The affected corneal surface, conjunctival tissues and eyelids should be thoroughly rinsed with copious amounts of saline as soon as possible, because destruction of the surface epithelium occurs rapidly, chemical residue elevates the risk of prolonged damage and severe inflammation and pain develop rapidly. Flushing of the ocular surface is best performed under general anaesthesia in veterinary patients, as prolonged (e.g. 20–30 minutes) irrigation may be required. Again, pH strips can be useful to assess the effectiveness of the flushing; irrigation should be maintained until the pH of the conjunctival sac returns to its normal value of around 7.5. For severe cases, particularly alkali burns, specialist advice should be sought. For thermal burns, supportive medical therapy is the same as that described for corneal ulcers.

Corneal degeneration: Corneal degeneration develops secondary to systemic disease or other local pathological changes within the cornea and involves lipid, calcium or a mixture of both. Corneal vascularization is often a feature and secondary corneal ulceration is common. The condition is seen in older dogs and usually represents progression of an underlying corneal disease such as corneal lipidosis or calcium keratopathy (see below). If the corneal degeneration is progressive or associated with chronic ulceration, keratectomy may be indicated, with or without conjunctival or CCT grafting.

Neurological disease:

Neurotrophic keratopathy: This develops when the afferent sensory output of the cornea is reduced or absent. It can be difficult to elucidate the exact cause of decreased corneal sensation, but it may be reduced to problems affecting the ophthalmic branch of the trigeminal nerve and its corneal trunks, or the trigeminal nerve itself. Recognized causes of neurotrophic keratopathy in humans include repeated trauma, corneal infection with herpesvirus, corneal surgery, the repeated, excessive use of topical anaesthetics, and conditions that cause peripheral nerve degeneration such as diabetes mellitus (Heigle and Pflugfelder, 1996). Corneal sensation in canine diabetic patients is also reduced (Good *et al.*, 2003). However, the effects of such problems are difficult to quantify in the canine population given the fact that corneal sensation can vary significantly depending on skull type (Blocker and van der Woerdt, 2001).

Cavernous sinus syndrome (middle cranial fossa disease) has been diagnosed in dogs, and can affect trigeminal nerve function (see Chapter 19). Decreased corneal sensation is usually associated with reduced reflex tear production and reduced blink rate. This, in turn, leads to an unstable tear film secondary to increased evaporative loss and the reduced cleansing effect of the reduced blink and overall surface dryness. Fluorescein may reveal a diffuse, superficial punctate uptake of the dye, but the condition can rapidly deteriorate and lead to ulcerative disease. Ulcers typically develop centrally and may involve the entire axial cornea within the interpalpebral fissure. Healing of the epithelium is likely to be delayed in animals with neurotrophic keratopathy, as it is in humans (Okada *et al.*, 2010).

Treatment is aimed at identifying and managing the primary cause where possible. In addition, the eye must be kept lubricated with the frequent application of a viscous tear substitute (ideally preservative free) and the use of a temporary lateral tarsorrhaphy (see Chapter 8 and Figure 12.23) may be considered in order to decrease the amount of corneal exposure and evaporative tear loss. A permanent tarsorrhaphy may be used in cases that are not expected to recover.

Neuroparalytic keratopathy: Facial nerve paralysis leads to eyelid akinesia and this predisposes the eye to exposure keratitis within the interpalpebral fissure (Figure 12.29). Natural, intermittent globe retraction into the orbit, a healthy tear response and the sweeping action of the third eyelid may prevent the development of keratitis in some cases, but more often than not, epithelial ulceration develops. Causes of facial nerve paralysis include otitis media, trauma, iatrogenic causes (e.g. following total ear canal ablation) and idiopathic facial neuropathy (see Chapter 19 for further details). Supportive management is similar to that described for neurotrophic keratopathy (see above). Recovery of function is variable and it may take weeks, or the condition may be permanent. Permanent lateral tarsorrhaphy is useful in cases where normal eyelid function is not thought likely to return.

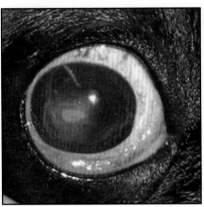

12.29 Superficial ulcer of the axial cornea within the interpalpebral fissure of a patient with neuroparalytic keratitis after total ear canal ablation surgery.

Less common causes of ulcerative keratitis:

Epithelial dystrophy in Shetland Sheepdogs: This uncommon problem is unique to the Shetland Sheepdog and is characterized by bilateral, superficial, multifocal, circular epithelial lesions 1–2 mm in diameter that can take up fluorescein centrally (Figure 12.30). In such cases, decreased tear film break up time (TFBUT; see Chapters 1 and 10) occurs with mild ocular discomfort shown by an increased blink rate and increased tearing. The aetiology remains unknown. Various treatments have been reported, from the application of mucinomimetic tear supplements, which is justified in cases with a rapid TFBUT, to the application of topical ciclosporin (0.2%) or the use of corneal debridement with bandage lens placement if topical therapy does not lead to the resolution of clinical signs.

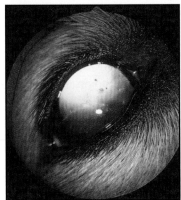

12.30 Epithelial dystrophy in a Shetland Sheepdog. (Courtesy of S Crispin)

Superficial punctate keratitis: This is a rare condition that presents as a diffuse but subtle bilateral punctate epitheliopathy which takes up fluorescein. A breed predisposition in the Miniature Longhaired Dachshund has been reported. Not all dogs affected are symptomatic, but those that are show mild to moderate signs of discomfort. There may be a link with poor tear film stability, although an immune-mediated aetiopathogenesis has also been suggested. The condition may therefore be multifactorial and include one or more of the following: immune-mediated disease; tear film instability; macropalpebral fissure; poor corneal sensation; and a low blink rate. It is important to: rule out eyelid diseases such as distichiasis, which can be the source of repeated microtrauma; assess completeness of the blink response and its rate; examine the tear film thoroughly by measuring tear production and the TFBUT; and, if possible, evaluate corneal sensation.

If a specific cause is identified an appropriate treatment plan can be selected. However, more often than not this is difficult, and different treatment options may be considered by the clinician. Tear supplements, such as mucinomimetics and lipid-containing preparations, may be of help. It is possible that, as with some epitheliopathies in humans, the long-term use of medications that contain preservatives may also play a synergistic role with other causative factors. For this reason, whenever possible, preservative-free viscous preparations should be selected over preservative-containing ones, especially for long-term use or when frequent application is advised. If an immune-mediated cause is suspected then topical therapy with ciclosporin may prove beneficial.

Endothelial dystrophy and degeneration: True dystrophy, affecting young animals of various breeds (including the Boston Terrier and Chihuahua), is relatively uncommon but age-related endothelial degeneration is more commonly encountered. It usually affects older animals and is slowly progressive. The cause is unknown but the pathogenesis involves gradual decompensation of the corneal endothelium, leading to progressive corneal oedema (Figure 12.31). This is often first seen in the temporal cornea before it progresses centrally to involve the entire cornea. The condition can lead to decreased vision and is generally non-painful in the early to moderately advanced stages. In advanced cases, subepithelial bullae (small accumulations of fluid arising within the anterior stroma) develop and these can spontaneously rupture, leading to the formation of small, superficial ulcers and intermittent bouts of pain. These small ulcers usually heal with supportive medical therapy, although healing may be protracted. Vascularization and pigmentation of the cornea may also be seen in advanced cases. Dense, diffuse oedema may lead to functional blindness in severely affected animals.

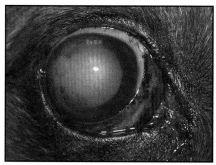

12.31

Diffuse corneal oedema in a patient with endothelial dystrophy.

The use of topical hypertonic saline ointment (5% NaCl) has been advocated by some as a means of decreasing the amount of oedema, but results are inconsistent at best. Advanced cases may benefit from placement of a very thin advancement conjunctival flap (Gunderson flap), which may slow the progression of the disease by absorbing fluid from the corneal stroma.

Thermokeratoplasty has been described for use in advanced cases with recurring ulcers and pain. In this technique, controlled micro-burns of the cornea create a superficial stromal scar and the contraction of thermally damaged corneal collagen fibres is theorized to prevent the formation of further bullae. Cases treated by this method are reported to heal faster and require supportive medication for shorter periods of time than cases treated by other methods (Michau *et al.*, 2003). However, the procedure may cause significant corneal opacity, which affects vision, and as such is only indicated in advanced, end-stage disease. Thermokeratoplasty should only

be performed by experienced ophthalmic surgeons and with the aid of an operating microscope.

Keratoprostheses have also been investigated for use in cases with vision loss due to severe corneal oedema and other causes of significant corneal opacification, with varying degrees of success (Allgoewer *et al.*, 2010; Isard *et al.*, 2010), but their use has not been widely adopted. Corneal collagen cross-linking with riboflavin and ultraviolet (UV)-A has recently been proposed as a promising treatment for the condition (Pot *et al.*, 2013).

Corneal sequestrum: This condition has been studied most thoroughly in cats, in which it is relatively common (see below). Although it has been reported in dogs (Bouhanna *et al.*, 2008), corneal sequestrum is considered extremely rare in this species. As with cats, canine corneal sequestra appear to be associated with corneal ulcerative disease and chronic irritation of the ocular surface.

Infectious keratitis: There are very few infectious agents that are considered primary corneal pathogens in dogs, and most are opportunistic invaders of the traumatized cornea. Corneal cytology, microbial culture and, in some instances, additional specific testing (see Chapter 3) may be necessary to identify the pathogen involved. Bacterial infections are more likely than fungal infections, which are rare, although they have been described in dogs. Leishmaniosis has been reported to cause severe keratitis as well as KCS in dogs, with localization of the parasite in many ocular tissues including the cornea. Dogs that live in or travel to endemic countries are at risk. In addition, natural infection with canine herpesvirus has been associated with superficial ulcerative disease in the dog (Ledbetter *et al.*, 2006, 2009).

Non-ulcerative keratitis

Chronic superficial keratitis: This common corneal disease is usually referred to as pannus or CSK and is characterized histopathologically by a lymphoplasmacytic infiltrate in the anterior stroma. The condition is idiopathic, although the nature of the cellular infiltrate and response to topical immunosuppressive therapy suggest an immune-mediated aetiology. There is a strong breed predisposition in the German Shepherd Dog, Belgian Shepherd Dog and the Greyhound (Bedford and Longstaffe, 1979). Increased exposure to UV light (e.g. during the summer months or when living at high altitude) is another risk factor for the development of CSK.

A typical lesion is characterized by a leading edge of cellular infiltrate that is accompanied by a prominent vascular response and, sometimes, pigment deposition. It has a tendency to develop in the temporal paralimbal cornea, but may involve other sectors of the cornea, and extends centrally with time (Figure 12.32). Later in the disease process, a secondary focus of cellular infiltrate may develop opposite the original lesion and extend centrally to join it. If the majority of the central cornea is

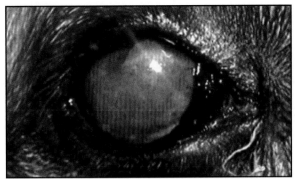

12.32 Chronic superficial keratitis infiltrate in a German Shepherd Dog.

affected, vision will also be compromised. In addition to corneal lesions, some patients also suffer from medial canthal erosion (see Chapter 9) and/or third eyelid lymphoplasmacytic infiltration (also known as plasma cell conjunctivitis or plasmoma; see Chapter 11). The condition is non-painful but may lead to progressive vision loss if untreated. A diagnosis is usually reached based on the characteristic clinical presentation, supportive history and response to treatment, although cytology may be used to confirm the diagnosis in equivocal cases.

Treatment: This consists of the application of an immune-modulating topical agent such as ciclosporin or a corticosteroid such as dexamethasone phosphate 0.1% eye drops. Although topical ciclosporin is considered the treatment of choice, both may be used in combination during the early part of the treatment course. Topical ciclosporin is applied twice daily. High frequency dosing with a topical corticosteroid (e.g. 4–6 times daily) may be required over the first 7–10 days, after which application frequency may be slowly reduced over a period of 6–8 weeks to a maintenance dose, such as once daily or every other day application. If both drugs are used at first, the corticosteroid may be slowly tapered off entirely in favour of the topical ciclosporin. It is important to ensure that the clinical signs do not worsen or recur when the frequency of medication is lowered.

Topical treatment is required for long periods of time, and lifelong maintenance therapy is generally necessary. Recurrence of the lesion is often associated with too rapid a reduction in use of the topical medication or its early withdrawal. Combination treatment with superficial keratectomy and radiotherapy using soft X-rays has also been described for advanced cases, but is not widely available (Allgoewer and Hoecht, 2010). Scar formation may be seen after regression of the primary corneal lesion (Figure 12.33). This is often worse in chronic cases and it may be associated with pigment deposition.

As the condition may be triggered or exacerbated by UV light, owners should be advised that it may worsen during the summer months. Precautions such as discouraging high exposure to UV light should be taken, although one study that treated affected corneas with UV-blocking bandage lenses found that blocking of UV light did not modify the course of the disease process (Denk *et al.*, 2011).

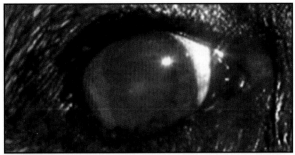

12.33 The cornea of the dog in Figure 12.31 following treatment with topical dexamethasone phosphate drops at a tapering dose (4 x daily for 1 week, then 3 x daily for 1 week, then 2 x daily for 1 week, then 1 x daily for 1 week) and ciclosporin (0.2%) (2 x daily for 8 weeks, then 1 x daily long term). Note the superficial scarring and pigment deposition that remains.

Pigmentary keratitis: In this common condition, chronic ocular surface irritation leads to the accumulation of surface pigment, which is progressive unless the source of irritation is identified and removed. Animals with a prominent band of pigment around the limbus or conjunctiva, such as Pugs, are more likely to be affected by superficial pigment proliferation in response to even minor ocular surface irritation. Corneal pigmentation may affect vision if it develops over the visual axis (Figure 12.34). This may be seen in patients with long-standing chronic superficial irritation, although in some breeds (such as Pugs), extensive pigmentation may develop as early as the first or second year of life either in association with medial canthal entropion, macropalpebral fissure and/or KCS, or may occur in the absence of significant inflammatory infiltrate. In the absence of clinical evidence of significant ocular surface inflammation in one cross-sectional study (Labelle *et al.*, 2013), the authors suggest the term 'pigmentary keratopathy' or 'corneal melanosis'. Corneal pigmentation is often difficult for owners to recognize in animals with dark hair coats and dark irises and so is frequently presented at an advanced stage. Common causes of proliferative pigmentary keratitis are listed in Figure 12.35.

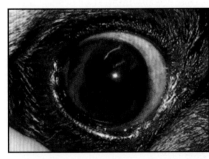

12.34 Pigmentary keratitis affecting the visual axis of a Pug.

• Medial canthal entropion (typically seen in brachycephalic breeds)
• Medial trichiasis (including nasal fold and caruncular trichiasis)
• Macropalpebral fissure (lagophthalmos)
• Keratoconjunctivitis sicca
• Chronic inflammatory conditions (e.g. chronic superficial keratitis)

12.35 Common causes of pigmentary keratitis in dogs.

Treatment: Topical corticosteroids and ciclosporin are seldom effective at reducing pigmentation if the underlying disease is not addressed. Pigment patches may be removed via lamellar keratectomy, but unless the specific cause or causes are identified and treated successfully they will quickly reform during the healing process (Whitley and Gilger, 1999). If the source of the chronic irritation is treated successfully, progression of pigmentation may be slowed or halted. However, the preferred approach is to limit corneal pigmentation in predisposed breeds such as the Pug through early recognition and treatment of predisposing factors. This may involve medical and/or surgical intervention, including:

- Long-term use of topical ocular lubricants
- Medial canthoplasty to shorten the palpebral fissure, improve blink and reduce trichiasis
- Nasal fold resection or treatment of medial entropion if indicated (see Chapter 9).

Corneal lipidosis: Corneal lipidosis is a 'catch-all' term that encompasses any disease in which corneal lipid deposition is a feature, including:

- Crystalline stromal dystrophy
- Lipid keratopathy
- Corneal arcus (arcus lipoides corneae).

Crystalline stromal dystrophy: This is a common hereditary condition that affects a variety of dog breeds, including the Cavalier King Charles Spaniel, Siberian Husky, Samoyed, Rough Collie, Beagle and Airedale Terrier. The pathogenesis remains unknown and there are several modes of inheritance suspected, from polygenic in Cavalier King Charles Spaniels to sex-linked recessive in Airedale Terriers. The stromal infiltrate has the appearance of finely ground glass and may appear refractile and 'sparkle' when light strikes it. It is commonly found in the central cornea in the form of a nebula or a circular to oval ring, and is most often confined to the superficial stroma (Figure 12.36). In some breeds, such as Huskies, the lesion may affect the deeper stroma (Figure 12.37) and presents in one of several possible patterns that are described elsewhere (Gilger, 2007).

Crystalline stromal dystrophy is most commonly seen in young adults and tends to be slowly

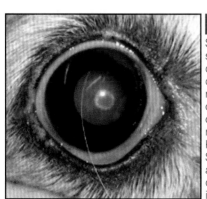

12.36

Subepithelial stromal lipid dystrophy with deposition of refractile lipid crystals in a characteristic ring in a Cavalier King Charles Spaniel. There is also an unrelated diabetic cataract in this eye.

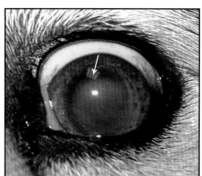

12.37

Diffuse superficial stromal lipid dystrophy in a Siberian Husky. The reflection of the overhead light on the cornea is arrowed.

progressive over time. In some bitches, the lesions may first appear or progress during oestrus. In all cases, there is no corneal pain and no uptake of fluorescein stain. There is no association with systemic lipid disorders, and serum lipid and cholesterol profiles of affected animals are normal (Crispin, 2002). Instead, it is most likely due to a local metabolic defect in the corneal fibroblast. The main types of lipid present are cholesterol and phospholipids, some of which are free within the stroma, whilst the remainder are trapped inside keratocytes that die at the site of lipid accumulation. Although uncommon, over time, the lipid liberated within the corneal stroma may lead to corneal vascularization in a process known as corneal degeneration, which is always secondary and may make it difficult to distinguish the condition from lipid keratopathy (see below).

There is no known treatment for crystalline stromal dystrophy. As the condition is not directly associated with serum lipid elevations, the instigation of low-fat diets is unlikely to affect progression. Lipid infiltrates rarely progress to the point of interfering with vision and hence their surgical removal is seldom indicated. In cases where lipid is removed, recurrence is likely.

Lipid keratopathy: This term refers to the deposition of lipid within the cornea of animals, secondary to other disease processes. It is always associated with corneal vascularization, which may precede or follow the lipid deposition (Crispin, 2002). It may develop as a sequel to corneal trauma, limbal masses, retained corneal foreign bodies and any condition that leads to chronic corneal vascularization. Lipid keratopathy is usually unilateral but may be bilateral, and may on occasion be associated with hyperlipoproteinaemia. Calcification and corneal degeneration may develop in established cases (see below).

Corneal arcus: This is a rare condition in dogs and describes bilateral lipid infiltration of the peripheral cornea (Crispin, 2002). A bilateral grey opacity develops perilimbally in the shape of an arc. This presents as an accumulation of lipid in the peripheral cornea, which follows the curvature of the limbus. There is usually a clear band of cornea (termed the lucid interval of Vogt) between the lesion and the limbus. In time, corneal vascularization may develop, making the condition difficult to distinguish from lipid keratopathy. Corneal arcus is always associated with hyperlipoproteinaemia and the work-up should include investigation of primary and secondary systemic lipid disorders such as primary hyperlipoproteinaemia, hypothyroidism, diabetes mellitus, hyperadrenocorticism, chronic pancreatitis and liver disease.

Calcium degeneration: This may be a primary condition or develop secondary to systemic disease, particularly in elderly animals. The corneal infiltrate in patients with calcium degeneration (calcium keratopathy) is usually associated with the development of corneal vascularization. It may be difficult to distinguish calcium deposition clinically from lipid and the differentiation can be challenging. Whilst lipid infiltrates have a sparkling, crystalline appearance and the lesions are not associated with epithelial disruption, calcific infiltrates tend to take on a more matt, chalky appearance. Calcific deposits may be associated with small epithelial defects that take up fluorescein, at which point they cause corneal discomfort (Figures 12.38 and 12.39).

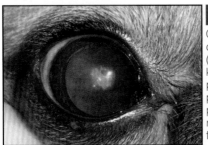

12.38
Calcium degeneration (calcium keratopathy) in a patient that presented with pain. The lesion retained fluorescein.

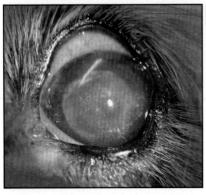

12.39
Calcium degeneration (calcium keratopathy) in a reticulated pattern.

Calcium degeneration can develop spontaneously in dogs with chronic inflammatory conditions such as keratitis, uveitis, glaucoma and severe hypotony, whether in the absence of obvious systemic abnormalities or in patients with increased calcium levels, hyperphosphataemia and hypovitaminosis D (Sansom and Blunden, 2010). Calcium deposits have also been reported to occur after parotid duct transposition for the management of KCS, but these more superficial deposits are of an entirely different nature, as they originate from saliva (see Chapter 10).

Treatment: Any underlying cause should be identified and managed if possible. Calcium deposits may progress to cause interference with vision and can be removed via superficial keratectomy, but the lesions might recur. EDTA is a chelating agent that, in theory, may aid removal of the calcium deposits. However, the lesion must be debrided first to remove the epithelium and allow the chelating agent to contact the calcium deposits. Complete lesion removal is rarely achieved in this manner and the results are often unpredictable, so this treatment is not indicated in most cases. Keratectomy with or without grafting is indicated if corneal degeneration is associated with painful ulceration.

Less common diseases:

Symblepharon: This is less common in dogs than in cats (see later) but may develop when there is severe destruction of the corneal and conjunctival epithelium; for example, following strong acid or alkali burns (see above). It leads to exposure of the corneal and conjunctival stroma, which form adhesions when they come into contact (e.g. during eye closure). Conjunctivalization of the de-epithelialized cornea often develops, leading to what is usually irreversible corneal opacification.

Posterior polymorphous dystrophy: This is a rare inherited condition of American Cocker Spaniels, which presents as multifocal opacities of the posterior cornea. Although the condition is thought to affect the endothelium, patients are usually asymptomatic.

Florida spots: These corneal lesions are multifocal, white to grey, small round opacities that vary in size and are located at the level of the superficial to mid-stroma in patients that are otherwise asymptomatic. Cases are reported to occur in tropical and subtropical climates and to date have not been described in Europe. There is no known treatment and the cause has not been definitively established.

Corneal masses

Epithelial inclusion cysts: These are smooth, round to ovoid superficial corneal lesions that are white to pink and are not associated with pain (Figure 12.40). Epithelial inclusion cysts are rarely associated with an inflammatory response of the cornea, which distinguishes them from corneal stromal abscesses. Their pathogenesis is not entirely understood. They may be congenital or form following accidental or surgical trauma that seeds healthy corneal epithelium into the superficial stroma where it continues to grow until it forms a cyst-like structure (Figure 12.41). Epithelial inclusion cysts are variable in size, but in most cases are relatively small when diagnosed (e.g. 2–4 mm in diameter).

Treatment: Complete surgical excision by keratectomy is the treatment of choice. This may require grafting of the cornea. Postoperative medical therapy is as for ulcerative disease of the cornea.

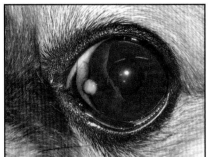

12.40

Epithelial inclusion cyst of unknown origin near the limbus in a Chihuahua.

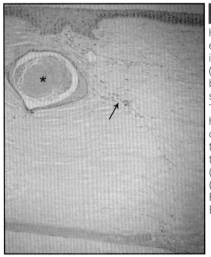

12.41

Histology of an epithelial inclusion cyst (✱) presumed to be secondary to surgical trauma. There is a linear, healed, surgical corneal incision to the right of the cyst (arrowed). (©Karen Dunn, FOCUS-EyePathLab)

Neoplasia: Tumours of the cornea are relatively rare in dogs. However, primary corneal squamous cell carcinoma has been described, with increasing frequency, in dogs with a history of chronic corneal irritation (Takiyama *et al.*, 2010). A study of 26 cases concluded the tumour was unilateral, that there was a predisposition in brachycephalic breeds with chronic keratitis secondary to KCS and a history of topical immunosuppressive therapy (Dreyfus *et al.*, 2011). Complete removal via keratectomy, with or without adjunctive therapy such as cryosurgery, is recommended to limit recurrence of the mass, together with ongoing conservative treatment of the keratitis. Corneal haemangiosarcoma has also been reported in the dog. Other corneal tumours include papillomas as well as melanocytic neoplasms that extend into the cornea. Other masses that develop near the limbus and may affect the cornea include dermoid, nodular episcleritis and scleritis, granulation tissue and staphyloma (see Chapter 13).

Feline conditions

Developmental abnormalities

Variations in corneal size and absence
These congenital abnormalities are probably as rare in cats as they are in dogs. In addition, acquired early-life infection with feline herpesvirus-1 (FHV-1) may be associated with severe ocular abnormalities within a litter of kittens that can involve other ocular structures as well as the cornea.

Corneal opacities
Transient early corneal opacities may be seen in kittens, as described for puppies, and it should dissipate soon after eyelid opening. Permanent, congenital corneal opacity occurs in cases where persistent pupillary membranes contact the corneal endothelium (Figure 12.42). As with dogs, these lesions may become more apparent over time if stromal oedema and fibrosis ensues. In addition, cats with lysosomal storage diseases, such as mannosidosis, gangliosidosis and mucopolysaccharidosis, may be affected by progressive opacification of the cornea as well as neurological disease.

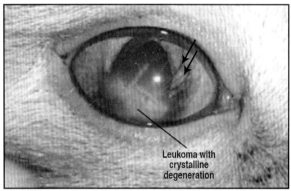

Leukoma with crystalline degeneration

12.42 Persistent pupillary membrane strands (arrowed) attaching to the posterior cornea in a cat, resulting in permanent, focal corneal opacity.

Non-developmental causes of progressive corneal opacification have also been reported in the cat, although they are much less common than in dogs, and the majority of these conditions cause corneal opacification through scarring. This is the case for eosinophilic keratitis, corneal sequestrum and herpetic keratitis. These conditions are covered in further detail below.

Dermoid
This condition shares many morphological similarities with its canine counterpart (see above). In the author's experience, these lesions are usually much smaller in cats than in dogs, seldom involve the cornea and may be found in a variety of locations ranging from the paralimbal bulbar conjunctiva to the bulbar surface of the third eyelid (Figure 12.43). Dermoids have been reported in Burmese cats, where an inherited basis is suspected (Christmas, 1992). As for dogs, removal of the entire lesion, including the hair follicles, via keratectomy and/or conjunctivalectomy is the treatment of choice.

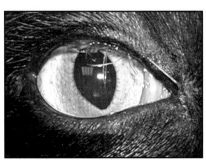

12.43

A conjunctival dermoid hidden under the upper eyelid of a cat is producing long hairs that irritate the ocular surface.

Acquired abnormalities

Ulcerative and non-ulcerative keratitis

The aetiopathogenesis of ulcerative keratitis in this species is similar to that in the dog. However, corneal ulcers secondary to adnexal, eyelid or lacrimal disease are seen less frequently in cats than in dogs. Although less common than in dogs, conditions such as distichiasis are likely to lead to keratitis in cats (Figure 12.44) and this may be ulcerative in some cases. Primary infectious agents (in particular, FHV-1) are a much more common cause of corneal ulceration in cats. Corneal sequestrum formation is also a significant cause of feline ulcerative keratitis. In addition, ulcerative keratitis may be seen accompanying upper eyelid agenesis (see Chapter 9) and eosinophilic keratitis. Conditions associated with feline ulcerative keratitis are given in Figure 12.45.

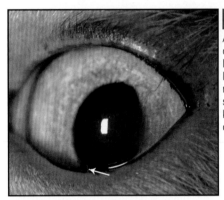

12.44 A single distichiasis lash in the lower eyelid, resulting in superficial keratitis in this cat.

Condition	Comments
Lateral lower eyelid entropion	Associated with corneal ulceration and sequestrum formation
Medial lower eyelid entropion	Brachycephalic breeds; frequently associated with sequestrum formation
Feline herpesvirus-1 (FHV-1) infection	Ulcerative keratitis; may predispose to sequestrum formation and symblepharon
Corneal sequestrum	Ulcers and various forms of chronic irritation are predisposing factors
Eosinophilic keratoconjunctivitis	Not primarily ulcerative but inflammatory plaques often appear to take up fluorescein
Keratoconjunctivitis sicca	Rare in cats; usually presumed to result from FHV-1-induced scarring of lacrimal excretory ductules secondary to severe conjunctivitis (see Chapters 10 and 11)
Trauma	Lacerations and abrasions (e.g. due to cat scratches, foreign bodies); careful assessment is needed to determine whether a penetrating injury has been sustained

12.45 Conditions commonly associated with feline ulcerative keratitis.

Treatment: The treatment of corneal ulcers in cats is as described for dogs. Generally, treatment is based on identifying and managing the specific underlying cause of the ulcer, where possible, supporting the healing process and increasing patient comfort. However, certain aspects of the treatment deserve a special mention. Surgical management of upper eyelid agenesis, entropion and corneal sequestrum is needed for resolution of ulcers related to these diseases. Medical management should take into consideration that cats are often averse to the bitter taste of many topically applied eye drops. Thus, atropine, for example, should preferably be applied as an ointment. If tolerated by the cat, gentle digital pressure on the lower eyelid at the medial canthus for a few seconds after the application of eye drops can limit this exaggerated response and systemic absorption of the drug, by occluding the lacrimal punctum.

Eyelid and adnexal disease:

Upper eyelid agenesis: This affects the upper lateral eyelid of cats and predisposes to the development of trichiasis and secondary keratitis, which can be ulcerative (see Chapter 9).

Lateral lower eyelid entropion: This may be seen spontaneously in young cats or in older cats in which weight loss is accompanied by a reduction in the retrobulbar fat volume and secondary enophthalmos. Lateral lower eyelid entropion may be associated with corneal ulceration and, as with other forms of entropion, it is exacerbated by the presence of eyelid spasm secondary to corneal pain. It is vital that any underlying sources of ocular pain are addressed.

Surgical correction with a simple Hotz–Celsus procedure may be sufficient to treat lateral lower eyelid entropion in cats. However, the condition may be associated with an overlong lower eyelid, necessitating eyelid shortening as an additional procedure (see Chapter 9 for further information). Patients with marked eyelid spasm preoperatively might suffer from recurring spasm postoperatively. This can be prevented with the use of a temporary lateral tarsorrhaphy that is left in place for 2 weeks, whilst the cornea heals with supportive medical therapy. Hotz–Celsus resection combined with permanent partial lateral tarsorrhaphy has also been described as treatment for feline lateral lower eyelid entropion (White *et al.*, 2012).

Feline herpesvirus:

In addition to causing feline upper respiratory tract disease, FHV-1 is a very common cause of conjunctivitis, and ulcerative and non-ulcerative keratitis in cats (see also Chapter 11). The virus replicates within the epithelial cells of the cornea, destroying them in the process and causing linear, branching superficial ulcers accompanied by conjunctivitis and signs of ocular pain (Figure 12.46). These linear 'dendritic' ulcers are considered pathognomonic for the condition, but are visible only in the early stages of the disease process with fluorescein or Rose Bengal stains; the former is preferred because it is less epitheliotoxic. The ulcerative process continues to give rise to larger superficial 'geographic' ulcers. FHV-1 infection is usually self-limiting and has a tendency to enter a period of quiescence in otherwise healthy cats until another episode of stress or immunosuppression

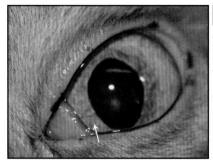

12.46

A superficial, thin, linear ulcer is seen stained with fluorescein in the cornea of this cat with active feline herpesvirus-1 infection (arrowed).

reactivates the virus. Immunocompromised patients can suffer from waxing and waning clinical signs and a high recurrence rate of ulcerative keratitis.

Some patients develop stromal keratitis, with deep corneal vascularization, haziness and pain. This is believed to be an immune-mediated response and may be recognized in the absence of demonstrable, active viral infection. Stromal keratitis is a frustrating condition that is often associated with marked recurrent ocular discomfort.

Diagnosis: The diagnosis of FHV-1 keratitis can be challenging. Plain conjunctival or corneal swabs (taken following the application of topical proxymetacaine to the ocular surface) can be sent for PCR testing (see Chapters 3 and 11). However, both false-negative results (due to insufficient sample collection or intermittent viral shedding) and false-positive results (due to viral shedding in clinically healthy cats, or detection of vaccinal virus) may occur. Before a diagnosis of FHV-1 infection can be made, other causes of ulcerative disease must be ruled out and the test results should be consistent with the clinical signs and supported by the patient's history.

Treatment: Medical treatment of FHV-1 infection can be frustrating. Anti-herpetic drugs are virostatic rather than virocidal, which means that very frequent topical applications are required. The majority of oral anti-herpetic drugs are fatal to cats. The only oral anti-herpetic drug that has been reported to be safe and effective in cats is famciclovir (Thomasy et al., 2011), which is excreted by the kidneys. There are anecdotal reports of successful outcomes over widely varying doses, but doses of 40–90 mg/kg three times daily have been shown to be safe and efficacious in published studies (Thomasy et al., 2011, 2012). The recommendation for humans with renal disease who take this drug is that the dose is adjusted accordingly, but such recommendations are not known for cats with renal disease. Although preliminary results of the effects of famciclovir in cats with FHV-1 infection seem promising, the drug is costly, and at the time of writing its use in cats is not approved and studies on the long-term effects in this species are lacking. Medical treatment of FHV-1 infection is discussed in more detail in Chapter 11.

Stromal keratitis related to FHV-1 infection is difficult to treat because the application of a topical corticosteroid will quickly reactivate the virus. The effects of topical ciclosporin on FHV-1 stromal keratitis or on viral reactivation have not been reported

to date. Other reported treatments for FHV-1 keratitis have included interferons (IFNs) and L-lysine. IFNs are virostatic immunomodulating agents produced by leucocytes during viral infections. Administered orally, they are expected to be destroyed by the conditions in the stomach and can exert their effect only if absorbed via the oropharyngeal mucosa. Despite *in vitro* studies showing the potential application of human and feline IFNs in the treatment of FHV-1 infection, a clinical study in which feline IFN-omega was applied topically in cats prior to experimental infection with FHV-1 found that there was no difference between treated and control cats in the development of the disease (Haid et al., 2007).

L-lysine is an amino acid that reportedly exerts its antiviral effect by lowering systemic levels of arginine, which inhibits viral replication. Arginine is a vital amino acid for cats and it is unclear how low its levels must be for L-lysine to exert its potential antiviral effects *in vivo*. Unfortunately, evidence shows that dietary lysine does not cause lysine–arginine antagonism in cats (Fascetti et al., 2004). Furthermore, oral administration of L-lysine to a colony of shelter cats had no effect on the incidence of upper respiratory tract or ocular disease (Drazenovich et al., 2009). The results of the controlled studies so far have shown that there is insufficient clinical or pharmacological data in favour of L-lysine or IFN to support their use, and that further controlled studies are needed.

Symblepharon: This condition is more commonly reported in cats than in dogs and develops when destruction of the epithelium of the conjunctiva and cornea allows stroma to stroma contact between the two tissues. This often leads to failure of normal corneal re-epithelialization and corneal conjunctivalization ensues. However, one important difference between dogs and cats is that the condition affects kittens at a very young age, as the development of this lesion is frequently associated with FHV-1 infection. If this infection occurs before 2 weeks of age, when the eyelids of kittens are still closed, it increases the risk of developing ophthalmia neonatorum, which is likely to lead to a more severe symblepharon that affects most if not all of the corneal surface (Figure 12.47). Fortunately symblepharon is not always symmetrical in the degree of severity and some cats may retain a transparent enough cornea in one of their eyes to provide useful vision.

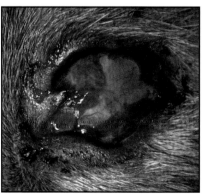

12.47

Extensive symblepharon in a cat.

Treatment: Symblepharon should be prevented if possible with early diagnosis and treatment of ophthalmia neonatorum and keratitis in young kittens. Otherwise, it may be treated surgically. However, surgical management of symblepharon is rather difficult and not usually successful due to a high rate of recurrence and scar formation. Consultation with a specialist is strongly recommended. Treatment consists of a superficial keratectomy and conjunctivectomy and supportive medical therapy. However, if there is little or no corneal limbal epithelium with regenerative capabilities, which is often the case, recurrence will rapidly develop. In addition, surgery may be complicated by extensive adhesions of the third eyelid conjunctiva to the corneal and other conjunctival surfaces, which leads to blockage of the lacrimal puncta and epiphora. Re-establishment of nasolacrimal duct flow requires reopening the puncta and temporary suture placement for a period of approximately 2 weeks.

Corneal sequestrum: This condition starts as a faint amber discoloration of the corneal stroma, which in most cases is not associated with discomfort, vascularization or ulcerative disease. Sequestra progress over a widely variable amount of time (days to months) to a darker and potentially larger and deeper plaque of denatured cornea, which elicits a vascular response and is often associated with loss of overlying epithelium and signs of ocular pain (Figures 12.48 to 12.50). Middle-aged to older cats are most commonly affected, although the condition has been documented in animals as young as 6 months of age. The cause remains unknown, although several predisposing factors have been proposed including chronic corneal irritation involving corneal surface overexposure (as seen in Persian and other brachycephalic cats), entropion, superficial grid keratotomy of ulcers, eosinophilic keratitis and, generally, a history of previous ulcerative disease or sequestrum development. FHV-1 infection has also been suggested to play a role in the development of corneal sequestra in cats.

Sequestra usually affect the central or paracentral cornea, although the location typically coincides with where irritation exerts its effects (e.g. centrally in brachycephalic cats or medially in the nasal cornea of patients with medial canthal entropion). It is worth noting that predisposed breeds might develop a sequestrum bilaterally. The nature of the discoloration remains unknown, with various authors proposing that it is pigment, iron or porphyrins (Featherstone *et al.*, 2004; Cullen *et al.*, 2005; Newkirk *et al.*, 2011). Although lighter coloured sequestra are typically expected to be more superficially located than darker ones, their depth varies from very superficial to close to full corneal thickness. Depth of corneal involvement can be very difficult to gauge, even for experienced examiners with expertise in slit-lamp biomicroscopy.

Treatment: Keratectomy is the treatment of choice for corneal sequestrum (Figure 12.51) and referral for this microsurgical procedure is strongly advised.

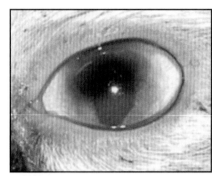

12.48 Corneal sequestrum showing brown discoloration of the left cornea.

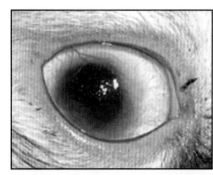

12.49 A more longstanding, dense sequestrum in the right eye of the same cat as in Figure 12.48. A dark plaque with no epithelial cover has developed.

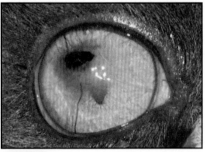

12.50 A dense black plaque is visible with this advanced, though small, corneal sequestrum, which has elicited a prominent vascular response.

Following this procedure, placement of a conjunctival pedicle graft or a corneoconjunctival transposition graft may be undertaken. Surgery should ideally be performed early in the course of disease, before the lesion becomes larger, deeper or more painful. Additional supportive medical therapy is as for other ulcerative diseases of the cornea and, in brachycephalic breeds, may include the long-term use of a viscous artificial tear preparation (ideally preservative free) 2–3 times daily to palliate the potential effects of central corneal overexposure.

Owners should be made aware of the potential for sequestrum recurrence postoperatively, with reported rates of 12% up to 38% (the latter in cases where an incomplete keratectomy was performed) (Featherstone and Sansom, 2004). It has been proposed that in order to reduce the recurrence rate, conjunctival pedicle grafts should not be transected postoperatively and that the use of conjunctival pedicle grafts and corneoconjunctival transposition grafts, which enhance the vascularity of the keratectomy site, are preferable to other grafting techniques. In addition, it is also important that potential underlying causes and contributing factors, such as entropion, are identified and treated.

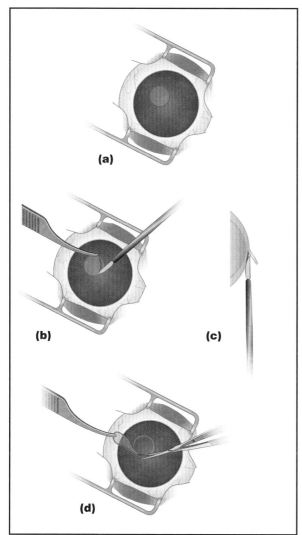

12.51 Lamellar keratectomy may be superficial or deep. Deep keratectomy requires tectonic support of the cornea and therefore grafting is recommended. Generally, keratectomy should be as superficial as possible, whilst at the same time attempting to remove the entirety of the lesion. The procedure should be performed with the aid of an operating microscope. **(a–b)** A partial thickness incision is made around the sequestrum with a diamond knife, beaver blade or a restricted depth blade. The edge of the lesion is then grasped with corneal forceps and either a lamellar dissector, beaver blade or diamond knife is used in a sweeping motion to undermine it at the required depth. **(c)** The surgeon must ensure that the corneal curvature is followed during the lamellar dissection so as not to progressively undermine the lesion at a much deeper level than intended and risk perforation. **(d)** Once the lesion has been completely undermined, resection of the undermined flap can be completed with corneal scissors.

Feline keratoconjunctivitis sicca: This disease is not as well documented in cats as it is in dogs, possibly owing to a much lower prevalence in the feline species or because the disease is overlooked due to its more subtle presentation in cats. KCS, as well as qualitative tear film disorders, is most often seen as a complication of FHV-1 infection in cats. KCS should be considered as a potential contributing factor in any cat presented with keratitis (Lim *et al.*, 2009; Martin, 2010) (see Chapter 10).

Treatment: Dry eyes generally benefit from supportive medical therapy with the use of viscous artificial tear preparations (preservative free, if possible) (see Chapter 10). Underlying FHV-1 infections should be addressed appropriately (see Chapter 11).

Superficial chronic corneal epithelial defects: These are persistent superficial ulcers that occur in one or both eyes and, although less common in cats than in dogs, have a similar clinical presentation and might have a similar aetiopathogenesis to SCCEDs in dogs (see above). The ulcers present as a rim of loose epithelium surrounding the denuded superficial stroma. Fluorescein aids the diagnosis as it highlights the exposed stroma and travels under the loose epithelium (Figure 12.52).

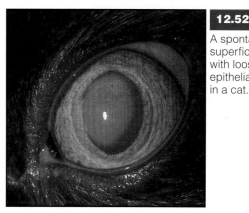

12.52 A spontaneous superficial ulcer with loose epithelial edges in a cat.

Treatment: As with dogs, the treatment options described for this type of ulcer include medical supportive therapy and debridement of loose epithelial tissue. A study by La Croix *et al.* (2001) found that besides a slower healing rate, patients that had undergone superficial grid keratotomy were more likely to develop corneal sequestrum. Based on these findings, superficial grid keratotomy or punctate keratotomy is generally considered to be contraindicated in cats.

Infectious keratitis: Aside from FHV-1, most other infectious organisms (bacterial and fungal) are secondary opportunistic pathogens of the traumatized or weakened cornea. There are very few infectious agents that are primary corneal pathogens. Keratitis secondary to fungal organisms has rarely been described in cats (Tofflemire and Betbeze, 2010).

Eosinophilic keratitis: This condition is believed to be immune-mediated in origin, based on cytology and response to treatment. A connection between FHV-1 and eosinophilic keratitis has also been suggested (Nasisse *et al.*, 1998). The typical cellular infiltrate comprises neutrophils, lymphocytes and plasma cells, as well as clusters of eosinophils. The latter may be largely outnumbered by other cell types in some cases, which highlights the importance of a thorough and systematic evaluation of the cytology slide. The corneal lesion typically comprises multiple, white to pale pink, slightly elevated spots that range between 0.5 and 2 mm in diameter. These small lesions may take up fluorescein and can coalesce to form a slightly raised plaque (Figures 12.53 and 12.54).

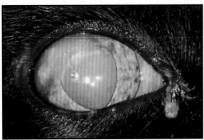

12.53

Eosinophilic keratitis in a cat.

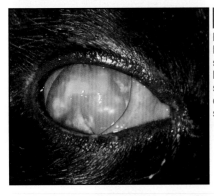

12.54

Eosinophilic lesions in the same cat as in Figure 12.50 showing uptake of fluorescein stain.

The lesion has a tendency to appear first in the superio-temporal paralimbal cornea and conjunctiva, and is accompanied by a vascular response as well as a variable amount of mucoid discharge and discomfort. As the lesion progresses centrally, so does the vascular response, patient discomfort and ocular discharge. Cats may be affected unilaterally or bilaterally, and in patients affected bilaterally the disease process may be far more advanced in one of the eyes. Patients that appear to be affected unilaterally should have the eye that appears healthy carefully examined. Diagnosis is based on lesion morphology and the presence of eosinophils on cytology. This is later confirmed with the response to treatment. Eosinophilic conjunctivitis without keratitis has been reported (Allgoewer *et al.*, 2001), but this is less commonly encountered than keratoconjunctivitis.

Treatment: The treatment for eosinophilic conjunctivitis and proliferative keratitis is as for eosinophilic keratoconjunctivitis. It consists of the topical application of a corticosteroid, such as dexamethasone phosphate 1%. High frequency dosing, such as 4–6 times daily, may be required for the first 7–10 days. After this time, applications may be slowly reduced over a period of 6–8 weeks to a maintenance dose, at which there is no recurrence of clinical signs, such as once daily or every other day applications. Maintenance dosing may be required for long periods of time, if not for life, because recurrence is often associated with too rapid a reduction of the topical medication or its early withdrawal. Topical ciclosporin has also been advocated as a successful treatment for eosinophilic keratoconjunctivitis

(Spiess *et al.*, 2009). However, some cats may find it irritating and will not tolerate it well for frequent or long-term use.

The use of a topical corticosteroid may induce reactivation of a latent FHV-1 infection. Cats with eosinophilic keratoconjunctivitis that have previously been diagnosed as, or that are under suspicion of being, FHV-1 carriers should therefore receive treatment for both conditions (see Chapter 11). Alternatively, in such cases, it may be preferential to use topical ciclosporin rather than a topical corticosteroid.

A small number of cases may prove refractory to treatment with topical corticosteroid or ciclosporin treatment. If so, systemic megestrol acetate may prove effective. Although this drug has a significant number of possible side effects (including transient diabetes mellitus, mammary gland hyperplasia and neoplasia, adrenal gland cortical suppression and temperament changes), these are more commonly associated with long-term use. Nevertheless, owners should be warned about the possible adverse effects prior to instigation of this drug, and its use should be reserved for patients that do not respond to topical therapy. A typical dosage regimen is 5 mg per cat orally for 5 days, then 5 mg every second day for 1 week, then 5 mg weekly as a maintenance dose.

Pigmentary keratitis: Cats typically have very little pigment in the limbus and conjunctiva compared with dogs and, therefore, rarely develop corneal pigment, which is only mild, at most, when present. Pigment deposition may be seen in association with chronic scarring or when the conjunctiva covers part of the cornea as a result of surgery or disease (e.g. following conjunctival pedicle grafting or symblepharon formation). It should be distinguished from corneal sequestrum formation (see above).

Florida spots: This rare condition (which is not recognized in the UK) as described for dogs, also affects cats. This is a disease of unknown aetiology and without known treatment. It appears to be self-limiting and non-painful in cats.

Corneal trauma: Feline corneal trauma may be blunt or sharp, penetrating, non-penetrating or chemically induced. Most of the aspects of traumatic injury described in the section dedicated to dogs apply to cats. Although the feline cornea may show a remarkable ability to regain clarity after injury, prompt, appropriate therapy is necessary to limit progressive corneal disease. In addition, corneal trauma in cats appears to predispose to sequestrum development. Cats that have sustained penetrating injuries, particularly cat scratches, may develop severe inflammation due to lens trauma. They should also be monitored long-term for the development of post-traumatic sarcoma (see Chapters 13, 14 and 16).

Lipid and calcium keratopathies: Secondary infiltration of the cornea in cats with lipid and/or calcium is uncommon and usually secondary to injury or disease. Dystrophic (primary) infiltration as described in the dog has not been reported in the cat.

Acute bullous keratopathy: This is a rapidly developing condition of the feline cornea, which can occur in cats of any age. It occurs when there is a sudden onset of stromal oedema and accumulation of fluid in the corneal stroma, leading to rapid and dramatic deformation of the cornea (Figure 12.55). The cause is unknown, although some affected cats have a history of systemic or topical corticosteroid use. In humans, the condition is associated with tears in Descemet's membrane, but these have not yet been identified in cats. The condition is usually unilateral but can be bilateral in some cases.

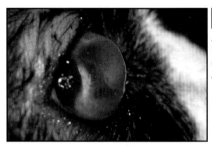

12.55

Acute bullous keratopathy in a cat. (Courtesy of J Mould)

Treatment: In the absence of large-scale studies on the treatment and follow-up of patients with acute bullous keratopathy, the most appropriate treatment has yet to be defined for feline patients. While conservative medical management is advocated in human patients with corneal hydrops, anecdotal evidence seems to suggest that early surgical treatment (including third eyelid flap or conjunctival pedicle grafting) may be of benefit (Allgoewer, 2012).

Neuroparalytic and neurotrophic keratopathies: The signs, aetiology and treatment of these conditions in cats are similar to those described in dogs (see above and Chapter 19).

Corneal masses

Epithelial inclusion cysts: The lesion in cats is very similar to that seen in dogs. The aetiopathogenesis is believed to be the same and the treatment, as for dogs, involves complete surgical excision.

Neoplasia: Tumours of the cornea in cats are rare. Primary haemangiosarcoma of the cornea of a cat has been described on its own, as well as in conjunction with a squamous cell carcinoma (Perlmann *et al.*, 2010; Cazalot *et al.*, 2011). Masses that develop near the limbus might affect the cornea and include dermoid, limbal melanocytoma, granulation tissue response and staphyloma (see Chapter 13).

References and further reading

Alfonso K, Kenyon KR, D'Amico DJ *et al.* (1988) Effects of gentamicin on healing of transdifferentiating conjunctival epithelium in rabbit eyes. *American Journal of Ophthalmology* **105**(2), 98–202

Allgoewer I (2012) Feline bullous keratopathy – a case series. *Proceedings of the European College of Veterinary Ophthalmologists*, p. 37. Trieste, Italy

Allgoewer I and Hoecht S (2010) Radiotherapy for canine chronic superficial keratitis using soft X-rays (15 kV). *Veterinary Ophthalmology* **13**(1), 20–25

Allgoewer I, McLellan GJ and Agarwal S (2010) A keratoprosthesis prototype for the dog. *Veterinary Ophthalmology* **13**(1), 47–52

Allgoewer I, Schäffer EH, Stockhaus C *et al.* (2001) Feline eosinophilic conjunctivitis. *Veterinary Ophthalmology* **4**(1), 69–74

Andrew SE, Tou S and Brooks DE (2001) Corneoconjunctival transposition for the treatment of feline corneal sequestra: a retrospective study of 17 cases (1990–1998). *Veterinary Ophthalmology* **4**(2), 107–111

Barnett PM, Scagliotti RH, Merideth RE *et al.* (1991) Absolute corneal sensitivity and corneal trigeminal nerve anatomy in normal dogs. *Progress in Veterinary and Comparative Ophthalmology* **1**, 245–254

Bedford PG and Longstaffe JA (1979) Corneal pannus (chronic superficial keratitis) in the German Shepherd Dog. *Journal of Small Animal Practice* **20**, 41–56

Befanis P, Peiffer R and Brown D (1981) Endothelial repair of the canine cornea. *American Journal of Veterinary Research* **42**, 590–595

Bentley E, Abrams GA, Covitz D *et al.* (2001) Morphology and immunohistochemistry of spontaneous chronic corneal epithelial defects (SCCED) in dogs. *Investigative Ophthalmology and Visual Science* **42**, 2262–2269

Bentley E and Murphy CJ (2004) Thermal cautery of the cornea for treatment of spontaneous chronic corneal epithelial defects in dogs and horses. *Journal of the American Veterinary Medical Association* **224**(2), 250–253

Binder DR, Sugrue JE and Herring IP (2011) Acremonium keratomycosis in a cat. *Veterinary Ophthalmology* **14**(S1), 111–116

Blocker T and van der Woerdt A (2001) A comparison of corneal sensitivity between brachycephalic and domestic short-haired cats. *Veterinary Ophthalmology* **4**(2), 127–130

Bouhanna L, Liscoët LB and Raymond-Letron I (2008) Corneal stromal sequestration in a dog. *Veterinary Ophthalmology* **11**(4), 211–214

Bromberg NM (2002) Cyanoacrylate tissue adhesive for treatment of refractory corneal ulceration. *Veterinary Ophthalmology* **5**(1), 55–60

Cazalot G, Regnier A, Deviers A *et al.* (2011) Corneal hemangiosarcoma in a cat. *Veterinary Ophthalmology* **14**, 117–121

Chan-Ling T (1989) Sensitivity and neural organization of the cat cornea. *Investigative Ophthalmology and Visual Science* **30**, 1075–1082

Christmas R (1992) Surgical correction of congenital ocular and nasal dermoids and third eyelid gland prolapse in related Burmese kittens. *Canadian Veterinary Journal* **33**, 265–266

Ciaramella P, Oliva G, Luna RD *et al.* (1997) A retrospective clinical study of canine leishmaniasis in 150 dogs naturally infected by *Leishmania infantum*. *Veterinary Record* **141**(21), 539–543

Clark JS, Bentley E and Smith LJ (2011) Evaluation of topical nalbuphine or oral tramadol as analgesics for corneal pain in dogs: a pilot study. *Veterinary Ophthalmology* **14**(6), 358–364

Cook SC (2007) Ocular embryology and congenital malformations. In: *Veterinary Ophthalmology*, 4th edn, ed. KN Gelatt, pp. 3–36. Blackwell Publishing, Iowa

Cooley PL and Dice PF 2nd (1990) Corneal dystrophy in the dog and cat. *Veterinary Clinics of North America: Small Animal Practice* **20**(3), 681–692

Crispin S (2002) Ocular lipid deposition and hyperlipoproteinaemia. *Progress in Retinal and Eye Research* **21**, 169–224

Cullen CL, Wadowska DW, Singh A *et al.* (2005) Ultrastructural findings in feline corneal sequestra. *Veterinary Ophthalmology* **8**, 295–303

Delgado E (2012) Symblepharon secondary to ophthalmomyiasis externa in a dog. *Veterinary Ophthalmology* **15**, 200–205

Denk N, Fritsche J and Reese S (2011) The effect of UV-blocking contact lenses as a therapy for canine chronic superficial keratitis. *Veterinary Ophthalmology* **14**, 186–194

Drazenovich TL, Fascetti AJ, Westermeyer HD *et al.* (2009) Effects of dietary lysine supplementation on upper respiratory and ocular disease and detection of infectious organisms in cats within an animal shelter. *American Journal of Veterinary Research* **70**(11), 1391–1400

Dreyfus J, Schobert CS and Dubielzig RR (2011) Superficial corneal squamous cell carcinoma occurring in dogs with chronic keratitis. *Veterinary Ophthalmology* **14**(3), 161–168

Fascetti AJ, Maggs DJ, Kanchuk ML *et al.* (2004) Excess dietary lysine does not cause lysine–arginine antagonism in adult cats. *Journal of Nutrition* **134**(8), 2042S–2045S

Featherstone HJ, Franklin VJ and Sansom J (2004) Feline corneal sequestrum: laboratory analysis of ocular samples from 12 cats. *Veterinary Ophthalmology* **7**, 229–238

Featherstone HJ and Sansom J (2004) Feline corneal sequestra: a review of 64 cases (80 eyes) from 1993 to 2000. *Veterinary Ophthalmology* **7**(4), 213–227

Filipec M, Phan MT, Zhao TZ *et al.* (1992) Topical cyclosporin A and corneal wound healing. *Cornea* **11**(6), 546–553

Flach AJ (2001) Corneal melts associated with topically applied non-steroidal anti-inflammatory drugs. *Transactions of the American Ophthalmological Society* **99**, 205–210

Galle LE (2004) Antiviral therapy for ocular viral disease. *Veterinary Clinics of North America: Small Animal Practice* **34**, 639–653

Garcia da Silva E, Powell CC, Gionfriddo JR *et al.* (2011) Histologic evaluation of the immediate effects of diamond burr debridement in experimental superficial corneal wounds in dogs. *Veterinary Ophthalmology* **14**(5), 285–291

Gilger BC (2007) Diseases and surgery of the canine cornea and sclera. In: *Veterinary Ophthalmology, 4th edn*, ed. KN Gelatt, pp. 690–752. Blackwell Publishing, Iowa

Gilger BC (2008) Immunology of the ocular surface. *Veterinary Clinics of North America: Small Animal Practice* **38**, 223–231

Gipson IK (2004) Distribution of mucins at the ocular surface. *Experimental Eye Research* **78**(3), 379–388

Good KL, Maggs DJ, Hollingsworth SR *et al.* (2003) Corneal sensitivity in dogs with diabetes mellitus. *American Journal of Veterinary Research* **64**(1), 7–11

Gosling AA, Labelle AL and Breaux CB (2013) Management of spontaneous chronic corneal epithelial defects (SCCEDs) in dogs with diamond burr debridement and placement of a bandage contact lens. *Veterinary Ophthalmology* **16**(2), 83–88

Grinninger P, Verbruggen AMJ, Kraijer-Huver IMG *et al.* (2012) Use of bandage contact lenses (Acrivet Pat D) for treatment of spontaneous chronic corneal epithelial defects (SCCED) in dogs. *Abstract No.7 ECVO Congress, Trieste, Italy*

Grundon RA, O'Reilly A, Muhlnickel C *et al.* (2010) Keratomycosis in a dog treated with topical 1% voriconazole solution. *Veterinary Ophthalmology* **13**(5), 331–335

Gum GG, Gelatt KN and Esson DW (2007) Physiology of the eye. In: *Veterinary Ophthalmology, 4th edn*, ed. KN Gelatt, pp. 149–182. Blackwell Publishing, Iowa

Haber M, Cao Z, Panjwani N *et al.* (2003) Effects of growth factors (EGF, PDGF-BB and TGF-β1) on cultured equine epithelial cells and keratocytes: implications for wound healing. *Veterinary Ophthalmology* **6**(3), 211–219

Hacker D (1991) Frozen corneal grafts in dogs and cats a report of 19 cases. *Journal of the American Animal Hospital Association* **27**, 387–398

Haeussler DJ, Munoz Rodriguez L, Wilkie DA *et al.* (2011) Primary central corneal hemangiosarcoma in a dog. *Veterinary Ophthalmology* **14**, 133–136

Haid C, Kaps S, Gönczi E *et al.* (2007) Pre-treatment with feline interferon omega and the course of subsequent infection with feline herpesvirus in cats. *Veterinary Ophthalmology* **10**(5), 278–284

Hakanson N and Merideth RE (1987) Conjunctival pedicle grafting in the treatment of corneal ulcers in the dog and cat. *Journal of the American Animal Hospital Association* **23**, 641–648

Hansen A and Guandalini A (1999) A retrospective study of 30 cases of frozen lamellar corneal graft in dogs and cats. *Veterinary Ophthalmology* **2**, 233–241

Heigle TJ and Pflugfelder SC (1996) Aqueous tear production in patients with neurotrophic keratitis. *Cornea* **15**(2), 135–138

Hirst LW, Fogle JA, Kenyon KR *et al.* (1982) Corneal epithelial regeneration and adhesion following acid burns in the rhesus monkey. *Investigative Ophthalmology and Visual Science* **23**(6), 764–773

Isard PF, Dulaurent T and Regnier A (2010) Keratoprosthesis with retrocorneal fixation: preliminary results in dogs with corneal blindness. *Veterinary Ophthalmology* **13**(5), 279–288

Khodadoust AA, Silverstein AM, Kenyon DR *et al.* (1968) Adhesion of regenerating corneal epithelium: the role of basement membrane. *American Journal of Ophthalmology* **65**(3), 339–348

La Croix NC, van der Woerdt A and Olivero DK (2001) Non-healing corneal ulcers in cats: 29 cases (1991–1999). *Journal of the American Veterinary Medical Association* **218**(5), 733–735

Labelle AL, Dresser CB, Hamor RE, Allender MC and Disney JL (2013) Characteristics of, prevalence of, and risk factors for corneal pigmentation (pigmentary keratopathy) in Pugs. *Journal of the American Veterinary Medical Association* **243**(5), 667–674

Landshamn N, Solomon A and Belkin M (1989) Cell division in the healing of the corneal endothelium in cats. *Archives of Ophthalmology* **107**, 1804–1808

Ledbetter EC, Kim SG and Dubovi EJ (2009) Outbreak of ocular disease associated with naturally acquired canine herpesvirus-1 infection in a closed domestic dog colony. *Veterinary Ophthalmology* **12**(4), 242–247

Ledbetter EC, Riis RC, Kern TJ *et al.* (2006) Corneal ulceration associated with naturally occurring canine herpesvirus-1 infection in two adult dogs. *Journal of the American Veterinary Medical Association* **229**(3), 376–384

Lewin GA (1999) Repair of a full thickness corneoscleral defect in a German Shepherd Dog using porcine small intestinal submucosa. *Journal of Small Animal Practice* **40**, 340–342

Lim CC, Reilly CM, Thomasy SM *et al.* (2009) Effects of feline herpesvirus type 1 on tear film break-up time, Schirmer tear test results, and conjunctival goblet cell density in experimentally infected cats. *American Journal of Veterinary Research* **70**, 394–403

Lin CP and Boehnke M (2000) Effect of fortified antibiotic solutions on corneal epithelial wound healing. *Cornea* **19**(2), 204–206

Maggs DJ and Clarke HE (2005) Relative sensitivity of polymerase chain reaction assays used for detection of feline herpesvirus type 1 DNA in clinical samples and commercial vaccines. *American Journal of Veterinary Research* **66**(9), 1550–1555

Maggs DJ, Nasisse MP and Kass PH (2003) Efficacy of oral supplementation with L-lysine in cats latently infected with feline herpesvirus. *American Journal of Veterinary Research* **64**(1), 37–42

Mallari PTL, McCarty DJ, Daniell M and Taylor H (2001) Increased incidence of corneal perforation after topical fluoroquinolone treatment for microbial keratitis. *American Journal of Ophthalmology* **131**(1), 131–133

Marfurt C, Murphy C and Florczak J (2001) Morphology and neurochemistry of canine corneal innervation. *Investigative Ophthalmology and Visual Science* **42**, 2242–2251

Marlar A, Miller P, Canton D *et al.* (1994) Canine keratomycosis: a report of eight cases and literature review. *Journal of the American Animal Hospital Association* **30**, 331–340

Martin CL (2010) Lacrimal system. In: *Ophthalmic Diseases in Veterinary Medicine*, ed. CL Martin, pp. 219–240. Manson Publishing Ltd, London

Matas M, Donaldson D and Newton RJ (2012) Intracorneal hemorrhages in 19 dogs (22 eyes) from 2000–2010: a retrospective study. *Veterinary Ophthalmology* **15**(2), 86–91

Michau TM, Gilger BC, Maggio F *et al.* (2003) Use of thermokeratoplasty for treatment of ulcerative keratitis and bullous keratopathy secondary to corneal endothelial disease in dogs: 13 cases (1994–2001). *Journal of the American Veterinary Medical Association* **222**, 607–612

Montiani-Ferreira F, Petersen-Jones S, Cassotis N *et al.* (2003) Early postnatal development of central corneal thickness in dogs. *Veterinary Ophthalmology* **6**(1), 19–22

Moodie KL, Hashizume N, Houston DL *et al.* (2001) Postnatal development of corneal curvature and thickness in the cat. *Veterinary Ophthalmology* **4**(4), 267–272

Morgan RV (1994) Feline corneal sequestration: a retrospective study of 42 cases (1987–1991). *Journal of the American Animal Hospital Association* **30**, 24–28

Morgan RV and Abrams K (1994) A comparison of six different therapies for persistent corneal erosions in dogs and cats. *Veterinary and Comparative Ophthalmology* **4**, 38–43

Morishige N, Komatsubara T, Chikama T *et al.* (1999) Direct observation of corneal nerve fibres in neurotrophic keratopathy by confocal biomicroscopy. *Lancet* **354**, 1613–1614

Nagasaki T and Zhao J (2003) Centripetal movement of corneal epithelial cells in the normal adult mouse. *Investigative Ophthalmology and Visual Science* **44**(22), 558–566

Nasisse MP (1990) Feline herpesvirus ocular disease. *Veterinary Clinics of North America: Small Animal Practice* **20**, 667–680

Nasisse MP, Glover T, Moore C *et al.* (1998) Detection of feline herpesvirus-1 DNA in corneas of cats with eosinophilic keratitis or corneal sequestrum. *American Journal of Veterinary Research* **59**, 856–858

Nasisse MP, Halenda RM and Luo H (1996) Efficacy of low dose oral, natural human interferon alpha in acute feline herpesvirus-1 (FHV-1) infection: a preliminary dose determination. *Proceedings of the 1996 Annual Meeting of the American College of Veterinary Ophthalmologists*, p. 79. Newport, Rhode Island

Newkirk KM, Hendrix DVH and Keller RL (2011) Porphyrins are not present in feline ocular tissues or corneal sequestra. *Veterinary Ophthalmology* **14**(S1), 2–4

Ofri R (2007) Optics and physiology of vision. In: *Veterinary Ophthalmology, 4th edn*, ed. KN Gelatt, pp. 183–219. Blackwell Publishing, Iowa

Okada Y, Reinach PS, Kitano A *et al.* (2010) Neurotrophic keratopathy: its pathophysiology and treatment. *Histology and Histopathology* **25**, 771–780

Ollivier FJ, Brooks DE, Van Setten GB *et al.* (2004) Profiles of matrix metalloproteinase activity in equine tear fluid during corneal healing in 10 horses with ulcerative keratitis. *Veterinary Ophthalmology* **7**, 397–405

Parshal CJ (1973) Lamellar corneal–scleral transposition. *Journal of the American Animal Hospital Association* **9**, 270–277

Peña MT, Naranjo C, Klauss G *et al.* (2008) Histopathological features of ocular leishmaniosis in the dog. *Journal of Comparative Pathology* **138**(1), 32–39

Perlmann E, da Silva EG, Guedes PM *et al.* (2010) Co-existing squamous cell carcinoma and hemangioma on the ocular surface of a cat. *Veterinary Ophthalmology* **13**, 63–66

Pot SA, Gallhofer NS, Walser-Reinhardt L, Hafezi F and Spiess BM (2013) Treatment of bullous keratopathy with corneal collagen cross-linking in two dogs. *Veterinary Ophthalmology* doi: 10.1111/

vop.12137

Prasse K and Winston SM (1996) Cytology and histopathology of feline eosinophilic keratitis. *Veterinary and Comparative Ophthalmology* **6**, 74–81

Rampazzo A, Euler C, Speier S *et al.* (2006) Scleral rupture in dogs, cats and horses. *Veterinary Ophthalmology* **9**(3), 149–155

Rodrigues GN, Laus JL, Santos JM *et al.* (2006) Corneal endothelial cell morphology of normal dogs of different ages. *Veterinary Ophthalmology* **9**(2), 101–107

Saito A and Kotani T (1999) Tear production in dogs with epiphora and corneal epitheliopathy. *Veterinary Ophthalmology* **2**, 173–178

Samuelson DA (2007) Ophthalmic anatomy. In: *Veterinary Ophthalmology, 4th edn*, ed. KN Gelatt, pp. 37–148. Blackwell Publishing, Iowa

Sanchez RF, Innocent G, Mould J *et al.* (2007) Canine keratoconjunctivitis sicca: disease trends in a review of 229 cases. *Journal of Small Animal Practice* **48**, 211–217

Sandmeyer LS, Keller CB and Bienzle D (2005) Effects of interferon-alpha on cytopathic changes and titers for feline herpesvirus-1 in primary cultures of feline corneal epithelial cells. *American Journal of Veterinary Research* **66**(2), 210–216

Sansom J and Blunden T (2010) Calcareous degeneration of the canine cornea. *Veterinary Ophthalmology* **13**(4), 238–243

Secker GA and Daniels JT (2009) Limbal epithelial stem cells of the cornea. In: *The Stem Cell Research Community*, StemBook, doi/10.3824/stembook.1.48.1, StemBook, ed. http://www.stembook.org.

Siebeck N, Hurley DJ, Garcia M *et al.* (2006) Effects of human recombinant alpha-2b interferon and feline recombinant omega interferon on *in vitro* replication of feline herpesvirus-1. *Journal of Veterinary Research* **67**(8), 1406–1411

Spiess AK, Sapienza JS and Mayordomo A (2009) Treatment of proliferative feline eosinophilic keratitis with topical 1.5% cyclosporine: 35 cases. *Veterinary Ophthalmology* **12**(2), 132–137

Stanley RG, Hardman C and Johnson BW (1998) Results of grid keratotomy, superficial keratectomy and debridement for the management of persistent corneal erosions in 92 dogs. *Veterinary Ophthalmology* **1**(4), 233–238

Stiles J, McDermott M, Bigsby D *et al.* (1997) Use of nested polymerase chain reaction to identify feline herpesvirus in ocular tissue from clinically normal cats and cats with corneal sequestra or conjunctivitis. *American Journal of Veterinary Research* **58**, 338–342

Stiles J and Pogranichniy R (2008) Detection of virulent feline herpesvirus-1 in the corneas of clinically normal cats. *Journal of Feline Medicine and Surgery* **10**(2), 154–159

Suzuki K, Saito J, Yanai R *et al.* (2003) Cell–matrix and cell–cell interactions during corneal epithelial wound healing. *Progress in Retinal and Eye Research* **22**, 113–133

Takiyama N, Terasaki E and Uechi M (2010) Corneal squamous cell carcinoma in two dogs. *Veterinary Ophthalmology* **13**(4), 266–269

Thomasy SM, Covert JC, Stanley SD and Maggs DJ (2012) Pharmacokinetics of famciclovir and penciclovir in tears following oral administration of famciclovir to cats: a pilot study. *Veterinary Ophthalmology* **15**(5), 299–306

Thomasy SM, Lim CC, Reilly CM *et al.* (2011) Evaluation of orally administered famciclovir in cats experimentally infected with feline herpesvirus type-1. *American Journal of Veterinary Research* **72**(1), 85–95

Tofflemire K and Betbeze C (2010) Three cases of feline ocular coccidioidomycosis: presentation, clinical features, diagnosis and treatment. *Veterinary Ophthalmology* **13**(3), 166–172

Tripathi RC, Raja SC and Tripathi BJ (1990) Prospects for epidermal growth factor in the management of corneal disorders. *Survey of Ophthalmology* **34**(6), 457–462

Van Horn D, Sendele D, Seideman S *et al.* (1997) Regenerative capacity of the corneal endothelium in rabbits and cats. *Investigative Ophthalmology and Visual Science* **16**, 597–613

Vanore M, Chahory S, Payen G and Clerc B (2007) Surgical repair of deep melting ulcers with porcine small intestinal submucosa (SIS) graft in dogs and cats. *Veterinary Ophthalmology* **10**(2), 93–99

Watté CM, Elks R, Moore DL and McLellan GJ (2014) Clinical experience with butyl-2-cyanoacrylate adhesive in the management of canine and feline corneal disease. *Veterinary Ophthalmology* **7**(5), 319–326

White JS, Grundon RA, Hardman C, O'Reilly A and Stanley RG (2012) Surgical management and outcome of lower eyelid entropion in 124 cats. *Veterinary Ophthalmology* **15**, 231–235

Whitley RD and Gilger BC (1999) Diseases of the canine cornea and sclera. In: *Veterinary Ophthalmology, 3rd edn*, ed. KN Gelatt, pp. 635–673. Lippincott Williams and Wilkins, Baltimore

Yamada N, Janai R, Inui M *et al.* (2005) Sensitizing effect of substance P on corneal epithelial migration induced by IGF-1, fibronectin or interleukin-6. *Investigative Ophthalmology and Visual Science* **46**(3), 833–839

13

The sclera, episclera and limbus

Natasha Mitchell

Anatomy and physiology

The cornea and sclera together comprise the dense fibrous tunic of the globe. Structurally, the sclera is similar to the cornea but it is not transparent because the scleral collagen fibres differ in diameter and shape, are not regularly spaced, and are oriented in different directions throughout the tissue. The sclera comprises an innermost layer containing mainly elastic fibres (the lamina fusca), a middle layer of dense, white fibrous tissue (the sclera proper) and an outer layer of loose connective tissue called the episclera, which forms the external boundary of the sclera. The episclera thickens anteriorly, where it blends with Tenon's capsule and the subconjunctival connective tissue towards the limbus.

The sclera is rigid and this provides resistance to intraocular fluid pressure (IOP) and maintains the globe as a sphere. It contains small channels to accommodate the long and short ciliary nerves, long posterior ciliary arteries, vortex veins and anterior ciliary vessels. It is through these channels that neoplastic or infectious disease processes can enter or leave the globe. There is also a larger sieve-like opening in the region of the exit of the optic nerve called the lamina cribosa. The intrascleral venous plexus is located in the anterior portion of the scleral stroma. It is a very important inter-connecting network of veins that receives aqueous humour from the angular aqueous plexus. It is well developed in the dog and cat, thus the anterior region is the thickest region of the sclera. In the dog and cat, the sclera is thinnest near the equator, especially at the points of insertion of the extraocular muscles, and thickest at the lamina cribosa and limbus.

The episclera is a thin collagenous and vascular tissue layer, which binds Tenon's capsule to the sclera anteriorly. Neighbouring tissues include the choroid, the cornea and conjunctiva, and these can be affected by any inflammatory process involving the sclera or episclera. The episcleral blood vessels lie beneath the superficial conjunctival vessels, and the two systems communicate. It is important to clinically distinguish hyperaemia of the conjunctival and episcleral vessels (Figures 13.1 and 13.2). Conjunctival hyperaemia may indicate conjunctivitis or keratitis, whereas episcleral hyperaemia may imply more serious intraocular disease. Congestion of the episcleral vessels occurs when venous outflow is impeded, as occurs with glaucoma or in the presence of an orbital space-occupying lesion. Uveitis also causes vascular congestion, resulting in dilatation of the episcleral vessels, which leads to the characteristic 'red eye' presentation. Due to the communication between the two systems, the conjunctival vessels become secondarily congested when the episcleral vessels are congested, but the reverse does not hold true.

Feature	Conjunctival vessels	Episcleral vessels
Position	Superficial	Deep
Width	Narrow; fine	Wide
Branching	Frequent; dichotomous	Occasional
Colour	Pink/red	Dark red
Pattern	Form loops; more tortuous; can be seen to cross the limbus if extend into adjacent cornea	Enter sclera and disappear from view just before the limbus; straight vessels
Mobility	Freely mobile	Fixed to globe
Individual vessels	Not distinct	Distinct
Response to topical 2.5% phenylephrine	Rapidly blanch	Blanch much more slowly

13.1 Distinguishing between conjunctival and episcleral blood vessels.

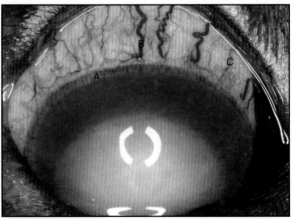

13.2 Glaucoma secondary to chronic cataractous lens luxation. There is a circumlimbal brush-border of blood vessels (A). The congested episcleral blood vessels (B) are very prominent. Conjunctival blood vessels (C) are much narrower.

The cornea and sclera merge in a transitional zone called the corneoscleral limbus. The limbus is usually clearly defined as a narrow pigmented region (Figure 13.3). The limbus contains the pluripotent limbal epithelium stem cells, which are essential for the health of the ocular surface because they amplify, proliferate and differentiate into corneal epithelium. These cells also act as a physiological barrier to the ingress of conjunctival cells across the cornea. Dysfunction (e.g. in some cases of multiple ocular defects) or destruction (resulting from chemical, thermal or inflammatory insults) of this stem cell 'barrier' at the limbus can lead to 'conjunctivalization' of the cornea (Figure 13.4).

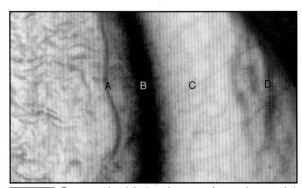

13.3 Corneoscleral limbus in a cat. A = major arterial circle of the iris; B = pigmented limbus; C = conjunctival blood vessels; D = deep scleral vessels.

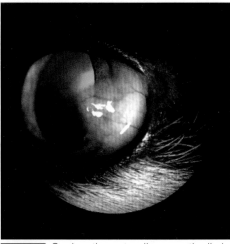

13.4 Conjunctiva extending over the limbus on to the cornea ('conjunctivalization' of the cornea) following a corneal/limbal injury in a 3-year-old Domestic Shorthaired cat. (Courtesy of D Gould)

Investigation of disease

Investigation of scleral, episcleral and limbal disease starts with a thorough clinical examination, assessing for evidence of trauma, tumour metastasis and signs of systemic disease. Only the most anterior aspect of the sclera and episclera may be visualized on a routine ocular examination, and these tissues lie beneath a layer of translucent bulbar conjunctiva. During fundus examination, it is not normally possible to see the sclera because the pigmented layers of the retina and choroid lie internal

to the sclera. However, in subalbinotic dogs and cats it may be possible to visualize the white innermost lamina fusca layer of the sclera behind the transparent retina and between the overlying spoke-like choroidal blood vessels.

Increased 'scleral show' may be present if there is a macropalpebral fissure, exophthalmos, proptosis, strabismus, microphthalmos or microcornea. The colour of the sclera is altered in some disease states; it may appear red if there is overlying conjunctivitis or episcleritis, yellow if the animal is jaundiced (Figure 13.5) or dark as a result of pigment accumulation (particularly if there is a melanocytic tumour or ocular melanosis). Episcleral hyperaemia or congestion may occur as a result of raised IOP, uveitis, episcleritis, scleritis, Horner's syndrome or orbital disease. Abnormal thickening may be present with episcleritis, scleritis and tumours; thinning may be present with glaucoma or staphyloma (see below). The contour may be altered if the sclera is ruptured. On fundus examination, an area may be out of focus if there is a coloboma (congenital absence of normal ocular tissue, which can affect multiple tissues including the sclera, retina and optic nerve) or scleral ectasia (thinning; see below and Figures 13.6 and 13.7).

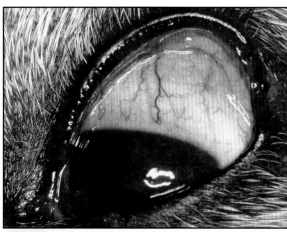

13.5 Jaundiced (icteric) sclera and conjunctivitis in a dog with leptospirosis.

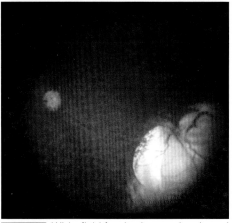

13.6 Wide-field fundus image showing a large peripheral region of scleral ectasia (equatorial staphyloma) in an Australian Shepherd with merle ocular dysgenesis. (Courtesy of NC Buyukmihci)

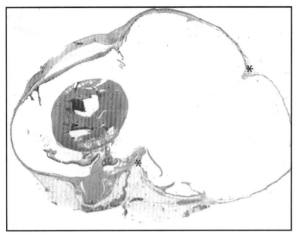

13.7 Subgross photomicrograph showing a large area of scleral outpouching (∗) in a dog with merle ocular dysgenesis. (Reproduced from Dubielzig *et al.*, 2010 with permission from the publisher)

Based on clinical and ocular findings, further diagnostic tests may be indicated, including tonometry and gonioscopy if glaucoma, melanosis or tumours are suspected. Ocular ultrasonography is useful in the diagnosis of scleral rupture. It is not always possible to image the rupture site directly, but a focal irregular contour with decreased echogenicity of the sclera in conjunction with intraocular haemorrhage is suggestive (see Chapter 2). Advanced imaging, such as magnetic resonance imaging (MRI) and computed tomography (CT), is useful in some cases (Figure 13.8).

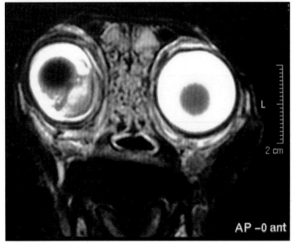

13.8 T2-weighted MR image of a cat that suffered blunt trauma showing interruption of the sclera nasally along with vitreal dislocation of the lens.

Canine conditions

Developmental abnormalities

Dermoid

An ocular dermoid (see also Chapters 11 and 12) is a congenital defect in which an island of haired skin is present in an abnormal location (e.g. on the cornea, conjunctiva or eyelids). The most common location is the temporal limbus, extending on to the

cornea. The condition may be familiar with breed predispositions noted in the Dachshund, Dalmatian, Dobermann, German Shepherd Dog, Shih Tzu and St Bernard. In cats, the Burmese breed is over-represented. Dermoids are typically circular, pigmented, raised hair-bearing areas (Figure 13.9). The presence of hair induces ocular irritation, presenting as epiphora or a mucopurulent ocular discharge and blepharospasm. The treatment of choice is surgical removal via superficial lamellar keratectomy and conjunctival resection. As the cornea is only about 0.5–0.6 mm thick, the use of an operating microscope is advised.

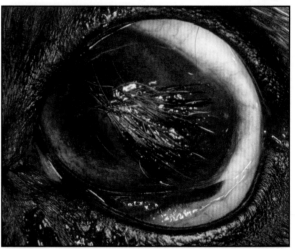

13.9 Epibulbar dermoid arising from the temporal limbus and affecting the temporal cornea in a 6-month-old crossbred collie.

Staphyloma

A staphyloma is defined as a thinned, bulging sclera with a lining of uveal tract. They occur most commonly at the posterior pole, where the optic nerve head is usually also involved, or at the equator of the globe. They may be a feature of Collie eye anomaly and Ehlers–Danlos syndrome, or form part of the multiple ocular abnormalities that occur with merle ocular dysgenesis (see Figures 13.6 and 13.7). Congenital anterior scleral staphyloma may also occur and manifests as an anteriorly protruding dark blue (due to the underlying uvea) mass with a cystic appearance. Staphyloma can be distinguished from uveal melanoma by gentle palpation (to determine the softness of the mass) and ocular ultrasonography. No treatment is indicated for posterior staphyloma. Focal anterior staphylomas may be repaired by reinforcement with a grafting procedure using a scleral autograft or xenograft, or other suitable tissue. However, this is a specialist procedure. Eyes with extensive anterior staphylomas are usually blind and, in these cases, enucleation may be indicated if the protrusion is preventing normal blinking.

Sclerocornea

Sclerocornea is a congenital, non-progressive condition in which the corneoscleral limbus is indistinct because there is extension of the sclera into the peripheral cornea (Figure 13.10). It is thought to arise from a disturbance of mesenchymal and

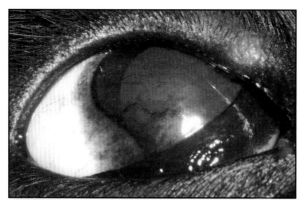

13.10 Sclerocornea in a 5-month-old English Cocker Spaniel with multiple ocular defects, including microphthalmia and persistent pupillary membrane. Note that the sclera has replaced the inferotemporal cornea.

surface ectodermal growth at the rim of the embryological optic cup. It may present in association with other congenital ocular defects and in the dog has been reported as a component of Ehlers–Danlos syndrome.

Acquired abnormalities

Inflammatory conditions

There are several inflammatory disorders that affect the episclera and sclera in dogs. These are a group of idiopathic, non-neoplastic, non-infectious diseases, which appear to represent a spectrum of disease pathology of variable but similar clinical presentation. They are considered to be immune-mediated on the basis of histological findings and the response to immunomodulatory medication. Breeds most commonly affected by episcleritis include the collie breeds, American Cocker Spaniel and Shetland Sheepdog, but any breed can be affected. Secondary episcleritis and scleritis may also occur as a result of deep fungal or bacterial ocular infection, infection with *Ehrlichia canis*, *Toxoplasma gondii*, *Leishmania* spp. or *Onchocerca* spp., systemic histiocytosis, chronic glaucoma or ocular trauma.

Episcleritis: Simple diffuse episcleritis is recognized by signs of generalized (Figure 13.11) or regional (Figure 13.12) episcleral vascular injection with thickening of the surrounding episclera. Usually, there is mild corneal oedema and peripheral neovascularization adjacent to the inflamed area. These clinical signs can be confused with glaucoma and, therefore, careful ocular examination and tonometry are indicated.

Nodular granulomatous episcleritis is the term most commonly used to describe several similar disease processes, including nodular fasciitis, fibrous histiocytoma, proliferative conjunctivitis, pseudotumour, limbal granuloma and collie granuloma. The condition presents as a unilateral or bilateral inflammatory disease, characterized by one or more discrete pink 'fleshy' nodular masses or thickened areas, most often located at the temporal limbus, in conjunction with hyperaemia of the episclera (Figure 13.13). It is common for adjacent tissues to be

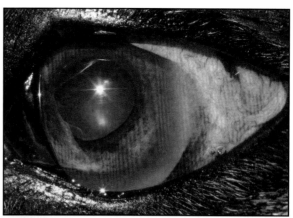

13.11 Diffuse episcleral hyperaemia associated with peripheral corneal oedema, stromal lipid deposition and neovascularization in a 5-year-old crossbred collie with generalized episcleritis.

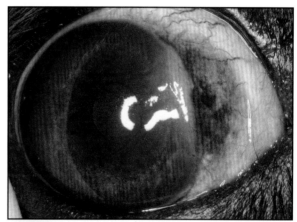

13.12 Focal thickening of the nasal episclera with extension into the adjacent cornea in a 2-year-old Cavalier King Charles Spaniel with regional episcleritis.

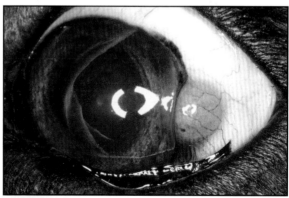

13.13 A focal nodular hyperaemic thickened region of episclera adjacent to the temporal limbus in a 4-year-old Border Collie with nodular granulomatous episcleritis.

inflamed, and additional presenting clinical signs may include any combination of conjunctivitis, keratitis, scleritis, blepharitis and chorioretinitis. The inflammation may result in lipid infiltration of the cornea (lipid keratopathy; see Chapter 12). The main differential diagnoses are the neoplastic diseases lymphoma, squamous cell carcinoma and amelanotic limbal melanoma. Thus, in some cases, biopsy is indicated.

Treatment:

- Topical corticosteroids, such as 1% prednisolone acetate or 0.1% dexamethasone, are the preferred first-line treatment. Initially, the recommended frequency of application is three to four times daily. This can be gradually reduced and, in some cases, withdrawn; although, a less frequent maintenance dose may be required to limit recurrence of the disease.
- Oral corticosteroids are indicated for cases that do not respond to topical corticosteroids alone.
- Subconjunctival or intralesional corticosteroids are administered in some situations.
- Azathioprine may be used alone or in combination with oral corticosteroids at a dose of 2 mg/kg q24h for 1 week, and then reduced to 1 mg/kg q24h for 2 weeks. Once the clinical signs have receded, the dose may be reduced to 1 mg/kg given 1–2 times weekly. Potential toxic effects include myelosuppression, hepatotoxicosis and gastrointestinal upset. Thus, routine biochemistry and haematology are indicated prior to treatment, and the blood count and liver function should be regularly monitored during treatment.
- An alternative systemic immunosuppressant is ciclosporin, administered at a dose of 5 mg/kg q24h for 30 days, possibly in conjunction with topical and oral corticosteroids. The dose may then be reduced to 2.5 mg/kg q24h or 5 mg every second day.
- Tetracycline together with niacinamide (a form of vitamin B3) may be administered orally three times a day at the recommended dose of 250 mg of each drug for animals <10 kg in bodyweight, and 500 mg of each drug for animals >10 kg in bodyweight.
- Surgical excision with lamellar keratectomy, debulking and cryosurgery, and beta radiation therapy have been used.
- If an infectious agent is identified or suspected as the causative agent (see above), specific aetiological diagnosis should be pursued and appropriate medical therapy instituted.

Scleritis: Canine scleritis is an uncommon, primary, idiopathic, immune-mediated disorder. It may present as a unilateral or bilateral condition. It may be classified as necrotizing or non-necrotizing based on the presence or absence of collagen necrosis on scleral biopsy. Non-necrotizing scleritis is a milder disease. It manifests as regional or diffuse thickening of the sclera with hyperaemia of the overlying conjunctiva and episclera. There is often ocular pain, lacrimation and photophobia, as well as involvement of the intraocular tissues. Severe or chronic disease, in particular, can lead to the involvement of the adjacent choroid and this can result in retinal detachment or chorioretinal degeneration along with vitreal exudates (Figure 13.14). Springer Spaniels and Cocker Spaniels may be predisposed.

Necrotizing scleritis is an aggressive, severe and painful disease that also affects the choroid, retina and episclera. Diagnosis may be achieved with a full

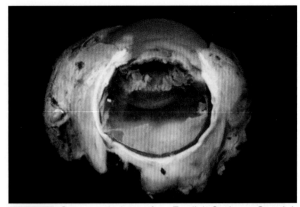

13.14 Gross pathology of an English Springer Spaniel with scleritis. There is tumour-like thickening of the episclera and sclera, extending from the limbus to the optic nerve. Note also the uveal thickening. (Courtesy of J Mould)

or partial thickness biopsy of the sclera, which can help determine the type, severity and extent of the inflammatory process. Due to the risk of globe perforation, this is a specialist procedure. Management of the condition is challenging and lifelong immunosuppression is generally required. Both inflammatory conditions are treated via systemic immunosuppression using corticosteroids or azathioprine. The overall prognosis is guarded, and the prognosis for retention of vision or the globe is poor. A systemic immune-mediated disorder may be present (Day *et al.*, 2008).

Trauma

Blunt trauma resulting in rupture of the sclera: Due to the force required to rupture the sclera, accompanying intraocular damage such as hyphaema, vitreous haemorrhage, lens luxation, lens capsule rupture, retinal detachment or protrusion of the uveal tract through the injury should also be expected (Figure 13.15). Corneal rupture is easily visualized, whereas scleral rupture can only be identified clinically if it occurs at the limbus (Figure 13.16) or if the globe is proptosed. However, many scleral ruptures in dogs and cats occur at the equator, posterior pole or close to the optic nerve (Rampazzo *et al.*, 2006; Dubielzig *et al.*, 2010). The most frequently reported clinical signs in the study

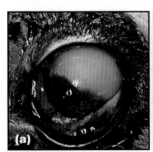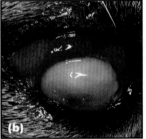

13.15 **(a)** Left and **(b)** right eye of a Labrador Retriever following a road traffic accident. (a) Note the blepharoedema, conjunctivitis, extensive corneal oedema and protrusion of the uvea through a large inferior scleral rupture at the limbus. (b) Note the blepharoedema, chemosis, conjunctivitis and pan-corneal oedema. Ultrasonography revealed rupture of the globe at the posterior pole.

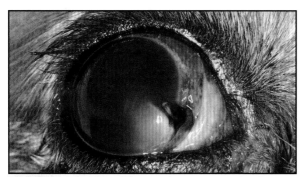

13.16 Laceration of the nasal cornea crossing the limbus to involve the adjacent sclera, resulting in protrusion of the underlying uvea, conjunctivitis and corneal oedema.

by Rampazzo *et al.* (2006) were hyphaema (80%), followed by subconjunctival bleeding (60%) and eyelid and conjunctival swelling (53%).

Assessment of the globe is facilitated by the application of topical anaesthesia. The presence of a menace response is a positive sign. In the absence of a menace response, a positive dazzle reflex indicates that there is still retinal and optic nerve function. The presence of a normal direct pupillary light reflex (PLR) does not confirm vision, but is a positive sign; absence of the PLR does not imply blindness. It is useful to check the consensual (indirect) PLR: constriction of the normal pupil when the traumatized eye is stimulated with light indicates that the retina and optic nerve are functioning. Ocular imaging is indicated if direct visualization of the intraocular structures is precluded by corneal damage, intraocular haemorrhage or lens opacity. This is especially important if surgical repair is being considered. Radiography may be indicated to assess the degree of damage to the bony orbit. Ocular ultrasonography may provide information about the position of the lens, vitreous haemorrhage or retinal detachment, and an interruption of the sclera may be appreciated at the site of the rupture. In some cases, CT or MRI provides a very useful view of the injuries present (see Chapter 2).

Simple scleral wounds near the limbus are suitable for surgical closure. For extensive injuries, more complex procedures such as phacoemulsification or scleral grafting may be required. If the trauma is severe, enucleation may be indicated.

Penetrating and perforating injuries: Penetrating injuries breach the fibrous tunic without an exit wound. They can occur as a result of the use of dental elevators during a dental procedure or a stick injury through the roof of the mouth. Perforating injuries, such as gunshot wounds, have both an entrance and an exit wound. Both types of injury may lead to intraocular infection (endophthalmitis) and damage to the intraocular structures (e.g. lens capsule rupture or retinal detachment). Treatment requires suture of the sclera, but may also involve lens removal, vitrectomy and scleral grafting. If there is extensive rupture or severe complications, such as endophthalmitis, phthisis bulbi and blindness, enucleation is usually indicated.

Glaucoma

Glaucoma affects the sclera in a number of ways:

- Episcleral congestion occurs when the normal flow of blood through the ciliary body to the vortex veins is impeded by raised IOP. This is one of the most common signs of increased IOP
- Hydrophthalmos occurs as prolonged raised IOP causes the sclera and cornea to stretch, resulting in an enlarged globe. Scleral ectasia is acquired thinning of the tissue due to dilatation, and the sclera appears slightly blue because the underlying uvea is partly visible. An increase in globe size occurs more readily and dramatically in younger animals because the sclera is more elastic (Figure 13.17)
- Optic nerve cupping occurs as the lamina cribosa is distorted and compressed posteriorly by increased IOP. This affects axoplasmic flow and reduces the blood supply to the optic nerve head, leading to optic nerve axonal death and blindness. This axon death, along with physical stretching, compression and alteration of the connective tissue in the lamina cribosa leads to clinically apparent optic nerve cupping (see Chapter 15).

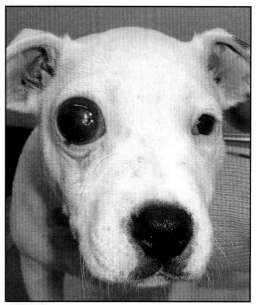

13.17 Gross enlargement of the right eye due to hydrophthalmos in a 12-week-old dog. Glaucoma occurred as a result of blunt trauma to the eye, and this led to exposure keratitis due to the inability to blink over such a large globe.

Neoplasia

Primary neoplasia of the sclera is uncommon, although intraocular and orbital tumours may invade the optic nerve and scleral vasculature. Neoplasia at the limbus is more common, probably because this is an area with high mitotic activity and the superotemporal aspect of the limbus is typically exposed to ultraviolet light. Types of neoplasm that may affect this region include melanoma, haemangioma, haemangiosarcoma, lymphoma and squamous cell carcinoma.

Melanoma: Limbal (epibulbar) melanoma is not uncommon in dogs. The typical appearance is a focally pigmented elevated mass at the limbus (Figure 13.18). There may be hyperaemia of the overlying conjunctiva, as well as infiltration and/or opacification of the adjacent cornea. Limbal melanoma can affect any breed, but the German Shepherd Dog, Golden Retriever and Labrador Retriever are over-represented. A genetic predisposition has been proposed in the latter two breeds (Donaldson *et al.*, 2006). These neoplasms arise from the pigmented cells (melanocytes) at the limbus. They are typically benign with a low metastatic potential, but can become quite large, and in younger dogs may grow more rapidly. Younger animals may benefit from full-thickness surgical resection or debulking, usually with an adjunctive treatment such as cryotherapy (Featherstone *et al.*, 2009). The deficit is repaired with a corneoscleral allograft, nictitans cartilage, commercially available sheets of porcine small intestinal submucosa or a conjunctival advancement flap. Photocoagulation with either a diode or neodymium:yttrium–aluminium–garnet (Nd:YAG) laser has also been successfully used by veterinary ophthalmologists (Sullivan *et al.*, 1996). The prognosis is very good.

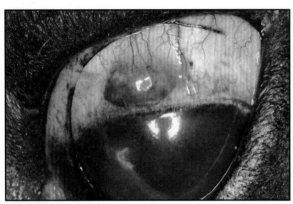

13.18 Raised dark focal area adjacent to the superior limbus, consistent with an epibulbar melanoma.

Care should be taken to distinguish limbal melanoma from malignant intraocular melanoma, which may occasionally penetrate the sclera. In these cases, orbital exenteration is indicated in an attempt to contain the spread of the tumour. Distinguishing the two conditions is not always straightforward and is achieved through history taking and careful clinical examination. Limbal melanomas are slow growing, discrete and typically do not penetrate the sclera or invade the adjacent iris and ciliary body. Malignant intraocular melanomas tend to grow rapidly and are larger and less well defined owing to invasion of the uvea and sclera. They may present with glaucoma and systemic signs if there is already metastasis. Ocular ultrasonography and gonioscopy might be required if the diagnosis is unclear.

Ocular melanosis: Ocular melanosis (previously called pigmentary glaucoma) is a condition in which excessive pigmentation of the uvea leads progressively to glaucoma (see also Chapters 14 and 15).

This condition mainly affects the Cairn Terrier, and in this breed an autosomal dominant mode of inheritance has been proposed on the basis of pedigree analysis (Petersen-Jones *et al.*, 2007). It is a bilateral condition, but not symmetrical. During the early stages, the periphery of the iris becomes thickened (an appearance that has been likened to a doughnut). As the disease progresses, the iris becomes darkened and pigment exfoliates into the anterior chamber. Multifocal dark patches of pigmentation become evident on the sclera and progressively enlarge (Figure 13.19).

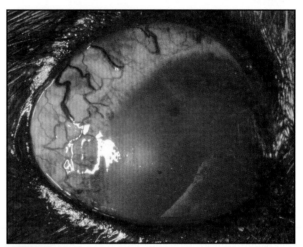

13.19 Multiple patches of dark pigment are visible within the sclera underlying the conjunctiva, along with episcleral congestion, corneal oedema and a dilated pupil in a Cairn Terrier with glaucoma secondary to ocular melanosis.

On gonioscopy, the angle is dark because of the presence of pigment and the cleft is narrow owing to the swollen iris periphery. Glaucoma develops as a result of occlusion of the drainage angle with melanocytes and melanophages, which obstruct aqueous outflow, and because of narrowing of the drainage angle caused by the thickened iris root. It is an insidious disease that responds poorly to medication, but topical carbonic anhydrase inhibitors may slow the onset and progression of glaucoma. In advanced stages, enucleation is indicated to control pain. Other breeds, such as the Labrador Retriever and Boxer, may also be affected by abnormal ocular pigment deposition and glaucoma (van de Sandt *et al.*, 2003).

Feline conditions

Developmental abnormalities

Ocular dermoids can occur in any breed of cat, but they are more common in the Birman and Burmese breeds, in which they may be inherited. They are typically situated at the lateral canthus or on the lateral limbus and involve the conjunctiva and cornea. As for dogs, the treatment of choice is surgical resection.

Congenital staphyloma can occur uncommonly in the cat. It may be accompanied by other ocular defects such as iris coloboma (Skorobohach and Hendrix, 2003).

Acquired abnormalities

Cats may be affected by many of the conditions that also affect dogs. However, compared with dogs, the inflammatory conditions episcleritis and scleritis are quite rare.

Trauma

Blunt trauma resulting in rupture of the sclera:
Blunt trauma may be a cause of scleral rupture. Road traffic accidents can cause skull fractures and scleral injury. The eyes present with chemosis, corneal oedema, hyphaema and aqueous flare, and are usually permanently blind owing to irreversible damage to intraocular structures such as the retina and optic nerve. Careful clinical assessment, with further evaluation using appropriate diagnostic imaging, should be conducted as described for dogs (see above). Initial treatment for the eye is conservative (pain relief and anti-inflammatory drugs) whilst the more serious injuries are addressed. Feline post-traumatic sarcoma is an uncommon but highly malignant tumour that can arise within the globe several years after the ocular injury, particularly to the lens, has been sustained. There is only a small risk of feline post-traumatic ocular sarcoma developing in the future, but because it has a potentially fatal outcome, it is one aspect to consider during the decision-making process regarding whether or not to enucleate an injured globe. It is reasonable to enucleate severely traumatized, irreversibly blind feline globes to prevent pain, and the prevention of sarcoma is another benefit.

Penetrating injuries: Penetrating trauma may be caused by cat scratch injury (Figure 13.20), which can result in scleral rupture. Iris prolapse adjacent to the limbus must be differentiated from epibulbar melanoma. Iris tissue protruding through a limbal or scleral laceration is usually covered by a thin layer of tan coloured clotted aqueous humour. The shape of the pupil is abnormal (dyscoria) because of the incarceration of iris tissue, and this becomes more obvious when testing the PLR. An epibulbar melanoma is covered by a layer of conjunctiva and the pupil is a normal shape.

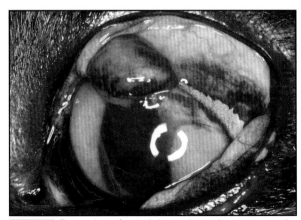

13.20 Protrusion of uveal tissue through a cat scratch laceration at the superior limbus. Note the fibrin and blood visible in the anterior chamber.

Iatrogenic injuries: Iatrogenic penetration of the sclera may occur during a dental procedure. The caudal maxillary tooth roots are anatomically in very close proximity to the orbit; they are only separated by a thin rim of alveolar bone. This type of injury occurs more commonly in cats because the bone is thinner compared with dogs, but can occur in both species. The injury is sustained if the dental elevator slips when force is applied in the direction of the globe. The instrument may penetrate the floor of the orbit and typically enters the globe at the 6 o'clock position (Mould and Billson, 2005). The posterior lens capsule is usually also penetrated (Figure 13.21). Ocular signs usually develop within days of the dental procedure, but occasionally can develop weeks later. Many cases require enucleation because of chronic uveitis and intraocular infection (endophthalmitis), which can lead to secondary glaucoma.

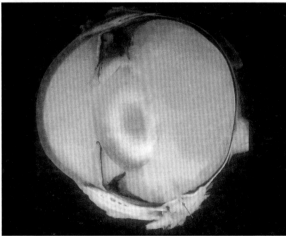

13.21 Gross pathology of a feline eye in which the sclera and lens were penetrated during a dental procedure. Features consistent with this form of penetrating trauma include the obvious scleral entry site (arrowed), dense infiltrate of inflammatory cells and protein exudation filling the anterior and posterior chambers and the vitreous cavity. Lens rupture was confirmed histologically. (Courtesy of J Mould)

Symblepharon

Symblepharon is the adhesion of the bulbar, palpebral or nictitating membrane conjunctiva to other ocular surfaces, most commonly the cornea. It is not common in dogs, but may be present in some microphthalmic eyes or may occur as a result of chemical injury, which damages the conjunctival and corneal epithelium. Symblepharon is much more common in cats, where it is usually a sequel to feline herpesvirus-1 infection (see also Chapters 11 and 12). The loss of limbal stem cells makes the surgical management of this condition very challenging and referral is recommended.

Neoplasia

In cats, limbal epibulbar (scleral shelf) melanomas (Figure 13.22) can occur, but are less common than in dogs. They are usually well circumscribed, benign and slow growing. Metastasis following surgical removal has been reported (Betton *et al.*, 1999) but is very uncommon. Regular monitoring is advised. If

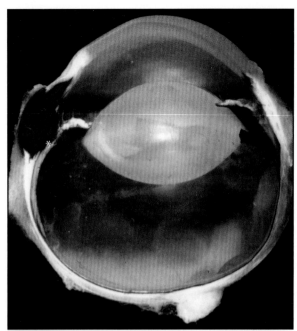

13.22 Gross pathology of a feline eye with a limbal (scleral shelf) melanoma. Note the outward extension of the pigmented mass and extension just into the iris base and angle. (Courtesy of J Mould)

the mass continues to increase in size, treatment with beta radiation, excisional biopsy followed by cryotherapy or diode laser photocoagulation may be indicated. The most common secondary tumour in this region is lymphosarcoma.

References and further reading

Barnes LD, Pearce JW, Berent LM *et al.* (2010) Surgical management of orbital nodular granulomatous episcleritis in a dog. *Veterinary Ophthalmology* **13**, 251–258

Betton A, Healy LN, English RV *et al.* (1999) Atypical limbal melanoma in a cat. *Journal of Veterinary Internal Medicine* **13**, 379–381

Breaux CB, Sandmeyer LS and Grahn BH (2007) Immunohistochemical investigation of canine episcleritis. *Veterinary Ophthalmology* **10**, 168–172

Day MJ, Mould JRB and Carter WJ (2008) An immunohistochemical investigation of canine idiopathic granulomatous scleritis. *Veterinary Ophthalmology* **11**, 11–17

Donaldson D, Sansom J and Adams V (2006) Canine limbal melanoma: 30 cases (1992–2004). Part 2: Treatment with lamellar resection and adjunctive strontium-90 beta plesiotherapy – efficacy and morbidity. *Veterinary Ophthalmology* **9**, 179–185

Donaldson D, Sansom J, Murphy S *et al.* (2006) Multiple limbal haemangiosarcomas in a Border Collie dog: management by lamellar keratectomy/sclerectomy and strontium-90 beta plesiotherapy. *Journal of Small Animal Practice* **47**, 545–549

Donaldson D, Sansom J, Scase T *et al.* (2006) Canine limbal melanoma: 30 cases (1992–2004). Part 1: Signalment, clinical and histological features and pedigree analysis. *Veterinary Ophthalmology* **9**, 115–119

Dubielzig RR, Ketring KL, McLellan GJ and Albert DM (2010) *Veterinary Ocular Pathology: A Comparative Review.* Saunders Elsevier, Oxford

Featherstone HJ, Renwick P, Heinrich CL *et al.* (2009) Efficacy of lamellar resection, cryotherapy and adjunctive grafting for the treatment of canine limbal melanoma. *Veterinary Ophthalmology* **12** (Supplement 1), 65–72

Grahn BH and Sandmeyer LS (2008) Canine episcleritis, nodular episclerokeratitis, scleritis and necrotic scleritis. *Veterinary Clinics of North America: Small Animal Practice* **30**, 1135–1149

Kanai K, Kanemaki N, Matsuo S *et al.* (2006) Excision of a feline limbal melanoma and the use of nictitans cartilage to repair the resulting corneoscleral defect. *Veterinary Ophthalmology* **9**, 255–258

Komnenou AA, Mylonakis ME, Kouti V *et al.* (2007) Ocular manifestations of natural canine monocytic ehrlichiosis (*Ehrlichia canis*): a retrospective study of 90 cases. *Veterinary Ophthalmology* **10**, 137–142

Mould JM and Billson FM (2005) Ocular penetration associated with dental extraction in the cat: 6 eyes. *Proceedings of the Winter Meeting of the British Association of Veterinary Ophthalmologists*

Peña MT, Naranjo C, Klauss G *et al.* (2008) Histopathological features of ocular leishmaniosis in the dog. *Journal of Comparative Pathology* **138**, 32–39

Petersen-Jones SM, Forcier J and Mentzer AL (2007) Ocular melanosis in the Cairn Terrier: clinical description and investigation of mode of inheritance. *Veterinary Ophthalmology* **10** (Supplement 1), 63–69

Petersen-Jones SM, Mentzer AL, Dubielzig RR *et al.* (2008) Ocular melanosis in the Cairn Terrier: histopathological description of the condition, and immunohistological and ultrastructural characterization of the characteristic pigment-laden cells. *Veterinary Ophthalmology* **11**, 260–268

Plummer CE, Kallberg ME, Ollivier FJ *et al.* (2008) Use of a biosynthetic material to repair the surgical defect following excision of an epibulbar melanoma in a cat. *Veterinary Ophthalmology* **11**, 250–254

Rampazzo A, Eule C, Speier S *et al.* (2006) Scleral rupture in dogs, cats and horses. *Veterinary Ophthalmology* **9**, 149–155

Skorobohach BJ and Hendrix DVH (2003) Staphyloma in a cat. *Veterinary Ophthalmology* **6**, 93–97

Smith MM, Smith EM, La Croix N *et al.* (2003) Orbital penetration associated with tooth extraction. *Journal of Veterinary Dentistry* **20**, 8–17

Sullivan TC, Nasisse MP, Davidson MG *et al.* (1996) Photocoagulation of limbal melanomas on dogs and cat: 15 cases (1989–1993). *Journal of the American Veterinary Medical Association* **208**, 891–894

van de Sandt RR, Boeve MH, Stades FC *et al.* (2003) Abnormal ocular pigment deposition and glaucoma in the dog. *Veterinary Ophthalmology* **6**, 273–278

Ward DA, Latimer KS and Askren RM (1992) Squamous cell carcinoma of the corneoscleral limbus in a dog. *Journal of the American Veterinary Medical Association* **200**, 1503–1506

Zarfoss MK, Dubielzig RR, Eberhard ML *et al.* (2005) Canine ocular onchocerciasis in the United States: two new cases and a review of the literature. *Veterinary Ophthalmology* **8**, 51–57

14

The uveal tract

Christine Watté and Simon Pot

The uveal tract is composed of continuous tissue that is anatomically subdivided into the iris, ciliary body and choroid (Figure 14.1). Pathological conditions that affect the uvea are commonly encountered in ophthalmic practice. This chapter covers a wide variety of conditions that affect the uvea, from normal variations, developmental abnormalities and age-related changes to acquired pathological processes. The anatomy, physiology and immune mechanisms are applicable to both dogs and cats. Thereafter, conditions are listed individually for each species. This chapter focuses on conditions that affect the anterior uvea (iris and ciliary body). Although diseases that also affect the choroid are mentioned, a more detailed description of abnormalities affecting the choroid can be found in Chapter 18.

Anatomy and physiology

The iris

When examined from the front, the iris can be subdivided into a peripheral ciliary zone and a central pupillary zone. The transition between these two zones is called the iris collarette (Figure 14.2) and is the typical site of emergence of persistent pupillary membranes (see later) when present. Pectinate fibres, comprising the pectinate ligament, originate from the peripheral iris to attach on to the sclera near the limbus (see Chapter 15 for more information on pectinate ligament anatomy). Viewed in cross-section, the bulk of the iris consists of stroma and its anterior surface is a modified stromal border layer, rather than an epithelial surface. Near the pupillary margin, the stroma contains the iris sphincter muscle, composed of smooth muscle fibres arranged in a circular (dog) or longitudinal fashion that interlace dorsally and ventrally (cat) to give the pupil its species-specific shape. The posterior stroma is lined by a bilayered posterior iris epithelium, which is continuous with the bilayered epithelium of the ciliary body.

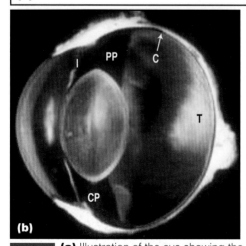

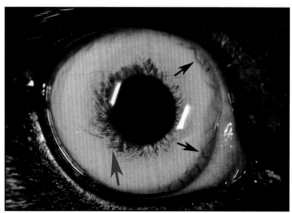

14.1 **(a)** Illustration of the eye showing the different parts of the uvea. **(b)** Canine eye showing the location of the uvea and its relative proportions. C = choroid; CP = ciliary process; I = iris; PP = pars plana; T = tapetum. (b, Courtesy of JR Mould)

14.2 Normal blue iris of a dog showing the major arterial circle in the periphery (black arrows) and position of the iris collarette at the border between the pupillary and ciliary zones of the iris (red arrow). The posterior iris pigmented epithelium is visible through the thinner pupillary zone of the iris, which therefore appears darker than the ciliary portion.

The posterior iris epithelium is darkly pigmented. The anterior iris epithelium is actually a myoepithelium that serves as dilator muscle.

The vascular supply to the iris is provided by an incomplete major arterial circle (see Figure 14.2) to which long posterior ciliary arteries (3 and 9 o'clock positions) and anterior ciliary arteries contribute. The major arterial circle branches off numerous radial arteries extending to the pupillary margin. Iridal veins drain into the anterior choroidal circulation. The primary function of the iris is to control the amount of light entering the eye. The balance between parasympathetic control of the constrictor muscle and sympathetic control of the dilator muscle provides the iris with dynamic control of the pupillary aperture. Various pathological conditions and pharmacological compounds can influence pupillary diameter and movement. Chapter 7 provides more information on pharmacological dilation of the pupil. Neurological control of the pupillary light reflexes (PLRs) is covered in Chapter 19.

The ciliary body
The iris is continuous posteriorly with the ciliary body, which has a roughly triangular structure on cross-section. The bulk of the ciliary body is composed of smooth muscle fibres (under parasympathetic control), connective tissue, blood vessels and nerves. Posterior to the pectinate ligament and juxtaposed to the sclera, the ciliary body harbours the uveal trabecular meshwork within the ciliary cleft. The inner, vitreal surface of the ciliary body is heavily folded anteriorly (pars plicata), constituting the ciliary processes that gradually smooth out posteriorly (pars plana) until the junction between the ciliary body and the retina is reached at the ora ciliaris retinae. Zonular fibres originate from the tips and valleys of the ciliary processes and insert near the lens equator, suspending the lens behind the iris and pupil. The vitreal surface of the ciliary body is covered by an inner non-pigmented epithelium and an outer pigmented epithelium. This double layer is continued anteriorly by the bilayered epithelium of the iris and blends posteriorly with the retina and retinal pigment epithelium at the ora ciliaris retinae.

The ciliary body vasculature is supplied mainly by the major arterial circle, and drains via the anterior choroidal veins to the vortex veins. By the balanced action of aqueous production and drainage (as described in greater detail in Chapter 15), the ciliary body contributes to the maintenance of a healthy intraocular pressure (IOP) that shapes the eye and provides the lens and inner cornea with nutrition. The ciliary body plays a predominant role in the production of aqueous humour, by diffusion, ultrafiltration and active secretion of solutes at the level of the non-pigmented epithelium. The ciliary body also participates in aqueous humour outflow at the level of the uveal trabecular meshwork. Contraction of the ciliary muscle may increase conventional aqueous outflow and provides accommodation (limited in dogs and cats) by moving the lens forward and increasing the lens curvature by releasing tension on the zonular fibres and lens equator.

The choroid
The choroid is the part of the uveal tract that extends from the ora ciliaris retinae to the optic nerve head. It is a highly vascular tissue, flanked on the outside by the sclera and lined on the inside by the retinal pigment epithelium. The choroid is composed of five main layers (from outside to inside): the suprachoroideae; large and medium vessel layers (which contain the tapetum where present); choriocapillaris; and Bruch's membrane. The anatomy of the choroid is described further in Chapter 18. The choroid is richly vascularized and has an extremely rapid blood flow, which ensures optimal nutrition and oxygenation of the outer retina. Short and long posterior ciliary arteries, as well as anterior ciliary arteries, supply the choroid and venous drainage is provided by the vortex veins.

Blood–ocular barrier and ocular immune privilege
The blood–ocular barrier serves to regulate retinal nutrition and the composition of intraocular fluids. The blood–ocular barrier can be roughly divided into a blood–aqueous and a blood–retinal barrier. The blood–aqueous barrier (Figure 14.3) is formed by tight junctions in the non-pigmented ciliary epithelium, iridal epithelium and non-fenestrated iris blood vessels. This barrier limits entry to the eye by many substances which would impair transparency and upset the osmotic and chemical balance of the aqueous. The non-pigmented ciliary epithelium plays a major role in this barrier because of the large surface area it covers on the ciliary processes. The blood–retinal barrier (Figure 14.3) is located at the level of the retinal pigment epithelium and in the retinal blood vessels. Both contain tight junctions that seal interepithelial spaces and tightly regulate the retinal microenvironment. The integrity of the barrier can be clinically tested by fluorescein angiography, although this is generally only used in a research setting in companion animals (see Chapter 1).

The eye is an immune-privileged site, which means it is protected from excessive inflammation and immunity. Multiple local and systemic mechanisms contribute to this status. In brief, these include mechanisms that limit the access of immune cells to the eye (such as the blood–ocular barrier, as well as the lack of direct lymphatic drainage), induce local immune suppression and suppress the systemic immune response to antigens introduced into the eye (Taylor, 2009). These multiple mechanisms, leading to the immune privileged status of the eye, serve to preserve vision, maintain a stable intraocular microenvironment and limit the ocular damage that would ensue with uncontrolled inflammation in the eye. However, ocular immune privilege is not a foolproof system as individual mechanisms can be overwhelmed, 'break down' and give way to inflammation, leading to the clinical signs of uveitis.

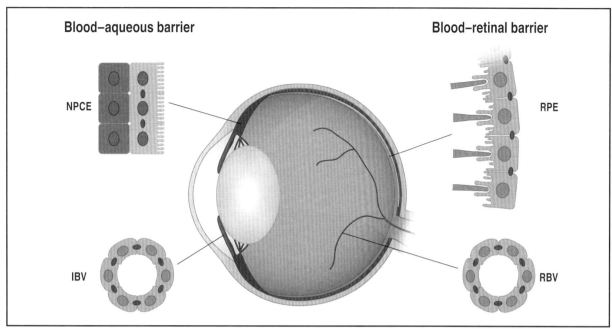

Blood–aqueous barrier

Blood–retinal barrier

NPCE

RPE

IBV

RBV

14.3 The blood–ocular barrier. The epithelial and vascular components of the blood–aqueous barrier are shown on the left, and the epithelial and vascular components of the blood–retinal barrier are shown on the right. IBV = iris blood vessel; NPCE = non-pigmented ciliary epithelium; RBV = retinal blood vessel; RPE = retinal pigment epithelium.

Canine conditions

Figure 14.4 provides an overview of uveal disease in dogs.

Developmental abnormalities
• Iris heterochromia • Subalbinism • Merle ocular dysgenesis • Aniridia, iris hypoplasia/coloboma • Persistent pupillary membranes/anterior segment dysgenesis • Iridociliary cysts
Acquired abnormalities
• Iris atrophy • Iris melanosis • Iridociliary cysts • Uveitis (see Figures 14.32 and 14.33) • Intraocular haemorrhage • Ocular melanosis • Neoplasia

14.4 Differential diagnoses of uveal disease in dogs.

Developmental abnormalities

Iris heterochromia

Iris colour is determined by melanin content and distribution. Heterochromia is a descriptive term and does not necessarily denote an abnormality. In complete heterochromia, the colour of the iris of one eye is different from that of the other (Figure 14.5). In partial or sectoral heterochromia only part of the iris is a different colour. Congenital iris heterochromia is commonly seen in dogs and should be distinguished from acquired causes of iris colour change, such as uveitis or neoplasia (discussed later). It may be the

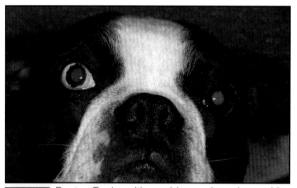

14.5 Boston Terrier with one blue and one brown iris. The blue eye lacks pigment in the choroid and retinal pigment epithelium, which results in a red fundic reflex. In addition, the blue eye also lacks a tapetum.

only expression of colour dilution or may be associated with colour dilution genes such as the Merle (see below) and piebald (e.g. Dalmatian) genes.

Subalbinism

Subalbinism refers to dilution of ocular pigmentation and is commonly encountered as a normal variant in association with colour dilution genes in many canine breeds. Melanin is absent from the iris stroma, but the posterior iridal epithelium is pigmented, conferring a blue appearance to the iris. Subalbinism may also be associated with iris hypoplasia, coloboma, corectopia (off-centre pupil), choroidal hypoplasia and a hypoplastic or absent tapetum. The effects of subalbinism on the ophthalmoscopic appearance of the fundus are described in detail in Chapter 18. In true albinism, the iris lacks pigment totally in the stroma and epithelium, and the iridal vasculature confers a reddish glow to the iris. Albinism has not yet been reported in dogs or cats.

Merle ocular dysgenesis

Multiple ocular abnormalities may be encountered in breeds that carry the Merle gene (such as the Australian Shepherd, Shetland Sheepdog, Great Dane, Old English Sheepdog and Rough and Smooth Collies). Animals that carry two copies of this dominant gene have an excessively white coat and the most severe ocular abnormalities. The condition has been particularly well documented in the Australian Shepherd. Uveal abnormalities may include iris heterochromia, iris hypoplasia, persistent pupillary membranes, corectopia, dyscoria (abnormal pupil shape), prominent iridal epithelium, iris coloboma, choroidal coloboma or hypoplasia and equatorial staphyloma (protrusion of uveal tissue through a defect in the sclera). Associated non-uveal abnormalities may include microphthalmos, cataract, scleral ectasia (thinning and outward bulging of the sclera), retinal dysplasia and retinal detachment. Ocular abnormalities may be encountered in eyes of either colour. Non-ocular abnormalities may include varying degrees of deafness.

Aniridia and iris hypoplasia/coloboma

These conditions reflect various degrees of incomplete iris development. True aniridia, a total lack of iris development, is a very rare condition in dogs. In most cases, a rudimentary iris base is still present. Iris hypoplasia, a congenital thinning of the iris visible on transillumination, is more commonly encountered. The condition is seen more often (but not exclusively) in blue eyes. A coloboma is a sectoral defect in the iris. Colobomas may manifest as a simple notch in the pupil, a focal lack of stromal development or may be a full-thickness defect resulting in pseudopolycoria (the appearance of an additional pupil (or pupils) not surrounded by sphincter muscle) (Figure 14.6). Typical colobomas occur at the 6 o'clock position and are due to incomplete closure of the embryonic optic fissure. Atypical colobomas may also be encountered in other locations. Colobomatous defects may also involve the ciliary

body. In such cases, the lack of development of a portion of the ciliary body and the resultant sectoral lack in ciliary processes and zonular fibres causes the adjacent lens periphery to be abnormally shaped, which is often incorrectly referred to as a 'lens coloboma' (see Chapter 16).

Anterior segment abnormalities

Persistent pupillary membranes (PPMs), Peters anomaly and anterior segment dysgenesis are developmental anterior segment abnormalities of increasing severity.

Persistent pupillary membranes: These are remnants of the anterior tunica vasculosa lentis and pupillary membrane, which provide nutrition to the lens and anterior segment of the eye during development. These vascular structures start regressing *in utero* and have usually disappeared by 6 weeks of age. However, in some animals these vascular remnants can persist beyond 6 weeks of age and continue to regress during the following months, or may persist throughout life. PPMs are recessively inherited in the Basenji breed, but also occur, and are presumed to be inherited, in many other breeds. Even with mildly affected dogs, breeding discretion should be advised because the offspring can be more severely affected.

Various PPM gradations exist. Minor PPM remnants may be seen relatively commonly on ophthalmic examination as pigmented dots confined to the central anterior lens capsule. They are of identical colour to the normal iris surface in the affected eye (Figure 14.7). Typical PPMs are string-like elevations coming off the iris surface, which originate at the iris collarette and are of identical colour to the adjacent normal iris. These vessel remnants either connect two or more portions of the iris (iris-to-iris PPM; Figure 14.8); span from the iris to the lens (iris-to-lens PPM); from the iris to the cornea (iris-to-cornea PPM; Figure 14.9); or have a free-floating end in the anterior chamber (Figure 14.10).

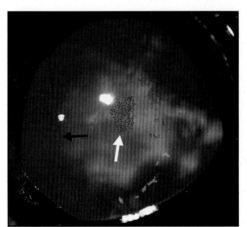

14.6 Heterochromic iris presenting a partial-thickness coloboma (arrowed). The overlying iris stroma is thin or absent, allowing direct visualization of the darkly pigmented iridal epithelium. Note the red fundic reflex, indicating a lack or paucity of fundus pigmentation and/or tapetal development. (Courtesy of BM Spiess)

14.7 Pupillary membrane remnants on the anterior lens capsule of a dog. Note the central location and light brown colouration of the pigment spots (white arrow). Although these pigment spots are a relatively common incidental finding in otherwise normal canine eyes, an iris-to-iris PPM remnant (black arrow) and a nuclear and cortical cataract were also present in this eye.

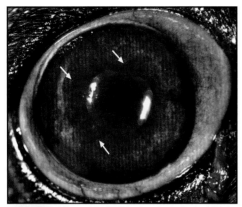

14.8 Iris-to-iris PPM remnants in a dog (arrowed). These strands originate at the iris collarette and not at the pupillary margin. Examination with a slit-lamp may be necessary to ascertain the origin and elevation of the PPM off the iris surface.

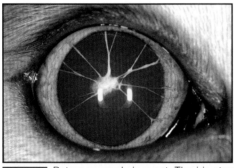

14.9 Peters anomaly in a cat. The iris strands all originate at the collarette region and have the colour of the normal yellow to light brown iris surface. The iris strands attach to a central corneal defect involving the posterior stroma, Descemet's membrane and endothelium. (Courtesy of the University of Wisconsin-Madison Comparative Ophthalmology Service)

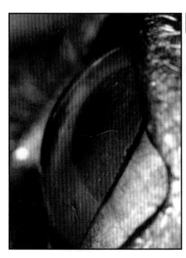

14.10 Free-floating PPM remnants originating at the iris collarette.

Free-floating and iris-to-iris type PPMs do not cause any problems and therapy is not indicated. Owing in part to traction on the corneal endothelium, focal endothelial absence/dysplasia and lens capsular pigment, iris-to-cornea and iris-to-lens PPMs can cause focal corneal opacity (oedema, fibrosis) or lens opacity (cataract). Vision can be affected, depending on the number, size and location of the PPM attachments to the cornea or lens.

If only minimal atrophy/rarefaction of the embryonal pupillary membrane takes place, a sheet of iris-like tissue, connected to the iris collarette, can persist in the pupillary aperture. The effect on vision depends on the density and completeness of the membrane, but is often significant. Medical therapy for corneal oedema and specialist surgical treatment of complete membranes and/or progressive cataracts can be indicated in certain cases.

Peters anomaly: If an iris-to-cornea PPM exists in combination with a defect in the posterior corneal stroma, Descemet's membrane and endothelium, a diagnosis of Peters anomaly can be made (see Figure 14.9). The most anterior corneal stroma may show signs of oedema, but is otherwise normal, as is the corneal epithelium. Iris hypoplasia and anterior cortical cataracts can also be observed.

Anterior segment dysgenesis: This is a term used for more severe forms of developmental malformation of the anterior segment and is often associated with microphthalmos. Both dogs and cats can be affected. Faulty separation of the various anterior segment structures can cause corneal, iris, lens and drainage angle abnormalities, including large sheets of iris tissue adhering to the cornea, a flattened anterior chamber, cornea–lens contact, lenticular malformations, cataracts and glaucoma.

Differential diagnosis: A prior traumatic episode, or other cause of globe rupture, should be a differential consideration in severe cases of iris-to-cornea PPMs, Peters anomaly or anterior segment dysgenesis. These aetiologies should be strongly suspected if there is a supportive history or indications of previous globe perforation or rupture are present.

Posterior synechiae caused by chronic or previous bouts of uveitis should be distinguished from iris-to-lens PPMs. Posterior synechia-associated pigment remnants (iris rests) on the anterior lens capsule are the most important differential diagnosis for pupillary membrane remnants on the anterior lens capsule. Iris-to-cornea PPMs and Peters anomaly need to be distinguished from anterior synechiae.

These lesions can be identified and differentiated on the basis of location and colour.

- Posterior synechiae initially form as a result of fibrinous adhesions between the iris and lens, and thus originate on the pupillary margin or posterior iris surface, but never on the anterior surface of the iris.
- Posterior synechiae and 'iris rests' on the anterior lens capsule are black (not the colour of the anterior iris stroma), owing to the involvement of the posterior iris pigment epithelium (Figure 14.11). They can be located anywhere on the anterior lens capsule, depending on the cause and the pupil size at the time of adhesion formation.
- Anterior synechiae are typically caused by perforating corneal trauma and incarceration of iris in the wound, and thus span from the pupil margin towards a full-thickness corneal scar.

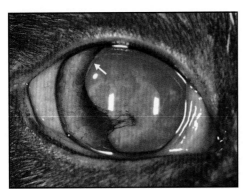

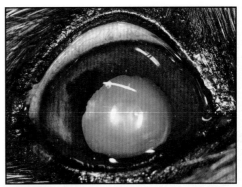

14.11 Posterior synechiae in a patient with chronic uveitis. Note the black colouration of the synechiae and how they originate at the pupillary margin. A complete cataract and subluxation of the lens (arrowed) have also developed as a result of the chronic uveitis.

14.13 Iris melanosis in a middle-aged dog. Note the irregularity of the pupillary margin as a result of concurrent iris atrophy. There is unrelated nuclear sclerosis and incipient anterior cortical cataract affecting the lens.

- Peripheral anterior synechiae are associated with a shallow peripheral anterior chamber and span from the peripheral iris surface to a relatively normal overlying cornea.

Acquired abnormalities

Iris atrophy

Iris atrophy occurs relatively frequently in dogs, most commonly as a result of ageing (senile iris atrophy; Figure 14.12). Clinically, the pupil may appear dilated, irregular and show reduced PLRs, leading occasionally to photophobia. Areas of thinning may be more obvious on transillumination and may progress to full-thickness holes in the iris. These lesions should be differentiated from iris hypoplasia and coloboma, which are congenital in nature. Iris atrophy may also occur following trauma, chronic uveitis and chronic glaucoma.

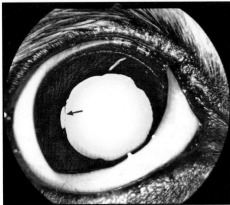

14.12 Senile iris atrophy. Note the relatively mydriatic pupil, irregular pupillary margin and strand of atrophied iris (arrowed). The hazy fundic reflex is due to nuclear sclerosis affecting the lens.

Iris melanosis

Iris melanosis is a descriptive term indicating focal spots of iris hyperpigmentation (Figure 14.13), whether these result from increased melanin content or an increased number of melanocytes. The hyperpigmented areas are flat, not raised relative to the adjacent tissue, and do not progress or progress only very slowly. Iris melanosis is of no clinical concern. However, care should be taken to differentiate iris melanosis from the more serious conditions of uveal melanoma and ocular melanosis leading to glaucoma (see below).

Iridociliary cysts

Iridociliary cysts originate from the posterior iris epithelium and ciliary body epithelium and can be variably pigmented, depending on the tissue of origin. In eyes that have undergone protracted episodes of uveitis, small dark cysts lining the pupillary margin may be observed. Diffuse hyperpigmentation of the iris as a result of chronic inflammation is often seen concurrently.

More typically, larger cysts of varying size and pigmentation are observed. These cysts are either attached to the posterior iris surface or to the ciliary body, or float freely in the anterior chamber (Figure 14.14) or, rarely, in the vitreous. If large enough, attached cysts can be observed through the pupillary aperture, especially when dilated (Figure 14.15). Smaller or more peripherally attached cysts can be difficult, if not impossible, to observe directly, especially through an undilated pupil. Large or numerous iridociliary cysts can become problematic if they cause obstruction of the pupil or iridocorneal angle. Large cysts that remain attached can impinge on the posterior chamber, causing forward displacement of the iris and localized narrowing of the iridocorneal angle. Their presence can be confirmed with ultrasonography. High frequency (>20 MHz) probes are ideally suited to this task (see Chapter 2).

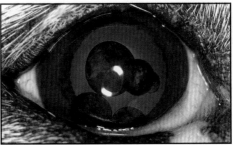

14.14 Free-floating, heterogeneously pigmented, iridociliary cysts in the anterior chamber of a dog. These cysts can be transilluminated and the tapetal reflection is observed through the cysts (retroillumination).

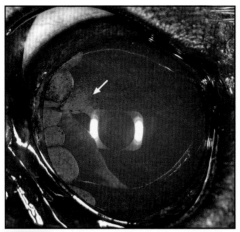

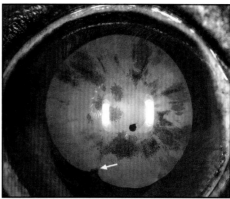

14.16 Radially oriented pigment deposits on the anterior lens capsule of an 11-year-old male neutered Golden Retriever. Note the inferior temporal posterior synechia (arrowed). This appearance is consistent with a diagnosis of 'pigmentary uveitis' in the Golden Retriever. (Courtesy of the University of Wisconsin-Madison Comparative Ophthalmology Service)

14.15 Multiple, transilluminating, iridociliary cysts observed through the dilated pupil of a 3-year-old neutered Golden Retriever bitch. The remains of one or more deflated cysts are visible as pigment remnants on the anterior lens capsule (arrowed). (Courtesy of the University of Wisconsin-Madison Comparative Ophthalmology Service)

Deflated cyst material can adhere to the lens, cornea and drainage angle structures, causing opacities or aqueous outflow impairment. Proteinaceous or haemorrhagic cyst contents can also contribute to aqueous outflow impairment, especially in patients with an already compromised angle.

Association with glaucoma: In Golden Retrievers and Great Danes, the occurrence of multiple, thin-walled, iridociliary cysts in combination with glaucoma has been described and is presumed to be an inherited disease. Most affected Golden Retrievers are middle-aged or older dogs. The condition remains relatively rare in Great Danes. However, particularly in the USA, Golden Retrievers frequently present with thin-walled iridociliary cysts (see Figure 14.15). A slow progression of cyst size and number is typically observed, which may lead to glaucoma during the lifetime of the dog. The actual incidence of secondary glaucoma remains undetermined in this breed.

Dispersion of pigmented cells in the anterior chamber and radial pigment deposits on the anterior lens capsule (Figure 14.16), presumably caused by rubbing of posterior iris cysts on the anterior lens capsule during pupil movement, are typical clinical findings at this stage of the disease. Spontaneous cyst rupture may release proteinaceous contents into the anterior chamber, which is recognized clinically as aqueous flare. In the later stages of the disease, additional clinical signs suggestive of uveitis, including posterior synechiae and even iris bombé formation and glaucoma, can be observed and need to be treated accordingly. It is difficult to predict the risk of developing pigmentary uveitis and glaucoma in affected Golden Retrievers.

Differential diagnosis: Iridociliary tumours are the main differential diagnosis for iridociliary cysts. Melanomas especially can mimic cysts. However, cysts can almost always be transilluminated with a bright light source, aided by retroillumination of the cysts using light reflected by the tapetum (see Figure 14.15). In addition, cysts are exquisitely round or ovoid in shape. Ultrasonography can help to differentiate a hollow cyst from a solid soft tissue tumour.

Treatment: Options include laser deflation, fine-needle aspiration or irrigation/aspiration of the cysts and cyst contents via the anterior chamber. These procedures require appropriate magnification and microsurgical expertise if serious adverse effects, such as lens trauma or intraocular haemorrhage, are to be avoided. These patients are therefore best referred to a specialist.

Uveitis

Uveitis is inflammation of any portion of the uvea. Theoretically, inflammation can be localized to the iris (iritis), ciliary body (cyclitis), pars plana (pars planitis) or choroid (choroiditis). However, owing to the anatomical continuity of the different intraocular structures, the terms anterior uveitis (or iridocyclitis) and posterior uveitis (or chorioretinitis) are more commonly used. This subdivision also serves a practical purpose, because it helps narrow down the list of potential aetiologies and has important implications regarding therapy.

The term endophthalmitis is used if the anterior and posterior chambers, vitreous cavity and retina are simultaneously involved in the inflammatory process. However, in patients with significant anterior and posterior uveitis, some involvement of these other compartments is unavoidable. In practice, the term endophthalmitis is reserved for patients with an uncontrollable and intensely painful intraocular inflammation, often presumed to be of infectious origin. The term panophthalmitis is used when the inflammatory process involves all the intraocular structures and the sclera. It is not unusual for panophthalmitis to be associated with orbital cellulitis as well. The following section concentrates on anterior uveitis and should be read in conjunction with Chapters 18 and 20.

Clinical signs: A wide variety of clinical signs associated with the hallmarks of inflammation (redness, swelling, pain, heat and loss of function) can be observed in eyes with uveitis. These signs are caused by the basic pathophysiological events of increased blood flow, increased vascular permeability and influx of inflammatory cells into the site of inflammation. The signs that accompany uveitis vary depending on the extent and severity of the inflammation, inciting cause, species and chronicity. They can be divided into specific and non-specific signs (Figure 14.17) and sequelae (Figure 14.18).

- In the acute stages of uveitis, vasodilatation and increased blood flow to the inflamed area can cause conjunctival, episcleral, perilimbal (ciliary flush) and iridal blood vessel congestion and hyperaemia.
- Increased vascular permeability disrupts the blood–aqueous barrier and allows extravasation of exudates, conjunctival swelling (chemosis), limbal corneal oedema, iris swelling (Figure 14.19) and granulomatous iris changes or iris nodules (Figure 14.20). Four types of exudate

Clinical sign	Type of response
Blepharospasm	General
Epiphora	General
Photophobia	Specific
Conjunctival and episcleral hyperaemia	General
Ciliary flush (perilimbal reddening)	General
Chemosis	General
Aqueous flare	Specific
Anterior chamber cells	Specific
Keratic precipitates	Specific
Corneal oedema	General
Hyphaema [a]	Specific
Fibrin in the anterior chamber	Specific
Hypopyon	Specific
Iris swelling	Specific
Rubeosis iridis (iris neovascularization)	Specific
Iris nodules [b]	Specific
Diffuse iris hyperpigmentation	Specific
Miosis [c]	Specific
Intraocular pressure decrease	Specific
Vitreal opacities (cells, protein, blood)	Specific
Pain	General
Decrease in vision	General

14.17 Clinical signs of uveitis in dogs. [a] Hyphaema is usually accompanied by uveitis. However, the list of differential diagnoses also includes coagulopathies/platelet disorders and systemic hypertension. [b] Nodular thickening of the iris can occur with various neoplastic diseases. However, lymphoplasmacytic and granulomatous nodules typically are distinguishable from neoplastic masses. [c] Miosis is also seen with Horner's syndrome (see Chapter 19).

- Persistent corneal oedema
- Bullous keratopathy
- Posterior synechiae
- Dyscoria
- Restricted movement of pupil
- Peripheral anterior synechiae
- Pigment on anterior lens capsule
- Preiridal fibrovascular membranes
- Ectropion uveae
- Iris bombé
- Pupil seclusion
- Glaucoma
- Iris atrophy
- Iris cyst formation
- Cataract formation
- Lens luxation
- Vitreal degeneration
- Retinal detachment
- Phthisis bulbi
- Blindness

14.18 Sequelae of uveitis in dogs.

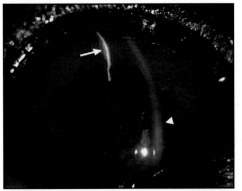

14.19 Slit-lamp image of the left eye of a dog with anterior uveitis. The slit beam is projected from the right towards the left side in this image and focused on the superior iris. Swelling of the ciliary zone of the iris is clearly observed as an elevation of the slit beam (arrowed). The cornea is out of focus (arrowhead). (Courtesy of the University of Wisconsin-Madison Comparative Ophthalmology Service)

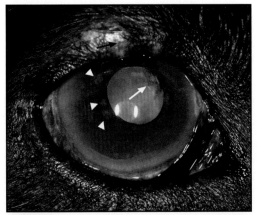

14.20 Granulomatous uveitis in a 4-year-old male crossbreed dog. Inflammatory nodules are present in the iris (arrowheads). Note the granulomatous upper eyelid lesion (black arrow), conjunctival hyperaemia, perilimbal corneal oedema, corneal neovascularization and the superionasal posterior synechia and pigment remnants on the anterior lens capsule (white arrow). The dog was diagnosed with leishmaniosis.

can be observed: serous (proteinaceous); fibrinous; sanguineous; and purulent. Within the eye, these exudates can be observed directly as aqueous or vitreous flare (Figure 14.21), fibrin clots (Figure 14.22), hyphaema (Figure 14.23), blood clots, cells in the aqueous or vitreous (Figure 14.24) or hypopyon (Figure 14.25). Protein in the aqueous humour causes light scattering in the anterior chamber, which is observed as a diffuse cloudiness or 'flare'. The intensity of the flare is directly correlated with the aqueous humour protein concentration and is graded by most ophthalmologists on a scale from 0 to 4 (0 = no flare; 4 = dense flare, approaching the observed density of the lens). The number of cells in the anterior chamber is also graded on a scale from 0 to 4 by some ophthalmologists (0 = no cells; 4 = >100 cells per fine slit-lamp slit beam) (Figure 14.24a; Hogan *et al.*, 1959). The precipitation of cells in the inferior anterior chamber results in a cell deposit with a horizontal demarcation line. Erythrocytes can form this in an eye with hyphaema. If caused by leucocytes, this is called hypopyon. Keratic

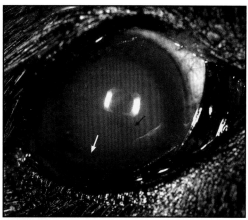

14.23 Hyphaema in a 12-year-old male neutered Labrador-cross dog. The precipitation of erythrocytes in the ventral anterior chamber is clearly demonstrated by the horizontal demarcation line (white arrow). The cell and protein content caused intense light scattering and reflection in the rest of the anterior chamber, which made observation of iris and lens details and fundus examination impossible. Blood deposits on the anterior lens capsule or corneal endothelium are visible as well (black arrow). This dog was affected bilaterally and was diagnosed with lymphoma. (Courtesy of the University of Wisconsin-Madison Comparative Ophthalmology Service)

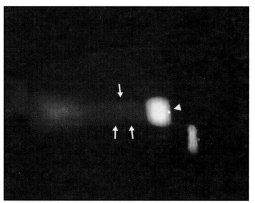

14.21 Anterior uveitis in a dog. A narrow beam of focused condensed light is projected from the right towards the left side in this image and focused on the aqueous flare in the anterior chamber. Note the diffuse scattering of light in the anterior chamber, which is best observed at the edge of the light beam (arrowed). This visible continuous beam of light resembles the appearance of car headlights in fog. The cornea is out of focus (arrowhead). This image was taken in a completely darkened room. (Courtesy of the University of Wisconsin-Madison Comparative Ophthalmology Service)

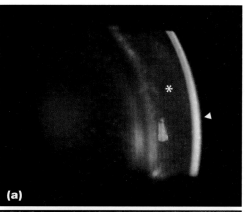

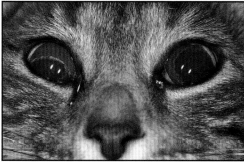

14.24 **(a)** Slit-lamp image of a 7-year-old male neutered Soft Coated Wheaten Terrier with anterior uveitis. The slit beam is projected from the right towards the left side in this image and focused on the anterior chamber cells and flare (*). Note the corpuscular nature of the material (cells) within the anterior chamber, resembling floating dust particles in a beam of light. Diffuse light scattering is present as well (flare). The cornea is out of focus (arrowhead). This image was taken in a completely darkened room. **(b)** Slightly less magnified view taken with the room lights on. Note how much more difficult it is to identify the anterior chamber flare and cells, let alone grade them.

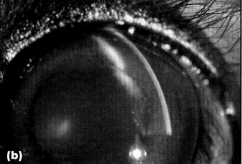

14.22 Bilateral fibrin and blood clots in the anterior chamber of a 10-month-old female European Shorthaired cat. No specific aetiology was identified and the cat was diagnosed with idiopathic uveitis.

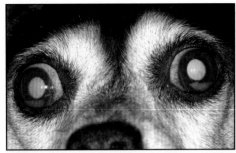

14.25 Bilateral hypopyon in a 6-year-old neutered Rat Terrier bitch. Note the horizontal demarcation lines. The rest of the anterior chamber also appears hazy owing to the cell and protein content, as evidenced by the loss of iris detail in both eyes. Small amounts of blood are also visible inferionasally in the anterior chambers. This dog was diagnosed with lymphoma. (Courtesy of the University of Wisconsin-Madison Comparative Ophthalmology Service)

precipitates (KPs) are deposits of inflammatory cells on the endothelial side of the cornea. They are recognized as fine, white to yellow spots on the cornea that are predominantly located inferiorly. Examination with a slit-lamp is necessary to confirm the endothelial localization of the deposits (Figure 14.26a). On retroillumination, KPs take on a darker, grey to brown colour (Figure 14.26b; see Chapter 1).

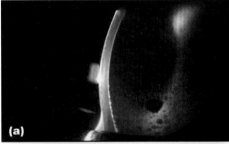

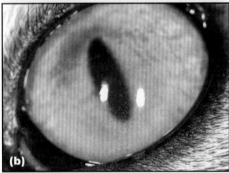

14.26 **(a)** Slit-lamp image of a Domestic Shorthaired cat with anterior uveitis. The slit beam is projected from the left towards the right side in this image and focused on the cornea. Under direct illumination in the slit beam, keratic precipitates (KPs) are visible as whitish deposits on the inferior, endothelial side of the cornea. With retroillumination (on the right-hand side of the slit beam) the KPs take on a grey–brown colour. The cat was found to be FIV-positive. **(b)** Appearance of KPs on the inferior cornea with diffuse illumination. With direct illumination (pupil as the background) the KPs are a yellow to tan colour; with retroillumination (iris as the background) they appear grey–brown. (Courtesy of the University of Wisconsin-Madison Comparative Ophthalmology Service)

- Pain is caused either directly by inflammation or as a result of ciliary muscle spasm. Signs of pain include blepharospasm, epiphora and photophobia.
- Miosis results from iris sphincter muscle stimulation by prostaglandins and other inflammatory mediators. Unilateral uveitis and miosis causes an unequal pupil size (anisocoria). This may be observed more easily in a dimly lit room using the technique of distant direct ophthalmoscopy (see Chapter 1). The response to pharmacological dilation (e.g. with 1% tropicamide) can be slow in uveitic eyes.
- A decrease in IOP occurs due to loss of function of the ciliary body epithelium and increased (prostaglandin-mediated) uveoscleral outflow. Chronic ocular hypotony can lead to globe shrinkage (phthisis bulbi).
- Chronic uveitis can cause diffuse hyperpigmentation of the iris, iris atrophy and iris cysts.
- Release of fibrogenic and pro-angiogenic growth factors leads to fibrosis and neovascularization, which can have several consequences:
  - Posterior synechiae result from fibrinous iris to lens adhesions that turn into fibrous adhesions. They originate from the pupillary margin or posterior iris surface (see Figure 14.11). When broken down by pupil movement, they may leave behind pigment deposits on the anterior lens capsule. Posterior synechiae can occur anywhere on the anterior lens capsule and can cause dyscoria and anisocoria. Pupil movement can be inhibited as well. Extensive posterior synechiae can occlude the pupil (pupil seclusion) and blind the patient. The flow of aqueous humour through the pupil can also be obstructed, which causes aqueous to accumulate in the posterior chamber and the iris to bulge forward (iris bombé; Figure 14.27), leading to secondary glaucoma (see Chapter 15)
  - Pre-iridal fibrovascular membranes (PIFVMs) are neovascular membranes covering the anterior surface of the iris (Figure 14.28). These should not be confused with congested, hyperaemic iridal vessels that have a radial orientation. PIFVM-associated vessels typically run a very irregular course and can even cover the anterior lens capsule and obstruct vision or, more commonly, cover the iridocorneal drainage angle and cause obstruction of aqueous outflow and thus secondary glaucoma. The presence of a PIFVM, described clinically as 'rubeosis iridis', is evidence of the chronic nature of the uveitis and is a poor prognostic indicator. Contraction of PIFVMs can cause a rolled-out appearance of the pupil margin (ectropion uveae), which is noteworthy because it points to the presence of a PIFVM
  - Corneal neovascularization can be observed as a result of chronic uveitis.

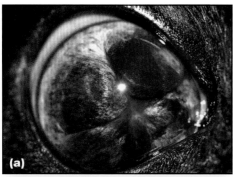

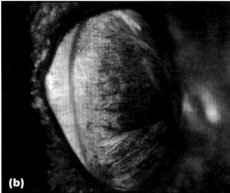

14.27 Pupil seclusion and iris bombé in an 8-year-old male neutered Domestic Shorthaired cat with chronic uveitis. **(a)** Front view. **(b)** Side view.

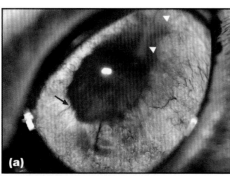

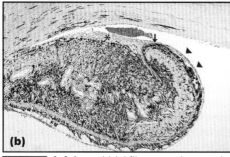

14.28 **(a)** A pre-iridal fibrovascular membrane (PIFVM) covering the anterior iris surface (rubeosis iridis) and anterior lens capsule in a 4-year-old female neutered European Shorthaired cat with chronic uveitis caused by an old corneal perforation. Note the irregular partially circumferential course of the blood vessels and blood vessels crossing from the iris surface on to the lens capsule (arrowed). The perforation wound had healed and left a corneal scar (arrowheads). **(b)** Histopathological cross-section of the iris and cornea of a dog with a thick PIFVM (asterisk and arrowheads) covering the anterior surface of the iris and causing ectropion uveae (arrowed). A history of ocular trauma was present. (Courtesy of Dr RR Dubielzig, Comparative Ophthalmic Pathology Laboratory of Wisconsin)

- Corneal endothelial decompensation and persistent corneal oedema can result from exudates in the anterior chamber, especially dense KPs and hypopyon, which can disrupt endothelial function. In extreme cases bullous keratopathy is seen. The reader is referred to Chapter 12 for further details.
- Cataracts may result from altered aqueous humour composition and flow rate. Weakening of the lens zonules due to chronic inflammation can cause lens luxation or subluxation. The reader is referred to Chapter 16 for further details.
- Chorioretinal inflammation may result in abnormalities that are visible on ophthalmoscopic examination of the fundus. The reader is referred to Chapter 18 for further explanation of the occurrence, diagnosis, treatment and prognosis of chorioretinitis, vitreal degeneration and retinal detachment in uveitic eyes.
- Vision can be temporarily impaired or irreversibly lost as a result of all the above-mentioned signs and sequelae.

Investigation of disease: The diagnosis of uveitis is relatively straightforward. However, determining the inciting cause can be challenging, partly because of the long list of diseases that can cause uveitis (see Figures 14.32 and 14.33), but also because of the common occurrence of idiopathic uveitis (Massa *et al.*, 2002).

Figure 14.29 presents a diagnostic approach to uveitis.

- Extensive history (geography, disease presentation, progression, response to medication, travel history and concurrent diseases)
- Complete ophthalmic examination of both eyes
- Complete physical examination
- Blood work:
  - Serology (*Toxoplasma, Neospora* ± others depending on vaccination status and history)
  - Haematology
  - Chemistry panel (protein values)
- Fine-needle aspiration (lymph nodes, masses, cutaneous nodules)
- Urinalysis
- Diagnostic imaging:
  - Thoracic radiography
  - Abdominal ultrasonography
  - Ocular ultrasonography
  - Advanced cross-sectional imaging (computed tomography, magnetic resonance imaging)
- Aqueocentesis
- Vitreocentesis
- Diagnostic enucleation with histopathology (blind eyes)

14.29 Diagnostic approach to uveitis.

With a long list of differential diagnoses, it is essential to narrow down the possible conditions to a list of likely or plausible diseases. This can be achieved by obtaining a detailed history, including geographical location, travel history, species, breed, gender, age, daily routine and behaviour, disease presentation, disease progression, response to medication and concurrent diseases (including those of other members of the household). In addition, every patient with uveitis needs to undergo both an ophthalmic and a thorough physical examination. Both eyes should be assessed completely, including a fundus examination if at all possible (the reader is referred to Chapter 1 for information regarding ophthalmic examination techniques).

The assessment of anterior chamber flare and cells is briefly discussed here. For the detection of anterior chamber flare, a narrow beam of focused, condensed light is needed (see Figures 14.21 and 14.24a). This is best achieved using the narrow and condensed slit of light projected by a slit-lamp (Figure 14.30). If a slit-lamp is not available, the finest direct ophthalmoscope spot setting (held very close to the eye) may allow identification of moderate to severe aqueous flare. The direct ophthalmoscope light beam should be observed from a different angle, rather than directly through the ophthalmoscope. The examination is best performed in a room that can be darkened completely. This is critical for the gradation of subtle flare in the anterior chamber (see Figure 14.24). Most degrees of flare, with the exception of the most subtle, can be detected in this manner. Slit-lamp biomicroscope magnification is usually needed to be able to detect and grade cells in the anterior chamber (see Figures 14.24a and 14.31).

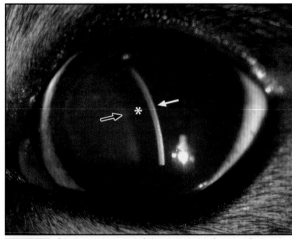

14.31 Slit-lamp image of the normal left eye of a 9-year-old male neutered Domestic Shorthaired cat, demonstrating the appearance of the anterior segment: the convex, bright corneal reflex (white arrow), completely dark anterior chamber (∗) and the somewhat dimmer, convex anterior lens capsular reflex (black arrow). The slit beam is projected from the right towards the left side in this image. (Courtesy of the University of Wisconsin-Madison Comparative Ophthalmology Service)

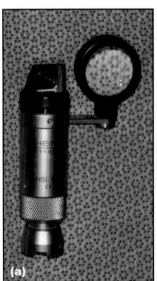

14.30

(a) In the hands of a reasonably experienced examiner, small handheld slit-lamps, whilst inferior to larger portable slit-lamps favoured by veterinary ophthalmologists, can be used by practitioners to perform a good anterior segment examination. (Courtesy of K Sherman) **(b)** Slit-lamp biomicroscopes provide the examiner with a binocular view and superior magnification. Advanced diagnostic training is needed to take full advantage of this instrument.

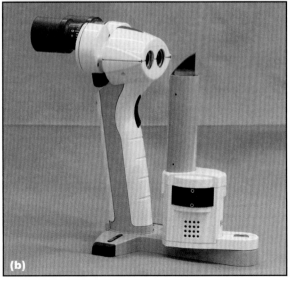

The decision to pursue a more thorough diagnostic work-up to assess for underlying diseases depends on the history and disease presentation, as well as the financial constraints of the owner. Further investigation is indicated in patients that present with:

- Bilateral uveitis, especially if the patient presents with an acute, symmetrical onset of disease. In these animals, until proven otherwise, a systemic disease is the most likely cause of the uveitis
- Abnormalities on physical examination that could indicate an underlying disease
- Posterior uveitis, for which a high probability of an underlying systemic infectious or neoplastic disease exists, especially in areas in which systemic mycotic, rickettsial and protozoal diseases are endemic. In the UK, a history of importation from an endemic area is important
- Severe uveitis, especially if treatment with systemic immunosuppressive medication is likely to be needed to control the inflammation
- Concurrent hyphaema, especially if a potentially life-threatening underlying coagulation or platelet disorder (immune-mediated, infectious) is suspected.

Further diagnostic steps are taken based on the shortlist of likely differential diagnoses. Clinical findings, such as lymphadenopathy, palpable masses or abdominal organ enlargement, can further guide the diagnostic process. Routine haematology, serum biochemistry and urinalysis, combined with geographically inspired serology, thoracic radiography and abdominal ultrasonography, are reasonable in the absence of a suspected aetiology. Ocular ultrasonography is indicated if opacification of normally transparent structures precludes a complete eye examination.

Cytological and histological sampling is guided by the clinical findings. Samples can also be submitted for culture and sensitivity testing. Serological and polymerase chain reaction (PCR) testing can be performed on aspirates obtained from the anterior chamber and vitreous (see Chapter 3 for further details on techniques). However, aqueocentesis and vitreocentesis are not without risk of complications, including intraocular haemorrhage or trauma to the lens and/or retina and therefore referral to a specialist is strongly recommended if either technique is contemplated. On cytology, lymphoma can generally be diagnosed readily; however, sometimes it can be difficult to distinguish lymphoma from a benign reactive proliferation of lymphocytes. Diagnostic enucleation with subsequent histopathological examination is typically reserved for blind eyes.

Differential diagnosis: Figures 14.32 and 14.33 list known causes of uveitis in dogs. Identifying the underlying disease causing uveitis in a patient is

Exogenous
• Septic keratitis
• Trauma (blunt or perforating)
• Drug-induced (miotic agents; prostaglandin analogues)
• Ionizing radiation
• Chemical injuries
Endogenous
Infectious
• See Figure 14.33
Immune-mediated
• Lens-induced:
– Cataract (phacolytic uveitis)
– Lens capsule rupture (phacoclastic uveitis)
• Immune-mediated vasculitis
• Immune-mediated thrombocytopenia
• Uveodermatological syndrome (also known as Vogt–Koyanagi–Harada (VKH)-like syndrome)
• Systemic lupus erythematosus (SLE)
• Granulomatous meningoencephalitis (GME)
Neoplastic
• Primary intraocular:
– Melanoma
– Iridociliary adeno(carcino)ma
– Medulloepithelioma
• Multicentric:
– Lymphoma
– Histiocytic neoplasia
• Metastatic
• Paraneoplastic (hyperviscosity syndrome)
Metabolic
• Hyperlipidaemia (e.g. Miniature Schnauzer)
Toxic
• Pyometra
• Abscess
Miscellaneous
• Idiopathic
• Pigmentary uveitis
• Scleritis

14.32 Differential diagnoses of canine uveitis.

Viral
• Infectious canine hepatitis (canine adenovirus-1, CAV-1)
Rickettsial
• Ehrlichiosis
• Rocky Mountain Spotted Fever
Bacterial
• Sepsis/bacteraemia (e.g. pyometra, abscess, periodontal disease)
• Leptospirosis
• Lyme borreliosis
• Brucellosis
• Bartonellosis
• Mycobacterial infection
Protozoal
• Leishmaniosis
• Toxoplasmosis
• Neosporosis
• Trypanosomiasis
Fungal
• Blastomycosis
• Cryptococcosis
• Coccidioidomycosis
• Histoplasmosis
• Aspergillosis
• Candidiasis
Algal
• Prototothecosis
Parasitic
• Ocular nematodiasis:
– Ocular larval migrans (*Toxocara*)
– Ocular filariasis (*Dirofilaria, Angiostrongylus*)
• Ophthalmomyiasis interna (Diptera)
• Onchocerciasis

14.33 Infectious causes of canine uveitis.

often essential for the effective treatment and long-term control of the uveitis. The most important initial question that needs to be addressed is whether an infectious or non-infectious disease is causing the uveitis, as this has immediate consequences for systemic symptomatic treatment. In a retrospective study of 102 dogs with uveitis, 58% of the dogs were diagnosed with immune-mediated or idiopathic uveitis, in 24% of the dogs a neoplastic aetiology was identified and in the remaining 18% of dogs an infectious cause for the uveitis was determined (Massa *et al.*, 2002). Causes of uveitis that are not related to primary intraocular or systemic diseases are considered to be exogenous and include septic keratitis and drugs.

Septic keratitis: Infectious processes in the cornea can cause secondary uveitis (see Chapter 12) mediated by an axonal reflex with effects on blood vessel dilatation, permeability and leucocyte chemotaxis. This axonal reflex can also cause uveitis in association with non-infectious corneal disease. Furthermore, minute amounts of endotoxins (i.e. bacterial cell membrane degradation products) may reach the anterior chamber and elicit an intense uveitis.

Clinically, this seems to be the case with infected ulcers caused by certain Gram-negative bacteria, such as *Pseudomonas* spp. (Figure 14.34). Aggressive treatment to control the infection, corneal degradation, pain and uveitis is essential to stabilize eyes with septic keratitis. If microorganisms gain entrance to the eye a septic endophthalmitis ensues. Eyes with endophthalmitis can rarely be saved.

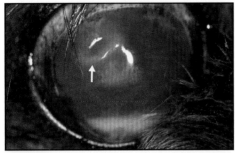

14.34 Septic keratitis and secondary hypopyon in a 9-year-old male neutered Shih Tzu. A white cell precipitate is clearly visible in the inferior anterior chamber. The edge of the corneal ulcer shows signs of melting (arrowed). *Pseudomonas* infection was identified on clinical microbiology.

Drug-induced uveitis: The topical application of direct-acting (pilocarpine) and indirect-acting (demecarium bromide) parasympathomimetic drugs can cause a transient increase in blood–aqueous barrier permeability. Prostaglandin analogues, such as latanoprost and travoprost, which are used extensively in the treatment of primary glaucoma in dogs, cause prominent miosis and can result in iris hyperpigmentation and even iritis. The effects of these drugs are most likely due to direct prostaglandin F (FP) receptor activation.

Viral infections: Viral causes of uveitis include infectious canine hepatitis. Canine adenovirus-1 (CAV-1) induced uveitis and endotheliitis has become a rare phenomenon as a result of an effective vaccination strategy using CAV-2 vaccine. Infectious canine hepatitis-induced keratouveitis should be suspected in unvaccinated young dogs presenting with uveitis that includes a distinct endothelial component (as evidenced by endothelial decompensation and dense corneal oedema: 'blue eye'). Symptomatic therapy may be indicated.

Rickettsial infections:

- **Canine monocytic ehrlichiosis (CME)** is caused by *Ehrlichia canis*, a widely distributed tick-borne disease that is relatively prevalent in (sub)tropical areas. A predilection may be present in the German Shepherd Dog. *E. canis* is an obligate intracellular microorganism that preferentially infects leucocytes and thrombocytes. Ocular signs are usually bilateral and include exudative anterior and posterior uveitis, panuveitis, intraocular haemorrhage, retinal detachment and optic neuritis. Up to 25% of patients with CME present with ocular involvement alone (i.e. with no apparent systemic disease).

The diagnosis is made by serological detection of *E. canis*-specific antibodies via an enzyme-linked immunosorbent assay (ELISA). This can be confirmed by demonstrating the presence of antigen via PCR testing on whole blood. Testing the patients for concurrent tick- or other vector-borne diseases may be relevant, depending on geography. The treatment of choice is doxycycline at 5 mg/kg orally q12h for at least 2–3 weeks. However, some cases require longer courses of doxycycline or imidocarb dipropionate treatment. In addition, the use of anti-inflammatory doses of systemic corticosteroids has been advocated and did not seem to have a negative effect on disease outcome in one study. A good response to treatment and subsequently a good outcome for vision can be expected in most dogs, especially those with only anterior uveitis signs. In two large recent case series, almost all patients with a poor response to treatment showed signs of panuveitis, panophthalmitis, posterior uveitis, necrotic scleritis or glaucoma (Leiva *et al.*, 2005; Komnenou *et al.*, 2007).

- **Rocky Mountain Spotted Fever (RMSF)** is caused by *Rickettsia rickettsii*, a tick-borne pathogen prevalent in the Americas (see also Chapter 20). The ocular signs are usually mild in comparison with CME. The diagnosis is based on seroconversion in paired titres. Various antibiotics can be used effectively (e.g. doxycycline at a dose of 5 mg/kg orally q12h for at least 2 weeks) (Davidson *et al.*, 1989). The spotted fevers are zoonotic diseases which cause similar clinical signs in humans and dogs. There are concerns about dogs being a reservoir host for the disease.

Bacterial infections: Septicaemia and bacteraemia can cause uveitis by dissemination of bacteria into the uveal tissues. Pyometra, localized abscesses and periodontal disease are examples of possible sources of infection. The circulation of endotoxins can also cause uveitis and, in addition, bacterial infection may result from penetrating or perforating ocular injury. Specific bacterial infections known to cause uveitis in dogs include leptospirosis, Lyme borreliosis, brucellosis and bartonellosis.

- **Leptospirosis.** The clinical signs of leptospirosis are the result of a vasculitis, which typically causes kidney and liver failure. Uveitis is relatively rarely observed as part of the disease complex. Anterior uveitis, evidenced by the presence of aqueous flare, hyphaema, vitreous flare and retinal detachments, has been reported. Vaccination has reduced the incidence of the disease. Vaccinations are usually not current in affected dogs, and a history of access to watercourses populated by rats is also common.

The diagnosis is based on the microscopic agglutination test (MAT), but there is considerable inter-laboratory variation in MAT results. Furthermore, the infecting serogroup cannot be accurately predicted by MAT. PCR assays can be used to confirm the diagnosis. Doxycycline (5 mg/kg orally or i.v. q12h for 2 weeks) is recommended as treatment for canine leptospirosis to clear the organism from the renal tubules. Alternatively, ampicillin (20 mg/kg i.v. q6h) or penicillin G (25,000–40,000 IU/kg i.v. q12h) may be used when adverse reactions preclude doxycycline administration. With early and aggressive treatment the prognosis is good. Since leptospirosis is a zoonotic disease, owners and hospital staff should be made aware of the tentative diagnosis and precautionary measures should be taken. Readers are referred to the 2010 ACVIM Small Animal Consensus Statement on Leptospirosis for a very thorough review of the diagnostics, epidemiology, treatment and prevention of the disease (Sykes *et al.*, 2011).

- **Lyme borreliosis** has been implicated as a possible cause of uveitis in dogs. However, although the organism is endemic in the UK, ophthalmic and systemic clinical disease appears to be rare. Typical systemic signs include lameness and lymphadenopathy. Doxycycline is recommended as a specific antimicrobial treatment.
- **Brucellosis.** *Brucella canis* can cause unilateral ocular signs including anterior uveitis, endophthalmitis, chorioretinitis, keratoconjunctivitis and hyphaema. Various serological tests for *B. canis* are available. Since sensitivity and specificity may vary with individual tests and disease stage, isolation or PCR confirmation is recommended for a definitive diagnosis. Brucellosis is a zoonotic disease and this should be pointed out to the owners of an affected animal. Owing to the intracellular nature of the microorganism, elimination of the organism is difficult to accomplish and treatment can be complicated, protracted and expensive (Ledbetter *et al.*, 2009). Canine brucellosis has not been reported in the UK.
- **Bartonellosis.** *Bartonella* species are considered to be emerging pathogens throughout the world. However, bartonellosis rarely causes ocular problems in dogs, and clinical cases have not been described in Europe.

Protozoal diseases: (The reader is referred to Chapter 20 for additional information.)

- **Leishmaniosis** is a protozoal disease that can affect multiple species, including dogs, cats and humans, in endemic areas. Leishmaniosis is caused by *Leishmania* spp., which are transmitted by feeding sandflies. The disease has been reported in the Mediterranean basin, parts of Africa, India and North, Central and South America. The incubation period may last several months to 3–4 years. Hence, obtaining a thorough travel history is essential. Ocular signs are common in infected dogs (see Figure 14.20) and are usually present in concert with signs of systemic disease.

The diagnosis is based on serology, PCR testing on blood, aspirates or biopsy specimens and cytological or histological identification of *Leishmania* amastigotes in skin scrapes/ impression smears, lymph node and bone marrow aspirates or skin or other organ biopsy samples. A favourable ocular and systemic response to treatment with systemic antiprotozoal and topical anti-inflammatory therapy can be expected, although long-term topical treatment is often needed to keep the uveitis under control. A combination of meglumine antimoniate (80 mg/kg s.c. q24h for 30 days) and allopurinol (10 mg/kg orally q12h for 6–12 months) is the most widely used therapy. Miltefosine and allopurinol is another recently described combination therapy. The use of a short course of anti-inflammatory doses of systemic corticosteroids has also been advocated. Relapses are not uncommon and can occur years after discontinuation of treatment (Peña *et al.*, 2000; Torres *et al.*, 2011).

- **Toxoplasmosis.** Dogs can be infected with *Toxoplasma gondii*, an obligate intracellular protozoan, by ingesting sporulated oocysts in cat faeces, or ingesting tissue cysts in other intermediate hosts or infected meat. Transplacental transmission is also possible. The infection is mostly subclinical in dogs and ocular toxoplasmosis is rare. However, reports of *T. gondii*-induced keratoconjunctivitis, (epi) scleritis, anterior uveitis, (chorio)retinitis, optic neuritis and polymyositis have been published.

  Serological testing for immunoglobulin (Ig)M and IgG antibodies, including paired samples and convalescent titres, may indicate an active *T. gondii* infection. Clindamycin is the antibiotic of choice and should be given twice daily at a dose of 12.5 mg/kg orally for 4 weeks. For detailed information on *T. gondii* prevalence, signs, diagnosis and treatment in dogs and cats, the reader is referred to an extensive review published by Dubey *et al.* (2009).
- **Neosporosis.** A single case series reports *Neospora caninum* as cause of ocular signs in dogs and *N. caninum*, therefore, seems to be a rare cause of uveitis in dogs.

Fungal infections: (The reader is referred to Chapter 20 for additional information.)

- **Blastomycosis** is caused by *Blastomyces dermatitidis*, which has a global distribution. However, blastomycosis remains largely a North American disease. After initial infection through inhalation of spores from the environment, a primary pulmonary infection occurs. The microorganism is thought to disseminate from the lungs via both haematogenous and lymphatic routes. Typical sites of involvement after dissemination include the skin, lymph nodes, bones, eyes (Figure 14.35), central nervous system (CNS) and testes.

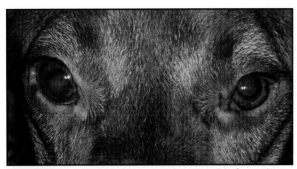

14.35 Endophthalmitis, posterior synechia formation, iris bombé and secondary glaucoma in the right eye of a 6-year-old male neutered Vizsla with blastomycosis. Note the yellow appearance of the pupil, due to chorioretinal granulomas and complete retinal detachment. The eye was enucleated as soon as the systemic condition of the dog had been stabilized.

In endemic areas, all dogs suspected of having systemic mycosis and all dogs with anterior uveitis should undergo fundic examination. The diagnosis is based on the history and clinical signs, thoracic radiography, serology and direct microscopic identification of the yeasts. A positive urine antigen test strongly supports the diagnosis. The diagnosis is confirmed through histological evaluation of tissue biopsy samples and cytological evaluation of smears or aspirates obtained from lymph nodes, skin lesions, urine, tracheal washes, aqueous humour or vitreous. Fungal cultures are not recommended owing to infection risks for laboratory personnel.

Treatment consists of supportive care and the administration of systemic antifungal medications. Various protocols exist, but itraconazole and fluconazole are typical first-choice medications (Foy and Trepanier, 2010). The uveitis should be treated aggressively with topical corticosteroids. The use of anti-inflammatory doses of systemic corticosteroids has been advocated as well. The enucleation of blind eyes to remove a potential nidus for reinfection has been a source of debate. Surgical removal of irreversibly blind eyes with uncontrollable uveitis or glaucoma is recommended. The prognosis for survival ranges from extremely poor to fair. The prognosis for vision depends on the extent and response to treatment of the posterior segment lesions. Eyes that develop glaucoma have an extremely poor prognosis. Systemic mycoses have zoonotic potential, but direct dog-to-dog and dog-to-human transmission is unlikely. The reader is referred to an extensive review by Bromel and Sykes (2005a).

- **Cryptococcosis** is caused by *Cryptococcus neoformans* and *C. gattii* (Trivedi *et al.*, 2011b). The nasal cavity is the suspected initial site of infection, from which the microorganisms are distributed throughout the body. The clinical signs largely resemble those seen with blastomycosis. Diagnostic, treatment and prognostic considerations are broadly the same as for blastomycosis. Serological tests for cryptococcal antigens are highly sensitive and specific, with few false-positive test results occurring. Cryptococcosis is a relatively rare but ubiquitous disease.

- **Coccidioidomycosis** is caused by *Coccidioides immitis* and *C. posadasii* and is most prevalent in the southwestern USA, Mexico and Central and South America. The clinical signs largely resemble those of blastomycosis. Diagnostic, treatment and prognostic considerations are broadly the same as for blastomycosis (Graupmann-Kuzma *et al.*, 2008).

- **Histoplasmosis** is a relatively rare disease in dogs, caused by various *Histoplasma* spp. The disease has a worldwide distribution. In the USA, the disease is most prevalent in the Ohio and Mississippi river valleys. The systemic and ocular clinical signs are similar to those seen with blastomycosis. Intestinal disease (diarrhoea with haematochezia or melaena) is common in dogs with histoplasmosis. Diagnostic, treatment and prognostic considerations are broadly the same as for blastomycosis (Bromel and Sykes, 2005b).

- **Aspergillosis.** Dogs with disseminated aspergillosis can develop ocular signs. The posterior segment is primarily affected. A panophthalmitis can ensue and septated hyphae are concentrated in the vitreous on histological examination. The prognosis for survival is poor for dogs with disseminated aspergillosis. A breed predilection exists in German Shepherd Dogs. Immunosuppression is thought to play a role because *Aspergillus* spp. are ubiquitous. The disease is very uncommon but has been reported in the UK.

Algal diseases:

- **Prototothecosis** is a rare disease caused by the algae *Prototheca zopfii* and *P. wickerhamii*. Patients initially present with haemorrhagic diarrhoea. After dissemination of the fungus, the clinical signs are mostly ocular and neurological. Ocular lesions resemble those seen with systemic mycoses. The diagnosis is based on culture and cytological or histological identification of the microorganisms. The prognosis for survival is poor and treatment attempts have been unsuccessful in the long term.

Parasitic diseases: (The reader is referred to Chapter 20 for additional information.)

- **Ocular nematodiasis and ophthalmomyiasis interna.** Parasitic uveitis is caused by the aberrant migration of nematode larvae (*Dirofilaria immitis, Angiostrongylus vasorum, Toxocara* spp.) or fly larvae of the order Diptera. *A. vasorum*-induced uveitis is not uncommon in endemic areas in the UK (including Wales and southwest England) and Ireland. *D. immitis* is found only in imported dogs. Fly larva-induced uveitis is rare. An inflammatory response is usually mounted to the presence of the parasite and its waste products. The uveitis can be exacerbated by killing the parasite. In selected cases, the clinician can monitor the parasite (*D. immitis*, *A. vasorum*, Diptera) and wait for spontaneous departure from the eye. However, in cases where the larvae are within reach, attempts should be made to remove them surgically without inflicting damage on the parasite. Referral to a specialist is strongly recommended for surgical parasite removal. Ocular larval migrans caused by *Toxocara* spp. is characterized by inflammatory changes in the vitreous and chorioretinitis and is not a surgical disease.

- **Onchocerciasis** has been observed in the Mediterranean basin and in the southwestern USA. Granulomatous, episcleral lesions containing parasites are found, and anterior and posterior uveitis are commonly seen in these patients. Surgical excision and anthelmintic therapy are recommended (Komnenou *et al.*, 2002).

Lens-induced uveitis: Lens pathologies are frequently associated with uveitis. Normal lens proteins are weakly antigenic, but fractionated proteins and the conversion of soluble to insoluble proteins (as with cataract development) stimulate the immune system. The inflammatory reaction most likely results from altered tolerance to lens proteins rather than a rejection phenomenon of sequestered proteins (van der Woerdt, 2000). The intensity of this reaction depends in part on the amount and type of protein to which the immune system is exposed.

In the presence of a complete or resorbing cataract, degraded lens cortex proteins can leak through an intact lens capsule and cause inflammation in the anterior and posterior segments of the eye. In this situation a *phacolytic uveitis* exists. With rapidly developing cataracts (e.g. diabetic cataracts), lens swelling may cause increased porosity of or microscopic tears in the lens capsule, allowing intact lens proteins to reach the ocular environment and engage the immune system.

- **Phacolytic uveitis.** Lens-induced uveitis is a very common condition in cataractous eyes and should be suspected *in all eyes with cataracts that show signs of redness and inflammation*. These eyes typically present with signs of anterior uveitis: reduced IOP, miosis, aqueous flare and cells, iris swelling, iridal blood vessel congestion and posterior synechiae (Figure 14.36). Hypopyon, hyphaema and fibrin are infrequently observed. If the IOP is elevated as a result of secondary glaucoma, the pupil may be mydriatic. Failure to recognize and treat lens-induced uveitis will either lower the success rate of cataract surgery or prevent the eye from being a candidate for cataract surgery at all (see Chapter 16).

  Aggressive anti-inflammatory treatment is indicated initially. Topical corticosteroids in combination with systemic non-steroidal anti-inflammatory drugs (NSAIDs) or corticosteroids

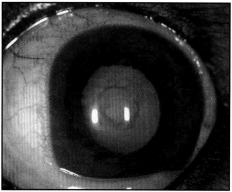

14.36 Lens-induced uveitis in a dog with a primary cataract. Note the conjunctival hyperaemia and peripheral corneal neovascularization (red eye), the mild perilimbal corneal oedema and the pigment rests on the anterior lens capsule due to previous iris-to-lens adhesions. (Courtesy of the University of Wisconsin-Madison Comparative Ophthalmology Service)

are often used. Most patients with lens-induced uveitis require some form of life-long anti-inflammatory treatment. Once the uveitis is under control, maintenance therapy can consist of topical NSAIDs or corticosteroids administered twice daily to once every other day. The use of systemic corticosteroids and the frequent administration of topical corticosteroids should be approached with caution in small patients with diabetic cataracts to avoid dysregulation of their glycaemic control. Topical NSAIDs are often used in diabetic dogs with early cataract formation to reduce the risk of lens-induced uveitis.

- **Phacoclastic uveitis.** In eyes that have sustained sharp or blunt trauma, the lens capsule may have been lacerated or ruptured. In these cases, large amounts of lens protein will overwhelm the immune system and elicit a severe uveitis. This is called a *phacoclastic uveitis*. All possible signs of uveitis can be observed. The presence of corneal oedema and blood, fibrin or hypopyon in the anterior chamber often precludes complete examination of the lens. Ocular ultrasound examination can be useful, but is not necessarily conclusive in these situations. Since most lens capsule lacerations are caused by cat scratches or bite wounds, either bacterial or fungal microorganisms are inoculated into the lens and a septic endophthalmitis can occur. Even with aggressive antibiotic and anti-inflammatory treatment, the inflammation in these eyes is often uncontrollable. Early surgical removal of the lens may help to control the problem (see Chapter 16). The prognosis is best, but still guarded, in eyes with recent trauma and no signs of endophthalmitis. The prognosis is poor in cases with severe, chronic uveitis or endophthalmitis. Early referral to a specialist is therefore recommended in cases of suspected lens capsule rupture.

Uveodermatological syndrome: This is also known as Vogt–Koyanagi–Harada (VKH)-like syndrome (see also Chapter 20). The condition is caused by immune-mediated destruction of melanocytes, and affects mainly the eyes and skin. Frequently observed ocular signs of this bilateral disease include: anterior uveitis; panuveitis; depigmentation of the iris, retinal pigment epithelium and choroid; retinal detachment; and retinal and optic nerve degeneration. Cataracts, posterior synechiae, iris bombé and glaucoma are common complications. Skin and fur depigmentation (vitiligo and poliosis, respectively) usually occur in later stages of the disease and are typically restricted to the face (the eyelids, nasal planum and lips). However, more generalized depigmentation may occur (Figure 14.37). The disease was initially described in the Akita, but has been diagnosed in many other dog breeds as well. Hereditary factors may play a role in the development of VKH-like syndrome in the Akita.

The diagnosis is based on the clinical signs and can be confirmed histologically with a skin biopsy (e.g. from the margin of the nasal planum). Owing to involvement of the entire uveal tract, including the choroid, topical and systemic treatment with immunosuppressive medications is indicated. Topical corticosteroids can be started with application at least 6 times daily, especially if severe uveitis is present. Systemic corticosteroids are initiated at an immunosuppressive dose of 2 mg/kg. This dose is gradually tapered once the uveitis is controlled. Systemic azathioprine, cyclophosphamide or ciclosporin can be used in combination with the corticosteroid treatment. Given the potential for ocular complications and the risk of treatment side effects, regular rechecks are recommended for these patients. The reader is referred to the section on treatment of uveitis for information on recommended dosages and blood work monitoring. The prognosis for vision is guarded and relapses are common after discontinuation of therapy. Life-long treatment should therefore be considered.

Neoplasia: Neoplastic diseases are a relatively common cause of blood–aqueous barrier breakdown in dogs. Multicentric neoplasms frequently infiltrate the uvea and cause intraocular haemorrhage, anterior chamber cells and flare, hypopyon and, potentially, even intraocular masses. Lymphoma is the most common secondary or multicentric neoplasm to affect the eyes and usually affects both eyes simultaneously (see Figures 14.23 and 14.25). Lymphoma often causes a surprisingly low level of discomfort when the severity of the ocular changes is taken into account (see Figure 14.25). Histiocytic tumours should be on the list of differential diagnoses if dogs of specific breeds present with sudden unilateral or (rarely) bilateral intraocular haemorrhage or uveitis. Middle-aged to older Bernese Mountain Dogs, Rottweilers and Golden, Labrador and Flat-coated Retrievers are predisposed to histiocytic neoplasia. More information can be found in the section on neoplastic diseases below.

Hyperlipidaemia: The combination of blood–aqueous barrier breakdown and elevated lipid levels in the systemic circulation can cause a sudden influx of lipids into the anterior chamber and a lipid-laden aqueous. This is observed as a very dense, milky flare (Figure 14.38). It is not clear whether the occurrence of uveitis and hyperlipidaemia is purely coincidental in these cases. A hyperlipidaemia-induced vasculitis and subsequent blood–aqueous barrier breakdown is a possible scenario in animals with a spontaneously occurring lipid flare. A recent history of ingestion of lipid-rich food or garbage seems to be a recurring theme. A diagnostic work-up for systemic diseases that can potentially cause elevated blood lipid levels may be indicated. Treatment of any underlying disease and symptomatic treatment of the anterior uveitis are necessary. Miniature Schnauzers with idiopathic hyperlipidaemia may be at increased risk, especially those with concurrent uveitis.

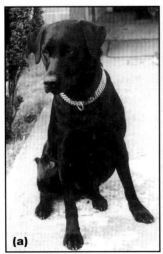
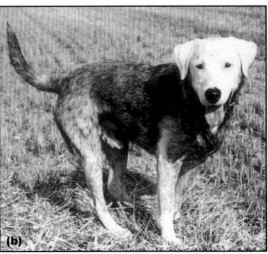
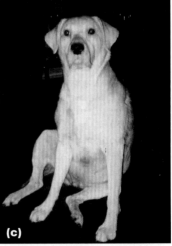

14.37 **(a)** Labrador Retriever with uveodermatological syndrome before overt onset of the disease. **(b)** Years later, depigmentation of the fur and eyelid margins is obvious. **(c)** Almost 6 years have passed between the first presentation and this recheck, during which almost complete pigment loss was observed. Note the progressive depigmentation around the edges of the nasal planum when comparing (b) and (c). At this time the dog had lost vision as a result of uveitis-induced cataracts. The uveitis was fairly well controlled with systemic corticosteroid therapy.

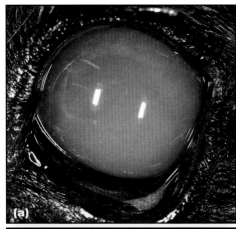

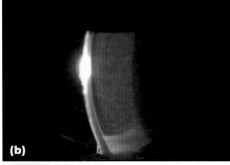

14.38 **(a)** Lipid-laden aqueous in a hypothyroid 5-year-old male neutered crossbreed dog. **(b)** Slit-lamp image of lipid-laden aqueous in a 5-year-old male neutered Cavalier King Charles Spaniel. The slit beam is projected from the left towards the right side in this image and focused on the dense, milky, lipid flare in the anterior chamber. Note the convection currents in the anterior chamber, caused by an upward movement of warmer aqueous close to the lens and a downward movement of cooler aqueous on the corneal side.

Pigmentary uveitis: The reader is referred to the section on iridociliary cysts for further information on this condition, which is presumed to be inherited in Golden Retrievers.

Scleritis: Necrotizing and non-necrotizing granulomatous scleritis can cause inflammation in adjacent tissues, including the orbit, extraocular muscles and uvea. In the anterior segment, this usually causes a non-granulomatous anterior uveitis. Therapy involves symptomatic anti-inflammatory treatment. Intralesional corticosteroids and systemic immunosuppressive medications may be necessary to control the scleritis. In selected cases, an infectious aetiology may be present. The reader is referred to Chapter 13 for further detailed description of the diagnosis and management of scleritis.

Idiopathic uveitis: Despite an extensive diagnostic work-up, the cause of canine uveitis remains undiagnosed in many cases. A default diagnosis of idiopathic uveitis is made in these situations. Symptomatic therapy is recommended for these patients. The clinician should realize that idiopathic uveitis is not a true diagnosis; it is merely a reflection of the fact that it has not been possible to identify the underlying cause. This can be due to false-negative test results, failing to test for the causative disease, or because the uveitis is caused by a 'new', unreported cause for this disease in dogs. As clinicians, we should not hesitate to reconsider our diagnostic steps, diagnosis and treatment if the response to therapy is not as expected.

Treatment: Every case of uveitis needs immediate anti-inflammatory therapy, regardless of the aetiology. The goals of anti-inflammatory therapy are to suppress inflammation, control pain and minimize the occurrence of adverse sequelae. The choice of anti-inflammatory medication, and which administration route to use, may depend on the suspected underlying disease. Once initiated, medications are usually tapered slowly. Many weeks to months of anti-inflammatory treatment may be needed. NSAIDs and corticosteroids can be used topically and systemically. Anterior segment structures can be medicated with appropriate topical therapy. Systemic medications are needed to achieve therapeutic concentrations in the posterior segment (see Chapter 7).

Topical corticosteroid treatment can be administered immediately if the cornea does not retain fluorescein stain. However, topical corticosteroids should not be used when corneal defects are present. The most commonly prescribed topical corticosteroids are 1% prednisolone acetate and 0.1% dexamethasone acetate because of their potency and availability. Lipophilic acetate preparations penetrate the cornea much better than polar phosphate preparations, owing to the fact that the lipid-rich epithelium is the most important barrier to intraocular penetration of topical drugs. The frequency of application depends on the severity of the uveitis. When clinical signs are mild, topical corticosteroids can be used two to three times daily; in severe cases topical drops can be given as often as every 2–4 hours, although care should be taken in smaller patients as a high frequency of topical corticosteroid application may induce systemic side effects. Topical NSAIDs can be given in addition to corticosteroids. Many different preparations are available and drops are usually given 2–4 times daily. Topical NSAIDs alone are safer to use in patients with corneal ulcers.

Systemic treatment with corticosteroids should only be instigated once any underlying infectious causes of the uveitis have been ruled out. If immediate systemic treatment with corticosteroids is necessary for the preservation or return of vision, blood should be collected from the patient and serum stored for diagnostic testing at a later time, and the patient should be carefully monitored for signs of disease progression.

For immune-mediated conditions, corticosteroid treatment can be started at immunosuppressive dosages (2–4 mg/kg daily in divided doses) and continued until the uveitis is under control. The dose is then tapered and the patient rigorously re-evaluated to ensure that the uveitis remains controlled with each successive reduction in the corticosteroid dose. Systemic corticosteroid treatment is discontinued as soon as it is no longer needed for uveitis control, when the underlying disease is cured and the uveitis controlled, or when the uveitis has been controlled by means of topical treatment alone or by means of another systemic immunomodulating medication. In some immune-mediated conditions, such as uveodermatological syndrome (see above), long-term systemic corticosteroid treatment may be required, at as low a dose as possible in order to maintain disease remission, either with or without additional immunomodulatory drugs. For non-immune-mediated or idiopathic aetiologies, anti-inflammatory doses of systemic corticosteroids (initial dose 0.5–1 mg/kg daily in divided doses) may be indicated, but should be used cautiously, especially in cases with known or suspected systemic infectious disease.

Systemic NSAIDs are usually a safe alternative to systemic corticosteroids. However, the fact that systemic NSAID use can cause inhibition of platelet function and may induce gastrointestinal and renal side effects should be taken into consideration.

Immunomodulating drugs may be necessary for the long-term control of uveitis, especially that due to immune-mediated disease. These drugs are used because of their favourable side-effect profile when compared with the long-term use of systemic corticosteroids. Typically, these drugs are started at their respective recommended dosages and given concurrently with systemic corticosteroids. The systemic corticosteroids are then tapered off, whilst the dose of the immunomodulating drug is maintained. After discontinuing the systemic corticosteroid, the immunomodulating drug is slowly tapered to the lowest effective dose.

- Azathioprine is initially administered orally at a dose of 2 mg/kg q24h. Potential side effects include vomiting and diarrhoea, bone marrow suppression and hepatotoxicity. Baseline haematology and serum biochemistry should be obtained and haematological and liver function parameters should be monitored every 2 weeks during the first few months, and at least every 4 months throughout the rest of the treatment.
- Cyclophosphamide, ciclosporin and methotrexate represent alternatives to azathioprine.

Mydriatics/cycloplegics are used to reduce the risk of posterior synechiae, reduce the pain associated with ciliary body spasm through relaxation of the ciliary musculature (cycloplegia) and stabilize the blood–aqueous barrier. Topical 1% atropine is a potent parasympatholytic with mydriatic and cycloplegic effects, which can be used to effect. In patients with moderate to severe uveitis, the initial frequency of application is usually 2–3 times daily. Tropicamide solution (0.5–1%) is a shorter-acting parasympatholytic with potent mydriatic but weak cycloplegic effects. Tropicamide can be used 2–3 times daily to keep the pupil moving and decrease the risk of posterior synechia formation in patients with little to no pain. Topical sympathomimetics (e.g. phenylephrine) can be used concurrently to enhance mydriasis; however, their cycloplegic effects are minimal. Mydriasis can lead to an increase in IOP.

Institution of appropriate therapy for glaucoma and repeated IOP measurements are indicated if a normal or increased IOP was observed initially during episodes of active uveitis. The reader is referred to Chapter 15 for guidelines regarding the treatment of uveitis-induced secondary glaucoma. Specific treatments for underlying diseases have been discussed in the relevant sections and should be administered as needed, in addition to the symptomatic treatments described above.

Recheck appointments are critical to ascertain whether control has been achieved over the uveitis and IOP. Recheck frequency depends on the severity of the uveitis and the response to treatment. Patients with severe uveitis are typically rechecked within a day or two of initiating therapy, and patients with moderate to mild uveitis are generally rechecked within 1–2 weeks. Owners should be advised of the need to contact the clinic without delay should clinical signs worsen despite treatment. Patients receiving long-term systemic immunosuppressive therapy need to be monitored at appropriate intervals throughout the course of treatment.

Trauma

Ocular trauma often involves pain, compromised globe integrity and/or loss of vision. Traumatic conditions affecting the globe and orbit are covered in Chapter 8; corneal and scleral injuries are covered in Chapters 12 and 13, respectively. Severe ocular trauma should be handled on an emergency basis, with prompt evaluation of the patient's systemic and ocular condition. Treatment should follow rapidly to avoid permanent damage to the eye or loss of vision. For painful conditions, or when ocular integrity is compromised, it may be safer to perform the eye examination under heavy sedation or anaesthesia, thereby limiting further ocular damage that may occur as a result of patient restraint. Exudates and haemorrhage can be gently flushed with warm sterile saline. The periorbital region should be examined for bruising and wounds. An ocular examination will determine whether a laceration or globe rupture is present. It should be noted, however, that scleral lacerations may not be readily visible and are more difficult to diagnose. Corneal lacerations may extend past the limbus, underneath a haemorrhagic conjunctiva. Clinical signs associated with blunt and perforating trauma are listed in Figure 14.39. When foreign bodies are suspected, the conjunctival fornices and both sides of the third eyelid should be examined. If the eye is perforated it should be determined, in consultation with a veterinary ophthalmologist, whether surgical repair is feasible or the eye is best enucleated (Figure 14.40).

Additional diagnostic work-up may include computed tomography (CT) or magnetic resonance imaging (MRI) of the head. CT is preferred if fractures or foreign bodies are suspected because the extent of the trauma can be assessed, fractures are more easily visualized and most foreign bodies

Blunt trauma
• Corneal oedema
• Flare, fibrin
• Hyphaema
• Iris laceration and drainage angle recession
• Lens luxation
• Lens capsule rupture
• Retinal detachment
• Choroidal detachment
• Scleral rupture and globe collapse

Perforating trauma
• Positive Seidel test
• Uvea coloured mound on the cornea
• Flare, fibrin
• Hyphaema
• Intraocular foreign body
• Collapsed anterior chamber
• Irregular anterior chamber depth
• Eccentric pupil or dyscoria
• Lens capsule rupture
• Extrusion of intraocular contents and globe collapse

14.39 Clinical signs associated with blunt and penetrating trauma.

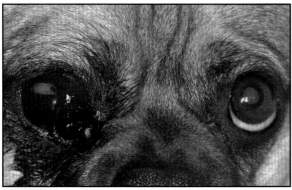

14.40 Traumatic rupture of the globe with extrusion of ocular contents (black material at the medial canthus). The eye was subsequently enucleated. (Courtesy of the University of Wisconsin-Madison Comparative Ophthalmology Service)

either show up directly or as an imaging void after contrast medium administration. MRI provides the best resolution to diagnose non-metallic intraocular foreign bodies, but is contraindicated for metallic foreign bodies because these may move during image acquisition and cause additional damage. Ocular ultrasonography is indicated when direct visualization of the intraocular structures is not possible. Chapter 2 provides a detailed discussion of ophthalmic imaging modalities.

Penetrating trauma: All penetrating wounds to the eye should be considered to be infected and treated accordingly with topical and systemic medication. Consultation with a veterinary ophthalmologist is indicated to determine the need for specialist intervention. The development of suppurative endophthalmitis is the most common reason for performing enucleation after penetrating trauma.

• **Small uncomplicated punctures** to the globe may seal rapidly, but are invariably associated with uveitis. A Seidel test (see Chapter 1) will determine whether aqueous humour is still leaking from the puncture site. Topical NSAIDs should substitute for topical corticosteroids for as long as the cornea is fluorescein-positive. A complete ocular examination should be performed with particular attention paid to lens integrity.

• **Penetrating trauma associated with lens damage.** Lens capsule rupture generally leads to intense phacoclastic uveitis, which requires prompt and aggressive intervention (see Chapter 16 and above for a more detailed discussion of this condition). Provided that the uveitis is treated early, small capsular rents may seal spontaneously with fibrin and result in focal cataracts only. If a large (>2 mm) capsular tear is present, or a significant amount of lens protein is present in the anterior chamber, prompt referral for early lens removal via phacoemulsification surgery is strongly recommended.

• **Perforating wounds with iris prolapse.** With larger perforations the iris may be carried forward into the wound by escaping aqueous. The appearance is that of uvea-coloured gelatinous mucus adhering to the cornea (Figure 14.41). Anterior chamber depth is lost or irregular, the chamber is often filled with blood or fibrin, and the pupil is eccentric or irregular. Depending on the duration and extent of the prolapse, the iris may be surgically repositioned and the globe surgically repaired (see Chapters 6 and 12).

• **Intraocular foreign bodies.** Surgical removal of intraocular foreign bodies depends on the nature, size and location of the foreign material, as well as the extent of associated tissue damage. Organic and reactive inorganic material (e.g. iron and copper) should be removed. The strategy for removal should be chosen so as to remove the foreign body completely, whilst avoiding further ocular damage in the process. Although not ideal, small inert inorganic foreign bodies (e.g. lead, glass, many plastics) may be left in place when limited finances, surgical skill or restrictions on referral ability do not allow for immediate surgical removal. Uveitis should be treated promptly and aggressively. Endophthalmitis may be a devastating

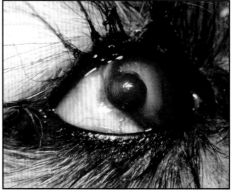

14.41 Perforation of the temporal cornea with protrusion of iris through the corneal defect in a young Shih Tzu.

consequence and occurs more commonly with organic foreign bodies.

- **Ocular perforation associated with oral disease.** Ocular perforation can be associated with injuries from the oral cavity that penetrate the orbit and perforate the globe. This can be seen in association with a foreign body. It can also occur following dental procedures for the removal of caudal maxillary tooth roots, when an inappropriately performed caudal maxillary nerve block or accidental slippage of dental instruments can perforate the globe (see Chapter 13).

Blunt trauma: Blunt trauma may cause severe damage to the head and eye (see Figure 14.39 and Chapter 8). Examination of the eye and palpation of the periocular bones should be performed after a general physical examination. Globe rupture associated with blunt trauma occurs more commonly at the equator and posterior pole, thus may not be directly visible. Suggestive clinical signs include hyphaema, subconjunctival haemorrhage, chemosis, globe collapse and a very low IOP. Ocular ultrasonography may show ill defined scleral borders, retinal detachment, echoic opacities in the vitreous and chambers (blood), lens luxation or cyclodialysis (separation of the iris and ciliary body from the sclera) (the reader is referred to Chapters 2 and 13 for specific features associated with these abnormalities). Lens capsule rupture may result from blunt trauma. Severe trauma to the uvea generally leads to phthisis bulbi and frequently secondary entropion. Therefore, severely traumatized blind eyes may be best managed by enucleation. A blind but comfortable globe with moderate pathology could be retained for cosmetic purposes.

Intraocular haemorrhage

Intraocular haemorrhage may diffusely fill the globe or may be more localized to the anterior chamber (hyphaema), vitreous or uveal tissue (e.g. iris stroma; Figure 14.42). Haemorrhage primarily affecting the posterior segment is discussed more extensively in Chapters 17 and 18. When investigating a patient with intraocular haemorrhage, local and systemic causes for the bleeding should be considered (Figure 14.43). Recurrent unilateral hyphaema in older dogs, especially if no abnormalities are found on the diagnostic work-up, should alert the clinician to the possibility of an intraocular tumour. An ocular ultrasound examination may be indicated, but is not always conclusive, as blood clots can resemble tissue masses. In these cases, Doppler ultrasonography or repeat ultrasound examinations to monitor the size of the mass can be useful. Systemic causes tend to affect both eyes, although possibly to varying degrees (Figure 14.44). See Chapter 20 for further discussion of systemic diseases that can cause intraocular haemorrhage.

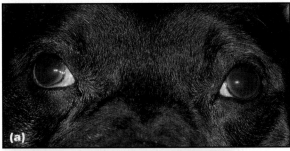

Local (eye-related) conditions
• Trauma (blunt or perforating)
• Uveitis/chorioretinitis
• Pre-iridal fibrovascular membrane
• Glaucoma (primary or secondary)
• Retinal detachment (congenital or acquired)
• Persistent hyaloid vasculature
• Neoplasia
Systemic conditions
• Thrombocytopenia/thrombopathies
• Coagulopathies
• Hyperviscosity/gammopathies (paraneoplastic)
• Systemic hypertension
• Vasculitis
• Polycythaemia
• Neoplasia
• Drug-induced/toxic
• (Profound anaemia)

14.43 Differential diagnoses of intraocular haemorrhage in dogs and cats.

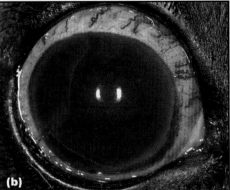

14.44 **(a)** Bilateral hyphaema associated with multicentric lymphoma in an 11-year-old American Staffordshire Terrier. **(b)** Close-up view of the right eye. (Courtesy of the University of Wisconsin-Madison Comparative Ophthalmology Service)

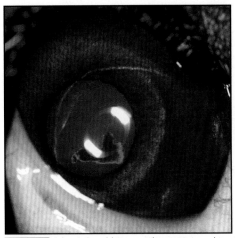

14.42 Iris stromal haemorrhage secondary to immune-mediated thrombocytopenia in a Great Dane.

When uncomplicated, small to moderate degrees of hyphaema may resorb quickly and uneventfully. Associated uveitis should be treated symptomatically with topical corticosteroids and mydriatic drugs. Systemic NSAIDs should be avoided because they increase blood clotting times and may be substituted with systemic corticosteroids if these are not contraindicated. In selected cases, an intracameral injection of tissue plasminogen activator (see Chapter 7) may be beneficial in dissolving fibrin that can entrap intraocular structures and lead to the formation of synechiae. Before resorting to this treatment every effort should be made to identify the underlying cause and prevent further bleeding.

Extensive, diffuse and recurrent hyphaema may hinder aqueous outflow (via accumulation of cells and fibrotic changes in the drainage angle) and subsequently lead to glaucoma. Fibrin deposits may also lead to extensive posterior synechiae (particularly when the concurrent uveitis is severe), limiting anterior movement of aqueous through the pupil, thereby causing iris bombé and further compromising the iridocorneal angle (see Chapter 15).

Ocular melanosis

Ocular melanosis is the abnormal accumulation of pigment within the uveal tissue to the extent that it interferes with ocular function (Petersen-Jones *et al.*, 2007). There is a predisposition for the Cairn Terrier to develop this condition bilaterally. Other breeds may also develop this condition, notably the Boxer and Labrador Retriever, but these cases often show only unilateral ocular involvement. Pigmented cells and free pigment granules exfoliate within the anterior chamber, become deposited on the lens and corneal endothelium and, most importantly, clog the drainage angle, impairing aqueous outflow and leading to glaucoma. At this stage, the condition has also been termed 'pigmentary glaucoma' (see Chapter 15). Accumulated pigment in the aqueous outflow pathways causes the development of black patches in the perilimbal sclera (Figure 14.45a). Initially, these are most noticeable in the inferior sclera. The choroid may also become diffusely infiltrated, leading to a progressive decrease in tapetal size (Figure 14.45b). The condition is typically slowly progressive regardless of treatment for either uveitis or glaucoma. Occasionally, melanocytic tumours also develop in affected eyes.

Uveal neoplasia

Neoplasia should always be considered in eyes with uveitis, haemorrhage, glaucoma, retinal detachment or intraocular masses.

Primary neoplasia: The majority of primary uveal neoplasms arise from the iris and ciliary body, rather than the choroid, and are usually benign in dogs. Melanocytic neoplasia most commonly affects the anterior uvea of the older, and occasionally also younger, dog. Rarely do these neoplasms originate in the choroid. Most of these tumours are benign melanocytomas (Figure 14.46) with little tendency to metastasize. However, they can be locally destructive by causing uveitis and glaucoma.

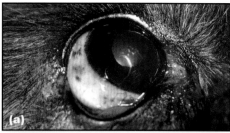

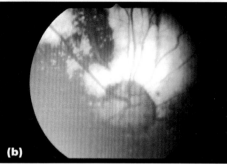

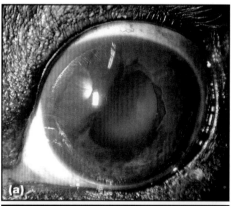

14.45 Ocular melanosis in a Cairn Terrier. **(a)** The iris is diffusely hyperpigmented and thickened. Pigment accumulation within the sclera results in the characteristic black patches. **(b)** Pigment also accumulates in the choroid, leading to infiltration of the tapetum. The fundic image is somewhat blurred owing to nuclear sclerosis.

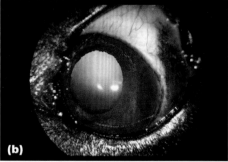

14.46 **(a)** Melanocytoma involving a large portion of the superior iris, leading to pupillary distortion. (Courtesy of BM Spiess) **(b)** Ciliary body melanocytoma extending into the sclera and temporal iris.

Malignant melanomas display histopathological features of malignancy, despite the fact that they are only rarely associated with systemic metastatic disease in this species. They occur less frequently and may actually arise from malignant transformation of melanocytomas. Amelanotic variants can be confused with other tumours on ophthalmic examination but may be differentiated on histopathology. Melanomas can also metastasize to the eye from distant sites, notably the oral cavity, skin and toes. Occasionally, extraocular extension of a melanocytic tumour may resemble an epibulbar melanoma (Figure 14.46b). The clinical distinction between epibulbar/limbal melanomas and intraocular melanocytic tumours is described in Chapter 13.

Iridociliary adenoma and adenocarcinoma represent the second most frequently encountered primary intraocular neoplasms in dogs, although their occurrence remains relatively uncommon. They present as pigmented or non-pigmented masses protruding through or distorting the pupil (Figure 14.47). Medulloepithelioma, a tumour of primitive neuroectodermal origin, is extremely rare in dogs and may resemble an iridociliary adenoma. Other uncommon primary intraocular tumours include spindle cell tumours of the iris in blue-eyed dogs, haemangioma/sarcoma and leiomyosarcoma.

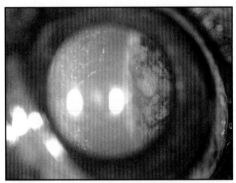

14.47 A ciliary body adenoma visible as a pink mass protruding into the pupil.

Treatment: Options for the treatment of primary uveal tumours depend on tumour behaviour, size, location, pigment content and visual potential of the eye. Some neoplasms may be amenable to diode or Nd:YAG laser photocoagulation by a specialist (Figure 14.48). Less often, small well circumscribed neoplasms can be managed by local excision; however, advanced ophthalmic microsurgical skills

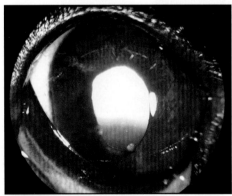

14.48 Appearance of the iris in a young Labrador Retriever that had undergone diode laser photocoagulation twice as treatment for a presumed iris melanocytoma involving the inferionasal quadrant in an otherwise comfortable and sighted eye. Note the mild dyscoria and iris atrophy at the 3 o'clock position. Two small iris cysts are also present.

are required and necessitate referral. With large tumours or when intraocular complications such as uveitis and glaucoma are present, enucleation is recommended. Orbital exenteration is warranted when extrascleral extension is noted. All enucleated globes and other excised tissues should be submitted for histopathological examination.

Secondary neoplasia: Lymphoma is the third most common intraocular neoplasm in dogs. At least one-third of dogs with multicentric lymphoma show ocular involvement (Krohne *et al.*, 1994). Generalized lymphadenopathy is usually present on physical examination. Ocular signs frequently involve the anterior uvea and include infiltration of the iris stroma by neoplastic cells, hyphaema and accumulation of neoplastic cells in the anterior chamber, mimicking a hypopyon. In the authors' experience, patients may show discordance between the severity of the ocular involvement and the moderate signs of inflammation (in terms of pain and episcleral congestion) (see Figures 14.25 and 14.44). An intravascular variant has also been described with ocular signs preceding signs of systemic involvement. The diagnosis is based on cytological or histological identification of neoplastic cells in peripheral blood samples, fine-needle aspirates of lymph node, organ or anterior chamber, bone marrow aspirates or tissue biopsy specimens. Lymphoma is responsive to various chemotherapy protocols, and the treatment of associated uveitis or glaucoma is symptomatic.

Histiocytic sarcoma is a systemic neoplasm in which unilateral ocular involvement may be the initial presentation. A thorough diagnostic work-up, including thoracic radiography, usually reveals other masses or systemic signs (see earlier discussion).

Metastatic tumours to be considered include haemangioma/sarcoma, adenocarcinoma, fibrosarcoma, rhabdomyosarcoma, osteosarcoma, chondrosarcoma, neurogenic sarcoma, phaeochromocytoma, malignant histiocytosis, seminoma, transmissible venereal tumour and oral and cutaneous melanoma.

Feline conditions

Developmental abnormalities
Several developmental uveal conditions may be seen in cats.

- Cats present with the same developmental uveal diseases as dogs. Merling is not a trait found in cats. Chediak–Higashi syndrome and agenesis of (the lateral portions of) the upper eyelids are cat-specific diseases.
- Cats with eyelid agenesis can present with iris colobomas as part of a colobomatous syndrome.
- The combination of a white coat colour, blue iris colour and deafness is found more often in cats than in dogs and resembles Waardenburg's syndrome in humans.
- These are relatively rare disease entities, which have been described elsewhere.

Iris and ciliary body cysts

Congenital iris and ciliary body cysts are occasionally seen in the cat (Figure 14.49). They have a smooth surface and are commonly very darkly pigmented, so can be difficult to transilluminate. In these cases, ocular ultrasonography may be helpful to confirm their cystic nature. Most cysts tend to remain attached to the iris or ciliary body; some are visible only after pupillary dilation. These cysts are usually non-progressive and do not seem to cause a threat to vision in cats.

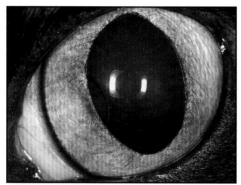

14.49 Multiple smooth-surfaced iridociliary cysts are visible behind the pupil in this cat.

White coat, blue eyes and deafness

White cats with blue eyes may show congenital deafness. This condition is transmitted through a dominant gene with complete penetrance for coat colour, and incomplete penetrance for eye colour and deafness. Hence, not all blue-eyed white cats are deaf.

Colobomatous syndrome

The most consistent abnormality in feline colobomatous syndrome is agenesis of the lateral upper eyelids (see Chapter 9). Concurrent intraocular abnormalities commonly include PPMs and, occasionally, uveal and optic nerve colobomas; retinal dysplasia is seldom seen.

Chediak–Higashi syndrome

This uncommon syndrome affects Persian cats with lightly coloured irides, hypopigmentation of the non-tapetal fundus and tapetal degeneration (see also Chapter 20). Affected cats also show bleeding tendencies and an increased susceptibility to infection. Ocular features may be caused by abnormal fusion of premelanosomes with lysosomes. Diagnosis is based on the clinical signs and finding enlarged melanin granules in the hair shafts.

Acquired abnormalities

Iris melanosis

Iris melanosis is a spontaneously occurring benign focal hyperpigmentation confined to the iris surface, which may be encountered in middle-aged to older cats. The hyperpigmented spots are not raised, do not alter the normal surface architecture of the iris, do not cause pupillary abnormalities or ectropion uvea, and are usually non-progressive or only slowly progressive (Figure 14.50). In cats it is particularly important to differentiate iris melanosis from early

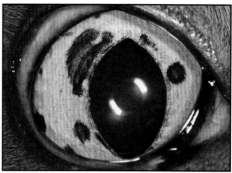

14.50 Multifocal iris melanosis in a middle-aged cat. (Courtesy of the University of Wisconsin-Madison Comparative Ophthalmology Service)

feline diffuse iris melanoma (FDIM; discussed later in the chapter). However, it may not always be easy to differentiate these two conditions. Therefore, apparently benign hyperpigmented lesions of the iris in cats should be continuously monitored for any sign of extension or tumour development.

Uveitis

Clinical signs: The clinical features of uveitis in cats are largely the same as those observed in dogs (see above). However, uveitis in cats tends to be of a more chronic, insidious nature than in dogs, with relatively mild signs. KPs, iris hyperpigmentation and hyperaemia are particularly common in cats with uveitis. Rubeosis iridis (or iris neovascularization) is not uncommon in cats with chronic uveitis and is more readily appreciable than in the brown iris of most dogs.

- In general, cats show the same clinical signs of uveitis as described in dogs. Uveitic cat eyes, however, generally appear less red and painful. Thus, uveitis in cats has a tendency to go unnoticed for relatively long periods of time.
- The presence of KPs, iris nodules, progressive iris hyperpigmentation and/or inflammation of the anterior vitreous (pars planitis or 'snow banking') are fairly typical signs of uveitis in cats.

Differential diagnosis: Figure 14.51 lists known causes of uveitis in cats. In a histopathological study, the most common causes were lymphoplasmacytic uveitis, feline infectious peritonitis (FIP), lymphoma, trauma and lens-induced uveitis (Peiffer and Wilcock, 1991). Other authors have found that infectious and neoplastic causes account for 40–70% of all uveitis cases.

Viral infections: Cats presenting with significant uveitis should be tested for feline leukaemia virus (FeLV), feline immunodeficiency virus (FIV) and FIP. All three viruses affect cats worldwide. The reader is referred to the European Advisory Board on Cat Diseases guidelines on FeLV, FIV and FIP for further details (Addie *et al.*, 2009; Hosie *et al.*, 2009; Lutz *et al.*, 2009; see also Chapter 20).

Exogenous
• Septic keratitis • Trauma (blunt or perforating) • Ionizing radiation • Chemical injuries

Endogenous

Infectious
• Feline immunodeficiency virus (FIV) • Feline leukaemia virus (FeLV) • Feline infectious peritonitis (FIP) • Toxoplasmosis • Leishmaniosis • Bartonellosis • Cryptococcosis • Histoplasmosis • Coccidioidomycosis • Blastomycosis • Candidiasis • Sepsis/bacteraemia/toxaemia (pyometra, abscess, periodontal disease) • Ophthalmomyiasis interna (Diptera)

Immune-mediated

• Lens induced:
  – Cataract (phacolytic uveitis)
  – Lens capsule rupture (phacoclastic uveitis)
• Immune-mediated vasculitis/periarteritis nodosa

Neoplastic

• Primary intraocular:
  – Melanoma
  – Iridociliary adeno(carcino)ma
• Post-traumatic sarcoma
• Lymphosarcoma (FIV/FeLV status?)
• Metastatic

Metabolic
• Hyperlipidaemia

Miscellaneous
• Lymphoplasmacytic uveitis • Idiopathic

14.51 Differential diagnoses of uveitis in cats.

- **FeLV** is a retrovirus that is transmitted vertically and horizontally via body fluids and faeces. Young cats living in a multi-cat household under poor hygiene conditions are at increased risk. Viraemic cats can develop a wide range of non-specific clinical signs years after infection. Clinical signs may result from immunosuppression, oncogenesis (development of lymphoma) and anaemia. Ocular signs include uveal, orbital and/or adnexal lymphoma, anterior uveitis with KPs, chorioretinitis, chorioretinal masses, retinal detachment, optic neuritis, spastic pupil syndrome (neuritis-induced) and CNS-related neuro-ophthalmological signs. A positive ELISA for FeLV antigen indicates exposure and persistent infection. If inconclusive, the diagnosis can be confirmed with a PCR test for proviral DNA. However, positive test results cannot be considered proof that the ocular disease is directly induced by the virus.

Palliative therapy can be provided and if accompanying medical problems and concurrent infections are managed, these cats can have a good quality of life. The effectiveness of systemic antiviral therapy is limited and some of the compounds can induce severe side effects in cats. In general, corticosteroids and other immune-suppressive or bone marrow-suppressive drugs should be avoided. FeLV-associated lymphoma can be treated with chemotherapy. However, the prognosis for these patients is poor. All cats with clinical signs of FeLV infection have a poor long-term prognosis.

- **FIV** is a human immunodeficiency virus (HIV)-related retrovirus with species specificity for cats. The virus is mainly transmitted through bite wounds via saliva. Older free-roaming male cats are at increased risk. Most clinical signs are not directly caused by the virus itself, but indirectly by opportunistic infections resulting from chronic immunosuppression. Oncogenesis and immunostimulation may play a role in the later stages of the disease. Ocular lesions are caused by opportunistic infections (e.g. toxoplasmosis), oncogenesis and direct virus-induced tissue damage. Cats with FIV can present with anterior uveitis (see Figure 14.26), pars planitis, chorioretinitis, intraocular lymphoma and CNS-related neuro-ophthalmological signs. A positive ELISA for FIV antibody indicates exposure and persistent infection, but does not necessarily correlate with clinical disease. Serology can be confirmed with Western blot. Treatment is palliative and the prognosis is poor.

- **FIP** virus is a mutated form of feline coronavirus (FCoV), for which multiple mutations are possible. FCoV infection is extremely common, especially in multi-cat households, where the seroprevalence may reach 100%. Up to 12% of FCoV-infected cats may develop and succumb to FIP. The majority of FIP-infected cats are <1 year of age.

The clinical signs of FIP are caused by immune complex disease and pyogranulomatous vasculitis. Signs of systemic disease include anorexia, lethargy, intermittent fever, weight loss, granulomatous lesions affecting multiple organ systems (the non-effusive or 'dry' form) and peritoneal and thoracic effusions (the effusive or 'wet' form). Ocular signs are typically bilateral and include anterior uveitis, fibrin exudation, hyphaema, prominent KPs (especially large granulomatous 'mutton fat' KPs), iris swelling and/or nodules, chorioretinitis, retinal vasculitis with perivascular accumulation of inflammatory cells (cuffing), exudative retinal detachment, optic neuritis and CNS-related neuro-ophthalmological signs. The development of panuveitis, or even panophthalmitis, with dense corneal oedema, is not uncommon.

The diagnosis cannot reliably be based on single tests. The analysis of any effusion is very useful and relatively non-invasive. Immunofluorescent staining of FCoV antigen in effusion macrophages is supportive of a diagnosis. If no effusion is present, biopsy of affected organs needs to be performed for a definitive diagnosis. A tentative diagnosis can be based on the patient history, typical clinical signs and corroborating bloodwork and serology results, including lymphopenia, hyperglobulinaemia, low albumin:globulin ratio, elevated FCoV titres (>160) and elevated acute phase proteins.

The treatment recommended for cats with FIP is the same as for cats with FeLV. However, the expected survival time for cats with FIP, especially with the effusive form, is much shorter than for cats with FeLV or FIV. Corticosteroids can be used in an attempt to control the immune-mediated disease.

Bacterial infections:

- **Bartonellosis.** *Bartonella henselae* and *B. clarridgeiae* are the species most often identified in cats. As with dogs, serology is the diagnostic method of choice, which makes it difficult to correlate the presence of the organism with clinical disease. An American Association of Feline Practitioners 2006 Panel Consensus Statement recommends the following criteria for the diagnosis of feline bartonellosis (Brunt *et al.*, 2006):
  - Presence of a disease syndrome reported to be associated with bartonellosis
  - Exclusion of other causes
  - A positive *Bartonella* test: serology, PCR, culture
  - Response to treatment.

The recommended treatment for *Bartonella*-positive cats with uveitis is doxycycline at a dose of 10 mg/kg orally q12–24h for 2–6 weeks. The administration of whole pills followed by water is recommended to avoid oesophageal irritation. As *Bartonella* spp. are transmitted by fleas, flea control is essential to minimize the risk of reinfection. Bartonellosis is a zoonotic disease, with *B. henselae* being the cause of cat scratch disease in humans. Immunocompromised individuals are especially at risk. For more in-depth information on the role of bartonellosis in feline uveitis, the reader is referred to a review by Stiles (2011).

Protozoal diseases:

- **Toxoplasmosis.** Cats are considered the only definitive host of *Toxoplasma gondii*. The most common route of infection is probably by ingesting intermediate hosts infected with bradyzoites in tissue cysts. However, cats can also become infected after ingesting faecal material contaminated with sporulated oocysts. Transplacental transmission of tachyzoites is also possible. The same routes of infection apply to humans.

Systemic toxoplasmosis can cause life-threatening disease in cats, and the clinical signs are diverse. Pulmonary, CNS, hepatic, pancreatic, cardiac and ocular signs are most commonly seen. Ocular disease occurs mostly, but not exclusively, in cats with systemic disease. The manifestations of ocular disease include anterior and posterior uveitis, retinal detachment, optic neuritis and extraocular myositis. Prenatal infection usually causes more severe disease signs than infection acquired during adult life. No conclusive evidence exists that concomitant infections aggravate the course of clinical toxoplasmosis.

The diagnosis can easily be missed when performing histological and cytological testing on various tissues, body fluids and faecal material. Serology too has its pitfalls, owing to the high prevalence of serum antibodies in cats worldwide. When performing serology, testing for IgM and IgG antibodies against *T. gondii* in paired samples is recommended. A tentative diagnosis of active toxoplasmosis can be made when:
- High IgM titres are present, which suggests a recent, active infection. IgM titres rise early in the course of disease and fall relatively quickly. However, IgM titres can remain significantly elevated for many months and not all cats with toxoplasmosis develop an elevated IgM titre
- A four-fold seroconversion of IgG or other antibody titres is demonstrated. The usefulness of convalescent titres is disputed as IgG titres can remain elevated for years (and IgM for months) following infection with *T. gondii*. In addition, the time between infection and the maximal IgG titre can be as short as 4 weeks, so it is possible to miss a rising titre if the patient is presented late in the disease course
- Other causes of the clinical disease have been excluded
- A beneficial clinical response to appropriate antiprotozoal treatment is observed.

Serology can yield false-positive test results due to persistently elevated titres. False-negative results are also possible because some clinically ill cats have low serum antibody titres. PCR tests may be used to confirm the presence of *T. gondii* DNA in sample material.

Clindamycin is the treatment of choice and should be given twice daily at a dose of 12.5 mg/kg orally for at least 4 weeks. Total clearance of the infection from the body is unlikely and, therefore, recurrence of the disease is possible. Whether the systemic use of corticosteroids induces reactivation of the disease is not known. Oocyst shedding does not seem to be induced by systemic steroid use.

Toxoplasmosis is a zoonotic disease with significant public health risks for pregnant and immunocompromised individuals. The reader is referred to Chapter 20 and to the review by Dubey *et al.* (2009) for more information regarding *T. gondii* prevalence, ocular and systemic disease signs, diagnosis, treatment and public health considerations.

- **Leishmaniosis:** Although dogs are the classical reservoir host for *Leishmania* spp., cats have also been implicated as potential hosts. However, actual cases of leishmaniosis have been reported only sporadically in cats. The skin and eyes seem to be the sites affected most often and the histologically identified parasite burden in affected tissues is quite high (Navarro *et al.*, 2010). As with dogs, this disease has geographical boundaries and is typically seen in (sub)tropical climates, e.g. the Mediterranean basin, southern USA and South America. *Leishmania infantum* is implicated most often, but other *Leishmania* spp. can also cause disease.

Fungal infections: The prevalence of systemic mycoses depends very much on geography. Cryptococcosis, caused by *Cryptococcus neoformans* and *C. gattii*, is the most common systemic mycosis of cats worldwide. The most likely route of infection is inhalation through the nasal cavity. The disease then disseminates to the skin, lungs, lymph nodes, CNS and eyes. The most common ocular signs are restricted to the fundus and include granulomatous chorioretinitis and optic neuritis.

Serological tests for cryptococcal antigens are highly sensitive and specific, but false-negative test results are possible in patients with localized disease. Histological evaluation of tissue biopsy specimens and cytological evaluation of smears or aspirates from lymph nodes, skin nodules, nasal discharge, aqueous humour and vitreous can be used to confirm the diagnosis. Systemic treatment with antifungal medications is indicated and can be successful, although long-term therapy may be necessary. The prognosis is variable and recurrence is possible. For extensive information on the prevalence, signs, diagnosis and treatment of cryptococcosis in cats, the reader is referred to work by Trivedi *et al.* (2011ab).

Blastomycosis, histoplasmosis, coccidioidomycosis and candidiasis have been reported in cats. These diseases are geographically confined and rare.

Lens-induced uveitis: Diagnostic testing, clinical decision-making and therapy of phacolytic and phacoclastic uveitis in cats follow the same principles as in dogs. In a recent report, *Encephalitozoon cuniculi* was identified as a cause of cataracts and secondary uveitis in cats (Benz *et al.*, 2011). The clinical signs of uveitis included aqueous flare, KPs and rubeosis iridis. The cataracts were described as immature or mature (sub)capsular and cortical cataracts with fingerlike processes extending towards the centre of the lens. All cats had elevated *E. cuniculi* antibody titres, which could be confirmed in aqueous humour or anterior lens capsule samples with PCR testing. The authors reported that conservative, symptomatic treatment of the uveitis was invariably associated with progressive disease. Uveitis was successfully controlled in all eyes, and

vision preserved in almost all eyes, when treated aggressively and specifically with lens removal by phacoemulsification, systemic fenbendazole, systemic NSAIDs and topical corticosteroids.

Lymphoplasmacytic uveitis: Despite an extensive diagnostic work-up, in many cases the cause of feline uveitis cannot be identified. Clinically conspicuous inflammatory iris nodules, which resemble lymphoid follicles on histopathology, are observed in many cats with chronic uveitis (Figure 14.52). In these patients, a diagnosis of lymphoplasmacytic uveitis can be made on exclusion of other causes. Lymphoplasmacytic uveitis is most likely a non-specific ocular immune response with an unclear aetiopathogenesis in cats. KPs, rubeosis iridis due to PIFVMs and inflammatory debris on the lens capsule and in the vitreous are commonly observed. Symptomatic anti-inflammatory therapy is recommended for these patients. However, this condition is relatively resistant to therapy and the long-term prognosis is therefore guarded. Secondary glaucoma is

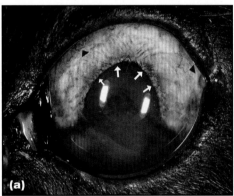

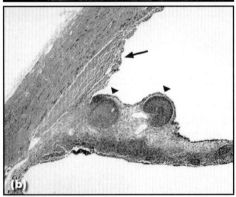

14.52 **(a)** Chronic lymphoplasmacytic uveitis in a 15-year-old cat. The branching mid to far peripheral blood vessels with an irregular course (arrowheads) are part of a pre-iridal fibrovascular membrane covering the anterior iris surface (rubeosis iridis). Note also the inflammatory nodules in the iris (arrowed). A clot of fibrin and blood is present in the ventral anterior chamber. **(b)** Histopathological cross-section of the iris, drainage angle and sclera of a cat with lymphoplasmacytic uveitis and secondary glaucoma. The clinically conspicuous lymphoplasmacytic inflammatory iris nodules are clearly visible (arrowheads). An inflammatory cell infiltrate fills and obstructs the drainage angle structures (arrowed). (Haematoxylin and eosin stain; original magnification x40) (Courtesy of Dr RR Dubielzig, Comparative Ophthalmic Pathology Laboratory of Wisconsin)

a relatively common complication of lymphoplasma-cytic uveitis and is caused by obstruction of the drainage angle by inflammatory infiltrates or PIFVMs. Lens luxation can also be observed as a secondary complication.

Treatment: In addition to specific antimicrobial therapy (see above), symptomatic treatment for uveitis is indicated as for dogs. Atropine (1%) is also used as a cycloplegic in cats but, whenever possible, it is best to use an ointment, owing to the intense salivation that occurs in reaction to the bitter taste of atropine. The use of systemic corticosteroids is usually not recommended for the treatment of feline uveitis because of the relatively high incidence of underlying infectious disease.

Intraocular haemorrhage

Causes of intraocular haemorrhage are listed in Figure 14.43. Systemic hypertension is a major cause of intraocular haemorrhage in older cats. Systemic blood pressure measurement should always be included in the diagnostic work-up of any older cat presented with intraocular haemorrhage (whether hyphaema, vitreal, iris stromal, preretinal, intraretinal or subretinal; Figure 14.53). Systemic hypertension is discussed in greater detail in Chapters 18 and 20.

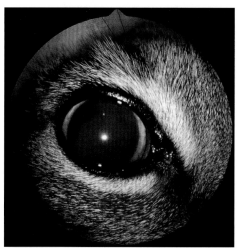

14.53 Vitreal haemorrhage in a cat with systemic hypertension.

Trauma

Most traumatic conditions discussed for the dog are applicable to cats, but some important particularities relevant to this species need to be taken into consideration:

- Cats tend to show less severe signs of uveitis with penetrating or perforating ocular trauma than dogs (Figure 14.54)
- Many penetrating injuries result from cat scratches. After a period of latency, these eyes may go on to develop a 'septic implantation syndrome' (characterized by suppurative and histiocytic inflammation) necessitating enucleation
- Malicious gunshot injuries may occur more frequently than in dogs

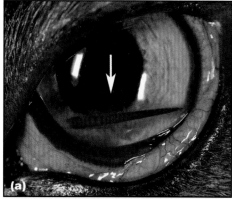

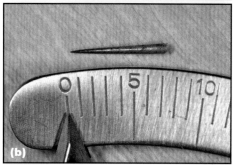

14.54 **(a)** A thorn lodged in the anterior chamber. There was surprisingly little discomfort and inflammation. Note the fibrin clot adhered to the intraocular portion of the thorn (arrowed). **(b)** Extracted thorn.

- Feline post-traumatic sarcoma is a highly malignant neoplasm that may develop several years after the initial trauma and is an important consideration in the decision to enucleate traumatized blind eyes in cats.

Uveal neoplasia

Feline diffuse iris melanoma: FDIM is the most frequently encountered primary intraocular neoplasm in cats. Lesions may start with focal or multifocal iridal hyperpigmented spots that gradually enlarge or spread. They locally alter the normal surface architecture of the iris or may acquire a slightly raised velvety surface and cause pupillary abnormalities (Figure 14.55). Atypical variations may be seen originating from the ciliary body or choroid, or may appear as solid localized masses rather than diffuse infiltration. Amelanotic variants can be confused with inflammation. The progression of FDIM may be highly variable, making it difficult to give clear advice on how best to manage these cases. These tumours often enlarge slowly over long periods of time with no associated ocular complications and no apparent metastatic disease. However, some tumours progress rapidly, leading to secondary uveitis, glaucoma and metastatic disease. Metastasis more commonly occurs to the abdominal organs than to the lungs.

Ocular signs that may indicate FDIM include:

- Pigmented (more rarely non-pigmented) spots with an altered surface architecture or a raised surface
- Pupil abnormalities (anisocoria, dyscoria) and

ectropion uveae
- Exfoliating cells in the anterior chamber
- Progression of the hyperpigmented areas
- Invasion of the drainage angle
- Associated signs of secondary uveitis and glaucoma.

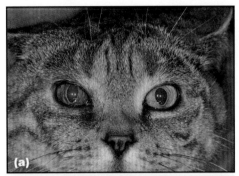

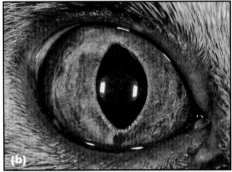

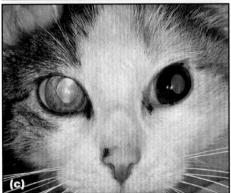

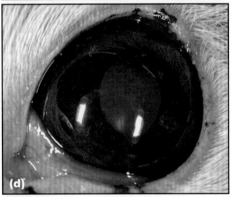

14.55 Different presentations of feline diffuse iris melanoma. **(a)** The right iris has developed a slightly darker shade. **(b)** Close-up view of the eye in (a) demonstrating the 'velvety' appearance of the iris surface. **(c)** The left iris in this cat is darkly pigmented. **(d)** Close-up view of the eye in (c) showing pigmented cell deposits on the anterior lens capsule (see also Figure 14.56).

Specialist advice should be sought when faced with any of these ocular signs, particularly in light of the life-threatening potential of FDIM. Following detailed ocular examination, the veterinary ophthalmologist may decide upon further tumour staging before choosing an appropriate therapeutic approach. Therapy for slowly progressive focal or multifocal melanomas may pose a dilemma, with some ophthalmologists advocating regular monitoring, laser ablation or early enucleation. Most ophthalmologists advocate enucleation if the masses are growing rapidly, if neoplastic cells are dispersed in the anterior chamber (Figure 14.56), if one or more masses are infiltrating the drainage angle structures and if secondary glaucoma is present. All enucleated globes should be sent for histopathological analysis because this provides helpful prognostic indicators for life expectancy. Melanomas that spread beyond the iris and trabecular meshwork have been associated with a shortened survival time (Kalishman *et al.*, 1998).

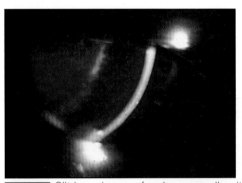

14.56 Slit-lamp image of melanoma cells within the anterior chamber of a cat. (Courtesy of BM Spiess)

Lymphoma: Uveal lymphoma is the second most common intraocular neoplasm in cats. The clinical appearance may range from refractory uveitis to nodular masses or diffuse infiltration of the anterior uvea (Figure 14.57). Ocular manifestations may precede signs of systemic involvement. The diagnostic work-up is the same as for dogs. Cats may also test positive for FeLV on PCR analysis of affected

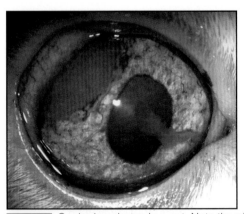

14.57 Ocular lymphoma in a cat. Note the pink nodular mass, iris neovascularization (rubeosis iridis), fibrin and inferior keratic precipitates. (Courtesy of BM Spiess)

tissues. In addition, primary intraocular lymphoma in cats can develop years after ocular trauma. This type of tumour, which is also known as the round cell variant of feline post-traumatic ocular sarcoma (FPTOS), tends to be more widely distributed within the globe and may be accompanied by lens rupture.

Feline post-traumatic ocular sarcoma: Neoplastic transformation may occur in feline eyes months to years following severe ocular trauma. In most cases, the lens capsule was ruptured during trauma. Other risk factors include chronic uveitis, possibly intraocular surgery and intravitreal gentamicin injections for the control of glaucoma. Clinically, the affected eyes may show refractory uveitis, glaucoma or a previously phthisical globe that has started to enlarge. There is usually extensive involvement of the intraocular structures. Extension through the sclera and optic nerve affects the orbital soft tissues and may lead to brain involvement.

Three main variants of FPTOS are recognized on histopathology.

- The spindle cell variant is the most common; it is more often associated with lens damage and shows the most invasive behaviour.
- A round cell variant of FPTOS may actually represent a variant of lymphoma.
- Osteosarcoma and chondrosarcoma are less frequently encountered.

The prognosis for cats with scleral extension of FPTOS is generally poor, even with exenteration, because most affected cats die from local extension and/or metastatic disease. In light of the particularly aggressive behaviour of FPTOS, prophylactic enucleation of traumatized blind globes is advised in cats, particularly when there is evidence of lens damage. All enucleated globes should be sent for histopathological analysis because this provides a valuable prognostic indicator. Traumatized but visual eyes should be continuously monitored.

Iridociliary epithelial tumour: This is the fourth most common intraocular neoplasm in cats. These tumours generally originate from the ciliary body, infiltrate the iris (Figure 14.58) and are almost always non-pigmented.

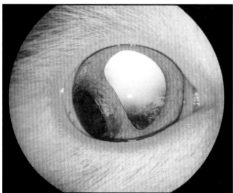

14.58 A feline iridociliary adenoma seen as a pink mass displacing the temporal iris and distorting the pupil.

Miscellaneous tumours: Feline ocular neuroglial tumours and medulloepithelioma are rare primary uveal tumours. Other metastatic uveal neoplasms (excluding lymphoma) that have been reported include metastatic carcinoma, squamous cell carcinoma, haemangiosarcoma and fibrosarcoma. These tumours may potentially affect one or both eyes. Bilateral ocular involvement is more common with angioinvasive neoplasms. They tend to localize more commonly to the posterior segment of the eye where they may induce a characteristic ischaemic chorioretinopathy (see Chapter 18).

References and further reading

Addie D, Belak S, Boucraut-Baralon C *et al.* (2009) Feline infectious peritonitis. ABCD guidelines on prevention and management. *Journal of Feline Medicine and Surgery* 11(7), 594–604
Benz P, Maass G, Csokai J *et al.* (2011) Detection of *Encephalitozoon cuniculi* in the feline cataractous lens. *Veterinary Ophthalmology* 14(Suppl. 1), 37–47
Bromel C and Sykes JE (2005a) Epidemiology, diagnosis and treatment of blastomycosis in dogs and cats. *Clinical Techniques in Small Animal Practice* 20(4), 233–239
Bromel C and Sykes JE (2005b) Histoplasmosis in dogs and cats. *Clinical Techniques in Small Animal Practice* 20(4), 227–232
Brunt J, Guptill L, Kordick DL *et al.* (2006) American Association of Feline Practitioners 2006 Panel report on diagnosis, treatment, and prevention of *Bartonella* spp. infections. *Journal of Feline Medicine and Surgery* 8(4), 213–226
Davidson MG, Breitschwerdt EB, Nasisse MP *et al.* (1989) Ocular manifestations of Rocky Mountain Spotted Fever in dogs. *Journal of the American Veterinary Medical Association* 194(6), 777–781
Dubey JP, Lindsay DS and Lappin MR (2009) Toxoplasmosis and other intestinal coccidial infections in cats and dogs. *Veterinary Clinics of North America: Small Animal Practice* 39(6), 1009–1034
Foy DS and Trepanier LA (2010) Antifungal treatment of small animal veterinary patients. *Veterinary Clinics of North America: Small Animal Practice* 40(6), 1171–1188
Gelatt KN, Gilger BC and Kern TJ (2013) *Veterinary Ophthalmology, 5th edn.* Wiley-Blackwell, Iowa
Graupmann-Kuzma A, Valentine BA, Shubitz LF *et al.* (2008) Coccidioidomycosis in dogs and cats: a review. *Journal of the American Animal Hospital Association* 44(5), 226–235
Hogan MJ, Kimura SJ and Thygeson P (1959) Signs and symptoms of uveitis. I. Anterior uveitis. *American Journal of Ophthalmology* 47(5, Part 2), 155–170
Hosie MJ, Addie D, Belak S *et al.* (2009) Feline immunodeficiency. ABCD guidelines on prevention and management. *Journal of Feline Medicine and Surgery* 11(7), 575–584
Kalishman JB, Chappell R, Flood LA *et al.* (1998) A matched observational study of survival in cats with enucleation due to diffuse iris melanoma. *Veterinary Ophthalmology* 1(1), 25–29
Komnenou A, Eberhard ML, Kaldrymidou E *et al.* (2002) Subconjunctival filariasis due to *Onchocerca* sp. in dogs: report of 23 cases in Greece. *Veterinary Ophthalmology* 5(2), 119–126
Komnenou A, Mylonakis ME, Kouti V *et al.* (2007) Ocular manifestations of natural canine monocytic ehrlichiosis (*Ehrlichia canis*): a retrospective study of 90 cases. *Veterinary Ophthalmology* 10(3), 137–142
Krohne SG, Henderson NM and Richardson RC (1994) Prevalence of ocular involvement in dogs with multicentric lymphoma: prospective evaluation of 94 cases. *Veterinary and Comparative Ophthalmology* 4, 127–135
Ledbetter EC, Landry MP, Stokol T *et al.* (2009) *Brucella canis* endophthalmitis in 3 dogs: clinical features, diagnosis and treatment. *Veterinary Ophthalmology* 12(3), 183–191
Leiva M, Naranjo C and Pena MT (2005) Ocular signs of canine monocytic ehrlichiosis: a retrospective study in dogs from Barcelona, Spain. *Veterinary Ophthalmology* 8(6), 387–393
Lutz H, Addie D, Belak S *et al.* (2009) Feline leukaemia. ABCD guidelines on prevention and management. *Journal of Feline Medicine and Surgery* 11(7), 565–574
Massa KL, Gilger BC, Miller TL *et al.* (2002) Causes of uveitis in dogs: 102 cases (1989–2000). *Journal of the American Veterinary Medical Association* 5(2), 93–98
Navarro JA, Sanchez J, Penafiel-Verdu C *et al.* (2010) Histopathological lesions in 15 cats with leishmaniosis. *Journal of Comparative Pathology* 143(4), 297–302
Peiffer RL, Jr and Wilcock BP (1991) Histopathologic study of uveitis in cats: 139 cases (1978–1988). *Journal of the American Veterinary Medical Association* 198(1), 135–138

Peña MT, Roura X and Davidson MG (2000) Ocular and periocular manifestations of leishmaniasis in dogs: 105 cases (1993–1998). *Veterinary Ophthalmology* **3**(1), 35–41

Petersen-Jones SM, Forcier J and Mentzer AL (2007) Ocular melanosis in the Cairn Terrier: clinical description and investigation of mode of inheritance. *Veterinary Ophthalmology* **10**(Suppl. 1), 63–69

Stiles J (2011) Bartonellosis in cats: a role in uveitis? *Veterinary Ophthalmology* **14**(Suppl. 1), 9–14

Sykes JE, Hartmann K, Lunn KF *et al.* (2011) 2010 ACVIM small animal consensus statement on leptospirosis: diagnosis, epidemiology, treatment and prevention. *Journal of Veterinary Internal Medicine* **25**(1), 1–13

Taylor AW (2009) Ocular immune privilege. *Eye (London)* **23**(10), 1885–1889

Torres M, Bardagi M, Roura X *et al.* (2011) Long term follow-up of dogs diagnosed with leishmaniosis (clinical stage II) and treated with meglumine antimoniate and allopurinol. *Veterinary Journal* **188**(3), 346–351

Trivedi SR, Malik R, Meyer W *et al.* (2011a) Feline cryptococcosis: impact of current research on clinical management. *Journal of Feline Medicine and Surgery* **13**(3), 163–172

Trivedi SR, Sykes JE, Cannon MS *et al.* (2011b) Clinical features and epidemiology of cryptococcosis in cats and dogs in California: 93 cases (1988–2010). *Journal of the American Veterinary Medical Association* **239**(3), 357–369

van der Woerdt A (2000) Lens-induced uveitis. *Veterinary Ophthalmology* **3**(4), 227–234

15

Glaucoma

Peter Renwick

Glaucoma in domestic animals presents as a group of well recognized pathological changes involving the globe. These may result from one or more ocular disorders whose common endpoint is elevation of the intraocular pressure (IOP) above normal limits, leading to impairment or loss of vision.

Disturbance to the optic nerve head, in terms both of its microcirculation and of the axoplasmic flow in its retinal ganglion cell axons, is the earliest and most significant effect of glaucoma. In dogs, these changes are accompanied by outer retinal necrosis, which occurs as a result of reduction in choroidal vascular perfusion, and this effect is greatest initially in the non-tapetal fundus. In an uncontrolled situation, these events may progress to complete and irreversible blindness in the affected eye.

The outlook for vision in cases of glaucoma is always guarded and, despite ongoing developments in glaucoma therapy, it remains one of the most challenging and potentially frustrating conditions for the clinician to manage. Early recognition of the problem followed by prompt, appropriate therapy is essential if sight is to be retained for as long as possible.

Physiological control of intraocular pressure

IOP is dependent upon a number of factors, including ocular rigidity and the volume of aqueous humour in the anterior segment of the eye. Constant production and drainage of aqueous is required to maintain both a formed globe and a steady state of physiological IOP. The aqueous is optically clear under normal conditions, a property which is important for visual function. Its continual flow is vital for the delivery of nutrients to, and removal of waste products from, the avascular structures it bathes (i.e. the lens, cornea and trabecular meshwork – a major part of the drainage apparatus of the eye).

Aqueous is produced from the processes of the ciliary body (Figure 15.1), primarily by active secretion and, to a lesser degree, by ultrafiltration. The ciliary processes are highly vascular and possess a double epithelial layer – the intercellular tight junctions of the inner, non pigmented cell layer form the ciliary body's contribution to the blood–aqueous barrier. These epithelial cells are responsible for the regulation of aqueous production, and the ciliary processes have a large surface area to facilitate

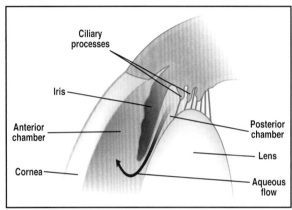

15.1 Aqueous humour is produced by the ciliary body and flows through the pupil into the anterior chamber.

their secretory function. Sodium ions are actively transported into the aqueous by a sodium/potassium adenosine triphosphatase (ATPase) pump mechanism, and bicarbonate ions enter the aqueous as a result of the reaction between water and carbon dioxide, which is catalysed by carbonic anhydrase. Entry of these solutes into the aqueous is accompanied by the ingress of water into the posterior chamber.

Once produced, aqueous traverses the posterior chamber, passes through the pupil and enters the anterior chamber (Figure 15.1). In order to maintain a steady IOP, aqueous must then drain out of the eye at the same rate at which it is produced. The majority of aqueous outflow in dogs and cats occurs through the drainage structures at the junction of the iris root, the base of the ciliary body and the corneoscleral tissue (Figures 15.2 and 15.3). This region is often termed the drainage angle (iridocorneal angle, filtration angle).

The major structures of the drainage apparatus are the pectinate ligament (Figure 15.4) and the ciliary cleft, which contains the sponge-like tissue of the trabecular meshwork. The bulk of the aqueous drains across these structures to the avascular aqueous plexus and thence to the scleral venous circulation (so-called 'conventional' outflow). In addition, there is also an 'unconventional' uveoscleral outflow route, which involves aqueous passing into the ciliary cleft and gaining access to the scleral venous circulation via the choroid and suprachoroidal space, bypassing the aqueous plexus. This

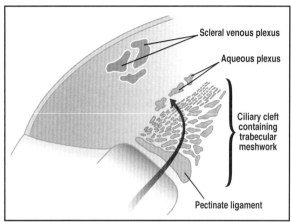

Scleral venous plexus

Aqueous plexus

Ciliary cleft containing trabecular meshwork

Pectinate ligament

15.2 Drainage of aqueous occurs primarily through the pectinate ligament and trabecular meshwork into the aqueous plexus, and thence to the scleral venous circulation.

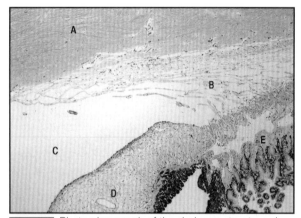

15.3 Photomicrograph of the drainage structures in the eye of a cat. A = sclera; B = trabecular meshwork within ciliary cleft; C = anterior chamber; D = iris; E = ciliary body. (Courtesy of E Scurrell)

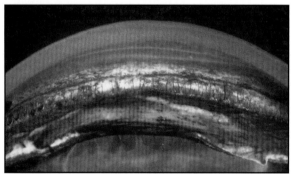

15.4 The fibres of the pectinate ligament viewed from within the anterior chamber. (Courtesy of JRB Mould)

route is believed to comprise approximately 15% of the total aqueous outflow in normal dogs and around 3% in normal cats.

Normal variations

IOP in normal dogs, as measured by applanation tonometry, is generally between 10 and 25 mmHg. Various factors may influence the reading obtained (Figure 15.5). When assessing a suspected case of glaucoma, it is important to bear in mind the possible

- Instrumentation used for measurement of IOP
- Age of dog – IOP is reported to decrease with ageing
- Patient positioning – a 'head back' posture, as required for Schiøtz tonometry, increases IOP
- Degree of restraint – vigorous restraint/pressure on the jugular veins increases IOP
- Forced lid opening and pressure on the globe increases IOP – exophthalmic/brachycephalic breeds are prone to this phenomenon during handling for tonometry
- Breed of dog – e.g. terrier breeds have been shown to have fluctuant IOPs
- Possibly other factors such as obesity and arterial blood pressure

15.5 Factors influencing IOP in normal dogs.

physiological parameters that may influence IOP. For example, the measured IOP can rise to around 30 mmHg when pressure is applied to the neck and immediately fall to <20 mmHg once the grip on the patient is relaxed. Likewise, manual extension of the eyelids (either by opening them or by extending them laterally) during tonometry measurement also causes significant increases in IOP (Klein *et al.*, 2011).

Investigation of disease

Tonometry

Almost all patients with glaucoma have elevated IOP on presentation, and the measurement of IOP is therefore fundamental to diagnosing the condition. It is also essential for monitoring the response to treatment; the IOP should be measured on every occasion that a patient undergoing treatment for glaucoma is presented. It is also a very useful aid in the diagnosis and management of cases of uveitis, because the IOP often falls as a result of anterior segment inflammation, and patients with uveitis are also at risk of developing secondary glaucoma. Various methods of IOP estimation are available and these are described in detail in Chapter 1.

Gonioscopy

Gonioscopy is a technique that allows visual inspection of the opening to the ciliary cleft. It is not normally possible to see the drainage structures using routine ophthalmic examination techniques, except to some extent in cats, where a limited and somewhat distorted view of the pectinate ligament can be obtained by viewing through the cornea at an oblique angle.

The technique of gonioscopy depends upon the use of a contact lens of some type. The Barkan and Koeppe lenses are the most common in veterinary use as they are both self-retaining, allowing the user to keep both hands free for restraining the patient and holding instruments (Figures 15.6 to 15.8). In the absence of a goniolens, a condensing lens gently pressed against the cornea offers a significantly less satisfactory alternative.

Magnification (e.g. with a direct ophthalmoscope, slit-lamp biomicroscope or fundus camera) is used to inspect the structures of the iridocorneal angle

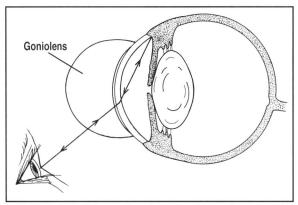

15.6 A goniolens alters the refraction at the corneal surface, allowing light that would normally be internally reflected to travel from the drainage angle to the viewer's eye.

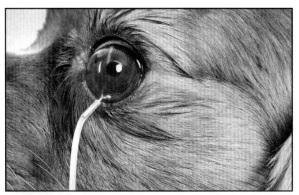

15.7 A Barkan goniolens applied to a topically anaesthetized cornea. This lens employs negative pressure, created by the column of saline within the attached silicone tubing, to maintain adherence of the lens to the globe. An improved view may be obtained by filling the chamber of the lens with artificial tears prior to placement on the cornea.

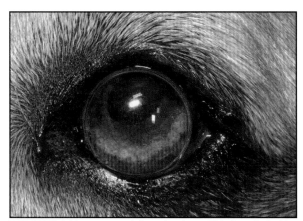

15.8 A Koeppe goniolens in place. This lens is held in place by a combination of surface tension on the corneal surface and the presence of a flange on the margin of the lens, which engages under the eyelids.

(Figure 15.9). Gonioscopy may reveal abnormalities, such as pectinate ligament dysplasia or closure/collapse of the ciliary cleft and pectinate ligament. Other changes in the area may also be identified (e.g. infiltration by neoplastic tissue, the presence of inflammatory swelling or deposits, abnormal pigment deposition and fibrovascular tissue ingrowth).

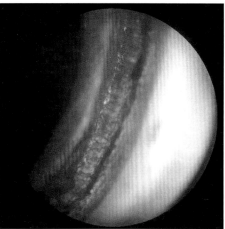

15.9 Gonioscopic view of normal pectinate fibres and ciliary cleft entrance in a Labrador Retriever.

Gonioscopy is indicated in any case of glaucoma where the cause of the IOP elevation is not immediately apparent. It is also a necessity when primary inherited glaucoma is suspected, particularly when an outwardly normal fellow eye may be inspected for abnormalities of the iridocorneal angle. Gonioscopy of the contralateral eye can be helpful in determining the diagnosis of glaucoma (the glaucomatous globe itself may be unsuitable for gonioscopy owing to the presence of corneal opacity, or secondary collapse of the entrance to the ciliary cleft may obscure pre-existing changes) and also provides useful information regarding the potential for predisposition to glaucoma in the normotensive globe.

The technique is not straightforward. The goniolens can be difficult to retain on the eye and the view obtained is not always clear, especially if the lens becomes contaminated with meibomian gland secretions or other debris. The positioning of the lens can be critical and slight alterations in this or in the viewing angle can lead to artefactual changes in the appearance of the entrance to the ciliary cleft. Practice is required in order to perform gonioscopy and interpret the findings reliably.

Gonioscopy is a very important technique for the diagnosis and management of glaucoma. If the clinician is presented with a case of suspected or confirmed glaucoma and the necessary equipment or expertise for performing and interpreting the findings of gonioscopy are lacking, immediate referral should be considered.

Clinical signs

The presenting signs of glaucoma vary, depending on a number of factors:

- Speed of onset
- Degree of elevation of IOP
- Duration of the problem
- Underlying cause
- Age of the animal (young animals have more distensible globes).

The special features of glaucoma in cats are discussed further at the end of the chapter. It is very important to appreciate that many of the clinical signs of glaucoma are common to numerous other ophthalmic disorders and in making a diagnosis of glaucoma, the importance of a comprehensive careful clinical examination (in association with a full assessment of the signalment and history) cannot be overemphasized. For convenience, the clinical signs are considered under the headings of 'acute' and 'chronic', but this division is somewhat arbitrary and not always clear cut in a clinical setting (e.g. some chronic cases may not be presented until an acute exacerbation draws the problem to the owner's attention).

Acute glaucoma

The major signs seen most often in the face of an acute rise in IOP are summarized in Figure 15.10.

Clinical sign	Description/comments
Pain	Increased lacrimation; blepharospasm; enophthalmos/third eyelid protrusion; head shyness
Corneal oedema	Especially with an acute rise in IOP >40–50 mmHg in dogs
Corneal vascularization	Deep 'brush-border' appearance in acute cases; may advance towards the central cornea at a rate of up to 1 mm per day
Mydriasis	Mid-dilated unresponsive pupil (the consensual PLR in the other eye should also be assessed to help to determine the presence/absence of potential visual function)
Episcleral congestion	Often accompanied by conjunctival congestion
Fundus	Optic nerve head swelling/haemorrhage may be seen in some patients
Vision loss	May not be noticed by the owner if the problem is unilateral at the time of presentation

15.10 Clinical signs of acute glaucoma.

Pain

In severe and very acute cases, especially where the IOP is >40–50 mmHg, the degree of discomfort may be so severe as to cause vocalization, head shyness and marked depression and/or inappetence. Blepharospasm, globe retraction with consequent third eyelid protrusion, increased lacrimation and epiphora may also result from discomfort (Figure 15.11). The signs may be less apparent in cases where the increase in IOP is less dramatic. The pain associated with glaucoma does not respond well to non-steroidal anti-inflammatory drugs (NSAIDs) and controlling the IOP is the main aim to provide pain relief.

Corneal oedema

The whole cornea may take on a 'steamy' bluish appearance, especially with a sudden elevation of IOP to >40–50 mmHg. The normal optical clarity of

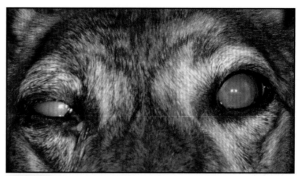

15.11 Acute-onset glaucoma secondary to endophthalmitis in a Greyhound. Marked corneal oedema was accompanied by signs of severe ocular discomfort in the right eye.

the cornea depends upon a number of factors. One of the most important is its state of deturgescence. This is primarily the result of the action of a pump mechanism in the corneal endothelial cells. Active transport of solutes from the cornea into the aqueous humour causes movement of water out of the corneal stroma down the resulting diffusion gradient. A marked elevation in IOP interferes with this phenomenon and oedema ensues (Figure 15.12). This sign is not found consistently; it tends to be less marked at low levels of IOP elevation and in chronic cases.

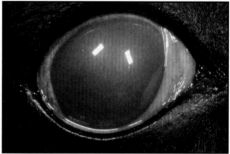

15.12 Corneal oedema due to high IOP in a 2-year-old English Springer Spaniel. Secondary glaucoma developed following intraocular haemorrhage.

Corneal vascularization

In acute cases, a fringe of blood vessels may invade the deep cornea from the limbus, usually through 360 degrees. The vessels may take on a 'brush-border' densely packed appearance at the leading edge, owing to the fact that they are constrained by the surrounding stromal collagen lamellae (Figure 15.13). Such vascularization is most commonly seen in association with marked corneal oedema and where the glaucoma is secondary to uveitis.

Mydriasis

A dilated or moderately dilated, poorly responsive pupil results from pressure-induced paresis or paralysis of the iris sphincter muscle (Figure 15.14). Absence of the direct pupillary light reflex (PLR) under such circumstances must not be presumed to equate with loss of vision; instead, other features should be used to gauge the potential for vision (e.g. the presence or absence of a menace response or dazzle reflex in the affected eye, or the presence or

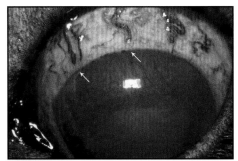

15.13 Deep corneal vascularization in a Labrador Retriever with primary glaucoma associated with goniodysgenesis. The vessels have invaded the cornea through 360 degrees and exhibit a 'brush-border' appearance at the leading edge. Deep vessels (arrowed) cannot be seen to cross the limbus in dogs (compare with the superficial vessels in Figure 15.21).

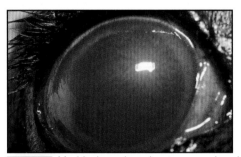

15.14 Mydriasis and moderate corneal oedema in a Basset Hound with acute-onset primary glaucoma associated with goniodysgenesis.

absence of a consensual PLR in the fellow eye when only the affected eye is illuminated). Mydriasis is not an invariable finding in glaucomatous globes, and in some cases of uveitis-induced glaucoma the pupil may even be constricted.

Episcleral congestion
Episcleral congestion (Figure 15.15) is a commonly encountered and useful diagnostic indicator in glaucoma cases. The engorged episcleral vessels run at right angles to the limbus, are frequently set against the white background of the sclera, and do not move in association with movement of the overlying lids and conjunctiva. The conjunctival vessels may also be distended, in which case the tissue between the episcleral vessels appears hyperaemic. The conjunctival vessels may be blanched rapidly by the application of topical 10% phenylephrine drops, allowing the

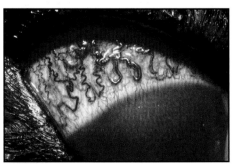

15.15 Episcleral congestion. Large vessels, which do not move with the conjunctiva, are seen against the scleral background.

episcleral vessels (which blanch less readily) to be assessed more accurately. It is important to appreciate that not all cases with episcleral congestion have glaucoma and *vice versa* (Figure 15.16).

* Glaucoma
* Uveitis/endophthalmitis/panophthalmitis
* Episcleritis (often localized in dogs)
* Retrobulbar space-occupying lesion (e.g. abscess, neoplasia)
* Horner's syndrome
* Hyperviscosity syndromes
* Excitement

15.16 Differential diagnoses of episcleral congestion and hyperaemia.

Vision loss
Loss of vision initially occurs as a result of damage to the ganglion cell axons in the region of the optic nerve head, due to the adverse effects of elevated IOP on both the vascular supply to the optic nerve head and axoplasmic flow within the optic nerve axons. These optic nerve head changes are accompanied in some acute-onset cases by retinal necrosis. In addition, the levels of glutamate within the vitreous and retina of dogs with glaucoma may increase, and this is turn has been suggested to cause retinal ganglion cell death due to 'excitotoxicity', mediated, at least in part, by an influx of calcium into the cells (Brooks *et al.*, 1999). Other substances such as endothelin-1 and nitric oxide have been shown to be increased in dogs with primary glaucoma, and these in turn may contribute to ganglion cell death (Kallberg *et al.*, 2007). In acute cases, the eye may become blind within hours of the onset of glaucoma and these changes rapidly become irreversible.

Whilst an observant owner may detect loss of vision in one eye, it is unlikely that partial visual field loss in only one eye will be noticed. By virtue of this fact, glaucoma affecting only one eye tends to present relatively late in the course of the disease and it is generally an alteration in the appearance of the eye, rather than altered vision, which prompts presentation. It is also relatively easy for the clinician to overlook the very important question of whether an abnormal, possibly glaucomatous, eye is visual or not, especially if the owners have not reported any historical evidence of blindness. A positive effort must therefore be made both during history taking and the examination to establish whether the eye is visual (Figure 15.17). This can not

* Loss of menace response in the affected eye
* Loss of dazzle reflex to a bright light shone in the affected eye
* Loss of consensual PLR: no constriction of the pupil in the contralateral eye when the affected eye is illuminated in a dimly lit room
* Re-dilatation of the pupil in the affected eye on a swinging flashlight test
* Absence of tracking response to cotton wool ball with the contralateral eye covered
* Inability to negotiate a maze with the contralateral eye covered

15.17 Clinical signs indicative of unilateral blindness in glaucoma.

only assist in making a diagnosis, but also has a major impact on the future management of the case. Those animals which have already lost vision in one eye tend to present as soon as the second eye is clinically affected, as a result of more overt effects on visual behaviour.

In the early stages of vision loss, optic nerve head damage and retinal ganglion cell dysfunction are potentially reversible, at least to some degree. In those cases which present with a very high IOP, or once the eye has been blind for more than a few days (or even hours in some instances), the prospects for the return of vision, even when the IOP is restored to normal, become more remote. It is therefore imperative that cases of acute-onset glaucoma are diagnosed accurately and as early in the course of the disease as the presentation allows.

Some patients with acute glaucoma develop swelling of the optic nerve head and this may be accompanied by the presence of small haemorrhages. However, the presence of corneal oedema and other potential intraocular changes may preclude examination of the fundus. Genuine acute-onset glaucoma constitutes an ocular emergency in those cases where there is the potential to preserve or restore vision. For those clinicians not fully familiar with both the diagnosis and treatment of the condition, it is advisable to offer urgent referral to a specialist.

Chronic glaucoma

Chronic glaucoma may arise as a sequel to an unsuccessfully controlled or misdiagnosed episode (or episodes) of an acute-onset nature, or it may develop insidiously and first present at a point where the eye is already showing signs of gross abnormality.

Many of the clinical signs seen with acute glaucoma are also present to a greater or lesser degree in more chronic cases, although some (e.g. pain and corneal oedema) tend to become less marked with increasing chronicity. In addition to the signs of acute glaucoma, chronic cases demonstrate various combinations of the signs summarized in Figure 15.18.

Globe enlargement

Enlargement of the globe (hydrophthalmos, bupthalmos) occurs due to pressure-induced stretching of the ocular tunics. It is often marked and relatively rapid in onset in young animals, because they possess less rigid globes than adults. Many of the clinical sigs of chronic glaucoma are the result of stretching of the globe. By the time globe enlargement is evident, most patients will already be blind in the affected eye(s). However, in young animals and cases in which the disease is very slowly progressive (e.g. primary open-angle glaucoma), it is possible for some useful vision to be retained even in the face of a quite marked increase in globe size. Exophthalmos, in which a normally sized eye is pushed forward by a retrobulbar space-occupying process such as an abscess or neoplasia, must be differentiated from buphthalmos (Figures 15.19 and 15.20).

- Fewer overt signs of pain/discomfort compared with acute glaucoma
- Globe enlargement:
  - Stretching of the ocular tunics, including the cornea, leads to many of the other changes listed below
  - Once the globe has enlarged, the prognosis is often very poor and enucleation is frequently indicated (with the possible exception of young animals and very slowly progressive cases – see text)
  - Every attempt should therefore be made to diagnose glaucoma well before this stage is reached
- Corneal neovascularization:
  - Often superficial branching vessels (unlike the 'brush-border' of acute cases)
  - Vessels may bring pigment into the superficial cornea
- Corneal ulceration due to exposure, resulting from an inadequate blink (lagophthalmos) and stretching and oedema of the corneal tissues
- Descemet's streaks (Haab's striae):
  - Grey streaks in the cornea, resulting from breaks in the Descemet's membrane due to stretching
- Equatorial staphyloma:
  - Scleral thinning seen as a bluish transilluminating bulge behind the limbus
- Iris atrophy:
  - Thinning allows easy transillumination and holes may develop
  - More commonly results from ageing change or uveitis
- Lens subluxation/luxation with resulting aphakic crescent:
  - Must be differentiated from primary lens luxation
- Cataract
- Intraocular haemorrhage:
  - More commonly seen in other disease states (see text)
- Optic disc cupping:
  - Posterior bowing of the optic disc due to scleral weakness at this point (lamina cribrosa)
- Retinal and optic nerve head atrophy
- Phthisis bulbi

15.18 Clinical signs of glaucoma associated with chronicity.

Feature	Buphthalmos	Exophthalmos
Third eyelid position	Pushed back towards medial canthus	Often (but not always) prolapsed across the globe
Corneal diameter	Increased	Normal
Pupil appearance	Often mid-dilated and unresponsive	Variable (may be normal)
Lens position	Often subluxated; aphakic crescent and stretched zonular fibres visible	Normal
Optic disc appearance	Cupped	Disc may be swollen or congested; not cupped
Oral examination	Normal	Swelling may be seen caudal to last upper molar tooth
IOP	Increased	Normal in most cases (any increase is typically modest)

15.19 Differentiation of buphthalmos from exophthalmos.

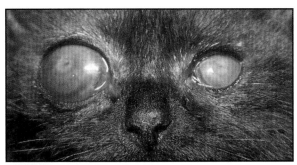

15.20 Buphthalmos in a kitten with congenital glaucoma.

Corneal changes

The diameter of the cornea increases as the globe enlarges. Blood vessels may invade the cornea from the limbus, often in a superficial arborizing pattern (Figure 15.21). Pigment is frequently deposited, having gained access to the cornea via the invading vessels. As the globe enlarges, the ability to blink and distribute the tear film becomes compromised. This, in turn, affects corneal health and may ultimately result in areas of epithelial irregularity and even frank ulceration, particularly of the central cornea.

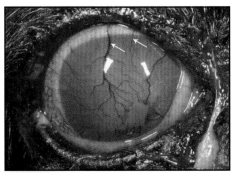

15.21 Superficial vascularization in chronic glaucoma. The vessels (arrowed) are branching and can be seen to cross the limbus (compare with Figure 15.13).

Grey opacities may develop within the cornea due to a number of factors, including:

- Disturbance to the normally regular arrangement of the collagen lamellae (e.g. by stretching, oedema or blood vessels)
- Scar tissue formation (e.g. following ulceration)
- Thickening/keratinization of the corneal epithelium secondary to exposure
- Breaks in the Descemet's membrane caused by stretching of the cornea (the grey streaks are also known as Haab's striae) (Figure 15.22).

Equatorial staphyloma

Scleral thinning and stretching may become marked at the equator of the globe, leading to the development of outward protrusion of the sclera and underlying uvea. This is seen as a bluish bulge some distance behind the limbus and is often obscured by the eyelids (Figure 15.23). The swelling must be differentiated from a solid mass; this may be achieved by transillumination – light shines through a staphyloma as a result of thinning of the tissues.

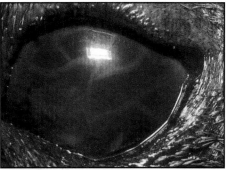

15.22 A Chow Chow with chronic glaucoma secondary to previous anterior uveitis. Descemet's streaks (Haab's striae) can be seen as blue-grey streaks across the cornea. They represent breaks in the Descemet's membrane, which occurs as a result of stretching of the ocular tunics.

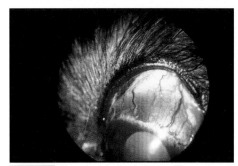

15.23 Equatorial staphyloma. Occasionally, pressure-induced thinning of the sclera may cause a bluish swelling posterior to the limbus. In contrast to a neoplastic mass, a staphyloma can be transilluminated because of thinning of the tissues. (Courtesy of PGC Bedford)

Lens changes

Luxation or subluxation: Enlargement of the globe results in stretching and tearing of the zonular fibres that support the lens. This results in subluxation and, in some instances, eventual luxation of the lens (Figure 15.24). The lens may come to lie in the anterior or posterior segment of the eye and is frequently seen to retain part of the zonular attachment around its equator (Figure 15.25). An aphakic crescent develops in cases of lens subluxation, where the lens comes to occupy a position away from the visual

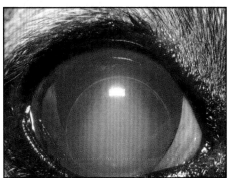

15.24 Primary open-angle glaucoma in a crossbred dog. The globe has enlarged, resulting in secondary lens luxation. The lens can be seen lying in the anterior chamber.

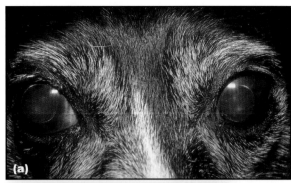

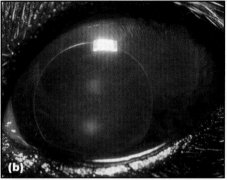

15.25 Primary open-angle glaucoma in a collie cross, resulting in bilateral globe enlargement. **(a)** Both lenses are suspended near the visual axes by the remaining zonular fibres. **(b)** The refractile lens equator can be seen and adjacent to this is an aphakic crescent. The cornea shows signs of breaks in the Descemet's membrane and corneal pigmentation has developed as a result of gross buphthalmos.

axis. The crescent is bordered by the pupil margin on one side and the equator of the lens on the other. In some patients, the fundus can be viewed through the aphakic region, by using either close direct ophthalmoscopy (with the lens in the ophthalmoscope set to approximately +12 dioptres) or a focal light source and naked eye examination, which often allows a limited view of the retinal vessels. In some cases with marked globe enlargement, the lens may remain approximately within the visual axis and a complete aphakic ring or penumbra may be seen between the lens equator and the pupillary margin. Luxation or subluxation of the lens may affect aqueous humour dynamics and further increase the degree of glaucoma present. Lens luxation may also develop as a primary event and it is therefore very important to determine whether the lens luxation is the cause or effect of glaucoma (see below).

Cataracts: Lens opacities often develop in cases of chronic glaucoma, especially when luxation has occurred (Figure 15.26). These probably result from alterations in lens nutrition and a build up of toxic products within the eye. The delivery of nutrients to, and removal of metabolic waste products from, the lens is hampered by alterations in aqueous humour dynamics. In addition, it is known that toxic levels of products such as glutamate build-up in the posterior segment of glaucomatous globes. Cataractous lenses may also cause glaucoma through a variety of mechanisms (see below).

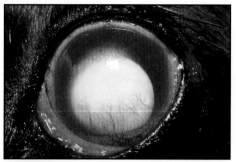

15.26 Globe enlargement in a case of chronic glaucoma, which has caused secondary lens luxation and cataract development. Chronic superficial corneal vascularization is also present.

Intraocular haemorrhage

Gross haemorrhage within the globe may develop as a result of glaucoma, but can also be related to the cause of the elevated IOP. Its presence may render accurate clinical diagnosis of the cause of the glaucoma difficult, or even impossible if it is present at the time of the first assessment of the case. Some of the differential diagnoses for intraocular haemorrhage that should be considered are listed in Figure 15.27.

- Trauma/surgery
- Intraocular neoplasia
- Uveitis
- Bleeding diathesis (numerous causes)
- Systemic hypertension
- Retinal detachment (numerous causes)
- Congenital abnormalities:
  - Collie eye anomaly
  - Retinal dysplasia
  - Persistent hyaloid artery
  - Persistent hyperplastic primary vitreous
- Chronic glaucoma

15.27 Causes of intraocular haemorrhage.

Optic disc cupping

Cupping of the optic disc is the phenomenon in which the optic nerve head becomes bowed outwards (Figures 15.28 to 15.30). This is a result of the effect of raised IOP on the relatively weak lamina cribosa (the perforated region of the sclera that allows optic nerve axon fibres to exit from the globe) and the loss of optic nerve fibres due to glaucoma. Cupping of the optic disc results in misalignment of the perforations within the lamina cribosa. This, in turn, results in shearing forces and mechanical damage to the optic nerve axons as they pass through the region, further exacerbating the effects of glaucoma on vision.

Optic disc cupping is perhaps most readily appreciated using stereoscopic indirect ophthalmoscopy, which provides a three-dimensional (3D) view of the fundus. However, if the ocular media remain sufficiently clear, it is also possible to gain an impression of the degree of cupping by using a direct ophthalmoscope. The retina is first brought into focus by dialling up the required lens in the ophthalmoscope (this may be a negative lens because

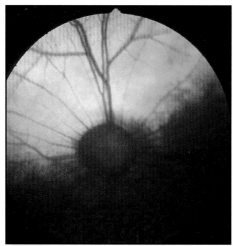

15.28 Primary open-angle glaucoma in a crossbred dog. The optic disc is severely cupped. The retinal vessels drop down over the rim of the cup where they are lost to view when the focus is in the plane of the retina.

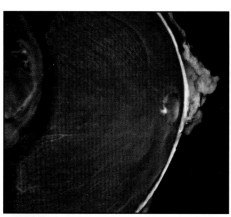

15.29 Severely cupped optic nerve head. (Courtesy of E Scurrell)

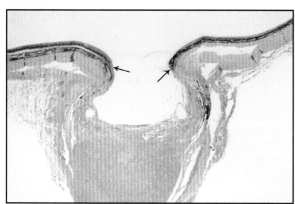

15.30 Histological section of a globe with chronic glaucomatous damage. The optic nerve head is cupped. The margins of the disc are denoted by the arrows. (Courtesy of JRB Mould)

of globe enlargement) and then the centre of the optic disc is focused upon by dialling in a negative lens of greater dioptre. The difference in the lens settings required gives an indication of the degree of optic disc cupping (each additional dioptre is approximately equivalent to 0.3 mm of cupping).

Retinal and optic nerve atrophy

With chronicity, the optic disc undergoes changes in its ophthalmoscopic appearance in addition to those of cupping. Typically, it takes on a chalky appearance due to the loss of vasculature, and may also become darkened owing to the loss of myelinated nerve fibres.

Tapetal hyper-reflectivity is another potential ophthalmoscopic finding. It results from retinal thinning, which allows increased reflection of light back from the tapetum (which lies within the choroid). In patients with glaucoma, this is often seen initially as shiny fan-shaped bands extending out from the optic nerve head (Figure 15.31). The bands of sectoral retinal necrosis and resultant retinal atrophy represent so-called 'watershed' lesions and result from pressure-induced effects on zones of choroidal vasculature (supplying the outer layers of the retina). As the disease progresses, the extent of tapetal hyper-reflectivity increases and the retinal vessels (supplying the inner retinal layers) become attenuated (Figure 15.32).

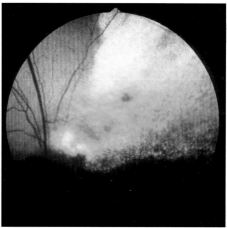

15.31 Sectoral retinal necrosis in a Basset Hound with primary glaucoma. The sharp demarcation between the hyper-reflective zone (indicative of retinal thinning) and the adjacent more normal area of reflectivity is known as a 'watershed' lesion.

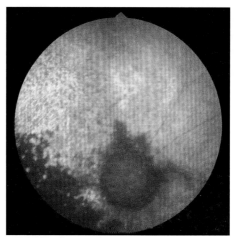

15.32 Chronic fundic changes in glaucoma due to goniodysgenesis in an English Springer Spaniel. The tapetal fundus shows generalized hyper-reflectivity and there is marked retinal vessel attenuation. The optic disc is severely cupped.

Phthisis bulbi

It is important to note that, in some cases, signs of chronic glaucoma may be present even though the IOP at the time of examination is normal. This occurs when a previously elevated IOP has caused pressure-induced atrophy of the ciliary processes, thus reducing aqueous production. In extreme cases, this may lead to a reduction in the size of the globe or phthisis bulbi.

Classification and causes of glaucoma

Glaucoma can be classified in a number of ways. In addition to whether the presenting signs are acute or chronic, it may be considered in terms of being congenital (rare in veterinary practice) or acquired, and in the latter case it may be further classified based on the underlying cause. The causes of glaucoma can be subdivided into two broad categories:

- Primary glaucoma – two major types:
  - Goniodysgenesis (closed-angle glaucoma)
  - Primary open-angle glaucoma
- Secondary glaucoma – numerous conditions may lead to a reduction in aqueous outflow.

Primary glaucoma

In cases of primary glaucoma, there is no other recognized antecedent ocular disease process and, almost invariably, there is the potential for elevation of the IOP to become bilateral. A number of breeds have been shown to be predisposed to the development of primary glaucoma. In some of these, the disease has been demonstrated to have a hereditary basis. The breeds vary between countries, but those recognized as more commonly affected are listed in Figure 15.33.

Goniodysgenesis
• English Cocker Spaniel • American Cocker Spaniel • English Springer Spaniel • Welsh Springer Spaniel • Basset Hound • Bouvier des Flandres • Labrador and Golden Retriever • Flat-coated Retriever • Great Dane • Welsh Terrier • Dandie Dinmont Terrier • Japanese Shiba Inu • Siberian Husky • Samoyed • Chow Chow • Shar Pei • Boston Terrier
Open-angle glaucoma
• Norwegian Elkhound • Beagle • Petit Basset Griffon Vendeen

15.33 Breeds predisposed to primary glaucoma.

Goniodysgenesis

Goniodysgenesis (acute primary closed-angle glaucoma) is the most common cause of primary glaucoma in dogs in the UK. The breeds in which it is most frequently seen are listed in Figure 15.33. In these cases, there is a developmental bilateral abnormality of the pectinate ligament termed pectinate ligament dysplasia (Martin, 1975; Bedford, 1980). Instead of the normal structure (see Figure 15.9), the dysplastic ligament comprises sheets of tissue which may be so extensive in some cases as to be perforated only by intermittent flow holes (Figure 15.34). The entrance to the ciliary cleft, spanned by the pectinate ligament, may also be narrowed in cases with goniodysgenesis (Ekesten, 1993) (Figure 15.35). In early life, these limited channels may allow sufficient passage of aqueous for the maintenance of a normotensive globe. After a variable period, usually in middle age, although earlier in adulthood in the Welsh Springer Spaniel, (Cottrell and Barnett, 1998), the flow becomes further compromised and glaucoma develops, often with an acute onset. In such cases, the normal drainage structures may not be visible (Figure 15.36). The precise mechanisms whereby aqueous

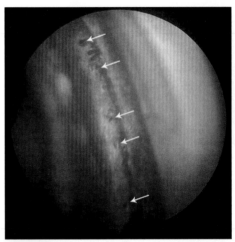

15.34 Gonioscopic view of goniodysgenesis in a Great Dane. The pectinate ligament comprises a sheet of tissue with only intermittent flow holes (arrowed) (compare with Figure 15.9).

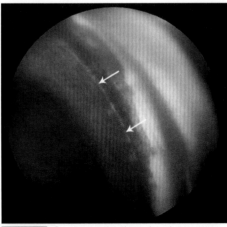

15.35 Gonioscopic view showing extreme narrowing of the entrance to the ciliary cleft (arrowed).

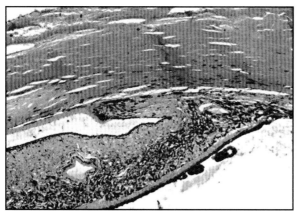

15.36 Histological section showing goniodysgenesis. The trabecular meshwork and other normal structures of the ciliary cleft (see Figure 15.3) are collapsed or not apparent. (Courtesy of E Scurrell)

drainage ultimately fails are not fully understood. Not surprisingly, those individuals that exhibit the greatest degree of pectinate ligament dysplasia have been shown to be the most likely to develop clinical signs of glaucoma (Read *et al.*, 1998).

Any dog of a breed listed in Figure 15.33 that presents with a sudden onset of a red or painful eye should be suspected of having closed-angle glaucoma, until proven otherwise. It is mandatory to carry out IOP measurement and gonioscopy in such patients. In addition, given that goniodysgenesis is a bilateral condition, the opposite eye is predisposed to developing glaucoma in the future. This may well influence case management and is very important information with respect to client education.

Chronic primary open-angle glaucoma

Primary open-angle glaucoma is seen in Norwegian Elkhounds and Petit Basset Griffon Vendeen (and occasionally other breeds and crossbred dogs) in the UK and in Beagles in the USA. Much research has been carried out on the condition in the Beagle, particularly because of its relevance to a very common disease in humans, but it is of limited importance in the veterinary clinical setting. The genetic mutation responsible for glaucoma in the Beagle has now been identified (Kuchtey *et al.*, 2011). The condition is bilateral and insidious in onset. Lens luxation or subluxation is not uncommon in affected eyes and may contribute to the development of glaucoma. Patients are often presented relatively late in the course of the disease, with enlarged globes and poor vision in both eyes. However, the optic nerve head appears to tolerate these prolonged, often marked, elevations in IOP better than in acute-onset forms of glaucoma. In some cases, useful vision can be retained through to the late stages of the disease, despite the presence of pronounced buphthalmos.

Secondary glaucoma

Secondary glaucoma Is the most commonly encountered type of glaucoma in both dogs and cats. It develops when antecedent ocular pathology reduces the circulation and drainage of aqueous, leading to an increase in IOP. Aqueous flow in secondary glaucoma may be impeded at the pupil or at the filtration angle (pectinate ligament and ciliary cleft structures). The site at which the major obstruction to aqueous circulation occurs may vary from one case to another. There are numerous possible causes of secondary glaucoma (Figure 15.37).

• Primary lens luxation (most common in terrier breeds)
• Lens luxation secondary to hypermature cataract
• Uveitis – including lens-induced uveitis due to lens rupture or hypermature cataract
• Neoplasia
• Intraocular haemorrhage (see Figure 15.27)
• Ocular melanosis (Cairn Terriers) – formerly described as pigmentary glaucoma
• Multiple iris cysts and uveitis (Golden Retrievers)
• Intumescence (swelling) of a cataractous lens – especially with diabetic cataracts
• Fibrovascular membrane formation in the drainage angle – secondary to retinal detachment, uveitis or neoplasia
• Vitreous prolapse after surgical lens extraction

15.37 Causes of secondary glaucoma.

Primary lens luxation

In the UK, primary lens luxation (see Chapter 16) is commonly seen in terrier breeds and Lancashire Heelers, and occasionally in Shar Peis and Border Collies. The lens may luxate into the anterior chamber, carrying vitreous humour with it. The flow of aqueous is then impeded by the presence of vitreous or lens within the pupil, causing pupillary block. The rise in IOP may also be associated with any prolapsed vitreous which comes to overlie the entrance to the ciliary cleft, and by the lens occupying a large proportion of the anterior chamber. Glaucoma may also be seen in cases where a luxated lens is resting within the posterior segment, and even in some instances where the lens is only subluxated. Once the IOP has been elevated for any length of time, the ciliary cleft may collapse and this change can rapidly become permanent due to the development of peripheral anterior synechiae. These are adhesions of the iris base to corneoscleral tissue, which effectively obliterate the ciliary cleft.

In some cases, it may be difficult to decide whether lens luxation is a cause or an effect of glaucoma. This distinction may have a profound influence on case management and will, to a certain extent, influence the prognosis. Establishing the order of events depends upon a careful assessment of the signalment, history and clinical findings. Gonioscopy, especially of the contralateral eye, may provide valuable information in this regard.

Uveitis

Inflammation of the uveal tract may result in secondary glaucoma through a variety of mechanisms:

- Accumulation of inflammatory debris within the structures of the filtration angle
- Damage to, and swelling of, the trabecular meshwork structures as a direct result of involvement in the inflammatory process (the ciliary cleft is composed of uveal tissue)

- The development of posterior synechiae (adhesions between the iris and the lens). If these adhesions become sufficiently extensive, aqueous is unable to flow from the posterior to the anterior chamber. This leads to a build-up of aqueous behind the iris, which then bulges forward (so-called 'iris bombé') (Figures 15.38 and 15.39). Initially, the obstruction to aqueous flow may be restricted to the pupil, but, with time, the forward displacement of the iris leads to collapse of the ciliary cleft. At this stage, the IOP remains elevated, even if the posterior synechiae are broken down or an alternative drainage channel through the iris is surgically created
- Fibrin clot material in the anterior chamber, impeding aqueous outflow, either at the pupil or at the drainage angle (Figure 15.40)
- Fibrovascular membrane formation over the pectinate ligament and entrance to the ciliary cleft (Figures 15.41 and 15.42). Fibrovascular membranes can also develop in response to neoplasia and retinal detachment (see below)
- Peripheral anterior synechiae. These may develop in disease states associated with inflammation:
  - Iris bombé, intumescent cataract or a luxating lens within the posterior chamber pushing the iris base forward
  - Anterior uveitis combined with a dilated pupil (e.g. with excessive use of atropine)
  - As a result of loss of the anterior chamber due to globe rupture.

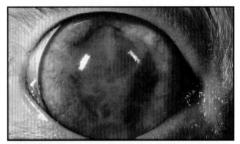

15.40 Extensive fibrin deposition within the pupil and anterior chamber as a result of blunt ocular trauma in a Persian cat.

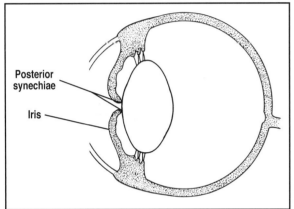

15.38 Iris bombé results when 360-degree posterior synechiae prevent flow of aqueous through the pupil.

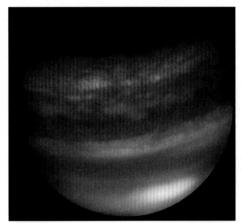

15.41 Gonioscopic view of fibrovascular membranes overlying the pectinate ligament and occluding the entrance to the ciliary cleft in a crossbred dog with uveitis.

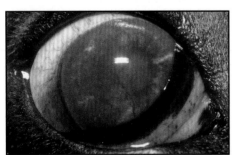

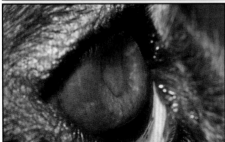

15.39 A Labrador Retriever was hit in the right eye by a golf ball 2 weeks previously. Glaucoma has developed as a result of uveitis and there has been considerable iris bombé formation. A cataract is also present and a small amount of haemorrhage can be seen in the pupil. The side view shows the iris bulging forward.

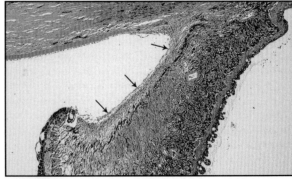

15.42 Histological section showing a pre-iridal fibrovascular membrane (arrowed) overlying the anterior face of the iris and extending across the entrance to the secondarily collapsed ciliary cleft. The iris is characteristically shortened and distorted by the membrane. (Courtesy of E Scurrell)

When dealing with any case of uveitis, it is important to monitor IOP, whether glaucoma is initially present or not. Both uveitis and glaucoma may present as a red, painful eye with a cloudy appearance. Tonometry is essential to distinguish the two condition. In addition, even initially uncomplicated uveitis may later become complicated by glaucoma and this may be overlooked until the situation is irreversible, unless a policy of routine IOP measurement is adopted in the management of patients with uveitis.

Neoplasia

Intraocular neoplasia may induce glaucoma by a variety of means:

- Direct involvement of the drainage angle in the neoplastic process
- A build-up of neoplastic cells from the aqueous within the trabecular meshwork
- Secondary blood–aqueous barrier breakdown, leading to debris within the trabecular meshwork
- Stimulation of fibrovascular membrane formation as a result of the release of angiogenic substances (Peiffer *et al.*, 1990).

The most common intraocular neoplasms are primary uveal melanoma (Figure 15.43), primary ciliary body adenoma/adenocarcinoma and lymphoma (usually with systemic involvement). Secondary intraocular neoplasia is also an occasional cause of glaucoma, with the commonest type in dogs being mammary adenocarcinoma (Figure 15.44). The diagnosis of intraocular neoplasia, especially when it is complicated by glaucoma, may not be straightforward. The cornea may exhibit marked oedema, neovascularization and pigmentation, all of which serve to obscure the view of the intraocular structures. Should any doubt exist as to the presence of an intraocular neoplasm, further investigation is required (Figure 15.45; see also Chapters 1, 2 and 14).

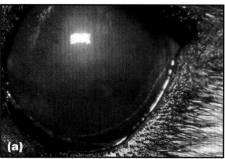

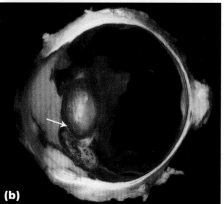

15.44 The left eye of an Anatolian Karabash bitch presenting with bilateral glaucoma secondary to metastatic carcinoma. The bitch had a history of recent mammary carcinoma resection. Thoracic radiography revealed the presence of multiple pulmonary metastases. **(a)** The left eye shows the presence of mild globe enlargement, corneal oedema, corneal vascularization and intraocular haemorrhage. Similar changes were evident in the right eye. **(b)** The section of the left globe shows evidence of invasion of the uveal tract by metastatic carcinoma (arrowed). The anterior chamber appears yellowish-white as a result of the post-mortem effect of the glutaraldehyde fixative in the presence of high protein levels, which have resulted from the antemortem breakdown of the blood–aqueous barrier.

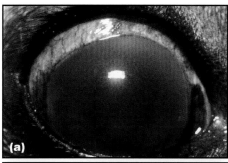

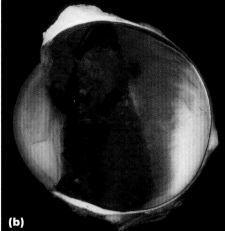

15.43 An 8-year-old Staffordshire Bull Terrier with a history of right ocular pain and discoloration. **(a)** The iris is dark and swollen dorsomedially, and the pupil is distorted. Corneal oedema is present. The diagnosis was one of glaucoma secondary to anterior uveal melanoma. **(b)** The cross-section of the globe shows that the bulk of the melanoma lies in the dorsal iris and ciliary body, but there is 'ring' spread to involve the entire anterior uvea. (b, Courtesy of JRB Mould)

- Full physical examination
- Ultrasonography of the globe and orbit
- Radiography of the thorax and abdomen
- Ultrasonography of the abdomen
- Lymph node aspiration or biopsy if lymphoma is suspected or lymphadenopathy is evident
- Blood samples for haematology and biochemistry
- Aqueous/vitreous centesis for cytological examination (probably best to refer the case if vision is still present)
- Enucleation and histopathology

15.45 Investigation of glaucoma where neoplasia is suspected.

Intraocular haemorrhage

This may occur for a number of reasons (see Figure 15.27). Even extensive haemorrhage may not lead to glaucoma, but in some instances the presence of blood and fibrin clots compromises aqueous outflow sufficiently to cause a rise in IOP (see Figure 15.12). Trauma cases often retain a low IOP in the face of severe intraocular haemorrhage; this may be the result of concomitant ciliary body damage or unsuspected scleral rupture, leading to a marked reduction in aqueous production. In addition to being a potential cause of increased IOP, intraocular haemorrhage may occur as a result of glaucoma in some chronic cases.

Ocular melanosis

This condition (also known as melanocytosis, pigmentary glaucoma and abnormal pigment deposition) involves the gradual accumulation of pigment-laden cells (primarily melanocytes but also melanophages) in the anterior segment structures, including the iris and ciliary body. It is seen in Cairn Terriers as an inherited defect (Petersen-Jones *et al.*, 2007, 2008) but can affect other breeds such as the Golden Retriever, Labrador Retriever and Boxer.

Ocular examination generally reveals both irises to be diffusely dark and thickened, and patches of pigment are visible in the sclera, especially ventrally (Figure 15.46a). Pigment accumulation can also be seen in the tapetal fundus and not infrequently over the region of the optic disc. As the condition progresses, it commonly leads to an insidious onset of glaucoma as a result of pigmented cell deposition in the ciliary cleft, the histological structure of which may become obliterated (Figure 15.46b).

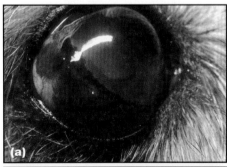

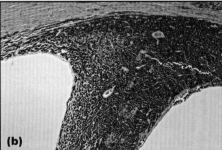

15.46 Ocular melanosis in a Cairn Terrier. **(a)** Heavy pigment deposition is evident within the sclera and at the limbus. The iris is dark and thickened.
(b) Histologically, the iris, drainage angle and areas of the sclera are shown to be heavily infiltrated with pigmented cells, the majority of which are melanocytes. (b, Courtesy of E Scurrell)

Iridociliary cysts

A syndrome involving the formation of multiple iridociliary cysts (see Chapter 14) and pigment dispersion, in association with glaucoma, has been described in Golden Retrievers (Deehr and Dubielzig, 1998; Esson *et al.*, 2009) and Great Danes (Spiess *et al.*, 1998). Whilst uveitis has been described as accompanying this condition, little or no histopathological evidence of uveitis was seen in the study by Esson *et al.* (2009). The exact mechanism whereby glaucoma develops in this condition is uncertain and management can be challenging.

Pathology of the lens

In addition to primary lens luxation (see above), glaucoma can develop as a sequel to a variety of pathological changes involving the lens:

- Lens-induced uveitis due to leakage of antigenic lens proteins into the aqueous humour:
  - Secondary to mature/hypermature cataracts
  - As a result of lens rupture, either due to trauma or associated with cataract formation
- Luxation of a hypermature cataractous lens
- Swelling (intumescence) of the lens. This is a relatively uncommon cause of glaucoma
- Retinal detachment secondary to a cataract, leading to fibrovascular membrane formation within the drainage angle (Figure 15.47).

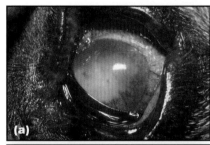

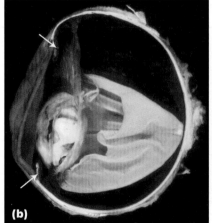

15.47 A Great Dane with a cataract, lens-induced uveitis, retinal detachment and pre-iridal fibrovascular membrane formation, which in turn has caused glaucoma. **(a)** Corneal oedema and corneal vascularization are present. Note also the obscured view of the cataract. **(b)** Post-enucleation specimen showing evidence of globe enlargement and total retinal detachment. The iris (arrowed) is shortened as a result of the pre-iridal fibrovascular membrane. (b, Courtesy of JRB Mould)

Vitreous prolapse

Large quantities of vitreous may enter the anterior chamber as a result of intraocular surgery (usually intracapsular lens extraction) or following lens luxation. Obstruction of aqueous flow subsequently occurs, either at the pupil or within the filtration angle. If vitreous presents in the anterior chamber during lens surgery, vitrectomy is necessary and reduces the likelihood of the subsequent development of glaucoma.

Treatment

The major aim in glaucoma management is to lower the IOP to a level at which vision no longer deteriorates. Setting a target IOP of ≤20 mmHg should help reduce the persistence of neurodestructive mechanisms that may otherwise continue to cause loss of vision, even after a grossly elevated IOP has been corrected.

Glaucoma therapy can be divided into medical and surgical approaches, although in many instances a combination of both will be required. In general terms, a reduction in IOP may be achieved by either reducing the production of aqueous or increasing the facility of aqueous outflow. Examples of both of these mechanisms can be found in the various medical and surgical approaches to glaucoma management. The management strategy in any individual case depends on a number of factors, including:

- The degree of vision present and the likelihood of its return. This is partly dependent on the duration of the condition. In acute-onset cases of only a few hours' or days' duration, where blindness is apparent, some return of vision may be achieved with rapid normalization of the IOP. Long-standing cases where the patient is blind, are unlikely to become sighted again, even with vigorous treatment. Signs of chronicity (e.g. buphthalmos and Descemet's streaks) do not necessarily preclude the presence of some useful vision. Young animals and patients with primary open-angle glaucoma may develop signs of globe enlargement well before optic nerve damage has caused total blindness. A careful evaluation of vision in any patient presenting with glaucoma is vital when formulating a treatment plan
- The underlying cause of the problem. For example, the approach to a case with uveitis that has led to secondary glaucoma will be entirely different from that to one in which neoplasia is the underlying cause. In some instances, the management of the contralateral eye is as important as that of the globe with elevated IOP (e.g. in cases of goniodysgenesis)
- The findings on gonioscopy. Medical therapy in uveitis or open-angle cases may be satisfactory if the appearance of the drainage structures suggests that a potentially adequate pathway remains for aqueous outflow. If gonioscopy shows marked pectinate ligament dysplasia due

to goniodysgenesis or closure of the entrance to the ciliary cleft, medical therapy alone may well be insufficient to achieve even short-term control of IOP. In many cases, especially those of a chronic nature, increased IOP generally results in the iris base being displaced anteriorly, leading to the development of peripheral anterior synechiae. Peripheral anterior synechiae and ciliary cleft collapse are often found, even at the first presentation, in domestic animals. They result in a severe reduction in the facility of aqueous outflow and in such circumstances, surgical therapy may be required to regain sustained control of IOP

- The initial response to therapy. If medical therapy is attempted and the initial response is excellent, surgical intervention may become less urgent
- If the contralateral eye is blind or absent, the need to preserve vision in the glaucomatous eye becomes more pressing to the majority of owners
- The age and general condition of the animal. Major surgery may be less justifiable in elderly or otherwise compromised patients
- Financial considerations, the wishes of the owner and the ease of access to a specialist.

Medical management

Osmotic diuretics

Acute glaucoma with high IOP (>40–50 mmHg) of very recent onset warrants the immediate use of osmotic diuretics to achieve a rapid reduction in IOP, especially if blindness is present. The drug in common use is intravenous mannitol (Figure 15.48). Oral glycerol (which may induce emesis as an unwanted side effect) may be supplied for emergency home use in dogs known to have a predisposition to primary glaucoma.

Therapeutic agent [a]	Class of agent	Dosage
Mannitol (10% or 20% solution)	Osmotic diuretic	1–2 g/kg i.v. over 20–30 min
Glycerol (50%)	Osmotic diuretic	1–2 ml/kg orally
Dorzolamide hydrochloride (2% drops)	Carbonic anhydrase inhibitor	3–4 times a day
Brinzolamide (1% drops)	Carbonic anhydrase inhibitor	2–3 times a day
Acetazolamide (tablets/solution)	Carbonic anhydrase inhibitor	10–25 mg/kg orally, i.v., i.m. q12h
Dichlorphenamide	Carbonic anhydrase inhibitor	5–10 mg/kg orally 2–3 times a day
Methazolamide	Carbonic anhydrase inhibitor	5–10 mg/kg orally 2–3 times a day
Latanoprost (drops)	Prostaglandin analogue	2–3 times a day

15.48 Drugs used to treat glaucoma. [a] Note that not all the agents listed may be commercially available. (continues) ▶

Therapeutic agent [a]	Class of agent	Dosage
Travoprost (drops)	Prostaglandin analogue	2–3 times a day
Pilocarpine (1% drops)	Miotic	2–3 times a day
Demecarium bromide (0.125% drops)	Miotic	1–2 times a day
Timolol (0.5% drops)	Beta-adrenergic blocker	1–2 times a day
Metipranolol (0.3% drops)	Beta-adrenergic blocker	2 times a day
Levobunolol (0.5% drops)	Beta-adrenergic blocker	1–2 times a day
Betaxolol (0.25% drops)	Beta-adrenergic blocker	2 times a day

15.48 (continued) Drugs used to treat glaucoma. [a] Note that not all the agents listed may be commercially available.

- Potassium depletion
- Metabolic acidosis
- Diuresis
- Anorexia
- Gastrointestinal disturbances (vomiting and diarrhoea)

15.49 Side effects of systemic carbonic anhydrase inhibitors.

Osmotic diuretics tend to be most useful for the management of patients with primary glaucoma or glaucoma secondary to lens luxation. They may also be used in cases with significant postoperative ocular hypertension following cataract surgery. However, they may be of less benefit in patients with glaucoma resulting from uveitis or intraocular haemorrhage. Care must be taken when using these drugs because they can cause a rapid reduction in circulating blood volume. In certain cases, this may induce prerenal azotaemia and even renal failure. If there is any doubt as to the renal or cardiovascular status of the patient, these parameters should be carefully assessed prior to the commencement of therapy. Whilst a rapid response may be seen with the use of mannitol, the effect is likely to be short-lived and further medical and/or surgical treatment is generally required to achieve long-term control of IOP.

Carbonic anhydrase inhibitors

Carbonic anhydrase inhibitors decrease the production of aqueous humour. Initially, their effect can be so dramatic as to reduce the IOP by up to 50%. They are available for both systemic and topical use; their therapeutic action is independent of their diuretic effects when used systemically. Traditionally, they are a mainstay of longer-term medical management of canine glaucoma.

The drugs of this class currently available in the UK are acetazolamide (which is used systemically) and dorzolamide and brinzolamide (which are topical preparations) (see Figure 15.48). Of these, the topical agents are the drugs of choice in dogs, as they appear to be as effective as acetazolamide but without the side effects encountered with the use of systemic carbonic anhydrase inhibitors (Figure 15.49). Brinzolamide is better tolerated than dorzolamide in some patients, possibly because of the relatively low pH of the latter drug. Both dorzolamide and brinzolamide are currently available in combination with timolol (a beta-blocker; see below), but these combination therapies should be used with caution

and reserved for refractory cases, owing to the potential systemic side effects of timolol (bradycardia and hypotension). Acetazolamide can be obtained in intravenous form for emergency use, although mannitol is more often used in these circumstances. Dichlorphenamide and methazolamide are systemic carbonic anhydrase inhibitors which can be used for the reduction of IOP in dogs, and appear to have a lower incidence of side effects than acetazolamide. However, they are not currently available in the UK.

Prostaglandin analogues

Latanoprost and travaprost are prostaglandin prodrugs which can be used topically to reduce IOP. Their mode of action in dogs is not entirely clear, but probably results from a combination of a reduction in the production of aqueous and an increase in its uveoscleral outflow. These drugs can have a profound and rapid effect on IOP in dogs (at least initially), even where the entrance to the ciliary cleft appears to be severely compromised on gonioscopy.

Prostaglandin analogues are generally applied twice daily, usually in addition to a topical carbonic anhydrase inhibitor. They appear not to be effective in reducing IOP in cats, but do cause miosis in both dogs and cats and the intensity of pupil constriction can cause discomfort and affect vision. Prostaglandin analogues also cause a degree of episcleral vasodilation, which can give treated eyes a red appearance. Their prolonged use may result in increased iris pigmentation in some species, although this has not been reported in dogs. The use of prostaglandin analogues in cases with uveitis is not recommended, especially in view of their miotic effect (increased risk of posterior synechiae formation and aggravation of discomfort due to iris spasm). They are also contraindicated in cases with anterior lens luxation and/or vitreous presentation in the anterior chamber, because the resulting miosis is likely to result in pupil block and consequent exacerbation of IOP elevation.

Miotics

The major indication for the use of miotics (such as pilocarpine) is in primary open-angle glaucoma. They cause an increase in aqueous outflow through their action on the ciliary muscles by opening up the trabecular meshwork. In cases where the ciliary cleft is permanently collapsed, or in cases of goniodysgenesis, there is little likelihood that these agents will prove effective. As these changes predominate in canine glaucoma, the routine use of miotics is probably not indicated. Miotics may be beneficial for patients in which the drainage angle remains open, but with the advent of agents such as dorzolamide and latanoprost, their use is rarely warranted. The use of miotics is contraindicated in cases of uveitis.

Pilocarpine is a direct-acting parasympathomimetic which is generally used as a 1% solution applied two or three times a day. It may cause location irritation. Demecarium bromide is commonly used as a miotic, but it is not currently available in a topical ophthalmic form in the UK. It is an anticholinesterase and a potent indirect-acting parasympathomimetic. It may cause the formation of iris cysts with long-term use.

Beta-adrenergic blockers

Beta-adrenergic blockers are used topically to reduce aqueous production (they may also increase outflow). Their effect at the concentrations commercially available is limited (Gum *et al.*, 1991) and as a result they are normally used in combination with a carbonic anhydrase inhibitor such as dorzolamide. Timolol maleate is the most commonly used of these agents. Metipranolol, levobunolol and betaxolol are other beta-blockers available. Potential systemic side effects include bradycardia and bronchospasm. Betaxolol causes less marked systemic side effects than timolol as a result of more specific beta-1 blocking activity.

Alpha-adrenergic agents

Sympathomimetics, such as 1% adrenaline (epinephrine) and the prodrug dipivefrin, are probably best avoided in the treatment of canine and feline glaucoma. They cause unwanted pupillary dilation, which may compromise aqueous outflow in all but open-angle glaucoma. It may be possible to reduce the pupillary effects by using these drugs in combination with a miotic such as pilocarpine.

Apraclonidine is an alpha-2 adrenergic agonist which is used in the short-term management of primary open-angle glaucoma in humans. It may be beneficial in some canine patients, but its effect is inconsistent and it can cause bradycardia. Due to its cardiovascular side effects, it is prudent to monitor any patient carefully for approximately 1 hour following the first application of apraclonidine.

Atropine

The use of atropine is contraindicated in all cases of glaucoma except those caused by early iris bombé. A potentially devastating cause of glaucoma, iris bombé must be dealt with very aggressively, ideally within hours of onset. In these circumstances, attempting to dilate the pupil may break down the posterior synechiae, allowing aqueous humour to escape from the posterior chamber. Topical phenylephrine (2.5% or 10%) may be used in addition to atropine in these circumstances in order to maximize the desired mydriatic effect.

Tissue plasminogen activator

Tissue plasminogen activator (TPA) causes the production of plasmin from plasminogen, and this in turn results in the lysis of fibrin. Amongst other indications for its use, TPA may be injected intracamerally (i.e. into the anterior chamber) when significant quantities of fibrin are contributing to an increase in

IOP. With the patient under suitable sedation or general anaesthesia, and following preparation of the eye for a sterile procedure, a small quantity (0.1–0.2 ml) of aqueous is removed by paracentesis and an equivalent volume containing 25–50 μg of TPA is injected into the anterior chamber. Clot lysis is normally complete within a few hours of injection. The patient should then be monitored over the following days and weeks for evidence of any recurrence of fibrin clot formation or intraocular haemorrhage, in addition to assessing other parameters (including IOP). Intracameral injection can result in significant ocular trauma if it is not performed properly; as a result it is primarily a specialist procedure.

Prophylactic treatment

There may be some benefit of prophylactic medical therapy in dogs with goniodysgenesis. These cases often present with glaucoma in one eye and an apparently normal contralateral eye. However, gonioscopy reveals the essentially bilateral nature of goniodysgenesis and, in these cases, it is possible that the onset of glaucoma in the contralateral eye may be delayed with the long-term use of topical medication. The evidence of the benefit of prophylactic treatment in such circumstances is limited; one study involved the use of either a topical beta-blocker or the miotic demecarium bromide in combination with a topical steroid (Miller *et al.*, 2000). However, it is possible that prophylactic treatment with a topical carbonic anhydrase inhibitor or a prostaglandin analogue may delay the onset of glaucoma in normotensive eyes with significant goniodysgenesis.

Neuroprotection

The major means by which the optic nerve head and the retinal structures can be protected from the effects of glaucoma is by lowering the IOP. However, other therapeutic strategies for neuroprotection are being researched, particularly with regard to improving survival of retinal ganglion cells and their axons. Despite earlier suggestions that cytotoxic levels of glutamate within the retina of glaucomatous eyes in dogs leads to an excessive influx of calcium into the retinal ganglion cells and a chain of events leading to apoptosis (Gelatt *et al.*, 2007), no clinically proven neuroprotective strategies have yet resulted from this finding. Investigations continue into drugs which may either help to reduce the rate of cell death in the retina in patients with glaucoma, or encourage regeneration of already damaged neural elements.

Surgical management

In many instances, particularly of primary glaucoma, medical therapy alone is not sufficient to reduce the IOP to a safe level. The decision-making process as to when to undertake surgery and what procedures may be indicated is not necessarily straightforward. If the patient is a potential surgical candidate, early (and sometimes urgent) referral to a specialist should be considered. Surgical approaches to glaucoma are aimed at either reducing aqueous production or creating an alternative pathway for aqueous drainage. The main techniques currently available for treating glaucoma are summarized in Figure 15.50.

- Lens extraction:
  - In cases of primary lens luxation
  - Infrequently indicated where lens luxation is secondary to glaucoma
- Procedures reducing aqueous production:
  - Laser cyclophotocoagulation (trans-scleral or endoscopic)
  - Cyclocryotherapy
- Procedures increasing aqueous outflow:
  - Drainage implant surgery
  - Scleral trephination and peripheral iridectomy
- Enucleation
- Evisceration and intrascleral prosthesis – only when there is a definitive diagnosis of primary glaucoma. Enucleation is the preferred option
- Pharmacological ablation of the ciliary body (intravitreal gentamicin injection) – only in blind eyes where enucleation or evisceration and intrascleral prosthesis are not viable options

15.50 Surgical techniques for the management of glaucoma.

Lens extraction

In the event of primary lens luxation, removal of the lens may be sufficient to allow return to a normal IOP. Lens extraction in such cases is most likely to be beneficial when the condition is detected early and treated promptly; the prognosis is probably optimal in cases of lens subluxation where the lens is extracted by phacoemulsification. It is very important that, at the time of lens extraction, any vitreal material which has prolapsed through the pupil is also carefully removed, preferably by mechanized anterior vitrectomy. Failure to do so may lead to persistence of pupillary block and glaucoma. In longer-standing cases of primary lens luxation, irreversible damage to the drainage apparatus may occur in the form of peripheral anterior synechiae. In these cases, lens extraction and anterior vitrectomy alone may fail to achieve the desired result of a normotensive globe. Thus, additional surgical procedures (such as laser cyclophotocoagulation; see below) are likely to be required to reduce the IOP to a safe level.

When lens luxation is secondary to glaucoma, lens removal is rarely indicated because the eye is often blind by this time; enucleation may be a better approach in these circumstances. However, if the eye is still sighted, lens removal combined with other glaucoma procedures and ongoing medical management may offer the best chance of controlling IOP and retaining useful vision.

Reducing aqueous production

The techniques for reducing aqueous production involve the destruction of a proportion of the ciliary body sufficient to decrease the IOP to within normal limits. Surgical cyclodestruction can be achieved through laser cyclophotocoagulation and (historically) cryotherapy or diathermy. These techniques were initially employed as an alternative to enucleation of blind eyes, but laser cyclophotocoagulation has become more frequently used in sighted eyes. A potential drawback of cyclodestruction is that many of the intraocular structures rely on aqueous circulation for maintenance of healthy function, and significantly reducing aqueous production may result in undesirable 'knock-on' effects. However,

this theoretical disadvantage is generally outweighed by the alternative of allowing the eye to succumb to the blinding and painful effects of uncontrolled glaucoma.

Laser cyclophotocoagulation: The most common type of laser in veterinary use for the treatment of glaucoma is the diode laser (Figure 15.51). The laser energy is aimed at and absorbed by the (generally) pigmented tissue of the ciliary body. This causes coagulative necrosis of the ciliary processes and surrounding tissues, resulting in a reduction in aqueous production.

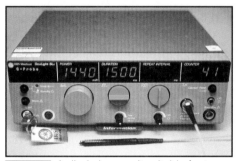

15.51 A diode laser unit suitable for trans-scleral cyclophotocoagulation.

The laser energy can be directed either through the sclera (trans-scleral laser cyclophotocoagulation; Figure 15.52) or from within the globe (endoscopic laser cyclophotocoagulation). The latter technique is under development and there are currently no published data regarding its efficacy and safety. The procedure involves introducing an endoscopic camera with a light source and laser delivery system via two limbal incisions, through the pupil and under the iris. The ciliary processes can then be visualized and the tissues photocoagulated (Figure 15.53). Satisfactory access to the ciliary processes generally requires prior lens extraction by phacoemulsification. The potential advantage of the procedure is that the damage caused to the ciliary processes is more controlled than that achieved by the trans-scleral approach. The potential disadvantages are that the procedure is invasive, requires significant training and expertise, is costly to perform, can result in significant postoperative uveitis, may involve demanding postoperative management regimes and has an as yet unproven success rate.

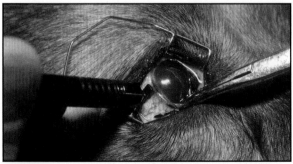

15.52 Trans-scleral laser cyclophotocoagulation in progress. The globe has been rotated so that the 9 o'clock position is away from the laser beam.

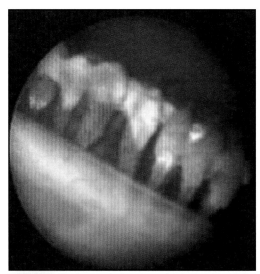

15.53 Endoscopic laser cyclophotocoagulation. The ciliary processes can be visualized during the procedure. Note that the processes have turned white at the photocoagulated sites. (Courtesy of D Wilkie)

Trans-scleral cyclophotocoagulation protocols vary, but commonly approximately 30–40 treatments are delivered trans-sclerally at multiple sites about 3–4 mm behind the limbus, avoiding the 3 and 9 o'clock positions (to prevent damage to the long posterior ciliary arteries). The total energy delivered is often about 80–120 joules. In a large series of cases of dogs with glaucoma, IOP was reduced to ≤30 mmHg in approximately 50% of patients 1 year after diode laser trans-scleral cyclophotocoagulation, although only 20% retained vision (Cook *et al.*, 1997). In another smaller study, patients had fewer sites (25 per eye) treated for longer but at a higher total energy level (125 joules). Of the 14 eyes followed up for 8–21 months, 50% regained or retained vision, although six cases developed cataracts (Hardman and Stanley, 2001). Trans-scleral laser cyclophotocoagulation has the advantages of being non-invasive and relatively quick to perform. However, management in the postoperative period can be problematical and the equipment is expensive. The complications of laser cyclophotocoagulation are listed in Figure 15.54.

- Immediate pressure spike after the procedure
  - May require aqueous paracentesis
  - Some veterinary ophthalmologists perform drainage implant surgery at the time of laser cyclophotocoagulation in anticipation of the pressure spike
- Intraocular fibrin formation/uveitis
- Intraocular haemorrhage
- Corneal ulceration
- Keratoconjunctivitis
- Cataract formation
- Inadequate control of IOP
  - Procedure may need to be repeated
  - Poorly pigmented eyes absorb less energy and respond less well
- Excessive drop in IOP leading to phthisis bulbi

15.54 Complications of laser cyclophotocoagulation.

Cyclocryotherapy: Freezing the ciliary body through the sclera can be performed to reduce IOP. A cryoprobe is placed over the ciliary body behind the limbus at several sites around the globe and the areas are frozen until the ice ball extends to the limbus. However, in addition to causing postoperative swelling and potentially significant discomfort, the IOP often increases for several days after the procedure and there is a risk of associated retinal detachment. The technique is infrequently used and, whilst it might be used in blind eyes as an alternative to enucleation, in the author's opinion it is preferable when dealing with an end-stage glaucomatous eye to perform a definitive procedure such as enucleation, hence obviating the need for ongoing management and the potential requirement for repeat general anaesthesia and surgery in the future.

Pharmacological ablation of the ciliary body: In blind eyes this can be achieved by an intravitreal injection of gentamicin (Moller *et al.*, 1986). The technique should only ever be used where:

- The patient is a dog
- The diagnosis of glaucoma is certain
- There is no evidence of neoplasia, infection or uveitis
- The eye is irreversibly blind and not suitable for enucleation due to patient factors.

Under general anaesthesia, a 20 gauge hypodermic needle is inserted approximately 1 cm into the vitreous from a point about 8 mm behind the limbus. The needle is directed towards the optic disc in order to avoid the lens. Approximately 0.5 ml of vitreous is aspirated (this has often undergone syneresis (liquefaction) and is easy to withdraw). Then 20 mg of gentamicin is injected, with or without 0.5 mg of dexamethasone. Gentamicin causes substantial damage to the ciliary body, thereby reducing its capacity to produce aqueous. Complications of the technique include:

- Severe uveitis
- Pain
- Corneal opacity
- Cataracts
- Phthisis bulbi.

However, many treated patients eventually require enucleation, primarily owing to the complications of severe uveitis and pain. Thus, the technique is not generally recommended and should definitely not be used in cats because they may develop ocular sarcoma in response to chronic inflammation and trauma (Dubielzig *et al.*, 1990). Enucleation is a more satisfactory surgical approach to end-stage glaucoma, particularly in patients in which the underlying cause of glaucoma has not been established.

Increasing aqueous outflow

In theory at least, the best prospects for retaining vision should be offered by techniques that improve aqueous outflow, given that it is the outflow of aqueous that is impeded in glaucomatous eyes. The techniques used in dogs all aim to create an outflow for aqueous that bypasses the drainage apparatus.

Scleral trephination and peripheral iridectomy:
This technique, which has become outmoded, involves the formation of a drainage hole through the sclera that enters the anterior chamber (Bedford, 1977). This allows aqueous to flow from the anterior chamber into a subconjunctival bleb, from which it is absorbed. A peripheral iridectomy adjacent to the sclerostomy site is designed to prevent it from becoming plugged with iris tissue and allows passage of aqueous from the posterior chamber to the anterior chamber (useful in cases of iris bombé). However, owing to complications such as uveitis and scarring of both the sclerostomy and the subconjunctival bleb, the technique frequently fails within the first few days, weeks or months.

Drainage implant surgery: The use of drainage implants for the treatment of selected canine patients with glaucoma has gained popularity in recent years, because these devices reduce the likelihood of early postoperative failure often seen with techniques such as scleral trephination (Gelatt *et al.*, 1987, 1992; Bedford, 1989). The use of various types of implant has been reported (Garcia *et al.*, 1998) and amongst the most common in use in the UK is the Joseph implant. A large silicone strap retained under the rectus muscles and covered by conjunctiva is joined to a silicone tube, which enters the anterior chamber at the limbus (Figure 15.55). Other implants available include the Molteno, Ahmed and Krupin–Denver devices, which have smaller strap arrangements and various inbuilt valves to reduce the risk of the IOP dropping too low.

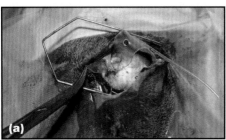

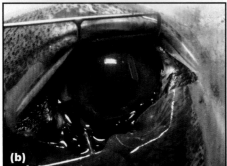

15.55 **(a)** A Joseph implant being placed in the left eye of a Flat-coated Retriever with primary glaucoma due to goniodysgenesis. The strap is passed under the rectus muscles and sutured to the sclera. **(b)** The Joseph implant tubing can be seen in the anterior chamber at the end of the procedure.

The placement of a drainage implant is a major procedure and should only be performed by specialist clinicians familiar with this type of surgery. Complications of the technique include:

- Intraoperative intraocular haemorrhage
- Postoperative uveitis
- Blockage of the tubing with fibrin in the immediate postoperative period. This often requires an intracameral injection of TPA
- Implant loosening or extrusion
- Scarring of the filtering bleb, reducing aqueous absorption. This process may be limited by the intraoperative use of anti-fibroblastic agents (e.g. mitomycin C or 5-fluorouracil). Failure often occurs at the 6- to 12-month stage because of scarring.

Implant surgery and laser cyclophotocoagulation currently offer the best prospects of medium- to longer-term control of IOP, particularly in dogs with primary glaucoma. Both procedures may ultimately fail, although both can be repeated if necessary. Both carry the risk of complications and patient management in the immediate postoperative period can be challenging. It is not uncommon for patients to have both laser cyclophotocoagulation and drainage implant surgery during the course of their glaucoma management, and there is some suggestion that combined therapy may offer advantages in terms of long-term IOP control compared with either procedure used alone (Bentley *et al.*, 1999; Sapienza and van der Woerdt, 2005). In most instances, superior postoperative control of IOP is afforded by continued lifelong medical therapy and associated monitoring by an ophthalmologist.

Enucleation
Despite attempts at therapy, cases of glaucoma may ultimately become end-stage, and enucleation (see Chapter 8) may be indicated. In some patients, this may be required bilaterally. Indications for enucleation include:

- A blind eye that requires unacceptable medication or surgery to control IOP
- Intractable pain
- Buphthalmos with persistent complications due to exposure
- Primary neoplasia.

Evisceration and intrascleral prosthesis (see Chapter 8) may be an alternative to enucleation, but this should only ever be performed where a definitive diagnosis of primary glaucoma has been reached, preferably by a specialist in veterinary ophthalmology. This technique should be avoided in any patients where secondary glaucoma has not been ruled out. In the author's view, any irreversibly blind eye in which the IOP cannot readily be kept <40 mmHg should be enucleated on the grounds that it may be causing the patient discomfort, of which both the owners and the veterinary surgeon may be unaware. Many owners report an improvement in their animal's demeanour postoperatively under such circumstances, suggesting that the patient may have been suffering undetected pain prior to surgery.

Glaucoma in cats

The majority of the previous discussion is applicable to both dogs and cats, but some features of feline glaucoma are worthy of note. For a detailed, comprehensive review of feline glaucoma, the reader is referred to McLellan and Miller (2011).

Aetiology

Primary glaucoma is rarely seen in cats, but it can appear sporadically in any breed (Ridgway and Brightman, 1989; Wilcock *et al.*, 1990; Trost *et al.*, 2007). It has been suggested that Siamese cats may be predisposed (Dubielzig *et al.*, 2010). An inherited congenital form has been identified in Siamese cats (McLellan and Miller, 2011) and primary glaucoma associated with pectinate ligament dysplasia has been reported in six Burmese cats in Australia (Hampson *et al.*, 2002).

Secondary glaucoma is not uncommon in cats and most frequently occurs as a result of uveitis or neoplasia (Wilcock *et al.*, 1990; Blocker and van der Woerdt, 2001; Dubielzig *et al.*, 2010). Iris melanoma (Figure 15.56) and intraocular lymphoma (Figure 15.57) are the commonest tumours to cause glaucoma in the cat. In glaucoma secondary to uveitis (Figure 15.58), the signs of the underlying disease can be extremely subtle in cats, and careful inspection of both eyes using slit-lamp biomicroscopy may

be necessary to establish that the glaucoma is indeed secondary to inflammation. Cases of uveitis should be investigated for potential systemic disease (see Chapter 14). Other causes of secondary glaucoma in cats include trauma and intraocular haemorrhage (the latter is often secondary to systemic hypertension).

One major difference between feline and canine glaucoma is the low incidence of primary lens luxation in cats (Olivero *et al.*, 1991). Lens luxation associated with glaucoma in a cat is usually secondary to underlying uveitis (sometimes with resultant cataract formation) or globe enlargement, or a combination of the two. Glaucoma may arise in cats as a result of aqueous misdirection syndrome (also known as malignant glaucoma in humans). The condition is generally seen in older cats and involves aqueous flowing into the vitreous, resulting in the vitreous face, lens and iris being pushed anteriorly (Czederpiltz *et al.*, 2005). The anterior chamber becomes uniformerly shallow, as does the drainage angle, and glaucoma may develop owing to a resultant decrease in aqueous outflow.

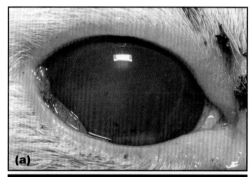
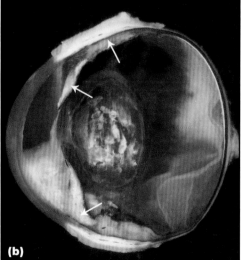

15.57 Glaucoma secondary to lymphoma in a Domestic Shorthaired cat with feline leukaemia virus. **(a)** The eye shows signs of conjunctival swelling and hyperaemia, corneal oedema and neovascularization. The iris is largely obscured due to the presence of fibrin, cellular effusion and haemorrhage in the anterior chamber. **(b)** The cross-section of the globe shows that the iris and ciliary body are heavily infiltrated by lymphoma tissue (arrowed). The aqueous appears opaque owing to the effect of fixative in the presence of high protein levels. (b, Courtesy of JRB Mould)

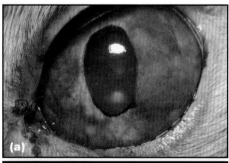
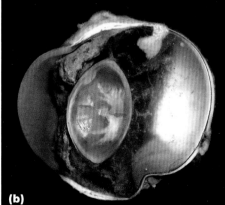

15.56 Diffuse iris melanoma in a Persian cat with secondary glaucoma. **(a)** The iris is thickened, discoloured and distorted. **(b)** A section of the affected eye. (b, Courtesy of E Scurrell)

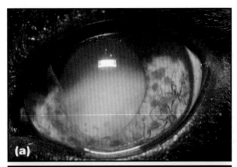

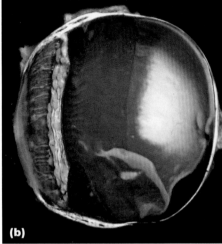

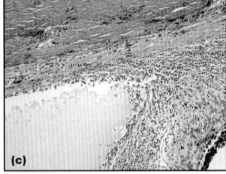

15.58 Lymphocytic-plasmacytic uveitis and secondary glaucoma in a cat. **(a)** Focal accumulations of inflammatory cells ('iris nodules'), iris neovascularization, keratic precipitates and a secondary cataract can be seen. **(b)** The gross section of the globe shows the cell infiltrates within the iris and obliterating the drainage angle. The lens has been removed. **(c)** Photomicrograph showing heavy infiltration of the iris and ciliary cleft by inflammatory cells. (b–c, Courtesy of E Scurrell)

Clinical signs

Feline glaucoma is very commonly insidious in onset. Signs of pain, corneal oedema and episcleral injection are frequently much less marked than in dogs. Alteration in the ophthalmoscopic appearance of the optic nerve head is less marked in cats with chronic glaucoma, compared with dogs, because of the normally smaller and darker appearance of the unmyelinated optic disc in cats (see Chapter 18). The first presenting signs may include suspected vision loss (although cats are extremely good at adapting to blindness) or, more often, a change in the appearance of the eye due to mydriasis, buphthalmos, uveitis or neoplasia (Figure 15.59).

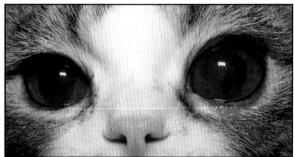

15.59 A 1-year-old Domestic Shorthaired cat with bilateral glaucoma secondary to uveitis caused by feline infectious peritonitis. The left eye is grossly enlarged and shows signs of a haemorrhagic inflammatory deposit on the corneal endothelium.

Any case of uveitis on long-term management should be carefully monitored for the possibility of glaucoma development, which can only be achieved by regularly measuring the IOP. This is of particular importance because topical steroids have been shown to cause elevation of the IOP in normal cats (Zhan *et al.*, 1992; Bhattacherjee *et al.*, 1999).

Treatment

The treatment of glaucoma in cats is similar to that in dogs, although as a result of the late presentation and the high incidence of secondary cases, the outcome is often disappointing. The primary aim is to treat the underlying cause of the glaucoma, and in cases with uveitis this may be sufficient to reduce the IOP to within normal limits. However, in some instances, the underlying uveitis may be low-grade and poorly responsive to medical therapy; in these cases, a relentless progression of the secondary glaucoma may occur, leading to blindness and end-stage disease.

There is the risk of adverse taste responses and systemic absorption when applying topical glaucoma medications in cats. In order to minimize these effects, it may be beneficial to occlude the lacrimal puncta temporarily by gentle digital pressure immediately after the medication has been applied. The topical carbonic anhydrase inhibitor dorzolamide has been shown to reduce IOP in the eyes of both normal cats (Rainbow and Dziezyc, 2003; Dietrich *et al.*, 2007) and those with glaucoma (Sigle *et al.*, 2011). It may be used 3–4 times daily for the treatment of cats with glaucoma. By contrast, brinzolamide has been shown to have no effect on the IOP of normal cats when applied twice daily (Gray *et al.*, 2003) and is likely to be less effective than dorzolamide in lowering IOP in glaucomatous cats. Cats tolerate systemic carbonic anhydrase inhibitors poorly, thus the use of acetazolamide in this species is not recommended.

The topical beta-blocker timolol was found to reduce the IOP in normal eyes (Wilkie and Latimer, 1991) and to be beneficial in reducing the IOP in one study of glaucomatous cats (Blocker and van der Woerdt, 2001) but not in others (Hampson *et al.*, 2002; G McLellan, personal communication). Latanoprost has been shown to have no effect on the IOP in normal cats, although it does cause marked miosis (Studer *et al.*, 2000). Its reported benefits in cats with glaucoma appear inconsistent to poor, and its use in cases of feline glaucoma is therefore not recommended.

All too often, medical treatment may ultimately prove to be ineffective in controlling glaucoma in cats. In some instances, there may be side effects, particularly with systemic therapy, which are not warranted, especially if vision has already been lost. Should the eye become irreversibly blind and if the IOP cannot readily be kept at <40 mmHg, enucleation may be the best management option. Intravitreal injections of gentamicin should not be used because chronically damaged feline eyes are at risk of developing intraocular sarcoma, and the underlying neoplasm may not be identified until a histopathological examination is carried out on the enucleated end-stage glaucomatous globe.

The surgical therapies described for dogs can be applied to cats. However, they are rarely performed as a result of the late presentation and secondary nature of a large proportion of feline cases. Lentectomy by phacoemulsification combined with extensive vitrectomy may be indicated in some cats with intractable glaucoma secondary to aqueous misdirection syndrome, although the majority of cases can be managed medically.

References and further reading

Barnett KC and Crispin SM (1998) Aqueous and glaucoma. In: *Feline Ophthalmology*, ed. KC Barnett and SM Crispin, pp. 104–111. WB Saunders, London

Barnett KC, Sansom J and Heinrich C (2002) Glaucoma. In: *Canine Ophthalmology*, pp. 99–107. WB Saunders, London

Bedford PGC (1977) The surgical treatment of canine glaucoma. *Journal of Small Animal Practice* **18**, 713–730

Bedford PGC (1980) The aetiology of canine glaucoma. *Veterinary Record* **107**, 76–82

Bedford PGC (1989) A clinical evaluation of a one-piece drainage system in the treatment of canine glaucoma. *Journal of Small Animal Practice* **30**, 68–75

Bentley E, Miller PE, Murphy CJ and Schoster JV (1999) Combined cycloablation and gonioimplantation for treatment of glaucoma in dogs: 18 cases (1992–1998). *Journal of the American Veterinary Medical Association* **215**, 1469–1472

Bhattacherjee P, Paterson CA, Spellman JM *et al.* (1999) Pharmacological validation of a feline model of steroid-induced ocular hypertension. *Archives of Ophthalmology* **117**, 361–364

Blocker T and van der Woerdt A (2001) The feline glaucomas (1995–1999). *Veterinary Ophthalmology* **4**, 81–85

Brooks DE (1990) Glaucoma in the dog and cat. *Veterinary Clinics of North America: Small Animal Practice* **20**, 775–797

Brooks DE, Komaromy AM and Kallberg ME (1999) Comparative optic nerve physiology: implications for glaucoma, neuroprotection and neuroregeneration. *Veterinary Ophthalmology* **2**, 13–25

Cook CS (1997) Surgery for glaucoma. *Veterinary Clinics of North America: Small Animal Practice* **27**, 1109–1129

Cook CS, Davidson M, Brinkmann M *et al.* (1997) Diode laser trans-scleral cyclophotocoagulation for the treatment of glaucoma in dogs: results of six and twelve month follow-up. *Veterinary and Comparative Ophthalmology* **7**, 148–154

Cottrell BD and Barnett KC (1988) Primary glaucoma in the Welsh Springer Spaniel. *Journal of Small Animal Practice* **29**, 185–199

Czederpiltz JMC, Croix NCl, van der Woerdt A *et al.* (2005) Putative aqueous humor misdirection syndrome as a cause of glaucoma in cats: 32 cases (1997–2003). *Journal of the American Veterinary Medical Association* **227**, 1434–1441

Deehr AJ and Dubielzig RR (1998) A histopathological study of iridociliary cysts and glaucoma in Golden Retrievers. *Veterinary Ophthalmology* **1**, 153–158

Dietrich UM, Chandler MJ, Cooper T *et al.* (2007) Effects of topical 2% dorzolamide hydrochloride alone and in combination with 0.5% timolol maleate on intraocular pressure in normal feline eyes. *Veterinary Ophthalmology* **10**, 95–100

Dubielzig RR, Everitt J and Shadduck JA (1990) Clinical and morphological features of post-traumatic ocular sarcomas in cats. *Veterinary Pathology* **27**, 62–65

Dubielzig RR, Ketring KL, McLellan GJ *et al.* (2010) The glaucomas. In: *Veterinary Ocular Pathology: A Comparative Review*, pp. 419–448. Saunders Elsevier, Oxford

Ekesten B (1993) Correlation of intraocular distances to the iridocorneal angle in Samoyeds with special reference to angle-closure glaucoma. *Progress in Veterinary and Comparative Ophthalmology* **3**, 67–73

Esson D, Armour M, Mundy P *et al.* (2009) The histopathological and immunohistochemical characteristics of pigmentary and cystic glaucoma in the Golden Retriever. *Veterinary Ophthalmology* **12**, 361–368

Garcia GA, Brooks DE, Gelatt KN *et al.* (1998) Evaluation of valved and non-valved implants in 83 eyes of 65 dogs with glaucoma. *Animal Eye Research* **17**, 9–16

Gelatt KN, Brooks DE and Källberg ME (2007) The canine glaucomas. In: *Veterinary Ophthalmology, 4th edn*, ed. KN Gelatt, pp. 753–811. Blackwell Publishing, Oxford

Gelatt KN, Brooks DE, Miller TR *et al.* (1992). Issues in ophthalmic therapy: the development of anterior chamber shunts for the clinical management of canine glaucomas. *Progress in Veterinary Ophthalmology* **2**, 59–64

Gelatt KN, Gum GG, Samuelson DA *et al.* (1987) Evaluation of the Krupin–Denver valve implant in normotensive and glaucomatous Beagles. *Journal of the American Veterinary Medical Association* **191**, 1404–1409

Gelatt KN, Peiffer RL, Gum GG *et al.* (1977) Evaluation of applanation tonometers for the dog eye. *Investigative Ophthalmology and Visual Science* **16**, 963–968

Gray HE, Willis AM and Morgan RV (2003) Effects of topical administration of 1% brinzolamide on normal cat eyes. *Veterinary Ophthalmology* **6**, 285–290

Gum GG, Larocca RD, Gelatt KN *et al.* (1991) The effect of topical timolol maleate on IOP in normal Beagles and Beagles with inherited glaucoma. *Progress in Veterinary and Comparative Ophthalmology* **1**, 141–149

Hampson ECGM, Smith RIE and Bernays ME (2002) Primary glaucoma in Burmese cats. *Australian Veterinary Journal* **80**, 672–680

Hardman C and Stanley RG (2001) Diode laser trans-scleral cyclophotocoagulation for the treatment of primary glaucoma in 18 dogs: a retrospective study. *Veterinary Ophthalmology* **4**, 209–215

Kallberg ME, Brooks DE, Gelatt KN *et al.* (2007) Endothelin-1, nitric oxide and glutamate in the normal and glaucomatous dog eye. *Veterinary Ophthalmology* **10**, 46–52

Klein HE, Krohne SG, Moore GE *et al.* (2011) Effect of eyelid manipulation and manual jugular compression on intraocular pressure measurement in dogs. *Journal of the American Veterinary Medical Association* **238**, 1292–1295

Kuchtey J, Olson LM, Rinkoski T *et al.* (2011) Mapping of the disease locus and identification of *ADAMTS10* as a candidate gene in a canine model of primary open angle glaucoma. *PLoS Genetics* **7**(2), e1001306

Lazarus JA, Pickett JP and Champagne ES (1998) Primary lens luxation in the Chinese Shar Pei: clinical and hereditary characteristics. *Veterinary Ophthalmology* **1**, 101–107

McLellan GJ, Kemmerling JP and Kiland JA (2012) Validation of the TonoVet® rebound tonometer in normal and glaucomatous cats. *Veterinary Ophthalmology* **16**(2), 111–118

McLellan GJ and Miller PE (2011) Feline glaucoma – a comprehensive review. *Veterinary Ophthalmology* **14**(Suppl. 1), 15–29

Martin CL (1975) Scanning electron microscopic examination of selected canine iridocorneal angle abnormalities. *Journal of the American Animal Hospital Association* **11**, 300–306

Miller P, Schmidt G, Vainisi S *et al.* (2000) The efficacy of topical prophylactic anti-glaucoma therapy in primary closed angle glaucoma in dogs: a multicenter clinical trial. *Journal of the American Animal Hospital Association* **36**, 431–438

Moller I, Cook CS, Peiffer RL *et al.* (1986) Indications for and complications of pharmacological ablation of the ciliary body for the treatment of chronic glaucoma in the dog. *Journal of the American Veterinary Medical Association* **22**, 319–326

Olivero DK, Riis RC, Dutton AG *et al.* (1991) Feline lens displacement: a retrospective analysis of 345 cases. *Progress in Veterinary and Comparative Ophthalmology* **1**, 239–244

Park Y, Jeong M, Kim T *et al.* (2011) Effect of central corneal thickness on intraocular pressure with the rebound tonometer and the applanation tonometer in normal dogs. *Veterinary Ophthalmology* **14**, 169–173

Peiffer RL, Wilcock BP and Yin H (1990) The pathogenesis and significance of pre-iridal fibrovascular membrane in domestic animals. *Veterinary Pathology* **27**, 41–45

Petersen-Jones SM, Forcier J and Mentzer AL (2007) Ocular

melanosis in the Cairn Terrier: clinical description and investigation of mode of inheritance. *Veterinary Ophthalmology* **10**, 63–69

Petersen-Jones SM, Mentzer AL, Dubielzig RR *et al.* (2008) Ocular melanosis in the Cairn Terrier: histopathological description of the condition, and immunohistological and ultrastructural characterization of the characteristic pigment laden cells. *Veterinary Ophthalmology* **11**, 260–268

Rainbow ME and Dziezyc J (2003) Effects of twice daily application of 2% dorzolamide on intraocular pressure in normal cats. *Veterinary Ophthalmology* **6**, 147–150

Read RA, Wood JLN and Lakhani KH (1998) Pectinate ligament dysplasia in Flat Coated Retrievers. I. Objectives, techniques and results of a PLD survey. *Veterinary Ophthalmology* **1**, 85–90

Regnier A (1999) Ocular pharmacology and therapeutics. Part 2. Antimicrobial, anti-inflammatory agents and anti-glaucoma drugs. In: *Veterinary Ophthalmology, 3rd edn*, ed. KN Gelatt, p. 336. Lippincott, Williams & Wilkins, Philadelphia

Ridgway MD and Brightman AH (1989) Feline glaucoma: a retrospective study of 29 clinical cases. *Journal of the American Animal Hospital Association* **25**, 485–490

Rusanen E, Florin M, Hassig M *et al.* (2010) Evaluation of a rebound tonometer (Tonovet) in clinically normal cat eyes. *Veterinary Ophthalmology* **13**, 31–36

Sapienza JS, Simo FJ and Prades-Sapienza A (2000) Golden Retriever uveitis: 75 cases (1994–1999). *Veterinary Ophthalmology* **3**, 241–246

Sapienza JS and van der Woerdt A (2005) Combined trans-scleral diode laser cyclophotocoagulation and Ahmed gonioimplantation in dogs with primary glaucoma: 51 cases (1996–2004). *Veterinary Ophthalmology* **8**, 121–127

Sigle KJ, Camaño-Garcia G, Carriquiry AL *et al.* (2011) The effect of dorzolamide 2% on circadian intraocular pressure in cats with primary congenital glaucoma. *Veterinary Ophthalmology* **14**(Suppl. 1), 48–53

Spiess BM, Bolliger JO, Guscetti F *et al.* (1998) Multiple ciliary body cysts and secondary glaucoma in the Great Dane: a report of nine cases. *Veterinary Ophthalmology* **1**, 41–45

Studer ME, Martin CL and Stiles J (2000) Effects of 0.005% latanoprost solution on intraocular pressure in healthy dogs and cats. *American Journal of Veterinary Research* **61**, 1220–1224

Trost K, Peiffer RL and Nell B (2007) Goniodysgenesis associated with primary glaucoma in an adult European Shorthaired cat. *Veterinary Ophthalmology* **10**, 3–7

Wilcock B, Peiffer RL and Davidson MG (1990) The causes of glaucoma in cats. *Veterinary Pathology* **27**, 35–40

Wilkie DA and Latimer CA (1991) Effects of topical administration of timolol maleate on intraocular pressure and pupil size in cats. *American Journal of Veterinary Research* **52**, 436–440

Zhan GL, Miranda OC and Bito LZ (1992) Steroid glaucoma: corticosteroid-induced ocular hypertension in cats. *Experimental Eye Research* **54**, 211–218

16

The lens

Robert Lowe

Embryology, anatomy and physiology

The lens is formed as a result of the development of the optic vesicle as the prosencephalon makes contact with and induces a thickening in the surface ectoderm. The surface ectoderm develops into the lens placode, which then invaginates. This invaginated ectoderm separates from the surface ectoderm to form the lens vesicle, which comprises a hollow monolayer of cells. The posterior cells of the lens vesicle elongate to form the primary lens fibres, whilst the anterior cells remain as the anterior lens epithelium (Figure 16.1). The anterior epithelial cells form secondary lens fibres throughout the lifetime of the animal. They divide at the lens equator and extend anteriorly and posteriorly to form the lens cortex.

Blood supply

The developing lens is supplied by the tunica vasculosa lentis, from the hyaloid artery posteriorly and from the pupillary membrane anteriorly. This vascular tunic regresses by 14 days postpartum in the dog. However, incomplete regression can be seen in the form of a persistent pupillary membrane (PPM), persistent hyaloid artery, persistent tunica vasculosa lentis or persistent hyperplastic tunica vasculosa lentis/persistent hyperplastic primary vitreous (see Chapter 17).

Structure of the adult lens

The lens is supported in the eye by the attachment of zonules, which originate from the ciliary body and insert in a criss-cross pattern on the lens capsule, anterior and posterior to the equator (Figure 16.2). It receives further support from its attachment to the anterior vitreous through the hyaloideocapsular ligament (see Chapter 17). Anteriorly, the lens provides support to the iris, which takes on its convex contour as it crosses the lens surface. The lens has excellent transparency due to the parallel orientation of adjacent fibres, minimal nuclei and interdigitation of the cell membranes with each other. The fibres are

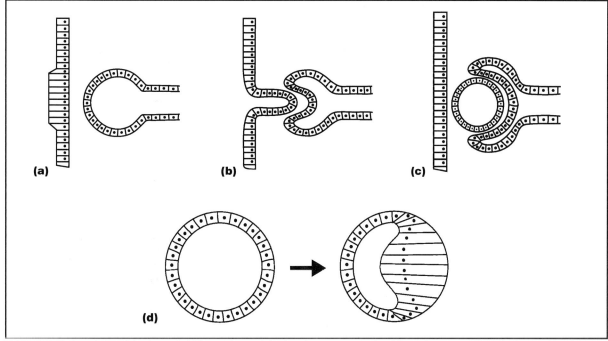

16.1 Embryology of the lens. **(a)** The optic vesicle develops as an outbudding of neurectoderm in the region of the developing forebrain. It induces a thickening of the overlying surface ectoderm to form the lens placode. **(b)** As the optic vesicle invaginates to form the optic cup, the lens placode invaginates from the surface ectoderm. **(c)** The lens vesicle consists of a hollow sphere with a single layer of cells. **(d)** The posterior cells of the lens vesicle elongate to form primary lens fibres, which obliterate the cavity forming the lens vesicle.

elongated, oriented in an anterior-to-posterior direction, and contain high levels of soluble protein (crystallins). They meet at their anterior and posterior poles along the suture lines. In the dog and cat, the suture lines form a Y shape anteriorly and an inverted Y shape posteriorly (Figure 16.3).

The lens is contained within the lens capsule, a basement membrane derived from the anterior and posterior epithelial cells. This acellular structure is transparent and allows diffusion of nutrients and waste across it, but is impervious to cellular migration. The lens capsule is of variable thickness, being at its thickest anteriorly (20 µm at birth), reducing to 8–12 µm at the equator and only 2–4 µm posteriorly.

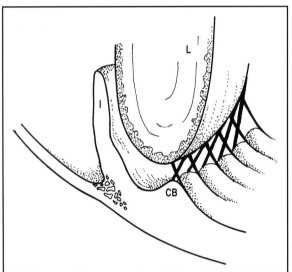

16.2 Zonular attachments to the lens. Note that zonular fibres arising from the peaks of the ciliary processes insert posterior to the lens equator, whilst those arising from the valleys between the processes insert anterior to the lens equator. CB = Ciliary body; I = Iris; L = Lens.

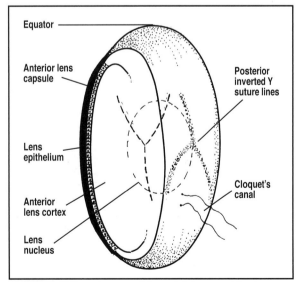

16.3 Different areas of the adult lens and the lens sutures. The anterior lens suture lines form a Y shape, whilst the posterior suture lines form an inverted Y shape. Cloquet's canal can often be seen as an optically clear space within the vitreous arising from the posterior lens surface.

The thickness of the anterior capsule increases throughout life by 5–8 µm/year (Bernays *et al.*, 2000). In contrast, because posterior lens epithelial cells are only present during early lens development, the posterior lens capsule does not thicken with age.

The lens has a high refractive index and as the ciliary muscles contract and relax (decreasing and increasing tension on the zonules, respectively) there is some limited change in lens curvature, which alters its focal length to allow objects at different distances to focus on the retina. This process is known as accommodation.

Physiology

As the mature lens lacks a blood supply, the supply of nutrients and oxygen to and waste removal from the adult lens are performed by the aqueous humour and to a lesser extent by the vitreous humour. Any disruption to normal aqueous or vitreous humour constituents and physiology may induce a change in the health of the lens epithelial cells. Any change in lens hydration, protein levels and structure, cell membrane permeability or cell metabolism can lead to precipitation of crystallins or disruption of the lens fibres in relation to one another. This leads to opacification within the lens and cataract formation. As the lens fibres are effectively lacking a nucleus and cellular organelles they have limited capacity for repair. There are protective mechanisms to counter this, such as high levels of antioxidants and ultraviolet (UV) filtering, but any damage is likely to be irreversible once it has led to cataract formation.

Investigation of disease

The normal lens is an optically transparent biconvex spheroid located deep to the iris and fixed in position by the lens zonules and the ligamentous attachment to the anterior vitreal face. Examination of the lens should assess primarily the position of the lens and its optical clarity. In an optically clear lens, it is only possible to identify the fluid–solid interface at the anterior and posterior capsules when magnification is used. Examination of the lens should be performed prior to and following pupil dilation (Figure 16.4; see also Chapter 1) and the clinician should remember to check the pupillary light reflex (PLR)

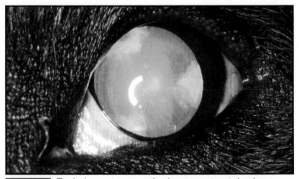

16.4 Early immature cortical cataracts at the lens equator with some minor cataract at the posterior suture lines. The majority of cataractous change in this lens would not be visible without pupil dilation.

prior to this. Dilation is normally achieved within 30 minutes of application of 1% tropicamide, but pharmacological dilation is generally contraindicated in eyes with suspected or confirmed glaucoma and in cases of suspected lens instability. In these cases, reliance on normal mydriasis during dim light examination by distant direct ophthalmoscopy may be preferable.

Distant direct ophthalmoscopy

Assessment of optical clarity is easily performed with distant direct ophthalmoscopy. By obtaining a tapetal reflection from the back of the eye, it is possible to identify any opacities within the visual axis that block the reflection of light back to the observer. Opacities appear as dark shadows against the background of tapetal reflection. Further localization of these opacities can be achieved using the technique of parallax (Figure 16.5). Observation of the opacity from directly in front of the animal locates the opacity at its position relative to the optical axis. As the observer moves to their right, whilst maintaining the tapetal reflection from the back of the eye, any opacities that are anterior to the centre of the lens appear to move to the left; whereas, opacities that are posterior to the centre of the lens appear to move to the right. The converse is true if the eye moves and the observer remains stationary. Opacities located at the centre of the lens (nucleus) appear stationary as the observer or eye moves. This technique allows ready identification and differentiation between any opacities that are either anterior or posterior to the centre of the lens. However, it does not necessarily mean that the opacities lie within the lens itself, because those opacities that appear to 'move' could be within the cornea, anterior chamber or vitreous. Distant direct ophthalmoscopy is described in more detail in Chapter 1.

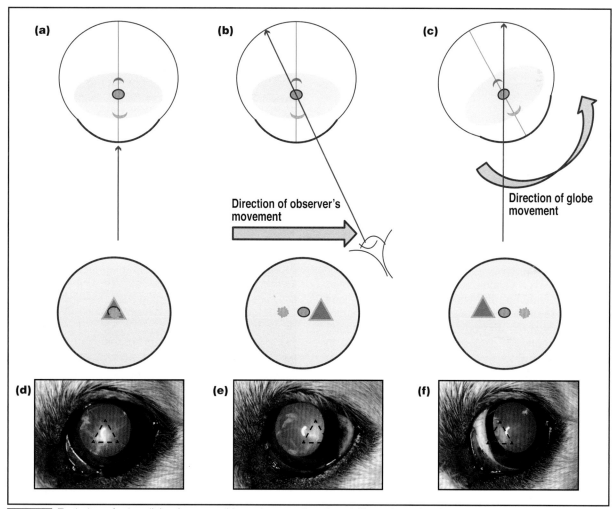

16.5 Technique for localizing lens opacities using parallax. **(a–c)** Illustrations showing three axial opacities at different levels in the lens that are (a) superimposed when viewed by an observer in front of the patient along the visual axis (blue line). (b) If the patient's eye remains stationary in a forward gaze and the observer moves to the side, opacities posterior to the lens nucleus will appear to move in the same direction as the observer, nuclear opacities will remain stationary and anterior opacities will appear to move in the opposite direction to the observer. (c) If the observer remains stationary and the patient shifts its gaze to the side, posterior opacities will appear to move in the opposite direction to the eye movement and anterior opacities will appear to move in the same direction. **(d–f)** This phenomenon is illustrated by the position of the dense white posterior lens opacity, which in (d) is seen at the centre of the visual axis, in (e) appears to move to the right as the observer moves to the right, and in (f) appears to move to the left when the animal directs its gaze to the right whilst the observer remains stationary. Other equatorial opacities in this patient are also located within the posterior lens in this patient. (a–c courtesy of G McLellan)

Direct ophthalmoscopy

A direct ophthalmoscope can be used to examine the lens with more magnification than the naked eye using the lenses available within the ophthalmoscope head. After adjusting for the observer's vision (refractive error), a setting of about +12 dioptres (D) provides a focal depth equivalent to the anterior lens capsule and a setting of +8 D provides a focal depth equivalent to the posterior lens capsule. Direct ophthalmoscopy is described in more detail in Chapter 1.

Slit-lamp biomicroscopy

The slit-lamp biomicroscope allows the observer to see a magnified binocular image of the lens. The use of the obliquely directed slit beam allows identification of the location of lesions with more accuracy than any other technique available to the veterinary ophthalmologist, as well as allowing assessment of the position of the lens within the eye. Slit-lamp biomicroscopy is described in more detail in Chapter 1.

Retinoscopy

Retinoscopy allows assessment of any refractive error and is discussed in detail in Chapter 1.

Ultrasonography

Ultrasonography is particularly useful where there is opacification or any abnormality of structures anterior to the lens, or opacification of the lens itself. The normal lens within a normal eye is difficult to identify with ultrasonography; only the central anterior and posterior capsules are readily apparent as hyperechoic lines because these acoustic interfaces lie perpendicular to the ultrasound beam. Abnormalities of the lens that can be identified include cataracts, lens capsule rupture, lens subluxation or luxation, persistent tunica vasculosa lentis or persistent hyaloid artery (although the latter may be more or less apparent depending on the imaging plane), lentiglobus or lenticonus, and posterior synechiae. Ocular ultrasonography is discussed in greater detail in Chapter 2.

Canine conditions

Congenital abnormalities

Persistent pupillary membranes and other mesenchymal remnants

In some cases of PPM, the membrane remains attached to the lens capsule, leading to focal opacification of the capsule and occasionally the subcapsular region. As the membrane is attached to the iris at the iris collarette, rather than at the pupil margin, it can be differentiated from posterior synechiae (Figure 16.6). Another type of mesenchymal remnant can be seen in the form of pigment spots on the central anterior lens capsule (Figure 16.7). English Cocker Spaniels are over-represented for this pathology, but it is not associated with cataract

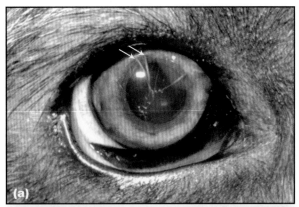

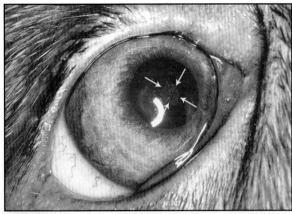

16.6 **(a)** Remnants of a persistent pupillary membrane (PPM) in a dog. Note how the strands arise from the iris collarette (mid-portion of the iris; arrowed). In this case, they insert on to the anterior lens capsule. **(b)** Posterior synechiae (adhesions from the posterior aspect of the iris to the anterior lens capsule; arrowed) and iris rests (pigment deposited on the anterior lens capsule from the posterior iris; arrowheads) secondary to penetrating corneal trauma in a dog. (Courtesy of D Gould)

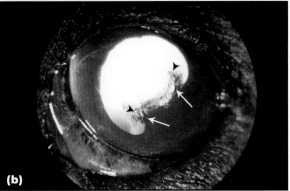

16.7 A 2-year-old Hungarian Vizla with mesenchymal remnants on the anterior lens capsule (arrowed). Compare the lighter colour and axial location with the appearance of the iris rests in Figure 16.6.

formation. The pigment spots can appear similar to iris rests (see Figure 16.6b), which are deposits on the lens capsule resulting from prior adhesion of the darkly pigmented posterior surface of an inflamed iris, but are generally lighter brown than iris rests, quite flat in profile and usually axial. One or both eyes can be affected. These abnormalities are described in greater detail in Chapter 14.

Cataracts

Congenital cataract is an autosomal recessive, inherited condition in the Miniature Schnauzer (see Chapter 4). These cataracts are bilateral, usually symmetrical and primarily involve the lens nucleus (Figure 16.8), although, on occasion they may extend into the lens cortex. These cataracts may also be associated with posterior lenticonus or microphakia. Other forms of congenital, but non-inherited, cataract are recognized sporadically and thought to result from presumed *in utero* insults (Figures 16.9 and 16.10).

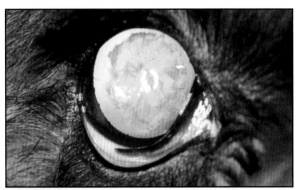

16.8 Nuclear cataract in a Miniature Schnauzer. (Courtesy of D Gould)

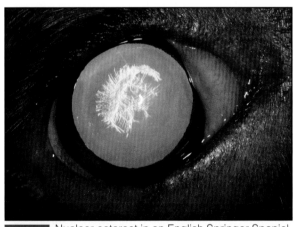

16.9 Nuclear cataract in an English Springer Spaniel with a feather-like appearance, which is unlikely to be progressive because of its nuclear position.

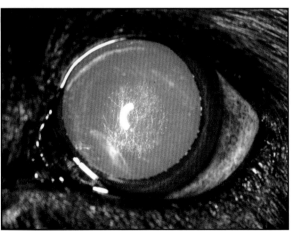

16.10 Pulverulent nuclear cataract in a 4-year-old Cocker Spaniel.

Congenital cataracts may also be associated with other ocular abnormalities such as PPM, persistent hyperplastic primary vitreous/persistent hyperplastic tunica vasculosa lentis (PHPV/PHTVL), retinal dysplasia, microphthalmos and an oscillating to rotatory type of nystagmus. These abnormalities may all be included in the suspected hereditary complex of multiple ocular defects (MOD). Breeds including the Cavalier King Charles Spaniel, English Cocker Spaniel, Golden Retriever, Old English Sheepdog and West Highland White Terrier may be affected by congenital cataract as part of the MOD complex.

Persistent hyperplastic primary vitreous/ persistent hyperplastic tunica vasculosa lentis

The vascular tunic that provides support to the developing lens should regress completely, but occasionally may undergo hyperplasia before incomplete regression to leave a variety of lesions. The main presenting sign is a posterior capsular fibrovascular opacity (Figure 16.11). There may also be other lens changes such as lentiglobus or a more extensive cataract. Occasionally, the lens may haemorrhage internally (intralenticular haemorrhage). This condition has been described as inherited in the Dobermann, Miniature Schnauzer and Staffordshire Bull Terrier but can also be seen in other breeds (see Chapter 17 for further details).

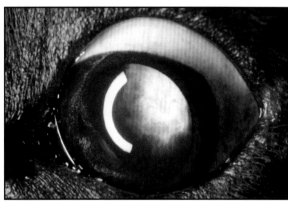

16.11 PHPV/PHTVL in a 2-year-old Cocker Spaniel. As the lesion was imaged from a lateral position, the posterior lens capsule opacity appears lateral rather than central. The presence of a vascular network indicates that this is more than a simple cataract.

Aphakia and microphakia

True absence of a lens (aphakia) is extremely rare because even the most malformed eyes often have some lens tissue present. An abnormally small lens (microphakia) may be seen as a feature of multiple congenital ocular abnormalities or as part of the PHPV/PHTVL disease complex (see Chapter 17). It may be associated with cataract formation but the lens may also be otherwise normal in appearance. The lens appears small within the pupil and may appear to have an aphakic crescent, similar to that seen with lens subluxation. However, there is little or no evidence of lens instability and the zonules appear to be normal in number but stretched to cover the extra distance between the lens and the ciliary body (Figure 16.12).

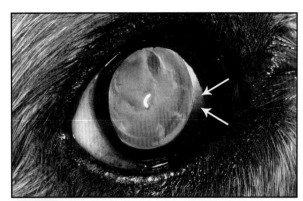

16.12 Microphakia and immature cataract in a 9-year-old Cavalier King Charles Spaniel. Note the presence of the stretched zonules medially (arrowed).

Spherophakia and coloboma

Spherophakia is defined as a developmental defect in which a smaller, more spherical lens develops, with partial or complete aplasia of the zonules. Lens coloboma is not a true coloboma, but rather is more accurately described as a focal absence or reduction of zonules, leading to poor lens growth adjacent to the zonule deficiency. The lens often demonstrates a flattened sector at its equator, rather than the normal curvature, at the site of the zonular deficiency (Figure 16.13).

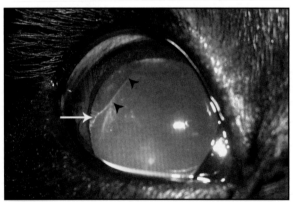

16.13 Lens/zonule coloboma. Deficit in the lens with a flat edge to the lens equator and a lack of zonules (arrowheads). Some stretched zonules (arrowed) can be seen laterally. (Courtesy of K Wendlandt)

Peters anomaly and anterior segment dysgenesis

An incomplete separation of the lens placode from the surface ectoderm may leave the lens confluent with the cornea. The cornea and lens are usually opacified at this location. These conditions are extremely rare (Swanson *et al.*, 2001) and are described in greater detail in Chapter 14.

Acquired abnormalities

Cataracts

The term 'cataract' describes any opacity of the lens or its capsule. Cataracts are commonly classified according to four criteria:

- Age of onset
- Aetiology
- Extent
- Position.

Age of onset: Cataracts can be described as congenital, juvenile or senile. There is no clearly defined or established distinction between juvenile- and adult-onset or senile cataracts, but a senile cataract is considered to be one seen first in middle-aged or old animals.

Aetiology: Acquired cataracts can be primary, such as hereditary or senile cataracts, or secondary to metabolic or nutritional diseases, external trauma, other intraocular diseases, electrocution or radiation.

Hereditary cataracts: The clinical features and morphological changes seen with hereditary cataracts vary across and within breeds. Figure 16.14 details the breeds affected, changes seen and modes of inheritance. A mutation in the gene encoding heat shock factor 4 (*HSF4*) causes early onset and progressive cataract in the Boston Terrier, French Bulldog and Staffordshire Bull Terrier. It is inherited as an autosomal recessive disease (Mellersh *et al.*, 2006). It should be noted that the Boston Terrier suffers from a second form of hereditary cataract as well. A base pair deletion in the *HSF4* gene is associated with a different hereditary cataract in the Australian Shepherd that is reported to be dominant

Breed	Age range	Location	Inheritance
Alaskan Malamute	6 months to 8+ years	Posterior polar subcapsular	Unknown
American Cocker Spaniel	2 months to 6+ years	Extremely variable	Probably autosomal recessive
Australian Shepherd	Variable	Posterior cortical and subcapsular	Probably dominant; *HSF4* gene
Belgian Shepherd Dog (all varieties)	6 months to 8+ years	Triangular or propeller-shaped posterior polar subcapsular with occasional progression to extensive and generalized cortical cataract	Unknown
Boston Terrier (early-onset)	8–12 weeks	Prominent suture lines, nuclear	Recessive; *HSF4* gene
Boston Terrier (late-onset)	4–8 years	Spokes or wedges from the equator towards the centre; usually anterior subcapsular	Unknown

16.14 Breeds known to be affected by hereditary cataract according to Schedule A of the BVA/KC/ISDS Eye Scheme. (continues) ▶

Breed	Age range	Location	Inheritance
Cavalier King Charles Spaniel	Thought to be 2 years	Progresses to become total	Possibly autosomal recessive
Chesapeake Bay Retriever	6 months to 8+ years	As for Belgian Shepherd Dog	Unknown
German Shepherd Dog	8 weeks to 4 months	Posterior suture line cataract	Autosomal recessive
Giant Schnauzer	6 months to 8+ years	As for Belgian Shepherd Dog	Unknown
Golden Retriever	6 months to 8+ years	As for Belgian Shepherd Dog	Unknown
Irish Red and White Setter	6 months to 8+ years	As for Belgian Shepherd Dog	Unknown
Labrador Retriever	6 months to 8+ years	As for Belgian Shepherd Dog	Unknown
Large Munsterlander	Thought to be 2 years	As for Belgian Shepherd Dog	Unknown
Leonberger	6 months to 8+ years	As for Belgian Shepherd Dog	Unknown
Miniature Schnauzer (congenital hereditary)	Congenital	Nuclear; may be associated with posterior lenticonus and microphthalmos	Recessive
Miniature Schnauzer (hereditary)	Thought to be 6 months to up to 2 years	Posterior cortex progressing to total	Recessive
Norwegian Buhund	Thought to be 3 months to 2 years	Large posterior polar	Unknown
Old English Sheepdog	7 months to 2 years	Cortical; may progress to total	Unknown
Siberian Husky	6 months to 8+ years	As for Belgian Shepherd Dog. Progression of disease is more likely in the Husky	Unknown
Staffordshire Bull Terrier	<18 months	Posterior suture lines with faint nuclear progressing to total	Recessive; *HSF4* gene
Standard Poodle	10 weeks to 3 years	Equatorial first, then posterior and anterior cortex	Unknown
Welsh Springer Spaniel	2–4 months	Peripheral posterior cortical vacuoles progressing to total	Unknown

16.14 (continued) Breeds known to be affected by hereditary cataract according to Schedule A of the BVA/KC/ISDS Eye Scheme.

with incomplete penetrance (Mellersh *et al.*, 2009). Another form of inherited cataract that is very commonly encountered in working breeds, including the Belgian Shepherd Dog, Golden Retriever and Labrador Retriever, is a characteristic posterior polar subcapsular cataract seen at the confluence of the suture lines (see Figure 16.20). This form of cataract seldom progresses to the extent of having a significant effect on vision; although, progression is more common in the Siberian Husky than in many other affected breeds. The underlying molecular genetic cause(s) of this type of cataract has not been established.

Senile cataracts: The age of onset of senile cataract is not well defined but senile cataracts show some typical changes. There is opacification of the nucleus, in addition to nuclear sclerosis and/or wedge-shaped or diffuse cortical cataract formation in the early stages (Figure 16.15). These cataracts are slowly progressive and as a result vision loss is usually only detectable months to years after onset. In a UK study, dogs aged 9.4 years old had a 50% chance of having some form of cataract; this increased to 100% at 13.5 years old (Williams *et al.*, 2004).

Metabolic cataracts: The overwhelming majority of metabolic cataracts in dogs are associated with diabetes mellitus. The main pathway for glucose

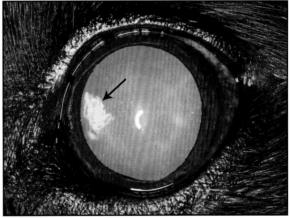

16.15 Incipient senile cortical cataract nasally (arrowed) with early nuclear sclerosis in an 8-year-old Miniature Poodle.

metabolism in the lens involves anaerobic glycolysis, and the rate of glycolysis is dependent on the enzyme hexokinase. Once glucose levels become too high relative to levels of hexokinase, an alternative pathway of glucose metabolism is invoked, catalysed by the enzyme aldose reductase. As glucose is metabolized by the aldose reductase pathway it produces sorbitol. This increases the osmotic potential of the lens, attracting water into the lens and causing coagulation of lens proteins. Typically, lenses of diabetic patients develop water clefts due to the increase in lens volume (intumescence) that occurs as fluid enters across the lens capsule. The clefting tends to occur along the suture lines because these are the weakest points of the lens structure (Figure 16.16). The use of a topical aldose reductase inhibitor has been shown to reduce or delay the onset of cataract formation in diabetic patients. However, once the cataract has formed it cannot be reduced medically (Kador *et al.*, 2010). Metabolic cataracts can also occur in dogs with hypocalcaemia (see Chapter 20).

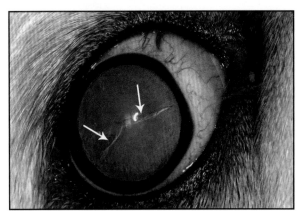

16.16 Early water clefting (arrowed) of an immature diabetic cataract in a 4-year-old crossbred dog.

Nutritional cataracts: Perinuclear cataract has been reported in puppies fed on certain types of milk replacement diet (Martin and Chambreau, 1982). These cataracts may be partially reversible. It has also been reported that diets deficient in proteins or vitamins can lead to cataract formation.

Traumatic cataracts: Trauma may occur in the form of blunt or sharp injury to the lens. Blunt or compressive trauma to the eye may induce cataract formation as a result of vibration injury to the lens material or lens instability due to damage to the lens zonules. In the most severe cases of compressive injury the eye may rupture, leading to expulsion of the entire lens. The most common causes of sharp or penetrating injury are thorns, claws and teeth. Penetrating injuries to the globe as a result of bite wounds tend to have a compressive component as well, so any injury that occurs to the lens is usually associated with more severe eye- and vision-threatening injury. Thorns and claws may cause what appear to be minor external injuries to the outer structures of the eye but have a devastating impact on the lens. All animals presenting with corneal injuries should have the lens assessed as part of the examination in case the lens capsule has been compromised. Even the smallest corneal wound can have more sinister internal ocular injuries. Pupil dilation is essential in these cases because the insult may have occurred to the periphery of the lens, even with a central corneal injury (Figure 16.17).

Penetrating corneal injury may cause penetrating or non-penetrating injury to the lens. Even if the lens capsule remains intact there may be a focal or complete cataract due to disruption of the lens

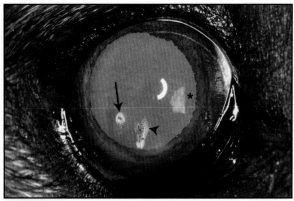

16.17 Corneal and lens penetration, which occurred 2 hours previously, in the right eye of a 6-year-old German Shepherd Dog. Note the corneal penetration temporally (arrowed), the lens laceration and iris rests inferiorly (arrowhead) and the free-floating clump of fibrin nasally (∗). The aqueous humour has cellular debris throughout.

epithelial cells deep to the capsule. More serious disease occurs when the lens capsule has been breached. If the capsule has been breached it is necessary to decide whether the lens needs to be removed completely, or whether the capsule will reseal and prevent any protein leakage. Usually the lens capsule tears significantly beyond the area originally damaged, making it unlikely that the capsule will reseal. The rupture allows or forces lens material outside the capsular bag. This can induce a very aggressive phacoclastic uveitis, probably due to a lack of immune tolerance to this large amount of liberated lens protein, or as a result of bacterial contamination (see also Chapter 14).

Early phacoemulsification surgery to remove the lens contents, performed in a similar fashion to cataract surgery (see later), is thought to offer a much better success rate than medical management alone and early referral of patients with suspected lens rupture is strongly advised. This type of surgery is technically more demanding than cataract surgery, owing to the presence of the corneal injury reducing visualization of the lens and a compromised lens capsule increasing the risk of the nucleus being lost into the vitreous, as well as precluding placement of a replacement intraocular lens in some cases. If it is decided to manage the rupture medically, then aggressive therapy with systemic and topical anti-inflammatory drugs needs to be instigated in addition to appropriate topical and systemic medical management of the corneal injury and intraocular bacterial contamination, respectively (see Chapters 12 and 14).

Cataracts secondary to other intraocular diseases: Any disease which changes the delicate physiological balance of nutrients in the eye, releases toxic metabolites or increases inflammatory mediators may lead to cataract development. Cataract is commonly associated with generalized progressive retinal atrophy (PRA; Figure 16.18), glaucoma, lens luxation and uveitis (Figure 16.19), although the exact mechanisms are poorly described.

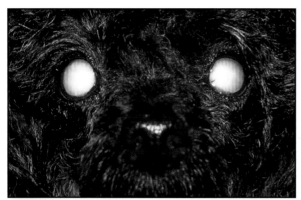

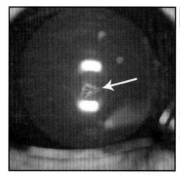

16.20 Typical appearance of an inherited posterior polar subcapsular cataract (arrowed) at the confluence of the posterior suture lines in a 4-year-old Labrador Retriever. (Courtesy of G McLellan)

16.18 Mature cataracts secondary to generalized PRA in a Miniature Poodle. The PLRs were sluggish and the pupils were dilated, implying underlying retinal disease (cataracts in the absence of concurrent intraocular disease should be associated with normal pupil size and PLRs). (Courtesy of D Gould)

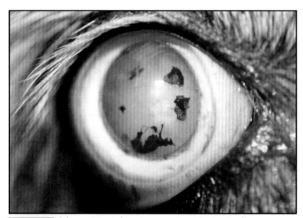

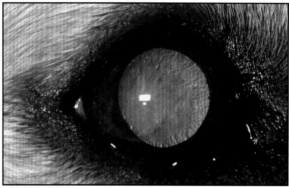

16.21 Immature (incomplete) cataract in a Labrador Retriever. The cataract involves the majority of the lens but a tapetal reflex is still present. (Courtesy of D Gould)

16.19 Iris rests and mature cataract secondary to prior uveitis in a Bearded Collie. The iris rests are distributed in a circular pattern, indicating previous miosis and pigment deposition. The eye also has secondary glaucoma.

dilated. This group can be further subdivided into early or late immature cataract, depending on the degree of opacity noted.

Mature (complete) cataracts: At this stage the visual axis is opaque with loss of the tapetal reflex and menace response (Figure 16.22). The lens may not be cataractous throughout its entire volume, but there is complete opacification of the lens apparent when viewed along the visual axis. The eye still retains a normal dazzle reflex and PLR, assuming that there are no other abnormalities, as the passage of light to the fundus is disrupted but not blocked.

Electrocution and radiation: These are relatively rare causes of cataract formation. Radiation may induce cataract formation in dogs undergoing radiation therapy where the eye is within or close to the treatment field.

Extent:

Incipient cataracts: An incipient cataract is defined as one involving <15% of the lens volume (see Figures 16.15 and 16.20). As a consequence they are rarely associated with any visual disturbance. Lens vacuoles may be seen and, although vacuoles are often cited as an indicator of cataract progression, they may persist for many years with no discernable change in lens opacity.

Immature (incomplete) cataracts: This term covers a range of cataracts from those just over 15% of the volume of the lens to almost complete cataract, but where the lens still has some transparency (Figure 16.21). The tapetal reflex can still be seen when examined by distant direct ophthalmoscopy. In less advanced cases, the fundus can still be examined using indirect ophthalmoscopy when the pupil is

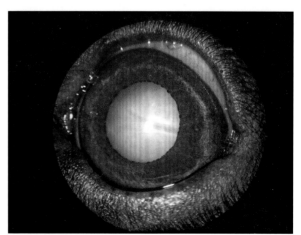

16.22 Mature (complete) cataract in a Springer Spaniel. The tapetal reflex is absent. Note the relatively normal iris surface architecture and colour, implying minimal lens-induced uveitis (compare with Figure 16.23). (Courtesy of D Gould)

Hypermature cataracts: As the mature cataract starts to liquefy and resorb, various changes occur. The lens may reduce in volume, develop clefts along the suture lines, leak lens protein through the lens capsule, develop dense white refractile plaques that adhere to the inner aspect of the lens capsule and start to develop wrinkling of the lens capsule. There may be a restoration of the tapetal reflex, which can make differentiation between immature and early hypermature cataracts difficult. In some dogs, the lens resorption may be sufficient to lead to a restoration of vision as the visual axis clears. However, this phenomenon seldom occurs in the absence of vision-threatening secondary problems such as uveitis, glaucoma or retinal detachment, so relying on this process to restore vision should not be recommended as a routine management option in patients that may be suitable candidates for cataract surgery.

Lens-induced uveitis

The leakage of lens protein associated with cataract progression and resorption may stimulate a phacolytic, lens-induced uveitis (van der Woerdt, 2000). Associated changes include mild episcleral hyperaemia, hyperpigmentation of the iris (Figure 16.23), reduced intraocular pressure (IOP) and iris rest formation. If left untreated, this may lead to more significant uveitis and associated problems such as glaucoma. There is also the risk of lens capsule rupture secondary to swelling of the lens (intumescence), which is often seen with rapid-onset cataract formation (e.g. in diabetes mellitus) (Wilkie *et al.*, 2006). Rapid-onset cataract formation without lens capsule rupture may also present in a similar fashion, with chronic or more acute uveitis developing. The reader is referred to Chapter 14 for further information on lens-induced uveitis and its treatment.

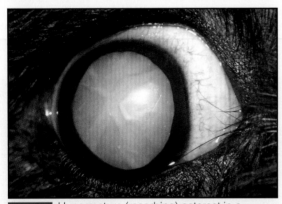

16.23 Hypermature (resorbing) cataract in a 4-year-old Tibetan Terrier. There is hyperpigmentation of the iris, indicating a lens-induced uveitis and some early fibrosis and wrinkling of the lens capsule.

Morgagnian cataracts: In this subset of hypermature cataract, there is significant resorption of lens material but a dense nuclear cataract remains which eventually falls into the inferior portion of the capsular bag (Figure 16.24).

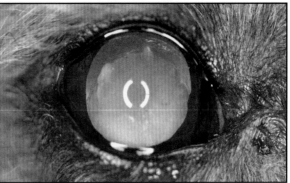

16.24 Morgagnian cataract in a Shih Tzu. In this case, resorption of the liquefied cortex of a hypermature cataract has led to partial clearing of the peripheral visual axis, but a dense nuclear cataract persists. The uveitis associated with the lens resorption has contributed to partial retinal detachment in this eye. (Courtesy of D Gould)

Position: Within the three-dimensional structure of the lens, it is possible to classify an incipient or immature cataract based on its position or positions, as determined by distant direct ophthalmoscopy with the use of parallax (see Figure 16.5) and/or slit-lamp biomicroscopy (see Chapter 1). The cataract can be identified by the layer or layers it affects within the lens (e.g. capsular, subcapsular, cortical or nuclear) (see Figures 16.3 and 16.25). The position of the cataract along the lens axis can also be specified (e.g. anterior cortical or posterior cortical), along with its location relative to the visual axis (e.g. axial, paraxial or equatorial). In addition, any association with other lens features, such as suture lines, can be used. An example of this would be the typical hereditary cataract in Labrador and Golden Retrievers, which is described in terms of its location as posterior polar subcapsular at the confluence of the suture lines (see Figure 16.20).

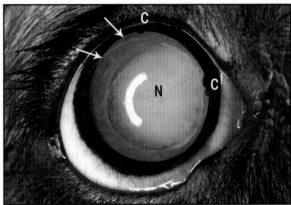

16.25 Dense nuclear cataract (N) with small areas of equatorial cortical cataract formation (arrowed) in a Labrador Retriever. Small iris cysts at the pupil margin (C) were an incidental finding.

Nuclear sclerosis

Nuclear sclerosis arises with age as the continual production of lens epithelial cells leads to compression of the lens nucleus. It takes on a change in refractive index, compared with the newer cortex, which makes the nucleus appear blue/grey when viewed with the naked eye (Figure 16.26). It is often mistaken by owners for cataract but can be easily differentiated using distant direct ophthalmoscopy to verify an absence of true lens opacity. In some cases, the nuclear sclerosis can become so severe that vision may be affected.

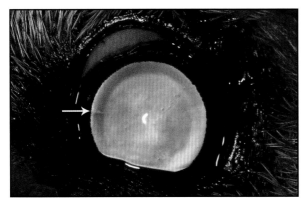

16.26 Nuclear sclerosis with a senile equatorial cortical cataract (arrowed) in a 12-year-old Chow Chow. The tapetal reflection is still visible through the lens nucleus, which has a circular outline.

Lens luxation/subluxation

Primary lens luxation has been described as a hereditary disease in many terrier breeds (Gould *et al.*, 2011), Border Collies and Shar Peis. It is a recessive condition for which a genetic test now exists in a number of breeds (see Chapter 4). Affected breeds typically present between 3 and 7 years of age, but clinical signs of subluxation can be detected earlier than this. It may also occur in other breeds such as the Springer Spaniel and German Shepherd Dog at a later age of onset. It is usually progressive and often leads to blindness as a result of acute glaucoma. Secondary lens luxation may occur as a result of chronic glaucoma due to stretching of the lens zonules as the eye enlarges. It is rarely necessary to remove the lens in cases of chronic glaucoma, and lensectomy alone is not an appropriate treatment for these cases. Lens luxation can also result from senile degenerative changes in the lens zonules in older dogs, or occur secondary to trauma, chronic uveitis or hypermature cataract. Differentiating between primary glaucoma with secondary lens luxation and primary lens luxation with secondary glaucoma can be difficult, and specialist advice should be sought in such cases (see also Chapter 15).

Primary lens instability is a bilateral disease, but one eye will often present earlier than the other. Care should always be taken to assess the contralateral eye for any signs of lens instability. Prior to dilation of the pupil, examination of the profile of the iris may give an indication as to whether the lens is supporting the iris, leading to an iris profile with normal convexity, or whether, owing to posterior subluxation, the iris is no longer supported by the anterior surface of the lens and has a change in its profile, becoming flattened or concave.

Other signs that lens zonule breakdown may be present include:

- Iridodonesis (subtle iris trembling movement when the globe moves)
- Phacodonesis (subtle lens trembling movement when the globe moves)
- Anterior displacement of vitreous through the pupil, which may be accompanied by pigment (Figure 16.27). (Anterior vitreal prolapse is not always pathognomonic for lens instability because it can be seen in some breeds and older dogs with vitreous degeneration without any evidence of lens instability (see Chapter 17), but its presence should prompt the clinician to perform a thorough assessment of the lens)
- Increased anterior chamber depth
- Loss of the anterior lens surface reflection (Purkinje image) from within the pupil
- An aphakic crescent between the pupil margin and equator of the lens (Figure 16.28).

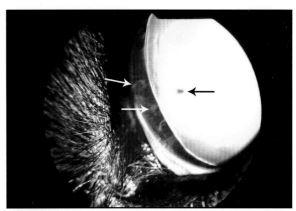

16.27 Vitreous prolapse associated with lens subluxation. The wisp-like strands of vitreous (white arrows) can be seen protruding within the aphakic crescent between the pupil margin and the lens equator. There is also some pigment dispersion from the posterior iris into the anterior chamber (black arrow). (Courtesy of D Gould)

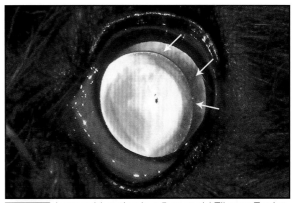

16.28 Lens subluxation in a 5-year-old Tibetan Terrier. Note the aphakic crescent and the lack of lens zonules (arrowed).

Complete lens luxation may be either anterior or posterior. Anterior luxation results in the lens moving forward into the anterior chamber and can be difficult to identify with the naked eye unless secondary signs are present or the lens is cataractous. Clinical signs associated with anterior luxation include glaucoma (scleral injection, raised IOP, blindness, diffuse corneal oedema), uveitis and focal corneal oedema due to the lens touching the corneal endothelium. Cases of anterior lens luxation (Figure 16.29) usually require immediate attention if vision is to be preserved. Posterior luxation is more difficult to identify because it is less likely to present with the same severity of clinical signs as anterior luxation. The most obvious changes are an increase in anterior chamber depth and iridodonesis.

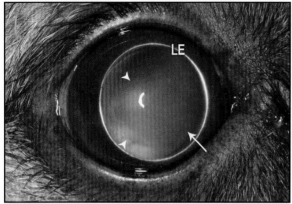

16.29 Anterior lens luxation in a 4-year-old terrier crossbreed. Note the edge of the pupil behind the lens (arrowed), the refractile edge of the visible lens equator (LE) and the subtle corneal oedema giving a steamy appearance to the cornea (arrowheads).

Treatment:

Surgical management: Surgical treatment for lens instability is required once anterior lens luxation has occurred, and prompt referral to a specialist is recommended. If the lens has completely luxated it is usually removed using an intracapsular technique, but some subluxated lenses can be removed by phacoemulsification (see below). Some surgeons also prefer to remove the lens from the contralateral eye prior to it developing complete luxation because the surgery is easier to perform and reduces the risk of acute glaucomatous or corneal damage to the eye by preventing anterior luxation.

Medical management: In some cases, it is possible to manage lens subluxation and posterior lens luxation (but never anterior lens luxation) medically. A topical prostaglandin analogue (e.g. latanoprost) is applied, usually twice daily long term, in order to induce a miotic pupil (see Chapter 7). In theory, this prevents anterior movement of the lens. However, there are significant risks associated with this medical approach.

- Care must be taken to ensure that the pupil remains permanently miotic. Topical prostaglandin analogues have a variable duration of action in animals, which may mean that an increased frequency of application is required in some dogs.
- If a treatment is missed and the lens moves anteriorly, then further application of a miotic is contraindicated because it will increase the risk of pupil block glaucoma.

- In older animals, iris atrophy may limit the efficacy of miotic therapy.
- The use of miotics in cases where there is vitreal presentation through the pupil (see Figure 16.27) risks causing vitreous entrapment within the miotic pupil. This leads to pupillary block and acute glaucoma.

For the above reasons, specialist advice should be considered before instigating medical management for posterior lens luxation or lens subluxation. There is no effective medical treatment for anterior lens luxation.

Hyperopia and myopia

The vast majority of canine eyes are emmetropic (i.e. have normal focus), but some may be hyperopic (long- or far-sighted) or myopic (short- or near-sighted). This deviation from the normal refractive state may be due to changes in the refractive power of the lens, or the corneal curvature or size (axial length) of the eye. Refractive errors can be assessed using retinoscopy (see Chapter 1). Retinoscopy is also used to assess the corrective power of synthetic intraocular lenses. Aphakic dogs have a refractive state of +14.4 D (extremely long-sighted) and their visual acuity decreases from a Snellen equivalent of 20/60 to 20/850. An intraocular lens placed within the capsular bag following lens extraction in dogs needs a power of 41.5 D in order to correct vision to within 1 D of emmetropia (Davidson *et al.*, 1993).

Feline conditions

The cat is much less frequently affected by lens disease than the dog, with most of the pathology seen as a result of other ocular diseases or trauma.

Congenital abnormalities

Persistent pupillary membranes

PPM is much less common in cats (Figure 16.30) than in dogs.

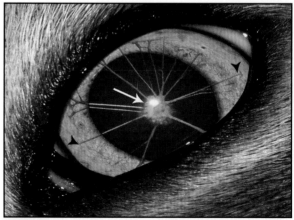

16.30 Persistent pupillary membrane (PPM) in a cat. The membrane remnants arise from the iris collarette (black arrows). Note the focal cataract (white arrow) at the attachment of the membrane to the anterior lens capsule.

Peters anomaly

The reader is referred to the section on canine congenital abnormalities (see above) and Chapter 14.

Persistent hyperplastic primary vitreous/persistent hyperplastic tunica vasculosa lentis

PHPV/PHTVL has been reported very sporadically in cats, but clinical manifestations are similar to the condition seen in dogs (Allgoewer and Pfefferkorn, 2001).

Aphakia and microphakia

Both of these conditions have been reported in the cat, but are considered to be very rare (Peiffer, 1982; Molleda *et al.*, 1995).

Macrophakia

Macrophakia has been described in three cats, in which the posterior pole of the lens was almost touching the retina. Although the condition was not proven to be congenital, all affected animals reportedly had visual disturbances from an early age. Other ocular abnormalities, such as retinal folds, were also described, but there was no cataract present at initial presentation (Benz *et al.*, 2011b).

Acquired abnormalities

Cataracts

Although much less common than in dogs, primary (presumed inherited) cataracts are seen in cats (Figure 16.31). However, the majority of clinically significant cataract formation in cats is secondary to other intraocular diseases (see below). Diabetic cataracts are occasionally seen in cats, but the extent of the lens changes is minor compared with those in dogs. This may be explained by the lack of aldose reductase activity in the lenses of cats >4 years of age (Richter *et al.*, 2002).

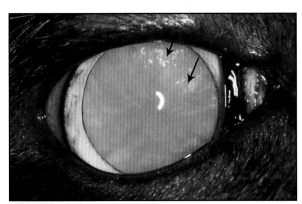

16.31 Hypermature primary cataract in a 4-year-old Domestic Shorthaired cat. Note the crystalline appearance associated with subcapsular plaques (arrowed).

Chronic uveitis is the most common cause of cataract in the cat (and is described in detail in Chapter 14), although these cases may also have glaucoma and lens subluxation (Figure 16.32), so it is not always possible to identify the precise pathological mechanism of the cataract formation.

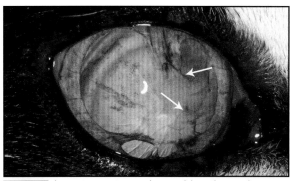

16.32 Immature cataract, lens subluxation and extensive posterior synechiae secondary to uveitis in a 12-year-old Domestic Shorthaired cat. Note the fibrovascular membrane covering the majority of the anterior lens capsule (arrowed).

Penetrating injury to the lens may not always induce a phacoclastic uveitis to the same degree as seen in dogs, but there is an association between lens injury and the development of intraocular sarcoma in the short or long term (Dubielzig *et al.*, 1990). As a consequence, regardless of whether early lens extraction surgery is performed on these cases, they should be monitored very closely in the long term. Recently, an association between *Encephalitozoon cuniculi* and cataract has been described in the cat (Benz *et al.*, 2011a).

Lens luxation/subluxation

In the majority of cases, lens luxation or subluxation is secondary to other ocular diseases. Lens luxation is often associated with chronic uveitis (Figure 16.33), although the signs of uveitis may be very subtle (see Chapter 14). Glaucoma may also cause lens subluxation due to expansion of the globe and tearing of the zonules (see Chapter 15), but lens luxation in cats is less likely to cause secondary glaucoma compared with dogs. Removal of the lens is only advised if anterior luxation is present, as an anteriorly luxated lens will cause dense, focal corneal oedema, become cataractous and may contribute to ongoing intraocular inflammation. Postoperative failure may result from ongoing uveitis,

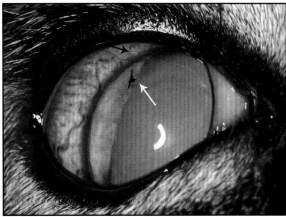

16.33 Anterior lens luxation in an 11-year-old Domestic Shorthaired cat secondary to chronic uveitis. Note the iris rubeosis/neovascularization (black arrow) and pigment deposition on the lens (white arrow).

glaucoma or retinal detachment. Primary lens instability has been reported in a closely related group of cats with a suspected dominant mode of inheritance. However, there was no association noted with the *ADAMTS17* gene responsible for most cases of primary lens instability in dogs (Payen *et al.*, 2011).

Lens surgery

Lens surgery invariably involves removal of the lens (the two most common approaches are detailed below). Lens surgery requires an operating microscope and specialist microsurgical training, and should only be attempted by veterinary ophthalmologists experienced in microsurgery.

Indications

The main indications for lens removal are the presence of a cataract or lens instability, but other possible indications include penetrating injury, foreign body removal and as part of a surgical approach to another part of the eye in retinal reattachment surgery, endocyclophotocoagulation for glaucoma or tumour removal.

Techniques

Surgical approaches can be classified as intracapsular or extracapsular. Intracapsular extraction involves removing the lens within the capsule; extracapsular techniques involve an incision into the capsule to remove the lens contents and include phacoemulsification and extracapsular lens extraction (ECLE). In modern veterinary ophthalmology, ECLE is a technique reserved for a tiny minority of cataract procedures where phacoemulsification is not possible owing to an excessively hard lens.

Phacoemulsification

Cataract is the most common reason to perform phacoemulsification. Given that it is usually an elective procedure, time needs to be spent thoroughly assessing the eyes (see below) and general health of the patient, and discussing the advantages and disadvantages of performing the surgery with the owner, as well as potential surgical complications and the need for ongoing postoperative medical therapy and regular re-evaluations.

Selection criteria: The early assessment of cataracts may allow the clinician to perform a thorough retinal examination. This can allow a more accurate assessment of other causes of visual disturbance, such as PRA, rather than relying on electroretinography alone. It also allows a larger window of time for monitoring progression before deciding to proceed with surgery. It is generally accepted that cataracts operated on at an immature stage have a better chance of long-term success because there is less pre-existing lens-induced uveitis and a softer lens, which reduces surgical time and the use of ultrasound energy. Early referral to a specialist is particularly important with diabetic patients because their cataracts can progress rapidly and develop a

significant phacolytic or even phacoclastic uveitis as the intumescent lens may cause capsular rupture. It is important that assessment is not delayed, even if the diabetes is not completely stable.

The ideal candidate for surgical intervention is an animal in good physical condition that has no existing or predisposition to other ocular diseases and has immature progressive cataracts. However, it is now possible to perform surgery on eyes with partial or complete retinal detachment and/or glaucoma because these conditions can be treated as part of the procedure, albeit with decreased success rates. Old age is not necessarily a contraindication as long as there are no other significant health issues. Therefore, the vast majority of patients with progressive, late immature or mature (complete) cataracts could be considered as possible candidates for surgery.

Diabetic patients are generally good candidates for phacoemulsification cataract surgery, assuming that their diabetes is fairly well regulated, but it should be remembered that diabetic cataracts can progress very quickly and that advanced cataracts are associated with a higher rate of postoperative complications. For this reason, early referral of diabetic cataract patients is generally advised whenever possible.

Preoperative assessment: In addition to a full clinical examination of the eye (including measurement of tear production and gonioscopy), it is necessary to perform ultrasonography to assess for lens capsule rupture, posterior lentiglobus or lenticonus, the presence and patency of the hyaloid artery, vitreous degeneration and vitreal or retinal detachment (see Chapter 2). None of these factors necessarily precludes surgery, but they may significantly alter the surgical approach and negatively impact surgical outcome. Whenever it is not possible to assess the retina ophthalmoscopically, or there is any concern about retinal function, electroretinography should be used to assess retinal function (see Chapter 18). Cataract is a common complication of PRA in breeds such as the Labrador Retriever, Poodle and Cocker Spaniel, and retinal function should be considered suspect if there is any history of night blindness or PLRs are slow and incomplete, and an inappropriate degree of pupil dilatation is recognized under normal lighting conditions. If a disease such as PRA is diagnosed, a decision needs to be made (in discussion with the owner) as to whether surgery is justified because some patients may still benefit from the short- to medium-term restoration of some visual capability.

Procedure: One- and two-handed approaches are used routinely, depending on surgeon preference. A two-handed approach to a cataractous lens without other complications is described here (and is broadly similar to the one-handed technique). The description below provides a general explanation of the technique and should not be considered as a guide to performing the surgery. Cataract surgery involves multiple steps that require extensive supervised training and a considerable investment in equipment to be able to be performed successfully. A small mistake at one stage will have a magnifying effect on the difficulty of the following stages and dramatically increase the failure rate of the surgery.

1. An initial incision (usually 2.5–3 mm wide) is made at the limbus (Figure 16.34a).
2. Injection of viscoelastic (hyaluronic acid) into the anterior chamber to maintain its depth is essential for formation of the second entry port and the anterior capsulorrhexis, and is necessary to protect the corneal endothelium from damage (Figure 16.34b).
3. A second incision is made in a similar fashion to the first, but is usually smaller in width.
4. Anterior capsulorrhexis is normally performed using a continuous curvilinear technique, and the aim is to create a smooth-edged circular hole of a similar or slightly smaller diameter than the optic of the synthetic lens in the centre of the anterior capsule (Figure 16.34c). This stage is technically very demanding and failure to complete this step correctly is likely to lead to an unsatisfactory surgical outcome. Staining the anterior lens capsule with trypan blue can aid in visualization of the capsule.
5. Phacoemulsification – there are many techniques described for the manipulation and physical breakdown of the lens, which are beyond the scope of this text. In broad terms, the phacoemulsification needle is advanced through the main entry port into the lens and, using a combination of irrigation, ultrasound vibration and vacuum, the lens material is broken down and aspirated from the eye (Figure 16.34de). A second entry port allows the use of a variety of manipulators or choppers to assist this process.

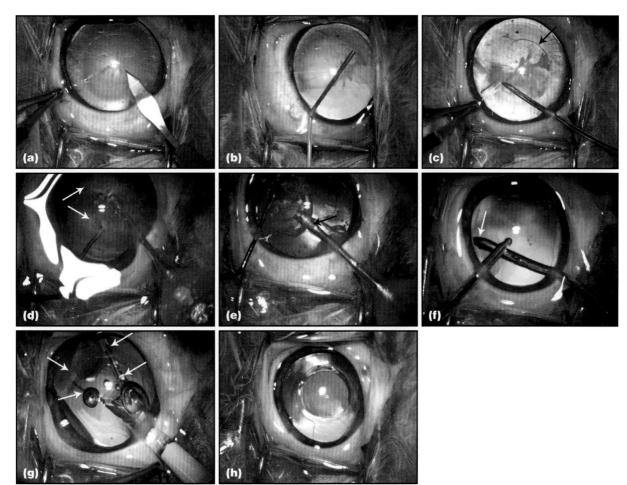

16.34 Phacoemulsification technique. **(a)** The main entry port is created with a slit knife through clear cornea adjacent to the limbus. **(b)** Injection of viscoelastic through a corneal entry port to maintain the anterior chamber and to protect the corneal endothelium. **(c)** Anterior capsulorrhexis (arrowed) is performed, creating a circular hole in the capsule. **(d)** The lens nucleus is divided into manageable sections. In this case, the lens is divided into two halves (arrowed) using a chop technique. **(e)** Lens material is phacofragmented and aspirated from the eye using a phacoemulsification needle (arrowed). The instrument on the left-hand side helps to position the material against the phacoemulsification needle. **(f)** The remaining lens cortex is aspirated from the eye, in this case using irrigation/aspiration handpieces. The instrument on the right-hand side is aspirating cortex from the lens equator inside the capsular bag (arrowed). **(g)** The intraocular lens (arrowed) is folded and injected through the main entry port into the lens capsule. **(h)** The intraocular lens within the capsular bag at the end of surgery. Both entry ports have been sutured.

6. Irrigation and aspiration – the remaining lens cortex is often attached to the lens capsule, especially at the equator. Irrigation/aspiration (I/A) handpieces, which have a rounded tip and no ultrasonic power, are used to reduce the risk of lens capsule rupture. The cortical material is aspirated from the capsular bag and the bag is 'polished' to remove as many of the remaining lens epithelial cells as possible (Figure 16.34f).
7. Synthetic intraocular lens placement – the capsule is re-inflated with viscoelastic and the folded intraocular lens is injected through the larger entry port into the capsular bag before being positioned completely within the bag using lens manipulators (Figure 16.34g).
8. The remaining viscoelastic is aspirated from the eye.
9. The entry ports are sutured and the eye re-inflated with a balanced salt solution (Figure 16.34h).

Figures 16.35 and 16.36 show the postoperative appearance in a cat and dog, respectively.

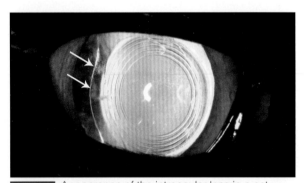

16.35 Appearance of the intraocular lens in a cat 1 week after cataract surgery. Note the opacities in the peripheral anterior lens capsule (arrowed).

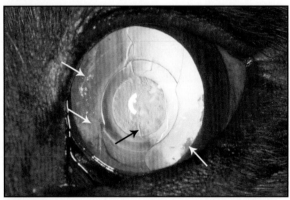

16.36 Appearance of an intraocular lens in a 9-year-old Labrador Retriever 3 years after surgery. Note the peripheral opacification of the lens capsule (white arrows) and some minor wrinkling of the posterior capsule deep to the lens optic (black arrow).

Postoperative management: In the immediate postoperative period, treated eyes can experience a raised IOP (postoperative ocular hypertension). Consequently, all lensectomy patients should have their IOP monitored closely in this period. All intraocular surgery induces a degree of uveitis and management of this is key to delivering acceptable long-term success rates. Topical and systemic corticosteroids or non-steroidal anti-inflammatory drugs (NSAIDs) are required to reduce postoperative uveitis and may need to be continued for life.

Failure rates (a totally blind eye) for the procedure are quoted at between 7.6% of eyes (cases reviewed 1–2 years post-surgery) and 10% of eyes (median follow-up time after surgery = 302 days) in two of the most recent studies (Sigle and Nasisse, 2006; Klein et al., 2011). Postoperative complications seen include glaucoma, retinal detachment, ongoing uveitis, posterior capsular opacification, corneal oedema, corneal ulceration, posterior synechiae between the iris and the lens capsule or synthetic lens, and endophthalmitis. Of these, glaucoma, retinal detachment and endophthalmitis are the most serious complications because they are vision-threatening and may necessitate enucleation of the eye owing to ongoing discomfort and total vision loss (Moore et al., 2003). Some breeds are more susceptible to these complications than others. For example, in one study, Labrador Retrievers had a 35% probability of developing postoperative glaucoma at 104 weeks post-surgery compared with 9% in other breeds (Moeller et al., 2011). Careful counselling of owners prior to surgery is essential in order to inform them of these risks.

Intracapsular lens extraction

Procedure: As for phacoemulsification, the description below is a general explanation of the technique and should not be considered as a guide to performing the procedure.

1. Initial incision – a half-depth corneal groove cut is created for 170 degrees adjacent to the limbus.
2. One end of this original groove is then incised completely, taking care not to penetrate the lens if it is anteriorly luxated.
3. Viscoelastic is injected anterior to the lens to protect the corneal endothelium and posteriorly to break down the hyaloidcapsular ligament.
4. The corneal incision is extended using curved corneal scissors along the length of the original cut.
5. The lens is removed using a lens loop or lens vectis forceps and any remaining vitreal attachments are cut away. An alternative approach involves cryofixation of the lens using a cryoprobe to secure the lens prior to removal from the eye.
6. Any anteriorly displaced vitreous is then cut away, ideally using automated vitrectomy, but manual vitrectomy using scissors and cellulose sponges is also effective.
7. The corneal incision is closed in a continuous pattern and the eye re-inflated with balanced salt solution.

Success rates of up to 70% of eyes retaining vision (mean time to last follow-up after surgery = 29 months) have been reported after intracapsular lens extraction with implantation and suture fixation of an intraocular lens (see below) (Stuhr *et al.*, 2009).

Other procedures

Posterior capsular opacification: This occurs after cataract surgery as a consequence of contraction of the capsule and/or posterior migration of epithelial cells. In dogs, it seldom causes clinically noticeable visual deficits, even in advanced cases. In patients with severe capsular opacification, the opacified capsule can be removed by excision or disrupted using laser capsulotomy. Yttrium–aluminium–garnet (YAG) laser capsulotomy has been described, but requires costly specialist equipment and carries the risk of damaging the lens optic owing to the proximity of the optic to the posterior capsule.

Suture-fixed lenses: During intracapsular lens extraction, or in some phacoemulsification cases, it is not possible to use the capsular bag to retain a synthetic lens implant. In these instances, it is possible to place a synthetic lens by suturing the haptics (arms) of the lens through the ciliary sulcus between the iris and ciliary body (Figure 16.37).

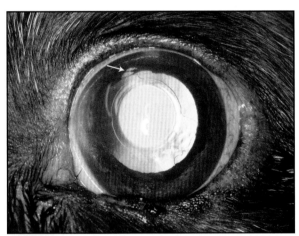

16.37 Suture-fixed intraocular lens in a 9-year-old English Springer Spaniel. Note the lack of lens capsule and unrelated minor iris atrophy (arrowed).

References and further reading

Allgoewer I and Pfefferkorn B (2001) Persistent hyperplastic tunica vasculosa lentis and persistent hyperplastic primary vitreous (PHTVL/PHPV) in two cats. *Veterinary Ophthalmology* **4**, 161–164
Benz P, Maaß G, Csokai J *et al.* (2011a) Detection of *Encephalitozoon cuniculi* in the feline cataractous lens. *Veterinary Ophthalmology* **14**, 37–47
Benz P, Walde I, Gumpenberger M *et al.* (2011b) Macrophakia in three cats. *Veterinary Ophthalmology* **14**(Supplement 1), 99–104
Bernays ME, Peiffer, RL Bernays ME *et al.* (2000) Morphologic alterations in the anterior lens capsule of canine eyes with cataracts. *American Journal of Veterinary Research* **61**, 1517–1519
Davidson MG, Murphy CJ, Nasisse MP *et al.* (1993) Refractive state of aphakic and pseudophakic eyes of dogs. *American Journal of Veterinary Research* **54**, 174–177
Dubielzig RR, Everitt J, Shadduck JA *et al.* (1990) Clinical and morphologic features of post-traumatic ocular sarcomas in cats. *Veterinary Pathology* **27**, 62–65
Gould D, Pettitt L, McLaughlin B *et al.* (2011) *ADAMTS17* mutation associated with primary lens luxation is widespread among breeds. *Veterinary Ophthalmology* **14**, 378–384
Kador PF, Webb TR, Bras D *et al.* (2010) Topical KINOSTAT™ ameliorates the clinical development and progression of cataracts in dogs with diabetes mellitus. *Veterinary Ophthalmology* **13**, 363–368
Klein HE, Krohne SG, Moore GE *et al.* (2011) Postoperative complications and visual outcomes of phacoemulsification in 103 dogs (179 eyes): 2006–2008. *Veterinary Ophthalmology* **14**, 114–120
Martin CL and Chambreau T (1982) Cataract production in experimentally orphaned puppies fed a commercial replacement for bitch's milk. *Journal of the American Animal Hospital Association* **18**, 115–119
Mellersh CS, McLaughlin B, Ahonen S *et al.* (2009) Mutation in *HSF4* is associated with hereditary cataract in the Australian Shepherd. *Veterinary Ophthalmology* **12**, 372–378
Mellersh CS, Pettitt L, Forman OP *et al.* (2006) Identification of mutations in *HSF4* in dogs of three different breeds with hereditary cataracts. *Veterinary Ophthalmology* **9**, 369–378
Moeller E, Blocker T, Esson D *et al.* (2011) Postoperative glaucoma in the Labrador Retriever: incidence, risk factors and visual outcome following routine phacoemulsification. *Veterinary Ophthalmology* **14**, 385–394
Molleda JM, Martin E, Ginel PJ *et al.* (1995) Microphakia associated with lens luxation in the cat. *Journal of the American Animal Hospital Association* **31**, 209–212
Moore DL, McLellan GJ and Dubielzig RR (2003) A study of the morphology of canine eyes enucleated or eviscerated due to complications following phacoemulsification. *Veterinary Ophthalmology* **6**, 219–226
Payen G, Hänninen RL, Mazzucchelli S *et al.* (2011) Primary lens instability in ten related cats: clinical and genetic considerations. *Journal of Small Animal Practice* **52**, 402–410
Peiffer RL (1982) Bilateral congenital aphakia and retinal detachment in a cat. *Journal of the American Animal Hospital Association* **18**, 128–130
Richter M, Guscetti F and Spiess B (2002) Aldose reductase activity and glucose-related opacities in incubated lenses from dogs and cats. *American Journal of Veterinary Research* **63**, 1591–1597
Sigle KJ and Nasisse MP (2006) Long-term complications after phacoemulsification for cataract removal in dogs: 172 cases (1995–2002). *Journal of the American Veterinary Medical Association* **228**, 74–79
Stuhr CM, Schilke HK and Forte C (2009) Intracapsular lensectomy and sulcus intraocular lens fixation in dogs with primary lens luxation or subluxation. *Veterinary Ophthalmology* **12**, 357–360
Swanson HL, Dubielzig RR, Bentley E *et al.* (2001) A case of Peters' anomaly in a Springer Spaniel. *Journal of Comparative Pathology* **125**, 326–330
van der Woerdt A (2000) Lens-induced uveitis. *Veterinary Ophthalmology* **3**, 227–234
Wilkie DA, Gemensky-Metzler AJ, Colitz CMH *et al.* (2006) Canine cataracts, diabetes mellitus and spontaneous lens capsule rupture: a retrospective study of 18 dogs. *Veterinary Ophthalmology* **9**, 328–334
Williams DL, Heath MF and Wallis C (2004) Prevalence of canine cataract: preliminary results of a cross-sectional study. *Veterinary Ophthalmology* **7**, 29–35

17

The vitreous

Christine Heinrich

The vitreous humour is a transparent hydrogel that occupies the posterior segment of the globe. Its function is not only to act as a clear medium for transmission of light between the lens and retina, but its viscoelastic properties also provide mechanical support and protection for the internal structures of the eye during movement and deformation of the globe. The vitreous contributes to intraocular metabolism and acts as a nutrient reservoir and metabolic waste repository for the retina and neighbouring tissues.

Embryology, anatomy and physiology

Embryology
The development of the vitreous has traditionally been divided into three stages.

- In the first stage, the relatively small retrolental space is filled by the primary vitreous, which consists of the hyaloid artery and its branches, providing nutrition to the developing lens via the tunica vasculosa lentis. The primary vitreous is thought to be of mixed ectodermal and mesenchymal origin. In addition to the vascular mesenchyme of the primitive ophthalmic artery, elements derived from the surface ectoderm, which surrounds the lens during invagination, contribute to its formation. Vitrosin (see below) may be of neuroectodermal origin. With the development of the iris and ciliary body, the need for a direct vascular supply is lost, so the hyaloid vasculature regresses. This begins at day 45 of gestation and is complete by 2–4 weeks postpartum in the dog.
- In the second stage, secondary or adult vitreous fills the increasing space of the posterior optic cavity. As it atrophies, the primary vitreous becomes condensed in the centre of the posterior segment and forms Cloquet's canal, which runs between the optic nerve head and lens. The area of previous attachment of the hyaloid artery to the posterior lens capsule remains visible in the adult dog as Mittendorf's dot. This mark can be seen ventromedial to the confluence of the posterior suture line; a fine remnant of the atrophied vessel is usually visible on slit-lamp examination within the anterior vitreous. The posterior remnant of the hyaloid artery, Bergmeister's papilla, is not usually visible on examination in the adult dog, but the area where the hyaloid artery originated

from on the posterior pole can be seen easily on ophthalmoscopic examination as the physiological pit on the surface of the optic nerve head. The origin of the secondary or adult vitreous remains unclear, but hyalocytes, ciliary epithelium, mesenchymal cells at the rim of the optic cup, hyaloid vessels during fetal development and retinal glial cells (Müller cells) are thought to contribute to its development (Forrester *et al.*, 1996).
- In the third stage, the collagen condensations of the vitreal base and lens zonular fibres are formed. As with the secondary vitreous, the exact origin of the tertiary vitreous is unclear, but it is suspected that the non-pigmented ciliary epithelium is involved in its formation.

The development and regression of the structures of the primary vitreous are of the utmost importance for normal ocular development; failure of the normal regression of these embryological structures gives rise to several congenital ocular abnormalities.

Anatomy and physiology
The vitreous is bound anteriorly by the lens, its zonules and the ciliary body, and posteriorly by the retina (Figure 17.1). Filling most of the posterior cavity of the globe, the vitreous is almost spherical

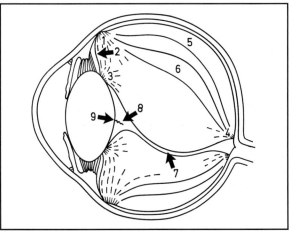

17.1 Globe and vitreous. 1 = vitreous base; 2 = anterior hyaloid face; 3 = hyaloideocapsular ligament; 4 = attachment to margin of optic nerve head; 5 = cortical vitreous; 6 = lamellae and tracts; 7 = Cloquet's canal; 8 = hyaloid vessel remnant; 9 = Mittendorf's dot.

in shape with a depression on its anterior face, the fossa hyaloidea, in which the lens rests. The vitreous can be divided into a cortical zone and a central zone. A further geographical description divides the vitreous into an anterior, an intermediate and a posterior zone.

The vitreous consists of approximately 99% water, with the remaining 1% comprising collagen, vitreal cells (hyalocytes), soluble protein and hyaluronic acid. Vitreous gel is approximately 2–4 times more viscous than water, the viscosity being largely dependent on the concentration of sodium hyaluronate. During ageing or pathological processes, this structure is lost and the vitreous becomes liquefied in a process known as syneresis. The hyaluronic acid molecules degrade and the collagen fibrils clump together, to form vitreal 'floaters' (see below).

The cortical vitreous is attached by the condensation of fine collagen fibrils to the peripheral retina and the pars plana (vitreous base), the posterior lens capsule (hyaloideocapsular ligament), the margins of the optic nerve head at the base of the hyaloid canal and the inner limiting membrane of the retina. Breakdown and disruption of the vitreous base is found in conditions such as primary lens luxation, although detachment of the vitreal face from the internal limiting membrane, where the attachments are the weakest, is more common. This condition, described as posterior vitreal detachment, can be demonstrated on ultrasonographic examination of the posterior segment and may predispose the eye to the development of retinal detachment.

Cellular elements

Although the vitreous is essentially acellular and avascular, a small number of macrophage-derived cells named hyalocytes are found within it; they are most numerous in the cortical zone. The function of these cells is not clear, but the high number of phagolysosomes indicates that they may be active phagocytes. It has also been shown that hyalocytes are able to produce hyaluronate *in vitro*, and it is suspected that hyalocytes contribute to the synthesis of vitreous humour.

Matrix

The vitreous contains vitrosin, a unique fibrous protein, which is similar to type 2 collagen, but differs from normal collagen in being inseparably linked with complex polysaccharides. Unlike type 1 collagen, which has weak interactions with only small amounts of proteoglycans and therefore presents as a compact fibril, vitrosin, in common with type 2 collagen, appears in extracellular matrices that are rich in proteoglycans and have strong collagen–proteoglycan interactions. Vitrosin fibrils form a skeleton for the vitreal gel by entrapping large coiled hyaluronic acid molecules, which, in turn, keep the collagen fibrils widely spaced. Electronegative charges of the hyaluronic acid triple helix are responsible for the hydrophilic character of the molecule.

Hyaluronic acid, a glycosaminoglycan molecule, is present in the gel and affects the flow of fluid within the vitreous. The transvitreal movement of substances is influenced by a number of mechanisms, such as diffusion, hydrostatic and osmotic pressure, convection and active transport. The strong electrostatic charges within the gel also affect electrolyte transport through the vitreous.

Glucose and other sugars are also present, suggesting that the vitreous could temporarily supply nutrients to the retina. Waste products of retinal and lenticular metabolism can accumulate within the vitreous, and increased intravitreal glutamate levels may be an indicator of retinal injury in glaucoma.

Light transmission

Light transmission in the vitreous occurs according to the same principles as in the cornea (i.e. vitreal collagen fibrils are thinner than half the wavelength of light) and the distribution of glycosaminoglycans between the fibrils reduces the effects of diffraction.

Canine conditions

Congenital and developmental abnormalities

Persistent primary vitreous

Persistent hyaloid artery: Failure of the normal regression of the hyaloid vascular system is a relatively uncommon and sporadic congenital ocular anomaly in the dog. Clinical signs vary in accordance with the part of the hyaloid artery structure that has persisted. The most common form is a small vascular remnant that protrudes from the posterior lens capsule into the anterior vitreous (Figure 17.2). A localized capsular opacity may be seen at the point of insertion of the vessel remnant on the posterior lens capsule, but the opacity is rarely progressive. The remnant does not usually carry blood, but a patent hyaloid artery may persist in rare cases, and haemorrhage from this vessel into the lens or vitreous may occur. Extensive cataract formation may ensue and persistent hyperplastic tunica vasculosa lentis (PHTVL)/persistent hyperplastic primary vitreous (PHPV) should be considered as a differential diagnosis (see below).

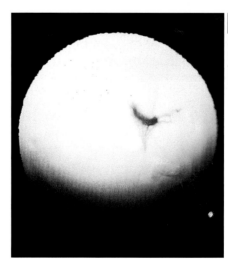

17.2

Small hyaloid remnant on the posterior lens capsule.

Persistence of the posterior part of the hyaloid artery is sometimes seen in collies affected with collie eye anomaly. The remnant of the glial sheath of the primitive hyaloid artery, Bergmeister's papilla, may in these cases give rise to a patent blood vessel with resulting vitreal haemorrhage.

Persistent hyperplastic tunica vasculosa lentis: Persistence of the posterior tunica vasculosa lentis in isolation is uncommon, but it does occasionally present on ophthalmoscopic examination as a fine filamentous web, or punctate or pigmented opacities, on the posterior lens capsule. It is rarely of any clinical significance, may be unilateral or bilateral and has a similar presentation to mild cases of PHTVL/PHPV.

Persistent hyperplastic tunica vasculosa lentis/ persistent hyperplastic primary vitreous: In this condition, the hyaloid system and tunica vasculosa lentis become hyperplastic during relatively early embryological development and continue to proliferate following birth. The extent of the lesions varies between affected animals. The degree of visual impairment that results depends on the degree of proliferation of the hyaloid system and the presence of complications, such as cataract formation and haemorrhage.

Clinically visible lesions vary in severity from fine pigment spots on the posterior lens capsule (Figure 17.3) to large fibrovascular plaques involving the posterior lens capsule. They may be accompanied by other abnormalities, including abnormal lens shape (lenticonus, lentiglobus or coloboma), cataracts, intralenticular haemorrhage (Figures 17.4 and 17.5), elongated ciliary processes, persistent hyaloid artery, persistent pupillary membrane and capsulopupillary vessels. These last vessels appear in the

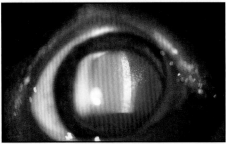

17.3 Fine opacities on the posterior lens capsule (Grade 1 PHTVL/PHPV).

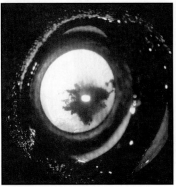

17.4 PHTVL/PHPV showing intralenticular haemorrhage and early cataract formation. (Courtesy of S Crispin)

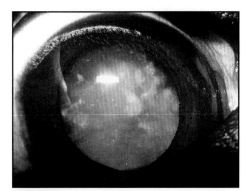

17.5 PHTVL/PHPV showing extensive cataract formation following intralenticular haemorrhage. (Courtesy of P Renwick)

form of pigmented strands or even patent vessels that originate from the retrolental plaque, course over the lens equator and, in most cases, insert on the anterior surface of the iris.

PHTVL/PHPV has been reported as a bilateral inherited trait in the Staffordshire Bull Terrier (Leon *et al.*, 1986), the Dobermann (Stades, 1980) and the Miniature Schnauzer (Grahn *et al.*, 2004). It has been studied extensively in the Dobermann, where an incomplete dominant mode of inheritance has been suggested (Stades, 1983a). A grading system has been suggested for the condition in the Dobermann, which allows clinical classification of the lesions:

* Grade 1 – very minor posterior capsular cataract and retrolental pigment dots
* Grade 2 – more intense central posterior capsular cataract with yellow/brown retrolental fibrous tissue and peripheral retrolental pigment dots. A persistent pupillary membrane is also commonly seen
* Grade 3 – persistent tunica vasculosa lentis– hyaloid system visible as retrolental meshwork and abnormalities as in Grade 2
* Grade 4 – lenticonus and abnormalities as in Grade 2
* Grade 5 – combination of Grade 3 and Grade 4 abnormalities
* Grade 6 – combination of former Grades associated with lens coloboma, microphakia and accumulations of pigment and blood.

Preventive measures, in the form of selective breeding (i.e. excluding severely affected dogs classed as Grade 2–6 from breeding programmes), have been successful in reducing the incidence of PHTVL/PHPV in the Dobermann in the Netherlands (Stades *et al.*, 1991). Unlike the Dobermann, where dogs with anomalies from Grades 2–6 develop progressive cataracts and blindness, extensive cataracts are uncommonly associated with the typical fibrovascular plaque on the posterior lens capsule seen in the Staffordshire Bull Terrier (Figure 17.6).

PHTVL/PHPV can occasionally occur in any breed of dog, and may be unilateral. When vision is severely impaired, but retinal morphology and function are unaffected, phacoemulsification with posterior capsulectomy and anterior vitrectomy can be

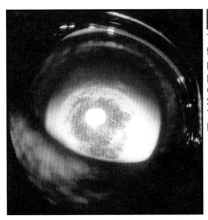

17.6
Typical fibrovascular plaque on the posterior lens capsule in a Staffordshire Bull Terrier with PHTVL/PHPV.

considered. The overall success rate in dogs with this condition is much lower than for uncomplicated cataracts because of the risks associated with vitrectomy and the potential for haemorrhage from a patent hyaloid artery (Stades, 1983b). Wet field cautery may be required to cauterize any patent hyaloid vessels, but is not without hazard.

Vitreoretinal dysplasia

Vitreoretinal dysplasia describes the abnormal development of the vitreous and neurosensory retina. Affected puppies have either retinal non-attachment (seen as a funnel-shaped, abnormally formed retina in the vitreal cavity) or develop early-onset detachment of an abnormally formed retina. Vitreal non-development is thought to be an important factor in the aetiopathogenesis of vitreoretinal dysplasia in the Bedlington Terrier and Sealyham Terrier. Vitreoretinal dysplasia due to non-allelic gene defects has been described in the Labrador Retriever and Samoyed (see Chapters 4 and 18). Animals homozygous for the gene defect have skeletal dysplasia in addition to vitreoretinal dysplasia. Heterozygous animals have multifocal retinal dysplasia (see Chapter 18). A syndrome of inherited retinal dysplasia and PHPV has been described in the Miniature Schnauzer (Grahn *et al.*, 2004). The condition is believed to be autosomal recessive and clinical findings in affected dogs range from multifocal retinal dysplasia to total retinal non-attachment with unilateral or bilateral PHPV in some cases.

Acquired abnormalities

Degeneration

Syneresis: As a result of ageing, or due to concurrent ocular disease (such as uveitis, vitreal haemorrhage or glaucoma), the vitreal collagen framework can break down, leading to vitreal liquefaction. Collagen fibrils that are clumped together are easily visible ophthalmoscopically as 'floaters' in the liquefied vitreous. This process is irreversible and can predispose the eye to the development of retinal detachment. There is some concern that a primary degenerative vitreal condition exists in certain breeds, including the Boston Terrier, Bichon Frise, Whippet and Italian Greyhound. Although vitreous

degeneration may predispose these breeds to retinal detachment, published data to support this direct association are currently lacking.

Asteroid hyalosis: This is a form of endogenous vitreal degeneration in which, in contrast to synchysis scintillans (see below), the vitreous does not become liquefied. Although the aetiopathogenesis of asteroid hyalosis remains unclear, it is thought that the dispersed particles consist of a lipid and calcium complex. The clinical diagnosis is straightforward because the presence of small refractile particles suspended throughout the vitreal framework is pathognomonic (Figures 17.7 and 17.8). The diagnosis can be confirmed with pen light examination alone in the majority of cases, and the condition is not thought to affect vision or give rise to other ocular diseases.

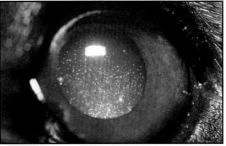

17.7 Asteroid hyalosis in a 3-year-old German Shepherd Dog. (Courtesy of P Renwick)

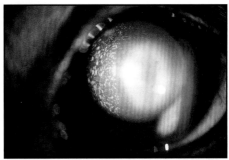

17.8 Asteroid hyalosis shown by slit-lamp examination in an 11-year-old crossbred dog.

Synchysis scintillans: In synchysis scintillans (also known as cholesterolosis bulbi), fine scintillating particles containing cholesterol are found in the liquefied vitreous. The particles settle ventrally if the eye is kept still, but following rapid ocular movement the particles become dispersed throughout the vitreous (Figure 17.9). This condition is not thought to

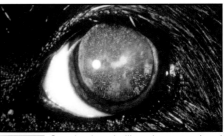

17.9 Synchysis scintillans in a crossbred dog. (Courtesy of S Crispin)

interfere with vision, but, because it is commonly the result of concurrent ocular disease, other abnormalities may be present. In humans, synchysis scintillans is usually the result of a previous intravitreal haemorrhage and, in such cases, the particles may be darker in colour.

Vitreal haemorrhage

As the vitreous is primarily avascular, vitreal haemorrhage is always the result of a pathological process affecting the neighbouring ocular tissue or associated with a congenital anomaly involving abnormal persistence of blood vessels (see above). It is commonly seen in cases of trauma and hypertensive retinopathy. Other causes include retinal detachment, neoplasia, coagulopathies, severe uveitis, glaucoma and optic neuritis. Vitreal haemorrhage can be severe and prevent a detailed ophthalmoscopic examination of the posterior segment. However, as many cases of vitreal haemorrhage are the result of an underlying systemic disease, careful examination of the patient as well as the other eye may suggest an aetiology.

Vitreal haemorrhage can be classified as preretinal (between the posterior vitreal face and the internal limiting membrane of the retina) or intravitreal. Whereas preretinal haemorrhages are usually keel-boat-shaped (Figure 17.10) and resorb rapidly, haemorrhage into the vitreal body is often diffuse (Figure 17.11) and clears only very slowly over weeks to months. Liquefaction of the vitreal gel is common following haemorrhage and condensations of vitreal collagen around the clot, with pseudocapsule and vitreal membrane formation, can occur. Severe vitreal haemorrhage can be deleterious to the retina, owing to the toxic effects of blood breakdown products or the formation of preretinal fibrous membranes and vitreoretinal traction bands (Figure 17.12). This may lead to rhegmatogenous retinal detachment (i.e. retinal detachment arising from a tear).

The treatment for vitreal haemorrhage is aimed at correcting any underlying disease. In humans, where vitreal haemorrhage is often associated with diabetic retinopathy, vitrectomy has become an established form of treatment. Vitrectomy is not, as yet, a commonly used treatment option for vitreal haemorrhage in veterinary patients.

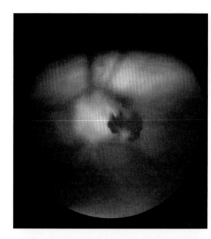

17.11 Small intravitreal haemorrhage in a 6-week-old Border Collie. (Courtesy of P Renwick)

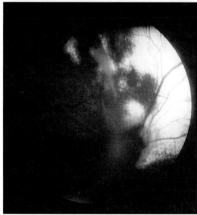

17.12 Vitreal haemorrhage and vitreoretinal traction band formation with a persistent hyaloid artery in a 1-year-old Welsh Terrier.

Vitritis

Being almost acellular, the vitreous is unlikely to mount an inflammatory response. However, involvement of the vitreous in inflammatory processes of the surrounding tissues is common and is described as vitritis or hyalitis. With intraocular inflammation, breakdown of the blood–ocular barrier occurs, allowing inflammatory cells and proteins, together with blood, to leak into the vitreous and destroy the gel structure. Vitritis presents clinically as a generalized 'blurring' of fundic detail on ophthalmoscopy, and severe vitritis may render fundic examination impossible. The most severe form of vitritis is seen in endophthalmitis or panophthalmitis, resulting from infections caused by penetrating injuries, intraocular surgery or spread from systemic disease. Potential bacterial and fungal aetiologies should be considered. Although rare in the UK, granulomatous endophthalmitis is commonly seen in other parts of the world as the result of ocular mycoses such as blastomycosis, cryptococcosis and histoplasmosis.

Foreign bodies

Vitreal foreign bodies are generally associated with severe ocular trauma. The most common intravitreal foreign bodies in dogs and cats are airgun pellets and lead shot. Thus, a gunshot injury must be considered in every case of sudden-onset ocular pain. Signs of ocular penetration, in the form of corneal or scleral wounds, should raise suspicion of the possible presence of a foreign body within the vitreal

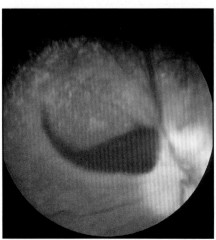

17.10 Keel-boat-shaped preretinal haemorrhage in a dog.

space. Ocular ultrasonography should be carried out if vitreal haemorrhage or opacification of the anterior segment prevents ophthalmoscopic assessment.

Although both lead shot and pellets are visible on radiographic examination, it is usually not possible to determine on radiographs alone whether the foreign body is situated within the vitreous or within the orbit. The use of ocular ultrasonography can aid in determining the exact location of the foreign body. Vegetable material that has penetrated the outer ocular coats is usually contaminated with microorganisms; thus, endophthalmitis is likely to result if a piece of vegetable material remains in the vitreous.

The prognosis for salvage of the eye is dependent on the extent of trauma at the time of entry of the foreign body, and especially on the involvement of the lens. Whether removal of a vitreal foreign body is attempted depends on whether the material is surgically accessible, as well as the type of material and its interactions with the intraocular tissues. Whereas high-quality glass, stone, high-quality plastics, stainless steel and other high-quality alloys are considered to be relatively inert and are probably best left *in situ*, other materials, such as organic matter, iron, copper, low-grade alloys and low-grade glass and plastics are known to be poorly tolerated (Belin, 1992). However, if a foreign body is retained intravitreally following ocular penetration or perforation, referral for a specialist assessment is advised.

Neoplasia

Primary vitreal neoplasia has not been reported, but involvement of the vitreous is seen with neoplasia of the adjacent tissues, either as a result of infiltration with neoplastic cells or displacement of the vitreous by solid tumours. Possibly the most common type of neoplastic vitreal involvement is seen with lymphoma, where neoplastic cells originating from the uveal tract infiltrate the vitreous. Exudate and haemorrhage from the leaky new blood vessels that often accompany intraocular neoplasia commonly lead to vitreal degeneration.

Clinically, vitritis, retinal detachment or masses within the vitreal cavity may be seen; further diagnostic tests, such as ocular ultrasonography (see Chapter 2) and vitreocentesis (see Chapter 3), should be considered. Cytology of a vitreal aspirate may aid in the diagnosis of systemic metastasis, especially if the primary tumour site has not been identified. However, the procedure is not without risk and, in sighted eyes, should be left to those experienced in the technique. The treatment depends on the type of tumour present, but most eyes with solid neoplasms within the vitreal space require enucleation.

Cysts

Uveal cysts can sometimes be found on examination of the vitreous. They present as variably pigmented, semi-transparent, spherical structures floating in the vitreous body. They can vary in size and usually have no impact on vision (Figure 17.13).

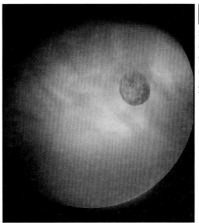

17.13 Small pigmented cyst within the vitreous. (Courtesy of the Animal Health Trust)

Parasites

Occasionally, aberrant parasites can be found in the vitreous on ocular examination (Figure 17.14). Reported parasites include *Toxocara canis*, *Dirofilaria immitis*, *Angiostrongylus vasorum* (Manning, 2007) and *Echinococcus* spp. Species of Diptera have also been seen in association with ophthalmomyiasis interna. Although some parasites can be eliminated with the use of systemic medication, surgical removal of larger parasites is indicated to avoid deleterious inflammatory reactions following parasitic death. However, surgical intervention is a skilled procedure and should only be performed by those with experience of posterior segment surgery.

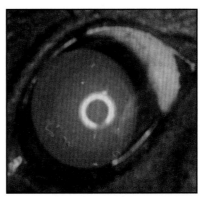

17.14 Intraocular larval migrans in a 5-year-old Staffordshire Bull Terrier bitch. (Reproduced from Manning, 2007 with permission from *Veterinary Record*)

Vitreal prolapse and herniation

Extraocular prolapse of the vitreous can be seen in traumatic ocular injuries with scleral or corneal lacerations or during some types of intraocular surgery. Herniation of degenerate vitreous through the pupil into the anterior chamber (Figure 17.15) is often the first sign of lens instability in dogs with primary lens luxation. As a result of zonular breakdown, the anchoring collagen fibril arrangements at the capsulohyaloid ligament weaken and the anterior vitreous undergoes syneresis. In severe cases, the herniated vitreous can cause pupil block or obstruct the iridocorneal angle, leading to an increase in intraocular pressure. Herniated vitreous is often present on first incision into the anterior chamber in cases of lens luxation; closure of the corneal incision should not be carried out until the prolapsed vitreous has been removed.

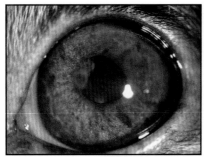

17.15
Degenerative vitreous within the pupil of a 5-year-old Jack Russell Terrier caused by lens zonule breakdown.

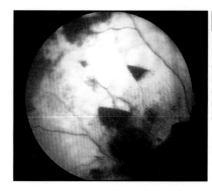

17.17
Retinal and vitreal haemorrhage in a cat with systemic hypertensive disease. (Courtesy of S Crispin)

Feline conditions

The embryology, anatomy and biochemistry of the feline vitreous are very similar to those of the canine vitreous, but there are minor differences: the cortical vitreous in the cat is more liquid and the central vitreous has a more solid nature.

Congenital abnormalities

Congenital abnormalities of the vitreous are extremely rare in the cat and published reports are limited to the presence of a persistent hyaloid artery (Ketring and Glaze, 1994; Barnett and Crispin, 1998). PHTVL/PHPV is very rare in the cat.

Acquired abnormalities

Chronic feline uveitis

Involvement of the vitreous in chronic feline uveitis is common; the extent of vitreal involvement is dependent upon the location of the uveitis (anterior, intermediate or posterior). An interesting phenomenon is the accumulation of inflammatory cells within the anterior vitreous with pars planitis (Figure 17.16). The clinical appearance of this change has led to the use of the descriptive term 'snowbanking'. It is thought to be associated with feline immunodeficiency virus infection. 'Snowbanking' is also occasionally seen with other causes of uveitis, including toxoplasmosis (see Chapter 14).

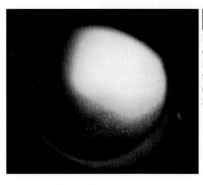

17.16
Pars planitis in a cat with feline immunodeficiency virus infection. (Courtesy of S Crispin)

Vitreal haemorrhage

Vitreal haemorrhage (Figure 17.17) is more commonly noted in the cat than in the dog and should alert the clinician to the possible presence of an underlying hypertensive chorioretinopathy (Barnett and Crispin, 1998; see Chapter 18). Vitreal haemorrhage can also be the result of head trauma and may be an indicator of the severity of the trauma, considering how well the feline globe is protected by the relatively deep orbit.

Vitreal interventions

Vitrectomy

As mentioned previously, herniation of vitreous into the anterior chamber is a common presentation in lens luxation. Vitreal prolapse through accidental tears in the posterior lens capsule is a major complication during phacoemulsification cataract surgery. Vitreous that prolapses into the anterior chamber as a result of posterior capsular defects or zonular breakdown during lens surgery should be removed. The prolapsed vitreous can impair aqueous drainage, potentially leading to glaucoma. If it is incarcerated in a corneal wound, it can lead to surface epithelial cell downgrowth into the anterior chamber, which may result in additional complications. If vitreous is left touching the corneal endothelium, it may lead to corneal endothelial dysfunction and corneal oedema.

Surgical removal of herniated or prolapsed vitreous (vitrectomy) can be carried out manually with cellulose sponges and scissors, or mechanically with automated vitreous cutting devices. These instruments are usually an integral part of the equipment required for phacoemulsification and can be used through a small corneal incision (approximately 2–3 mm). If removal is carried out manually, great care must be taken not to exert excessive traction on the adherent vitreal gel, to avoid retinal detachment.

Vitrectomy can also be carried out as a diagnostic procedure in cases of endophthalmitis, with samples obtained for microscopic examination, as well as bacterial and fungal culture. It must be emphasized that vitrectomy is a challenging procedure with severe potential complications and should only be performed by experienced veterinary ophthalmologists.

Therapeutic intravitreal injection

Adequate treatment with antibiotics and anti-inflammatory drugs is of the utmost importance for the outcome in cases of hyalitis and endophthalmitis. Topical application of any drug is rarely able to achieve therapeutic levels in the vitreous, especially in cases of bacterial endophthalmitis. As the vitreous is avascular, the systemic delivery of drugs is limited by the blood–ocular barrier and only lipid-soluble drugs (such as chloramphenicol) are likely to reach a significant concentration following systemic administration. With the breakdown of the blood–ocular barrier in uveitis, adequate levels of other drugs may also be achieved within the vitreous following systemic administration.

However, the most efficient way to achieve adequate levels of medication in the vitreous is by intravitreal injection. The drugs administered by intravitreal injection are usually antibiotics and corticosteroids, and recommended intravitreal doses of antibiotics have been extrapolated from use in rabbits, primates or humans. It must be remembered that intravitreal injection is associated with significant risks, such as lens injury, haemorrhage, infection and retinal detachment, and that the drug itself can have a deleterious effect on vitreous gel structure and other intraocular tissues, such as the retina. For this reason, intravitreal injections should only be carried out by experienced veterinary ophthalmologists.

References and further reading

Barnett KC (1990) *A Colour Atlas of Veterinary Ophthalmology*. Wolfe, London
Barnett KC and Crispin SM (1998) Vitreous. In: *Feline Ophthalmology: An Atlas and Text,* ed. KC Barnett and SM Crispin, pp. 144–145. WB Saunders, Philadelphia
Belin NW (1992) Foreign bodies and penetrating injuries to the eye. In: *Ocular Emergencies*, ed. RA Catalano, pp. 197–213. WB Saunders, Philadelphia
Forrester JV, Dick AD, McMenamin P and Lee WR (1996) *The Eye – Basic Sciences in Practice*. WB Saunders, Philadelphia
Grahn BH, Storey ES and McMillan C (2004) Inherited retinal dysplasia and persistent hyperplastic primary vitreous in Miniature Schnauzer dogs. *Veterinary Ophthalmology* **7**(3), 151–158
Ketring KL and Glaze MB (1994) Vitreous. In: *Atlas of Feline Ophthalmology*, ed. KL Ketring and MB Glaze, pp. 201–207. Veterinary Learning Systems, New Jersey
Leon A, Curtis R and Barnett KC (1986) Hereditary persistent hyperplastic primary vitreous in the Staffordshire Bull Terrier. *Journal of the American Animal Hospital Association* **22**, 765–774
Manning SP (2007) Ocular examination in the diagnosis of angiostrongylosis in dogs. *Veterinary Record* **160**, 625–627
Stades FC (1980) Persistent hyperplastic tunica vasculosa lentis and persistent hyperplastic primary vitreous (PHTVL/PHPV) in 90 closely related Doberman Pinschers: clinical aspects. *Journal of the American Animal Hospital Association* **16**, 739–751
Stades FC (1983a) Persistent hyperplastic tunica vasculosa lentis and persistent hyperplastic primary vitreous in Doberman Pinschers: genetic aspects. *Journal of the American Animal Hospital Association* **19**, 957–964
Stades FC (1983b) Persistent hyperplastic tunica vasculosa lentis and persistent hyperplastic primary vitreous in Doberman Pinschers: techniques and results of surgery. *Journal of the American Animal Hospital Association* **19**, 393–402
Stades FC, Boeve MH, van der Brom WE and van der Linde-Sipman JS (1991) The incidence of PHTVL/PHPV in the Doberman and the results of breeding rules. *Veterinary Quarterly* **13**, 24–29

18

The fundus

Gillian J. McLellan and Kristina Narfström

The term 'fundus' describes the part of the posterior segment of the eye that is viewed with an ophthalmoscope. Structures that contribute to the ophthalmoscopic appearance include the optic nerve head (ONH; also known as the optic disc or optic papilla), the retina and its vasculature, the underlying choroid and, in some animals, the sclera (Figure 18.1). Due to the intimate anatomical relationships between these structures, disease conditions seldom affect one component of the fundus in isolation. For example, inflammatory disease of the choroid will typically involve the retina and its vasculature, and may also extend to involve the optic nerve. A general understanding of the underlying anatomy facilitates the interpretation of the ophthalmoscopic features of the fundus in health and disease. As these features are very similar between dogs and cats, both species are considered together in the sections on normal anatomy and disease conditions in this chapter.

Embryology, anatomy and physiology

The retina develops from the two layers of neuroectoderm that constitute the optic cup. The optic cup develops from an evagination of the primitive forebrain, known as the optic vesicle. Together, the retina and optic nerve may be regarded as an extension of the forebrain and are therefore part of the central nervous system (CNS). The neurosensory layer of the retina forms from the inner, non-pigmented layer and the retinal pigment epithelium (RPE) from the outer, pigmented layer of the optic cup (Figure 18.2). In the dog and cat, development of photoreceptor cells occurs in the first 1–16 days postnatally, and organization of the retinal layers may not be completed until the 40th day of life.

The neurosensory retina is continuous anteriorly, at the ora ciliaris retinae, with the non-pigmented epithelium of the ciliary body, and the RPE is continuous with the pigmented epithelium of the ciliary body. In the dog, the ONH represents the commencement of myelination of the retinal ganglion cell axons as they converge to form the optic nerve and exit the globe through the lamina cribrosa of the sclera before continuing to the brain via the optic chiasm.

Histologically, the retina is a highly organized tissue that may be described in terms of ten 'layers'

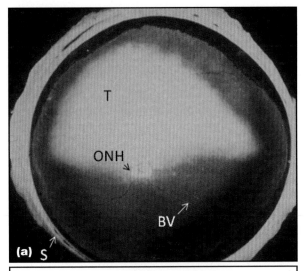

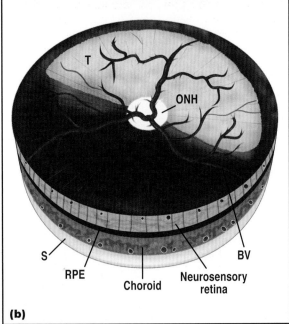

18.1 **(a)** Gross photograph of the posterior part of the eye and **(b)** accompanying illustration demonstrating the anatomical structures that contribute to the ophthalmoscopic appearance of the typical canine and feline fundus. These structures include the optic nerve head (ONH) and the neurosensory retina, within which lie the retinal blood vessels (BV). The retinal pigment epithelium (RPE), choroid and sclera (S) may also contribute to the fundic appearance, depending on their degree of pigmentation and the presence or absence of a tapetum (T) within the inner choroid.

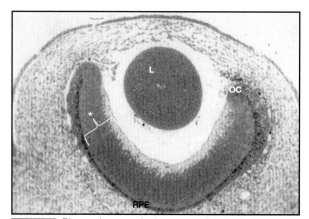

18.2 Photomicrograph demonstrating both the inner (neurosensory) layer (*) and the outer, retinal pigment epithelial layer (RPE) of the optic cup (OC) as the eye forms from an outpouching of the forebrain in a canine embryo. The developing lens (L) is also shown.

(Figure 18.3). The outer layer, closest to the choroid, is the RPE and the remaining layers constitute the neurosensory retina. The outermost layer of the neurosensory retina is the photoreceptor layer, which contains the outer segments of the rod and cone photoreceptor cells. In dogs and cats, the photoreceptor layer consists mainly of rod photoreceptors. In both species, an area of greater cone density (known as the area centralis) exists as an oval area extending horizontally, dorsal and lateral to the ONH. Rod photoreceptors are slender and cylindrical in profile and function more effectively in dim light than do cones, and are thus more suited to night vision. However, the visual acuity produced by the rod photoreceptors is lower than that of cones. Photoreceptor outer segments consist of stacks of membranous discs, which undergo constant shedding and renewal. Photoreceptor inner segments contain large numbers of mitochondria and other organelles and are highly metabolically active. The photoreceptor inner segments are separated from

their nuclei, within the outer nuclear layer, by a very thin outer limiting membrane.

Progressing inwards, towards the vitreous, the outer plexiform layer consists of the terminal branches of the photoreceptor cell axons and their synapses with the horizontal and bipolar cells. The cell bodies of the horizontal and bipolar cells, and the amacrine cells, together with those of the Müller cells, which serve as supportive cells extending through the neurosensory retina, are located in the inner nuclear layer. The horizontal, bipolar and amacrine cells, which maintain connection between the photoreceptors and ganglion cells, are involved in the modification and integration of stimuli. The inner plexiform layer, which is thicker than the outer plexiform layer, represents a region of synapses between the bipolar and amacrine cells and the ganglion cells. Functionally, this layer accentuates contrast in the retinal image and enhances detection of motion.

The ganglion cell layer contains retinal ganglion cell bodies, the axons of which gather in the nerve fibre layer. These axons pass centripetally, without branching, to form the optic nerve. To maintain retinal transparency, allowing light to pass to the photoreceptors, the nerve fibres are typically not myelinated until they reach the ONH. The nerve fibre layer also contains some neuroglial cells and the innermost tips of the Müller cells. Retinal blood vessels lie within the nerve fibre, ganglion cell and inner plexiform layers. The inner limiting membrane of the retina is formed by the fused terminations of the Müller cells.

The outermost layer of the retina, the RPE, consists of a single layer of cells, which play a vital role in the maintenance of the overlying neurosensory retinal tissue. The RPE is responsible for control of metabolite movement to and from the outer retina, and phagocytoses and processes spent photoreceptor outer segment debris. The RPE also plays an important role in the metabolism of vitamin A, which is vital to normal photoreceptor function. Although elsewhere they are normally densely

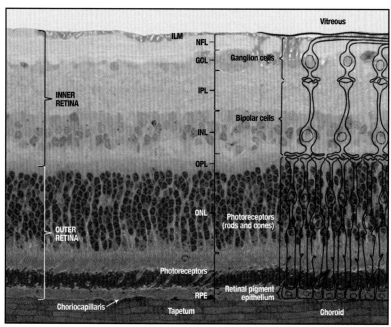

18.3 Histological detail of the retina and choroid in a normal dog showing the tapetum and choriocapillaris within the choroid, the retinal pigment epithelium (RPE) and the cells of the neurosensory retina. The neurosensory retina consists of the photoreceptor layer, the outer nuclear layer (ONL), the outer plexiform layer (OPL), the inner nuclear layer (INL), the inner plexiform layer (IPL), the ganglion cell layer (GCL), the nerve fibre layer (NFL) and the inner limiting membrane (ILM). The structures that are considered to represent the outer retina lie closer to the RPE and those of the inner retina lie closer to the vitreous. (Original photomicrograph courtesy of W Beltran)

pigmented, the RPE cells which overlie the tapetum (see below) lose their melanin granules as the tapetum develops (a process that occurs in the first few weeks of life in dogs). Numerous microvilli extend from the inner surface of the RPE cells and surround the photoreceptor outer segments. These microvillous processes increase the surface area available for metabolite exchange and transport, facilitate phagocytosis of photoreceptor material and promote adhesion between the RPE and the neurosensory retina. Separation between these RPE microvilli and their overlying photoreceptors is the anatomical location of most forms of retinal detachment that are recognized in veterinary patients.

External to the RPE lies the choroid, a highly vascular pigmented tissue which represents the posterior extension of the uveal tract. Thus, the spectrum of disorders that can affect the uveal tract (see Chapter 14) may be manifest in the choroid and in turn can have an impact on the appearance and function of the fundus. The choroid also consists of a number of distinct layers. Immediately underlying the RPE is a thin capillary layer, the choriocapillaris, beneath which, in the superior portion of the fundus, lies the highly reflective tapetum. The presence of a tapetum increases visual sensitivity in dim light by reflecting incident light back through the photoreceptors. In dogs and cats, the cellular tapetum consists of layers of polyhedral cells, which contain reflective crystals (of differing chemical composition between species) within a regular array of membrane-bound rodlets. Beneath the tapetum lie medium-sized and large vessel layers and, in turn, the elastic, pigmented connective tissue of the suprachoroidea, which represents a transition between the choroid and sclera (Samuelson, 2007). Small blood vessels penetrate the tapetum to connect the medium-sized vessel and choriocapillaris layers.

Investigation of disease

There are three components of the ocular examination that are fundamental to the initial investigation of disorders of the fundus in dogs and cats:

- Testing of visual behaviour
- Dazzle and pupillary light reflexes and menace response
- Ophthalmoscopy.

Practical aspects of these techniques have been described in detail in Chapter 1. Further ancillary diagnostic tests pertinent to the assessment of the structure and function of the fundus are also discussed below.

Behavioural tests
The ability to 'follow' moving objects (e.g. cotton wool balls) and to negotiate obstacles and stairs should be tested in both photopic (bright) and scotopic (dim) lighting conditions. However, the subjective nature of these tests can be problematic and visual deficits associated with focal disease may not be readily identifiable using conventional behavioural testing.

Reflexes
Pupillary light reflexes (PLRs), menace response and dazzle reflexes may allow a crude assessment of visual capability. However, the PLR and dazzle reflex are subcortical reflexes that do not require conscious perception of visual stimuli. Thus (as discussed in detail in Chapters 1 and 19), these neuro-ophthalmological tests have significant limitations as a means of assessing both retinal function and vision.

Ophthalmoscopy
Both indirect and direct ophthalmoscopy (see Chapter 1) are central to any investigation of disease that affects the retina and choroid. Both techniques are employed to facilitate a thorough evaluation of the fundus: indirect ophthalmoscopy provides an overview, and direct ophthalmoscopy allows a more detailed, magnified image of specific regions to be obtained.

Normal features of the canine and feline fundus
Marked variation in the ophthalmoscopic appearance of the fundus exists both within and between species. The degree to which the appearance of the fundus may vary amongst normal individuals within a species can be dramatic. In dogs, in particular, differences can be very striking, whilst the basic anatomical 'blueprint' (Figure 18.4) remains consistent. The degree of variation in the appearance of the fundus between individual normal cats is far less than among dogs. It is imperative that the clinician is familiar with the spectrum of normal variation in each species if incorrect diagnosis is to be avoided. An understanding of the histological basis for the ophthalmoscopic appearance of the fundus is also helpful (see below).

Anatomical structure/layer	Ophthalmoscopic appearance
Inner limiting membrane	Imparts a 'sheen' to the inner surface of the retina
Neurosensory retina	Translucent (like a thin layer of 'dust')
Retinal vasculature (within the neurosensory retina)	Venules darker red and generally larger than arterioles
Retinal pigment epithelium (RPE)	Degree of pigmentation variable and often related to iris/coat colour. Transparent over the tapetum
Tapetum (within the inner choroid)	Bright, shiny sweep of colour over a variable extent of superior fundus. May be small islands of pigment in the tapetum or islands of tapetum within the non-tapetal fundus

18.4 Summary of the anatomical structures responsible for the ophthalmoscopic appearance of the fundus. Structures are listed from innermost (closest to the vitreous) to outermost (closest to the sclera) (see also Figures 18.1, 18.3, 18.5, 18.7 and 18.13). (continues) ▶

Anatomical structure/layer	Ophthalmoscopic appearance
Choroid (medium-sized and large vessel layers of pigmented, vascular structure)	Degree of pigmentation is variable and often relates to iris/coat colour. Blood vessels are large, approximately radial (spoke-like) in orientation and lighter in colour (more orange–red) than the overlying retinal blood vessels. Where tapetum is present or choroid or RPE pigment very dense, these may obscure blood vessels in the choroid
Sclera (collagenous, outer coat of the eye)	May be seen as a white or pale pink background to choroidal blood vessels in subalbinotic animals that lack pigmentation in the overlying choroid and RPE, where the tapetum is absent

18.4 (continued) Summary of the anatomical structures responsible for the ophthalmoscopic appearance of the fundus. Structures are listed from innermost (closest to the vitreous) to outermost (closest to the sclera) (see also Figures 18.1, 18.3, 18.5, 18.7 and 18.13).

Tapetal fundus: In most dogs and cats, a bright, shiny sweep of colour, roughly triangular in shape, occupies the superior part of the fundus. In this region, the RPE lacks pigment and there are tapetal cells present within the choroid, beneath the choriocapillaris (Figure 18.5). Although the normal thickness of the retina does slightly attenuate light reflected from the underlying tapetum, its effects on the ophthalmoscopic appearance may be considered to resemble a thin 'layer of dust'. As the neurosensory retina is virtually transparent, the ophthalmoscopic appearance is of retinal blood vessels against a background of tapetum. The small blood vessels within the choroid connecting the medium-sized vessel and choriocapillaris layers may be observed 'end-on' as they penetrate the tapetum (Figures 18.6 and 18.7). These appear as multiple dark spots known as 'stars of Winslow'. This ophthalmoscopic feature is less obvious in dogs than in some cats and many herbivores.

The colour of the tapetal fundus differs greatly between individuals, although it is typically yellow, orange, green or blue. The tapetal colour often differs slightly at its margins; for example, a yellow tapetum may have a blue/green border. The margins of the tapetum may be clearly demarcated or irregular and broken up (the latter appearance being particularly prevalent in longhaired breeds of dog). Islands of pigment may be visible within the tapetal fundus and islands of tapetum may be visible within the non-tapetal fundus. A transient phenomenon may be recognized in cats at the onset of funduscopy whereby the area centralis takes on a grey, granular appearance. However, this should not be considered to indicate underlying pathology unless the appearance persists for more than a few seconds.

Typically, the tapetum extends to the level of the ONH in dogs and generally slightly inferior to the ONH in cats. The extent of the tapetum can be quite variable in dogs, tending to be small in the toy breeds (Figure 18.8). The tapetum may be absent, particularly in subalbinotic cats and dogs (Figure 18.9), with no clinically appreciable, detrimental

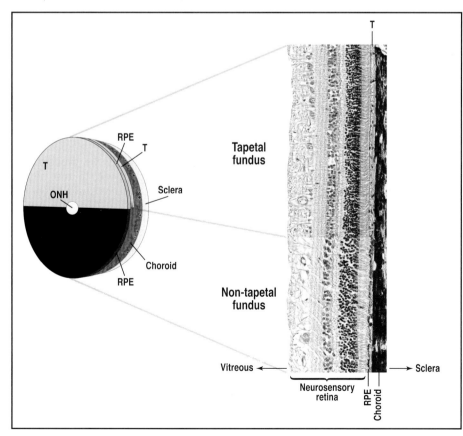

18.5

Illustration relating the appearance of the ocular fundus to the underlying histological features. In this case, the neurosensory retina with retinal blood vessels has been removed from the image. The tapetum is a bright, shiny sweep of colour in the superior fundus and, on histological section, the retinal pigment epithelium (RPE) is non-pigmented where the tapetum (T) has developed within the inner choroid. The arrowheads indicate the relative locations of the vitreous and the outermost sclera. ONH = optic nerve head.

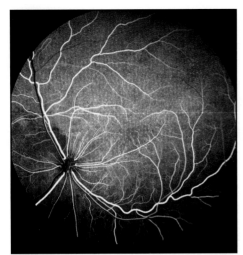

18.6 Image of the fundus in a normal adult cat taken using special filters during fluorescein angiography. The arterial vasculature is highlighted by the injection of fluorescein. When viewed 'end-on' in cross-section, the small connecting vessels that traverse the tapetum appear as small, dark dots on ophthalmoscopy and are visible throughout the tapetal fundus. In this case they appear as white dots owing to the fluorescent dye.

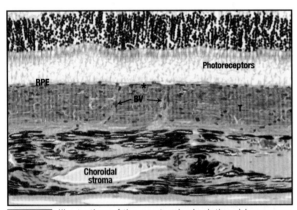

18.7 Illustration of the anatomical relationship between the tapetal tissue (T; comprising cells in an orderly alignment) and the small connecting blood vessels (BV) that traverse it. These connecting blood vessels from the vascular choroidal stroma supply the choriocapillaris (∗), which nourishes the outer retina (RPE and photoreceptors). (Courtesy of J Mould)

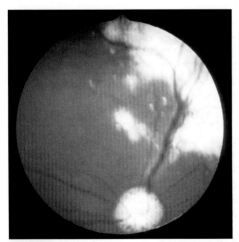

18.8 Normal adult canine fundus in a Chihuahua showing the limited tapetal development that is commonly encountered in toy breeds.

effect on vision. It should be borne in mind that tapetal development is incomplete in puppies up to 12–14 weeks of age. In very young puppies, the future tapetal region first appears dark grey, changing to violet/lilac (Figure 18.10) and then bright blue before achieving its definitive adult coloration.

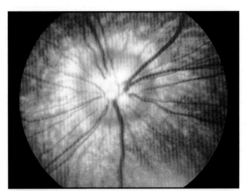

18.9 Normal adult canine fundus in an Old English Sheepdog (right eye with blue iris). The tapetum is absent, which is a common feature in subalbinotic eyes, and choroidal pigment is sparse.

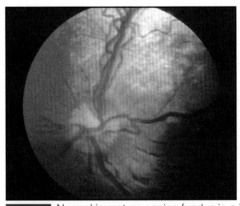

18.10 Normal immature canine fundus in a 7-week-old puppy. The tapetum has not yet fully developed within the superior part of the fundus.

Non-tapetal fundus: The non-tapetal fundus, ventral to the ONH and peripheral to the tapetum, typically appears dark grey, brown or black (Figure 18.11). This appearance is due to the presence of melanin within the RPE cells beneath the neurosensory retina, with retinal blood vessels observed against a dark background of RPE and dense choroidal pigment (see Figure 18.5). However, degrees of pigment dilution in the RPE and choroid lead to variations, ranging from a reddish tan (e.g. in dogs with a chocolate or liver coat colour and pale yellow iris; Figure 18.12) to a striped appearance (characteristic of subalbinotic animals with blue irides; see Figures 18.9 and 18.13). The choroidal vessels have a more orange appearance than the retinal vasculature and are oriented approximately radially. The striped appearance is due to an absence of pigment in the RPE, exposing the underlying choroidal blood vessels, which are observed against a background of limited choroidal pigmentation (Figure 18.13). The 'tigroid', striped appearance is accentuated in animals that lack any choroidal pigment, as the choroidal vessels are viewed against the white background of the underlying sclera (Figures 18.14 and 18.15). This appearance is most commonly associated with a merle or white coat colour and with blue and heterochromic irides.

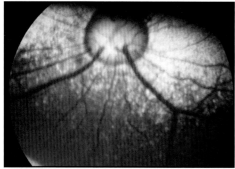

18.11 Normal adult canine fundus. The inferior, non-tapetal fundus is generally darkly pigmented.

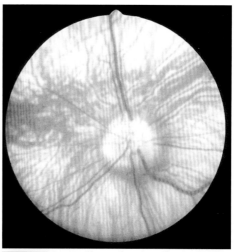

18.14 Image illustrating the effects of extreme pigment dilution on the appearance of the fundus in the blue eye of a normal merle Shetland Sheepdog.

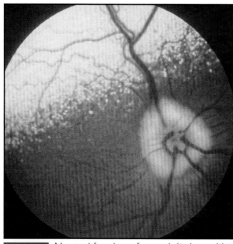

18.12 Normal fundus of an adult dog with a light brown iris. Dilution of pigment in the RPE and choroid lend a red–brown appearance to the non-tapetal fundus. (Courtesy of S Crispin)

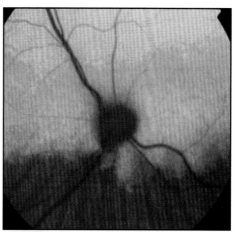

18.15 Normal subalbinotic fundus in a Siamese cat. The lack of pigment in the RPE and choroid lend a characteristic striped or 'tigroid' appearance to the non-tapetal fundus, as the choroidal vessels are seen against a background of white scleral tissue.

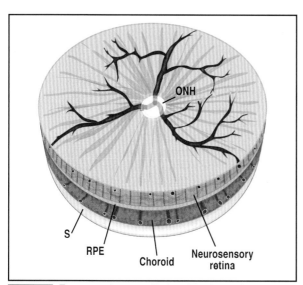

18.13 Extreme pigment dilution. The lack of choroidal and RPE pigment exposes choroidal vasculature against a background of sclera. ONH = optic nerve head; RPE = retinal pigment epithelium; S = sclera.

Optic nerve head: The normal canine ONH appears white or pale pink, owing to myelination of nerve fibres as they converge to form the optic nerve (Figure 18.16). In contrast, the feline optic nerve generally remains unmyelinated until posterior to the globe, so the ONH in cats appears small, circular and dark grey or dark pink (Figure 18.17). Although the canine optic nerve is also circular in cross-section, the shape of the canine ONH may vary as a result of myelin extending into the nerve fibre layer of the retina beyond the margins of the ONH. It is not uncommon for the ONH to have an oval, triangular or irregular outline in dogs. This excessive myelination is frequently exaggerated in Golden Retrievers and German Shepherd Dogs and is termed 'pseudopapilloedema' (Figure 18.18). This may be distinguished from pathological swelling of the ONH by observing the course of the retinal blood vessels, which, in normal dogs, should not be deviated over the surface of the ONH, and by identification of the normal physiological pit (a small grey spot at the centre of the ONH; see Figures

18.16 and 18.18). Occasionally, a small glial remnant of the hyaloid vasculature (known as 'Bergmeister's papilla') may be observed at the centre of the ONH. Some dogs have a hyper-reflective crescent around the ONH, known as 'conus' (the only instance of 'normal' hyper-reflectivity; Figure 18.19), whilst others demonstrate a ring of pigment around the ONH. Pronounced 'conus' is relatively uncommon in cats; however, it is not unusual to see a thin ring of pigment or a narrow margin of hyper-reflectivity surrounding the ONH in cats, which typically lies entirely within the more extensive feline tapetum.

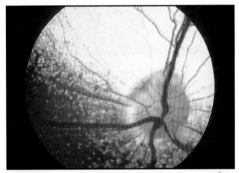

18.16 Normal adult canine fundus in a Cocker Spaniel. The ONH appears pale pink/almost white as a result of myelination of the nerve fibres as they converge before exiting the globe. Major retinal blood vessels form an almost complete circle on the surface of the ONH in dogs.

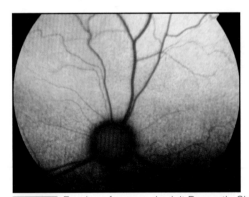

18.17 Fundus of a normal adult Domestic Shorthaired cat showing the typical appearance of the unmyelinated feline ONH. There is no anastomosis of blood vessels on the surface of the ONH.

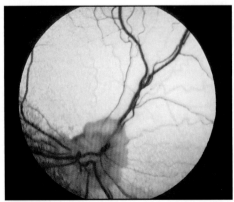

18.18 Normal adult canine fundus in a Golden Retriever. Note the extensive myelination of the ONH.

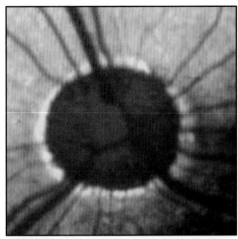

18.19 Normal adult canine ONH. There is a narrow rim of hyper-reflectivity at its margins. This 'conus' is the only example of 'normal' hyper-reflectivity. (Courtesy of C Heinrich)

Retinal vasculature: Dogs and cats both possess a holangiotic retina, in which the inner neurosensory retina receives a direct blood supply. The number of major retinal blood vessels may vary. Typically, three to five major veins are visible, which converge at the ONH. In dogs, these veins may anastomose on the ONH surface to a variable degree. Slightly narrower diameter and more numerous retinal arterioles (around 10–20 in dogs, fewer in cats) emerge at the margin of the ONH and the major arterioles follow the course of the retinal veins. These major retinal blood vessels branch as smaller venules and arterioles throughout the fundus. The vasculature tends to curve around, rather than traverse, the area centralis, dorsolateral to the ONH. Tortuosity of the retinal vasculature may be a normal feature in some individuals (Figure 18.20).

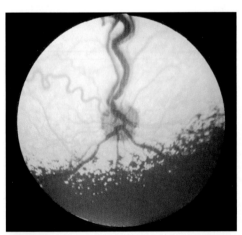

18.20 Normal adult canine fundus demonstrating tortuous retinal vasculature and a small ONH (micropapilla).

Common abnormalities

Documentation of the appearance of fundic lesions forms an important part of the medical record for ophthalmic patients and drawings can be particularly helpful when evaluating lesions for progression over time. The abnormal ophthalmoscopic findings outlined below and summarized in Figure 18.21 are suggestive of underlying pathology and warrant careful evaluation. The location of these lesions should be described using terms such as central, peripheral, superior, nasal, temporal, inferior and 'peripapillary' (the latter indicating lesions adjacent to the ONH). The extent of the lesions should be described as focal, multifocal or generalized/diffuse. It is customary to relate the size of fundic lesions to the size of the ONH, as well as indicating the distance from the ONH in 'disc diameters'.

Altered tapetal reflectivity: Tapetal reflectivity may be altered by conditions that affect the thickness of the overlying neurosensory retina (Figure 18.22). Tapetal hyper-reflectivity signifies a thinning (e.g. due to atrophy/degeneration) of the neurosensory retina. The tapetum is viewed through a thinner layer of retinal tissue ('less dust') than normal and consequently appears brighter with a more 'metallic' sheen, owing to a reduction in the degree of attenuation of reflected light. As the tapetum represents a 'curved mirror', the amount of light reflected back from its surface will depend on the viewing angle and will not be consistent in appearance in the moving globe of non-sedated dogs and cats. Tapetal reflectivity may be reduced by disease processes which are associated with thickening of the retina

(e.g. due to oedema, cellular infiltration, folding or detachment of the neurosensory retina). In addition, deposits within the RPE and infiltrates within the choroid itself may reduce tapetal reflectivity.

Altered pigmentation: Lesions within the pigmented region of the fundus, which result in thickening, oedema or exudates within the neurosensory retina will appear as paler areas against the background of RPE pigment. Proliferation, migration and aggregation of RPE cells and choroidal melanocytes within either the tapetal or non-tapetal fundus, represent a non-specific response to insult, such as inflammation, injury and degenerative processes. Black/dark brown melanin pigment should be distinguished from the lighter brown/tan lipopigment which accumulates within the RPE of animals affected by retinal pigment epithelial dystrophy.

Vascular changes: Attenuation of retinal vasculature occurs secondary to retinal degeneration, and is most readily observed in the peripheral fundus and affecting the smaller arterioles around the ONH. The major venules 'disappear' only in very advanced retinal degeneration, although their calibre may be reduced earlier in the degenerative process. Perivascular cuffing with inflammatory cell infiltrates may be observed in chorioretinitis.

Ophthalmoscopic abnormality	Underlying pathology	Figure examples
Hyper-reflectivity of the tapetum	Thinning of overlying neurosensory retina (less 'dust on mirror') (e.g. in PRA)	18.35, 18.39–41, 18.54, 18.56, 18.62–65
Reduced tapetal reflectivity	Thickening of neurosensory retina by oedema or infiltrates	18.30, 18.33, 18.42, 18.46, 18.49–53, 18.57–59
Altered tapetal colour	May indicate choroidal damage with disruption of tapetal structure or RPE disease	18.66, 18.68
Pigment alterations	Migration, loss or clumping of RPE cells, which is often patchy. Thickening of overlying neurosensory retina by oedema or infiltrates (e.g. 'more dust') will appear as pale areas against the dark background of the underlying RPE and choroid	18.31, 18.36, 18.43, 18.54–55
Vascular abnormalities	Changes in blood vessel calibre (dilatation or attenuation), orientation (displaced by underlying infiltrate or detachment) or increase in tortuosity	18.33–43, 18.53, 18.57–60
Distinct, bright to dark red lesions: • Keel-shaped • Flame or brush-like • Dot–blot • Darker, diffuse	Haemorrhages may be: • Preretinal (trapped between the retinal surface and posterior vitreous face) • Within the nerve fibre layer • Within the retina • Subretinal	18.23, 18.57–60, 18.72

18.21 Examples of ophthalmoscopic abnormalities and the associated underlying pathology. PRA = progressive retinal atrophy; RPE = retinal pigment epithelium.

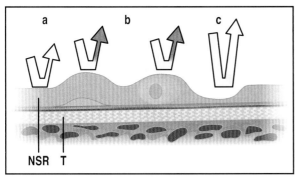

18.22 The effects of lesions that increase or decrease retinal thickness on the amount of light reflected by the underlying tapetum (T) during ophthalmoscopy relative to **(a)** normal. **(b)** Lesions that increase the thickness or opacity of the neurosensory retina (NSR) (such as subretinal exudates, infiltrates or disorganization), reduce the amount of reflected light from the tapetum and will appear dull (hyporeflectivity). **(c)** Lesions that lead to thinning of the neurosensory retina (such as retinal degeneration or retinal tears), increase the amount of reflected light (hyper-reflectivity).

Changes may also be observed in the retinal vasculature in response to systemic disease processes such as anaemia, hyperviscosity syndrome, systemic hypertension and hyperlipoproteinemia (see later and Chapter 20).

Haemorrhage: The appearance of retinal haemorrhages depends on their relative position/depth within the retina (Figure 18.23).

• Preretinal haemorrhages may assume a 'boat-keel' shape as erythrocytes settle under gravity, trapped between the inner limiting membrane of the retina and the posterior vitreous face.
• Superficial retinal haemorrhages appear as radial, flame-like streaks, reflecting the course of axons within the nerve fibre layer.
• Intraretinal haemorrhages appear as small dark round spots.
• Subretinal haemorrhages generally appear very dark red and are often diffuse and ill defined.

Over time, retinal haemorrhages darken and may come to resemble melanin pigment. Haemorrhage can be distinguished from melanin using the red-free filter (i.e. green light source) on the direct ophthalmoscope. When viewed with red-free light, haemorrhages and blood vessels appear black, whereas ocular melanin still appears dark brown.

Ancillary diagnostic tests

Ultrasonography

Ultrasonography is particularly useful in those cases in which opacity of the ocular media precludes ophthalmoscopic examination of the fundus (see Chapter 2). It may aid in the diagnosis of focal or total retinal detachment, vitreous haemorrhage or degeneration, and may be used to detect the presence of subretinal infiltrates or exudates.

Fluorescein angiography

Fluorescein angiography is used infrequently in the clinical investigation of fundus disorders in dogs and cats owing to the requirement for specialist instrumentation to obtain photographs in rapid sequence. However, it is particularly helpful in the investigation of retinal vascular disease, although tapetal auto-fluorescence combined with an absence of RPE melanin within the tapetal fundus may mask visualization of capillaries in this region (see Figure 18.6).

Advanced high-resolution imaging

These techniques, which include optical coherence tomography (OCT), have transformed the clinical evaluation of retinal disease in humans; however, their use in companion animals remains largely restricted to a research setting. Chapter 2 provides further information on advanced fundus imaging and OCT.

Electrodiagnostic testing

In contrast to most other aspects of the clinical examination of the fundus, this is an objective and non-invasive method designed to detect changes in physiological function rather than changes in structure associated with ocular disease. Electro-retinography (ERG), once largely restricted to use in academic research, has become more widely available in recent years in clinical veterinary ophthalmology practice, with relatively economical systems now designed for portability and ease of use. ERG provides a measure of the electrical response of the retina to a light flash or pattern stimulus and is dependent on photoreceptor activity. Measurement of visually evoked potentials (VEPs) allows the evaluation of gross electrical activity elicited in the occipital cortex of the brain in response to a light stimulus, and thus gives a more accurate indication of visual perception. However, this technique requires general anaesthesia or

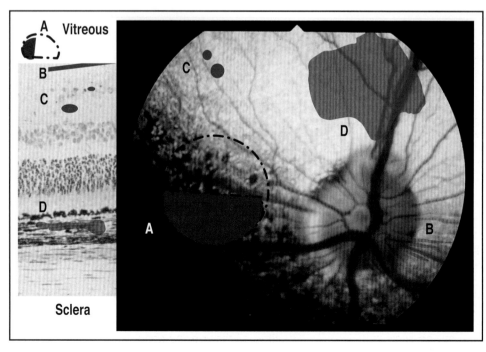

18.23 Characteristic ophthalmoscopic appearance and relative retinal depth of **(a)** preretinal, **(b)** nerve fibre layer, **(c)** intraretinal and **(d)** subretinal haemorrhages.

heavy sedation and is rarely used in the clinical investigation of disorders of the ocular fundus in dogs and cats.

Indications for electroretinography: The most common indication for performing ERG in veterinary clinical practice is to assess retinal function in animals with mature cataract, *prior to cataract surgery*. ERG is invaluable in patients presented for investigation of *sudden-onset blindness*, allowing differentiation between retinal (e.g. sudden acquired retinal degeneration syndrome (SARDS); discussed later) and CNS causes of vision loss (e.g. brain or optic nerve disease). Simple, short scotopic ERG protocols (conducted in response to bright white light stimuli, after a period of dark adaptation) are frequently used to screen patients for adequate photoreceptor function prior to cataract surgery and may be performed in conscious or lightly sedated patients. Short scotopic protocols are also employed in the diagnosis of SARDS, which results in extinguished photoreceptor responses and a 'flat line' trace on the electroretinogram.

In animals with *suspected retinal dystrophy or degeneration*, ERG can enable a diagnosis of retinal disease to be made early in the course of the disease, when clinical signs of abnormal visual behaviour or ophthalmoscopic abnormalities may be subtle or imperceptible. ERG can aid in the more precise localization of the disease process within the retina and even provide information on the cell type affected (e.g. cone *versus* rod photoreceptors) and has played a major role in acquiring information that has transformed our understanding of inherited retinopathies in companion animals and humans. However, detailed investigation of these retinal diseases requires more complex and time-consuming protocols, which generally necessitate sedation or anaesthesia to accomplish. Consequently, these 'long' protocols are much less commonly conducted in clinical practice.

Components of the response: The electroretinogram is a composite waveform that represents the sum of the electrical responses elicited from a number of different cells in the retina in response to a light stimulus. These responses occur both consecutively and concurrently, thus responses of individual cell types and/or layers within the retina can be difficult to assess under a single set of test conditions. Typical normal canine waveforms recorded in response to different stimuli are shown in Figure 18.24.

In simple terms:

- The *a wave* mainly reflects photoreceptor electrical activity, as the cells hyperpolarize in response to a bright flash of light which interrupts the 'dark current'
  - By varying the intensity and frequency of the stimulus and the degree of dark or light adaptation, the responses of the rod and cone photoreceptors may be evaluated.

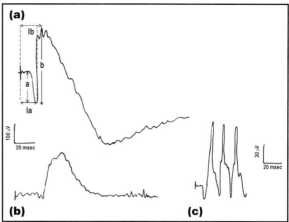

18.24 **(a)** Typical waveform showing a scotopic mixed rod–cone response to a bright 1 Hz flash in a non-sedated dog that had been dark-adapted for 20 minutes (short protocol). The a wave and b wave, along with the locations at which to measure their respective implicit times/peak latencies (Ia and Ib) and amplitudes (a and b), are indicated on the trace. **(b)** Rod responses (dim flash presented in a dark-adapted animal) are characterized by a relatively large b wave with longer implicit time/latency and a minimal or absent a wave. **(c)** Cone responses (light-adapted responses to a bright flash) are characterized by a relatively large a wave, shorter implicit time/latency and a prominent negative response after the b wave (photopic negative response), and cone flicker (shown here) at a frequency of 30 Hz that largely eliminates any rod contribution.

Prior light adaptation, intense stimuli and rapid flicker rates (e.g. 30 Hz) favour detection of cone responses. Use of very dim stimuli in dark-adapted animals at low rates of stimulus presentation favours detection of rod responses
- The *b wave* reflects bipolar cell activity and associated changes in the electrical potential of glial cells
  - *Oscillatory potentials* on the b wave and the negative wave that follows the b wave provide information on the electrical activity within the inner retina
- The c wave reflects mainly RPE activity; however, this component is not usually detected using routine ERG protocols because brighter stimuli of longer duration are required, together with alterations to the standard recording equipment (Aguirre and Acland, 1988).

Recording the electroretinogram: Three electrodes are used to record the signal following pupil dilation with tropicamide. The *active* (or positive) electrode is most commonly a monopolar corneal contact lens electrode (e.g. ERG Jet), or occasionally a Dawson Trick Litzkow (DTL) fibre electrode or bipolar electrode (e.g. Burian-Allen). The *reference* (or negative) electrode is generally a subdermal needle electrode (although bipolar electrodes (e.g. Burian-Allen) that combine active and reference electrodes may be used). The typical position for the reference electrode is just posterior to the lateral canthus of the eye (by about 3–4 cm). The *ground* electrode is another subdermal needle electrode, often placed at the occiput. The impedance (opposition of material to a moving charge) of the three electrodes should be low and must also be balanced/similar in each electrode.

The difference between the responses recorded by the active and reference electrodes represents the eye's response to the stimulus, whereas 'noise' common to both electrodes will be rejected (*common mode rejection*). The signal that remains is then amplified, filtered and digitized and displayed on a screen. For a given stimulus/stage of dark adaptation, each trace (sweep) is recorded and then averaged by the ERG software. The light stimulus is critical and 'ganzfeld' (i.e. full field, diffuse illumination of the fundus) is optimal because it stimulates all photoreceptors simultaneously. Use of a 'ganzfeld' or 'mini-ganzfeld' stimulus also allows for provision of a background illuminating light for light-adapted (photopic) recordings. Alternatively, a light-emitting diode (LED) stimulus may be incorporated into the contact lens electrode.

Important practical considerations include the extent of pupil dilation, eye position and the effect of sedatives and anaesthesia on the amplitude and implicit times/latencies of the response, in addition to the breed and age of the animal. The degree of dark adaptation, which may in turn be affected by the history of prior light exposure (including ophthalmoscopy and fundus photography), can also alter response thresholds and amplitudes.

Evaluation of the response: The best time to conduct an initial critical evaluation of the response is at the time of data collection. This allows for sources of artefacts to be identified and corrected and for the reproducibility of any abnormality to be verified. The operator should consider whether the waveform is appropriate for the species and stimulus conditions, with a and b waves of appropriate amplitude (μV) and implicit time/latency to peak (milliseconds). The waveform should then be compared with the results obtained in normal subjects of similar breed, age and sex. The results should be considered in the context of the clinical history and examination findings (i.e. whether they support or contradict a clinical suspicion). If the waveforms are abnormal, it should be determined whether the abnormalities are consistent with the suspected disease or unexpected (Figure 18.25). If the latter, the data should be carefully reviewed to identify any potential artefacts and their sources.

The retina and choroid

Developmental and inherited conditions

Inherited disorders of the fundus are relatively commonly encountered in dogs in clinical practice but remain much less common in cats; however, several conditions have been identified and characterized in specific cat breeds. In recent years, advances in our understanding of the molecular genetic basis of many of these disorders have facilitated the development of DNA-based tests (see Chapter 4). These

Flat trace
• Sudden acquired retinal degeneration syndrome (SARDS)
• Light stimulus failure/too dim/insufficient dark adaptation
• Electrodes not connected to the correct ports in the amplifier (i.e. inadvertently recording from the unstimulated eye)
• Equipment failure (can a response be elicited in another, presumed normal, animal?)
• Very high intraocular pressure (IOP; e.g. ≥70 mmHg) will extinguish the trace – if short term, this effect with be transient

Electrical noise and unstable traces
• Ensure all electrodes are properly positioned and that the recording electrode is in good contact with the cornea (i.e. no bubbles). Relocate reference electrode
• Ensure that electrodes are clean, free of corrosion and not excessively long. Check that impedance of the three recording electrodes is low (<5 kΩ) and balanced
• Switch off non-essential electrical equipment in the room. If available, electrically isolate the animal (e.g. in a Faraday cage)
• Ensure adequate sedation (instability and muscle activity is expected when recording from non-sedated animals, but efforts should be made to minimize this, e.g. by limiting eyelid movement). Apply topical anaesthetic to the cornea
• Avoid extraneous audible noise that may stimulate patient movement/blinking
• Employ a 50 (or 60) Hz notch filter (only use if absolutely necessary)

Abnormal waveform/low amplitude
• Is there a clinical suspicion of photoreceptor disease or intraocular inflammation?
• Ensure full field illumination of retina by ensuring that pupils are well dilated, eyes are centrally positioned and third eyelid protrusion is not restricting illumination of the retina
• Signal amplitudes may be reduced by inadequate dark adaptation (dark adaptation state can be negatively impacted by prior exposure to bright light, e.g. from indirect ophthalmoscopy or fundus photography)
• Check placement of reference electrode (not too close to the eye) and recording electrode (poor contact between active electrode and ocular surface, air bubbles or excessively viscous ionic contact medium)
• Avoid excessive signal averaging (fewer than five responses)
• Avoid use of 50 (or 60) Hz notch filter, if possible
• Evaluate all waveforms that have been averaged and eliminate those that do not resemble a typical waveform or that show evidence of excessive muscle activity or other artefacts
• Ensure adequate sedation if possible (instability and muscle spiking activity is expected when recording from non-sedated animals, but efforts should be made to minimize this, e.g. by limiting eyelid movement)
• Most anaesthetic drugs will adversely affect amplitude and alter latency of the waveform, as will hypoxia and hypothermia
• Cardiac artefact (reposition reference electrode)

18.25 Sources of common electroretinogram abnormalities and common recording artefacts.

tests increasingly offer a means of effectively eradicating many disabling inherited ocular disorders. However, as new disorders continue to emerge in previously unaffected breeds, these tests must be considered an adjunct to diagnosis rather than a replacement for diligent clinical examination.

Specific inherited disorders of the fundus (both developmental/congenital and acquired) are addressed in the following sections. Whilst the most commonly affected breeds are discussed in the text, exhaustive lists of affected breeds and the molecular genetic basis of disease in each breed are outwith the scope of this chapter. To facilitate the recognition of developmental and inherited diseases of the fundus, the key clinical features are summarized in Figure 18.26. For further detailed information about disease conditions in specific breeds, molecular genetic tests and additional online resources, the reader is directed to Chapter 4.

Collie eye anomaly

This congenital disorder is most prevalent in the collie breeds, in particular the Rough and Smooth Collie and the Shetland Sheepdog. The clinical prevalence of this disorder in collie breeds is high, with the reported percentage of affected dogs of these breeds ranging from approximately 40% to >75% depending on geographical location, the age group examined and criteria employed in the interpretation

of disease status (Roberts, 1969; Bedford, 1982b; Bjerkås, 1991; Wallin-Håkanson *et al.*, 2000ab). The prevalence of the disease in the Border Collie appears to be much lower (Bedford, 1982a). Collie eye anomaly (CEA) may also be seen in other breeds, notably the Australian Shepherd (Rubin *et al.*, 1991), Lancashire Heeler (Bedford, 1998) and Nova Scotia Duck Tolling Retriever.

Clinical and pathological features: The characteristic lesion of CEA is an area of choroidal hypoplasia temporal to the ONH. Choroidal hypoplasia appears on ophthalmoscopy as a pale patch temporal to the ONH, within which abnormal choroidal vessels can be seen against a white scleral background (Figures 18.27 and 18.28). Abnormal choroidal vessels may be recognized by their altered

Ophthalmoscopic abnormality	Disorder	Commonly affected breeds	Figure examples
Pale patch lateral to the ONH with abnormal choroidal blood vessels visible. May be accompanied by coloboma of ONH. Intraocular haemorrhage and retinal detachment are uncommon complications	Collie eye anomaly/ choroidal hypoplasia	Border Collie; Lancashire Heeler; Rough and Smooth Collie; Shetland Sheepdog	18.27–29
Distinct grey curvilinear and small circular lesions	Multifocal retinal dysplasia	American Cocker Spaniel; Cavalier King Charles Spaniel; English Springer Spaniel; Hungarian Puli; Labrador and Golden Retriever; Rottweiler	18.30–31
Large, circumscribed circular to horseshoe-shaped areas with altered tapetal pigmentation, colour and reflectivity	Geographical retinal dysplasia	Cavalier King Charles Spaniel; English Springer Spaniel; Golden Retriever	18.32
Retinal detachment ± chondrodysplastic dwarfism	Total retinal dysplasia/ oculoskeletal dysplasia	Bedlington and Sealyham Terrier; Labrador Retriever; Samoyed	18.33
Diffuse tapetal hyper-reflectivity, narrowing of retinal blood vessels and reduced number of smaller arterioles visible	Generalized progressive retinal atrophy	English and American Cocker Spaniel; Labrador Retriever; Miniature and Toy Poodle; Miniature Schnauzer Abyssinian; Bengal; Persian; Siamese; Somali	18.35–36, 18.38–40
Multiple grey to tan bullous lesions throughout fundus	Canine multifocal retinopathy	Coton du Tulear; Great Pyrenees; Mastiff breeds	
Tan/brown pigment spots and patches within tapetal fundus	Retinal pigment epithelial dystrophy/vitamin E deficiency	English Cocker Spaniel	18.66

18.26 Summary of clinical features of inherited disorders of the fundus. ONH = optic nerve head.

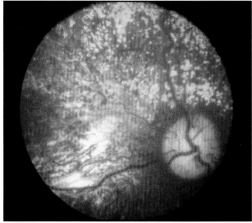

18.27 Choroidal hypoplasia in the right eye of a Rough Collie with CEA. Note the pale patch lateral to the ONH. (Courtesy of SR Hollingsworth)

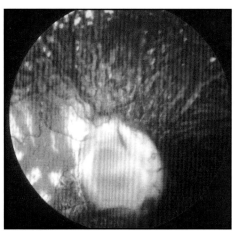

18.28 Choroidal hypoplasia and ONH coloboma in the right eye of a Shetland Sheepdog. (Courtesy of PGC Bedford)

diameter and irregular distribution, which departs from the normal radial pattern of the choroidal vasculature. Within this region, the choroid is thinner than normal, has a poorly developed vascular bed and lacks pigment (Roberts, 1969). Embryological studies have implicated faulty obliteration of the optic vesicle and abnormal differentiation of the RPE in the process of impaired development of mesenchymal (i.e. choroidal and scleral) tissues (Latshaw *et al.*, 1969).

Choroidal hypoplasia may be accompanied by other ocular abnormalities, including optic nerve or peripapillary colobomas (Figures 18.28 and 18.29; see also later in the chapter). Retinal detachment and intraocular haemorrhage may also occur as secondary complications. In a study of the incidence of CEA in collies in the UK, 34% of dogs with choroidal hypoplasia had concurrent colobomas, 6% had retinal detachment and approximately 1% had intraocular haemorrhage (Bedford, 1982b). Retinal detachment and intraocular haemorrhage are generally recognized within the first few years of life. CEA is typically a bilateral condition, but the severity of the ocular lesions can differ greatly between the two eyes of affected individuals. Minor lesions of choroidal hypoplasia have little effect on vision, but very large colobomatous defects, extensive areas of retinal detachment or intraocular haemorrhage may lead to blindness. Fortunately, bilateral blindness as a result of CEA is not common.

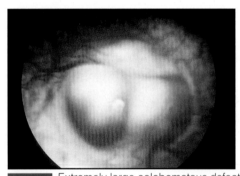

18.29 Extremely large colobomatous defect involving the ONH in a Border Collie with CEA. (Courtesy of R Elks)

Heritability and disease control: CEA is a complex, pleomorphic trait with simple autosomal recessive inheritance of choroidal hypoplasia (Yakely *et al.*, 1968; Bedford, 1982b). The mutation responsible for choroidal hypoplasia has been identified and is common to all affected breeds tested to date (Parker *et al.*, 2007). However, there is a wealth of evidence to suggest that peripapillary coloboma (for which the underlying genetic basis has not yet been clearly defined) may not be inherited directly along with choroidal hypoplasia, and that the combination of choroidal hypoplasia and coloboma is polygenic (Wallin-Håkanson *et al.*, 2000ab).

Historically, control of CEA by selective breeding has proved difficult for several reasons. Reliance on ophthalmoscopic diagnosis in mature dogs may be masked, confounded by the 'go normal' phenomenon, in which regions of the choroidal hypoplasia

are obscured by postnatal tapetal maturation in a proportion of affected dogs. Although these animals are neither genetically nor phenotypically normal and the choroidal hypoplasia remains, it becomes impossible to detect the abnormal phenotype by ophthalmoscopy. For this reason, screening of litters of puppies at approximately 6–7 weeks of age, prior to tapetal development, has traditionally been advised. However, ophthalmoscopic diagnosis of small areas of choroidal hypoplasia may prove challenging in dogs with a subalbinotic fundus, particularly in merle animals. Nonetheless, clinically affected dogs, regardless of how mildly affected, should not be included in breeding programmes. The high prevalence of this disease in the Rough and Smooth Collie and Shetland Sheepdog means that an extremely large proportion of the breeding stock are genetically affected. However, molecular genetic testing allows carrier animals to be bred to genetically unaffected animals (see Chapter 4).

Retinal dysplasia

Retinal dysplasia may be defined as abnormal retinal differentiation with disorderly proliferation and disorganization of the retinal layers. In dogs, retinal dysplasia most frequently occurs as a primary genetic disorder. However, it may arise spontaneously or may be acquired as a result of external insults to the developing retina, such as systemic infection (e.g. canine herpesvirus), X-ray irradiation, vitamin A deficiency or a range of intrauterine insults (Percy *et al.*, 1971; Narfström and Petersen-Jones, 2007). The condition is characterized histopathologically by folding and rosette formation within the neurosensory retina (O'Toole *et al.*, 1983). The lesions of retinal dysplasia may occur in isolation or in conjunction with other congenital ocular defects, such as microphthalmos or persistent hyperplastic primary vitreous (Grahn *et al.*, 2004). They may also be associated with systemic abnormalities, such as oculoskeletal dysplasia, as reported in Labrador Retrievers and Samoyeds with short-limbed dwarfism (Meyers *et al.*, 1983; Carrig *et al.*, 1988) or in association with deafness and other lesions of merle ocular dysgenesis in homozygous merle animals (see Chapter 14).

Retinal dysplasia in cats is not commonly encountered in clinical practice but may be recognized following perinatal infection with feline leukaemia virus (FeLV) or panleucopenia virus, or as a component of feline colobomatous syndrome (the most common manifestation of which is eyelid agenesis; see Chapter 9).

Clinical features: Individual affected dogs of breeds that segregate inherited retinal dysplasia can demonstrate lesions across a spectrum of disease that ranges from mild to severe. Retinal dysplasia lesions may be unilateral or bilateral. Clinically, three major forms of retinal dysplasia are recognized:

- Focal or multifocal retinal dysplasia
- Geographical retinal dysplasia
- Total retinal dysplasia

Focal or multifocal retinal dysplasia: In the mildest form, focal or multifocal retinal dysplasia, dysplastic lesions appear as single or multiple greyish, vermiform, linear streaks and small circular lesions which are most frequently observed as regions of reduced reflectivity within the tapetal fundus dorsal to the ONH (Figure 18.30). Lesions of retinal dysplasia are generally observed in the region of the superior retinal blood vessels, although occasionally, dysplastic lesions may be visible within the pigmented non-tapetal fundus (Figure 18.31). The lesions of focal or multifocal retinal dysplasia generally remain static, although occasionally, the lesions become less obvious with time or may become more clearly demarcated by hyper-reflectivity or hyperpigmentation as dysplastic foci undergo degeneration.

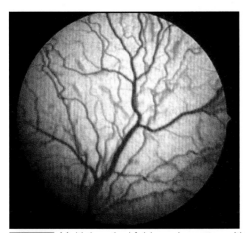

18.30 Multiple retinal folds and rosettes within the tapetal fundus of an American Cocker Spaniel with multifocal retinal dysplasia. (Courtesy NC Buyukmihci)

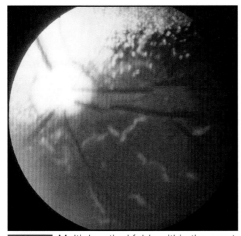

18.31 Multiple retinal folds within the non-tapetal fundus associated with multifocal retinal dysplasia in an English Cocker Spaniel.

Geographical retinal dysplasia: In geographical retinal dysplasia, larger circumscribed horseshoe-shaped or approximately circular areas are typically observed within the tapetal fundus, generally in close association with the dorsal retinal vasculature. The abnormal dysplastic areas may include regions of retinal detachment, tapetal hyper-reflectivity and hyperpigmentation (Figure 18.32). Breeds in which these more

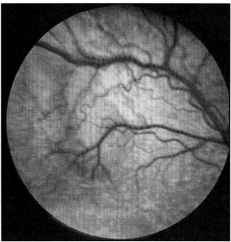

18.32 Area of geographical retinal dysplasia within the tapetal fundus of an adult English Springer Spaniel.

extensive geographical lesions are commonly seen include English Springer Spaniels, Labrador and Golden Retrievers and Cavalier King Charles Spaniels. As with multifocal retinal dysplasia, the appearance of these lesions may alter throughout life. Generally, geographical lesions become more obvious with the passage of time as the degenerative changes contribute to greater distinction between dysplastic and adjacent normal retinal tissue. In addition, focal or total retinal detachment or intravitreal haemorrhage may occur within the first few years of life as infrequent complications of geographical retinal dysplasia (Lavach *et al.*, 1978). As chorioretinal scars (see below) may mimic lesions of geographical retinal dysplasia and *vice versa*, controversy exists as to whether lesions with this appearance represent post-inflammatory changes or are caused by focal areas of choroidal or retinal ischaemia/necrosis, rather than true dysplasia.

Total retinal dysplasia: In the most severe form, total retinal dysplasia, there is congenital infundibular detachment or non-attachment of the retina, which is seen as greyish folds floating behind the lens (Figure 18.33).

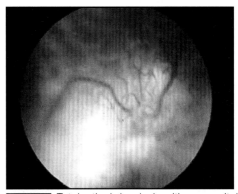

18.33 Total retinal dysplasia with congenital non-attachment of the retina in a Labrador puppy with oculoskeletal dysplasia. The neurosensory retina lies just posterior to the lens and is visible through the dilated pupil as grey folds. (Courtesy of NC Buyukmihci)

Implications for vision: The clinically appreciable effect on vision depends on lesion severity and whether one or both eyes are affected. In its mildest form, retinal dysplasia does not noticeably affect vision. However, extensive multifocal or geographical retinal dysplasia may lead to significant visual impairment, and total retinal dysplasia invariably results in blindness which is frequently associated with a 'searching' nystagmus. Secondary complications associated with retinal dysplasia include intraocular haemorrhage, cataract and secondary glaucoma.

Heritability and disease control: Primary retinal dysplasia may occur sporadically in any breed; however, those breeds in which the disease is frequently encountered include the Labrador Retriever, American Cocker Spaniel, English Springer Spaniel and the Cavalier King Charles Spaniel (Figure 18.34). In most affected breeds which have been adequately studied, the condition is considered to be recessively inherited (Rubin, 1968; MacMillan and Lipton, 1978; Schmidt *et al.*, 1979; Meyers *et al.*, 1983; Carrig *et al.*, 1988; Long and Crispin, 1999). However, recent unpublished studies in Golden Retrievers indicate that geographical retinal dysplasia is not inherited in a recessive manner (C Mellersh, personal communication) and the inherited basis of geographical retinal dysplasia remains somewhat controversial.

Form of retinal dysplasia	Breeds affected
Focal/multifocal	**American Cocker Spaniel** **Cavalier King Charles Spaniel** **English Springer Spaniel** **Golden Retriever** Hungarian Puli **Labrador Retriever** [a] Rottweiler
Total	Bedlington Terrier Sealyham Terrier **Labrador Retriever** [a] (OSD) Samoyed (OSD)

18.34 Breeds affected by inherited retinal dysplasia according to the BVA/KC/ISDS eye scheme. Breeds in which retinal dysplasia appears to be common are indicated in bold text. [a] Note that multifocal retinal dysplasia in the Labrador Retriever, although common, does not appear to be related to the genetic mutation responsible for oculoskeletal dysplasia (OSD) in the UK. In other countries in which oculoskeletal dysplasia is more prevalent, heterozygous animals may demonstrate only multifocal or focal retinal dysplasia.

Distinct genetic mutations responsible for oculoskeletal dysplasia in Labrador Retrievers and Samoyeds have been identified and molecular genetic tests are commercially available (see Chapter 4). In these breeds, it has been shown that heterozygotes may demonstrate a relatively mild spectrum of ocular disease, ranging from vitreous strands and focal or multifocal retinal dysplasia to more severe geographical regions of dysplasia, but they do not demonstrate skeletal abnormalities (Goldstein *et al.*, 2010). However, this genetic mutation does not appear to be prevalent in the UK dog population and multifocal retinal dysplasia

probably represents a separate disease entity in the British Labrador Retriever.

As with many forms of retinal disease, problems exist in the interpretation of ophthalmoscopic findings. In particular, areas of focal, multifocal or geographical retinal dysplasia associated with tapetal reflectivity and hyperpigmentation may prove difficult to distinguish from post-inflammatory lesions. In breeds known to be affected by inherited forms of retinal dysplasia (e.g. the English Springer Spaniel), lesions of this type should be viewed with suspicion, especially if bilateral (although unilateral lesions are common), and particularly if the lesions are closely associated with the superior retinal vasculature. Transient retinal folds may be observed in immature dogs of any breed, possibly as a result of disparity between the rates of growth of the tissues of the neurosensory retina and the outer layer of the optic cup, and disappear with age. Results of an investigation conducted in a number of affected breeds in the USA suggested that lesions of retinal dysplasia, in particular the so-called geographical form, may not be ophthalmoscopically visible until the animal is 6–18 months old (Holle *et al.*, 1999). However, as previously discussed, multifocal forms may become less obvious as the animal matures. The screening of puppies has therefore been recommended at 4–6 and 10–12 weeks old (Crispin *et al.*, 1999), together with later examination which may help distinguish mismatched growth of fundus layers from genuine dysplasia and may help ensure that lesions of retinal dysplasia do not go undetected.

Generalized progressive retinal atrophy in dogs
This is an important cause of inherited blindness in pedigree dogs. Generalized progressive retinal atrophy (GPRA) is a broad, general term encompassing a range of different diseases in which rod and/or cone photoreceptors either fail to develop normally (photoreceptor dysplasia) or degenerate prematurely following normal postnatal photoreceptor maturation (photoreceptor dystrophy or degeneration). Although genotypically and phenotypically heterogeneous, the vast majority of these disorders are characterized by bilateral degeneration of the neurosensory retina with gradual loss of vision, ultimately progressing to complete blindness.

Clinical features: Typically, GPRA is first recognized as night blindness (nyctalopia) with subsequent progression to complete blindness, even under bright lighting conditions. Much rarer are forms of inherited day blindness associated with pure cone degeneration, in which vision in dim light is preserved and affected animals demonstrate photophobia and become day blind early in life. Both the age of onset of clinical signs and the rate of progression of loss of vision differ amongst breeds as well as affected individuals. Specific breed-related differences in clinical presentation have been reviewed in detail elsewhere (Curtis, 1988; Millichamp, 1990; Clements *et al.*, 1996; Narfström and Petersen-Jones, 2007) and detailed descriptions are beyond the scope of the chapter.

Characteristic ophthalmoscopic findings, irrespective of the form of GPRA, include retinal vascular attenuation and diffuse tapetal hyper-reflectivity (Figure 18.35). Progressive attenuation of the superficial retinal vasculature, initially recognized as a reduction in the number and narrowing of retinal arterioles, proceeds to a loss of retinal venules in the later stages of the disease process. In the early stages of the degenerative process, altered tapetal granularity or altered coloration, often in a radial or striated pattern, may be noted within the peripheral tapetal fundus. Subsequently, tapetal hyper-reflectivity develops as a result of thinning of the neurosensory retina. Although the primary defect in GPRA lies within the photoreceptors, RPE atrophy or hypertrophy with intraretinal migration of RPE cells may be observed in very advanced stages of the disease. This leads to a mottled appearance of the non-tapetal fundus (Figure 18.36). Ultimately, secondary optic atrophy may also be observed (Figure 18.35).

PLRs may be reduced and the pupils of affected dogs frequently appear relatively dilated under normal lighting conditions. However, it should be borne in mind that PLRs may be retained long after functional vision has been lost. Secondary cataract formation is a common finding in advanced cases of GPRA and several of the breeds commonly affected by GPRA also exhibit forms of inherited cataract (see Chapters 4 and 16). Hence, ERG (see above) plays a vital role in evaluating retinal function, particularly in 'at risk' breeds, prior to embarking on cataract surgery.

Breed incidence and disease control: In the UK, GPRA is most commonly encountered in the Toy and Miniature Poodle, the Labrador Retriever and the English Cocker Spaniel. However, a wide range of breeds and even crossbreeds such as the Cockapoo and Labradoodle are known to be affected by GPRA in the UK and worldwide. Although dominant and X-linked forms of PRA have been described, most forms of GPRA encountered in clinical veterinary practice demonstrate a simple autosomal recessive mode of inheritance. In recent years, significant advances have been made in the understanding of the molecular genetics of canine GPRA, many mutations have been identified and molecular genetic tests are now available to facilitate control of GPRA in a number of affected breeds (see Chapter 4 for further details).

Feline progressive retinal atrophy

An autosomal dominant form of early-onset retinal degeneration has been established within a breeding colony and extensively characterized in the Abyssinian cat (Barnett and Curtis, 1985). Affected individuals already show abnormal photoreceptor development at 22 days of age and at 4–6 weeks dilated pupils and an intermittent rotary nystagmus may be observed. At approximately 8 weeks of age, ophthalmoscopic changes appear in the central parts of the fundus primarily, and these spread peripherally within another few weeks. The disease leads to generalized complete retinal degeneration, usually within the first 3–4 months of life. Further characterization of the dystrophy has demonstrated that the photoreceptors never develop normally, and the disease has therefore been designated as a rod–cone dysplasia (and designated *Rdy*) with early-onset degeneration of both the cones and rods (Leon and Curtis, 1990). The molecular genetic basis for *Rdy* has now been elucidated (Menotti-Raymond *et al.*, 2010b; see Chapter 4). Extensive screening of cat breeds from all over the world has failed to detect any other domestic feline breeds with the disease allele.

Another congenital feline retinal disease has been described in Persian cats (Rah *et al.*, 2005). This is also a rod–cone dysplasia, but the disease demonstrates an autosomal recessive mode of inheritance. Affected individuals show clinical signs of disease 2–3 weeks after birth and clinical blindness at 16 weeks of age. The photoreceptors in affected individuals never reach full maturity. The molecular genetic defect for this disorder has not as yet been elucidated.

An autosomal recessive disease, with the gene symbol *rdAc*, has been thoroughly studied over three decades, mainly in Scandinavia, but it has

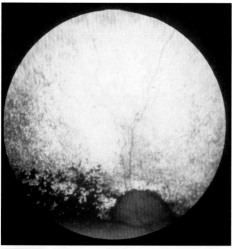

18.35 Advanced GPRA in a Miniature Poodle with pronounced attenuation of the retinal vasculature.

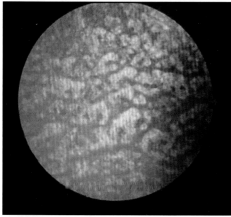

18.36 Mottled pigmentation within the non-tapetal fundus of a dog with advanced GPRA. (Courtesy of NC Buyukmihci)

been shown that the disease occurs worldwide in Abyssinian and Somali cats (Narfström *et al.*, 2009). The molecular genetic basis of *rdAc* has been established (Menotti-Raymond *et al.*, 2007). Further, it has been shown that the gene mutation is prevalent in many other breeds of cat (Menotti-Raymond *et al.*, 2010a) and specifically in the Siamese, in which a high allele frequency has been observed (approximately 33%). This indicates that breeding between Abyssinians and Siamese cats probably occurred in the past.

At birth, cats affected with the *rdAc* mutation have a normal fundus appearance (Figure 18.37) and vision, but by 1.5–2 years of age they develop early funduscopic changes (Figure 18.38; Narfström, 1985). Affected cats demonstrate significantly reduced retinal function by 7 months of age, as determined by ERG (Kang-Derwent *et al.*, 2006; Padnick-Silver *et al.*, 2006), and rod photoreceptor outer segments exhibit the first signs of disorganization at around the same age (Narfström and Nilsson, 1989). Progression of the disease results in further degeneration of the rods, followed by disruption of the cone photoreceptors, until end-stage disease is

typically reached by 3–5 years of age, with generalized photoreceptor degeneration and retinal atrophy (Figures 18.39 and 18.40) leading to complete blindness. In a large population genetic survey of 846 cats, the *rdAc* mutation was found in a total of 34% of 41 cat breeds examined and there was significant distribution of the mutation in both the USA and Europe (Menotti-Raymond *et al.*, 2010a).

A hereditary retinal degeneration has also been observed, through clinical and morphological studies at the University of California-Davis, in the Bengal cat population (Narfström *et al.*, 2010). The disease is under further investigation but appears to be an early-onset primary photoreceptor disorder, leading to blindness within the first year of life. Genetic mapping and further characterization of the presumed genetic disorder are in progress.

Canine multifocal retinopathy
This is an unusual retinopathy, characterized by the appearance of multifocal well circumscribed grey to tan lesions throughout the fundus of puppies and young dogs. The lesions may have a slightly raised, bullous appearance. These lesions rarely progress

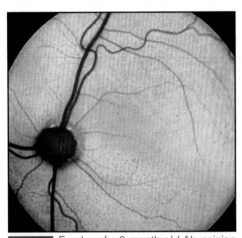

18.37 Fundus of a 6-month-old Abyssinian homozygous for the *rdAc* PRA mutation. Note that the fundus still has a normal appearance.

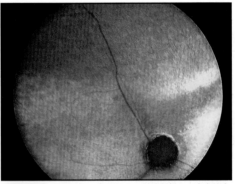

18.39 Fundus of a 6-year-old Abyssinian homozygous for the *rdAc* PRA mutation. The disease is at an advanced stage. Note the generalized hyper-reflectivity and discoloration of the tapetal fundus and the severe vascular attenuation.

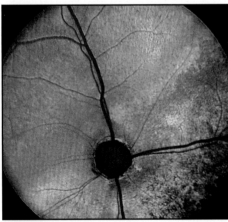

18.38 Fundus of a 2-year-old Abyssinian homozygous for the *rdAc* mutation. The disease is at a moderately advanced stage with generalized discoloration of the tapetal fundus and slight vascular attenuation. (Reproduced from Narfström *et al.*, 2011 *Veterinary Ophthalmology* **14**(Supple.1) 30–36 with permission)

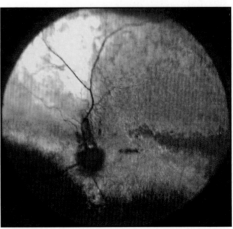

18.40 Fundus of an 8-year-old Siamese homozygous for the *rdAc* PRA mutation. The disease is at an advanced stage. Note the generalized hyper-reflectivity and discoloration of the tapetal fundus and the severe vascular attenuation. (Reproduced from Narfström *et al.*, 2009 *Veterinary Ophthalmology* **12**(5) 288–291 with permission)

beyond 1 year of age or reach a degree of severity that has a significant impact on vision in companion animals, although they may be associated with variable degrees of focal degeneration of the neurosensory retina. The lesions of canine multifocal retinopathy (cmr) should be differentiated from chorioretinal scars and retinal dysplasia, both of which have a similar clinical appearance. The condition is inherited as an autosomal recessive trait. Mutations in the *bestrophin* gene (designated *cmr1* and *cmr2*) have been identified as being responsible for this retinopathy in a number of breeds, including the Great Pyrenees and Mastiff breeds and the Coton du Tulear, respectively (Grahn and Cullen, 2001; Grahn *et al.*, 2008; Zangerl *et al.*, 2010).

Retinal dystrophy in Briards

Congenital hereditary retinal dystrophy, characterized by night blindness and variable day blindness, has been described in Scandinavian Briards (Narfström *et al.*, 1994) with sporadic reports of the disease in Briards in the USA and France. Low amplitude or non-recordable electroretinograms are diagnostic for this disease in 5-week-old puppies (Narfström *et al.*, 1994). However, no distinctive ophthalmoscopic changes are observed in this disease until the animal is at least 2–3 years old. Often, a subtle alteration in the tapetal colour or sheen is observed, which may be followed by the development of focal yellow–white spots throughout the fundus (Narfström, 1999). Although there generally appears to be little clinical evidence of deterioration in vision in affected animals (and the disease is also known as congenital stationary night blindness or CSNB), histological changes have been shown to be progressive. The disease shows an autosomal recessive mode of inheritance but with varying expression. A mutation in the *RPE65* gene, which codes for a protein involved in RPE retinoid metabolism, has been identified as the cause of this form of retinal dystrophy (Veske *et al.*, 1999).

Although not commonly encountered in clinical veterinary practice, the canine disease has been extensively studied as a model for a human disease associated with a similar mutation. The model is of particular importance because it provided the first successful demonstration of retinal gene therapy as a means to restore visual function in eyes comparable in size to those of humans with a similar disease (Narfström *et al.*, 2003; Acland *et al.*, 2005).

Acquired conditions

Sudden acquired retinal degeneration syndrome

Sudden acquired retinal degeneration syndrome (SARDS) refers to a canine clinical syndrome that is quite commonly recognized in middle-aged and older dogs, in which an acute onset of blindness is associated with a complete absence of photoreceptor activity on ERG. In SARDS-affected dogs, vision is usually lost within days or, at most, within a few weeks of the owner first observing that their pet is visually impaired. Most affected dogs demonstrate moderately dilated pupils under normal lighting conditions, with slow, incomplete PLRs to intense blue light stimuli and absent PLRs to red light and weak white light sources (Grozdanic *et al.*, 2007). In the early stages of the disease process, the fundus appears normal on ophthalmoscopy, although, over a period of months, vascular attenuation and alteration of tapetal reflectivity become apparent. Ultimately, in SARDS-affected dogs, degeneration of the neurosensory retina leads to an ophthalmoscopic appearance which becomes indistinguishable from advanced retinal degeneration associated with other disorders such as GPRA. In the early stages, prior to the development of funduscopic changes, SARDS may be distinguished from other causes of acute-onset blindness in which there are no funduscopic abnormalities (e.g. retrobulbar optic neuritis or CNS disease) using ERG (Montgomery *et al.*, 2008). In SARDS, because the photoreceptors are no longer functioning, the electroretinogram trace is extinguished.

SARDS typically affects middle-aged or older dogs (van der Woerdt *et al.*, 1991). Dogs of any breed or sex may be affected; however, affected animals are often obese or have a recent history of weight gain. In addition, many SARDS-affected dogs have a history of polyuria and polydipsia. It is not uncommon for affected dogs to demonstrate haematological or serum biochemical abnormalities, such as neutrophilia, lymphopenia and elevations in serum liver enzyme values. A proportion of dogs also show abnormal responses to adrenocorticotropic hormone stimulation or dexamethasone suppression tests, which suggests an association between SARDS and hyperadrenocorticism (Holt *et al.*, 1999). Serum levels of cortisol and sex hormones were found to be elevated in a significant number of dogs with SARDS in a recent study (Carter *et al.*, 2009).

It has been demonstrated that the initial retinal morphological abnormalities in SARDS are restricted to the photoreceptor layer, with subsequent degeneration of other layers of the neurosensory retina only occurring very late in the course of the disease (Miller *et al.*, 1998). However, the diagnosis of SARDS may encompass a spectrum of retinopathies. Although an immune-mediated attack on photoreceptors has been implicated in at least some cases, and intravenous or intravitreal immunoglobulin therapy (which is not without the risk of very serious complications) has been proposed, the underlying cause of the photoreceptor loss observed in SARDS remains unclear in the majority of cases. Unfortunately, there is currently no treatment for this disorder which has proven to be consistently safe and effective, and the majority of affected animals remain permanently blind (Spurlock and Prittie, 2011). Fortunately, with time most animals learn to compensate for their sudden loss of vision and maintain an acceptable quality of life.

Retinal detachment

Clinical and pathological features: The neurosensory retina is only firmly attached at the ONH and the ora ciliaris retinae; between these points the attachment is relatively weak, relying on the close apposition between the photoreceptors and the microvillous processes of the underlying RPE and the support of the vitreous. Thus, detachment almost always reflects separation of the neurosensory retina from the RPE, rather than detachment of the entire retina from the posterior globe. In cases with giant retinal tears and total detachment of the retina, the neurosensory retina may become disinserted from the ora ciliaris retinae peripherally, only remaining attached at the ONH (Figure 18.41).

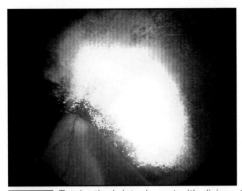

18.41 Total retinal detachment with disinsertion from the ora ciliaris retinae in a 9-year-old Shih Tzu with vitreous degeneration. The detached neurosensory retina hangs inferiorly, draped over the ONH. Absence of neurosensory retina from the superior fundus results in pronounced tapetal hyper-reflectivity.

On ophthalmoscopy, areas of detachment may appear as focal grey areas within the tapetal fundus (with local reduction in tapetal reflectivity; Figure 18.42) or non-tapetal fundus (where they appear paler than the surrounding area). More extensive retinal detachments are no longer observed within the normal plane of the retina and appear as greyish billowing folds, with surface blood vessels appearing progressively out of focus as they billow towards the observer (Figure 18.43). In tapetal regions of the fundus where the neurosensory retina is absent as a result of tearing, holes or disinsertion, hyper-reflectivity may be noted.

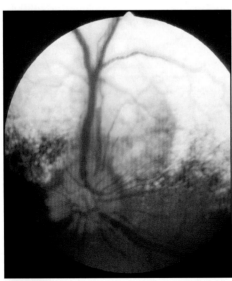

18.42 Focal area of exudative retinal detachment superior to the ONH in a dog.

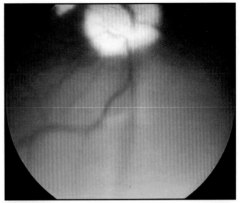

18.43 Idiopathic extensive serous/exudative detachment involving most of the inferior retina, which remains attached at the ora ciliaris retinae and ONH, in a German Shepherd Dog. No underlying infectious cause was identified and the detachment resolved in response to immunosuppressive corticosteroids.

Retinal detachment may be classified according to the extent of retinal involvement as focal, multifocal or total. Focal areas of detachment may not be associated with clinically appreciable visual impairment, but total detachment is inevitably associated with blindness and reduced or absent PLRs (in all but the most acute cases) in the affected eye. Potential secondary complications of retinal detachment include preretinal and intravitreal haemorrhage or hyphaema, cataract and glaucoma. Glaucoma following retinal detachment (or retinal detachment surgery) may occur for a number of reasons. Haemorrhage, inflammatory cells or free photoreceptors may obstruct the aqueous outflow pathways (Smith *et al.*, 1997), as may the preiridal fibrovascular membranes that form in response to retinal hypoxia (Dubielzig *et al.*, 2010a).

Causes of detachment: The causes of retinal detachment are summarized in Figure 18.44. Congenital retinal detachment (or non-attachment)

Predisposing factor	Examples
Congenital malformation	Collie eye anomaly; coloboma; staphyloma; retinal dysplasia
Choroidal and/or subretinal infiltrates and exudates	Chorioretinitis; neoplasia
Vasculopathy	Hypertension; hyperviscosity; vasculitis
Trauma	Blunt or penetrating trauma
Vitreoretinal traction	Posterior segment inflammation; vitreous dysplasia or degeneration; vitreal haemorrhage
Lens disease	Luxation; hypermature cataract
Retinal thinning	Peripheral cystoid degeneration; generalized progressive retinal atrophy
Globe/retinal stretching	Chronic glaucoma
Idiopathic	Serous retinal detachment

18.44 Causes of retinal detachment.

may be recognized in association with disorders such as retinal dysplasia or CEA (see above). Acquired retinal detachment may also be classified in terms of the pathophysiology of the detachment.

Exudative or serous detachment: This is caused by the accumulation of fluid or cellular infiltrates within the potential 'subretinal space' which exists between the neurosensory retina and the RPE, and thus separates the two layers. This may occur as a result of choroidal inflammatory and vascular disease and is the most common form of retinal detachment encountered in small animal patients. Causes of exudative or serous retinal detachments include:

- Chorioretinitis
- Vascular disease related to hypertension, hyperviscosity syndrome, diabetes mellitus and coagulopathies (see below and Chapter 20)
- Neoplasia
- Idiopathic.

Idiopathic serous retinal detachments are generally bilateral and appear to occur more commonly in German Shepherd Dogs and their crossbreeds than other canine breeds. This form of serous retinal detachment often responds favourably to immunosuppressive therapy (Andrew *et al.*, 1997). Occasionally, more solid detachments are observed due to elevation of the retina by dense infiltrates of granulomatous inflammatory or neoplastic cells from the choroid or retrobulbar space (see Figure 18.53).

Rhegmatogenous detachment: This is caused by tears in the neurosensory retina which allow fluid (e.g. liquefied vitreous) to enter the potential 'subretinal space'. The subretinal fluid is then responsible for dissecting the neurosensory retina from the underlying RPE. Rhegmatogenous detachment is relatively common in dogs (Hendrix *et al.*, 1993) and may occur as a result of trauma or tearing of the thinned neurosensory retina in cases of advanced retinal degeneration. Displacement, movement or fibroblastic changes within the vitreous body may contribute to the formation of rhegmatogenous retinal detachments. Rhegmatogenous retinal detachment is not uncommon in dogs with hypermature cataract or lens luxation and may occur as a postoperative complication following cataract surgery (see Chapter 16). Tearing of the neurosensory retina may occur in dogs with colobomatous lesions of the fundus, and these tears have been implicated in the development of retinal detachment in cases of CEA (Vainisi *et al.*, 1989).

Giant retinal tears (i.e. those involving >25% of the circumference of the ora ciliaris retinae) are frequently encountered in the Shi Tzu. In this breed, vitreous degeneration and liquefaction, peripheral and generalized retinal degeneration and cataract are all common predisposing factors (Vainisi and Packo, 1995; Itoh *et al.*, 2010). Peripheral cystoid degeneration, which is a common finding at the ora ciliaris retinae of elderly dogs (Figure 18.45), may lead to the formation of splits within the neurosensory retina with separation occurring between the

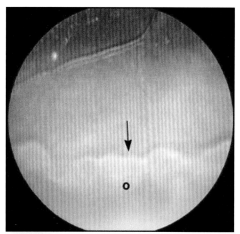

18.45 Peripheral cystoid retinal degeneration (arrowed) involving the ora ciliaris retinae (o) in an elderly dog. (Courtesy of RW Bellhorn)

retinal layers (retinoschisis). This predisposes to tearing of the peripheral retina.

Traction retinal detachment: This occurs when bands comprising inflammatory and/or fibrotic tissue form within the vitreous and subsequently exert anterior traction forces on the neurosensory retina (Figure 18.46). Traction retinal detachments are less common in small animal patients, although they may follow trauma, intraocular haemorrhage or posterior segment inflammation, as a result of the organization of inflammatory infiltrates within the vitreous. Unfortunately, this form of retinal detachment is rarely amenable to medical or surgical therapy in dogs or cats.

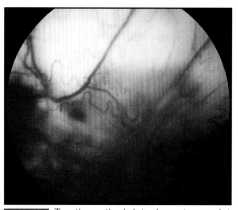

18.46 Traction retinal detachment associated with a migrating vitreoretinal foreign body (grass awn) in a Border Collie.

Treatment and implications for vision: Provided that the underlying cause of detachment is addressed (e.g. by specific treatment of infectious chorioretinitis or systemic hypertension) and that retinal tears have not occurred, areas of serous detachment may reattach. If no specific local or systemic disorder can be identified following a very thorough clinical evaluation, oral prednisolone therapy may be instituted at an immunosuppressive dose (2 mg/kg q24h). Although the time that elapses prior to reattachment of the neurosensory retina may be prolonged, some degree of useful vision may still be regained in dogs, regardless of the subsequent development of ophthalmoscopic signs of multifocal or diffuse retinal degeneration. However, a variable degree of degeneration of the neurosensory retina is to be expected when photoreceptors are separated from the underlying RPE for more than a few days. The prognosis for restoration of vision is poor when there is evidence of significant cellular infiltrate or haemorrhage underlying the detached neurosensory retina (which may be identified on ocular ultrasonography; see Figure 2.17) or within the vitreous.

Surgical repair of rhegmatogenous retinal detachment with retinal disinsertion is possible, but is seldom undertaken in veterinary patients at present, owing to the requirement for advanced microsurgical skills and costly instrumentation (Vainisi *et al.*, 2007). Nevertheless, an increasing number of veterinary ophthalmologists have the facility to perform vitreo-retinal surgery. However, despite advances in the field, outcomes in veterinary patients remain variable and are often disappointing to owners, who are faced with high costs and high rates of postoperative complications, ranging from corneal ulcers and intraocular inflammation, to intraocular haemorrhage, glaucoma and persistent retinal detachment with blindness. Use of prophylactic diode laser retinopexy at the margins of retinal tears is more widespread in specialist veterinary ophthalmology practices, whether delivered through the sclera or using an indirect ophthalmoscope, and this can help to prevent the propagation of retinal detachment in selected patients. Prophylactic retinopexy may be considered in dogs with lens luxation, as an adjunct to lensectomy. Prophylactic retinopexy has also been recommended by some veterinary ophthalmologists prior to performing cataract surgery in the Bichon Frise, a breed that may have a relatively high incidence of postoperative retinal detachment in the USA (Schmidt and Vainisi, 2004). However, a recent study suggests that retinal detachment may not be a significant concern following cataract surgery in the Bichon Frise in the UK (Braus *et al.*, 2012).

Chorioretinitis

Owing to the intimate anatomical relationship between the retina and underlying choroid, inflammatory disease processes rarely affect either structure in isolation. Generally, inflammation affects both the choroid and the retina concurrently and often the inflammatory process within the choroid is predominant, as reflected in the term *chorioretinitis*. As the choroid is also continuous with the structures of the anterior uveal tract, chorioretinitis is often recognized in association with a degree of anterior uveitis, and has a similar range of causes (see Chapter 14). Causes of chorioretinitis in dogs and cats include:

- Many systemic infectious diseases (Figures 18.47 and 18.48)
- Trauma
- Foreign bodies

- Immune-mediated disorders (such as uveodermatological syndrome)
- Neoplasia.

Viral
Canine distemper virus Canine herpesvirus Infectious rhinotonsillitis
Bacterial
Any generalized bacteraemia/septicaemia Leptospirosis Brucellosis Lyme disease
Protozoal
Toxoplasmosis Neosporosis Leishmaniosis
Parasitic
Toxocariasis Angiostrongylosis Ophthalmomyiasis interna posterior (dipteran larvae)
Rickettsial
Ehrlichiosis Rocky Mountain spotted fever
Mycotic
Cryptococcosis Blastomycosis Coccidiodomycosis Histoplasmosis Aspergillosis Geotrichosis
Algal
Protothecosis

18.47 Infectious causes of chorioretinitis in dogs.

Viral
Feline infectious peritonitis (caused by feline coronavirus) Feline panleucopenia virus Feline leukaemia virus Feline immunodeficiency virus
Bacterial
Generalized bacteraemia/septicaemia Mycobacteriosis Bartonellosis
Protozoal
Toxoplasmosis
Parasitic
Ophthalmomyiasis interna posterior (dipteran larvae)
Mycotic
Cryptococcosis Blastomycosis Histoplasmosis Coccidioidomycosis Candidiasis

18.48 Infectious causes of chorioretinitis in cats.

Specific disorders associated with canine and feline chorioretinitis are reviewed in greater detail in Chapters 14 and 20 and elsewhere (Cullen and Webb, 2007ab; Narfström and Petersen-Jones, 2007; Stiles and Townsend, 2007).

Clinical and pathological features: Chorioretinitis may be unilateral or (as is more often the case with systemic infectious disorders) bilateral. However, the lesions of chorioretinitis are rarely bilaterally symmetrical. In the acute stages of chorioretinitis, ophthalmoscopic findings may include irregular greyish, ill defined areas of inflammatory cell infiltrates. These lesions may be focal, multifocal or perivascular in location (Figures 18.49 to 18.52). Cellular infiltrates and more diffuse areas of retinal oedema may be recognized as areas of reduced reflectivity within the tapetal fundus and as pale, greyish areas within the non-tapetal fundus (Figure 18.52). A variable degree of detachment of the neurosensory retina may occur where inflammation and exudation are severe (see above), leading to impairment of vision. Severe inflammation may also lead to retinal or intravitreal haemorrhage (see Figure 18.72), and secondary vitreal involvement may lead to vitreous haze or the accumulation of inflammatory material within the vitreous, with subsequent vitreous degeneration

and liquefaction. Chorioretinitis may also be associated with inflammation of the optic nerve (see below). Particularly in mycotic diseases, well demarcated raised subretinal granulomas with deviation of the overlying retinal vasculature may be observed (Figure 18.53). However, with the possible exception of cryptococcosis (Figure 18.50), systemic mycoses are very unlikely to be encountered in dogs and cats in the UK.

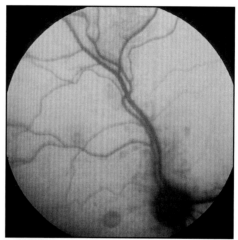

18.51 Multifocal chorioretinal inflammatory lesions with subretinal effusion in a Domestic Shorthaired cat with toxoplasmosis. (Courtesy of S Crispin)

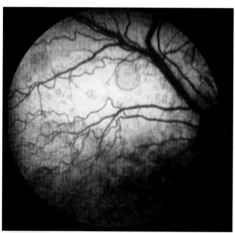

18.49 Active chorioretinitis in a dog with distemper. (Courtesy of NC Buyukmihci)

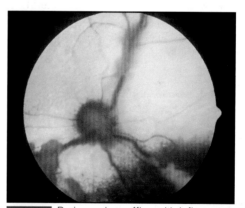

18.52 Perivascular cuffing with inflammatory infiltrates in a 14-month-old cat with feline infectious peritonitis. (Courtesy of S Crispin)

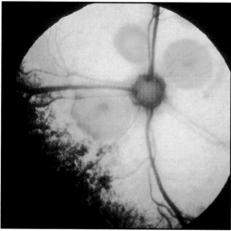

18.50 Multifocal circular areas of active chorioretinitis in a cat with *Cryptococcus neoformans* infection.

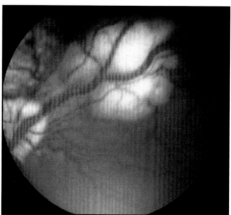

18.53 Large white subretinal granuloma superior to the ONH in a dog with ocular and systemic blastomycosis. (Courtesy of NC Buyukmihci)

In the more chronic stages of chorioretinitis, degeneration of the neurosensory retina may lead to regions of tapetal hyper-reflectivity, often associated with well demarcated hyperpigmented foci due to hypertrophy and migration of RPE cells (Figure 18.54). Within the non-tapetal fundus, areas of depigmentation may be observed. More extensive depigmentation of the retina and choroid may be encountered in animals with uveodermatological syndrome (Figure 18.55). Small, localized, focal post-inflammatory lesions are rarely associated with clinically appreciable impairment of vision and may be observed as an incidental finding in dogs and cats with no history of prior ocular or systemic disease (Figure 18.56). However, widespread degeneration of the neurosensory retina in more severely affected patients can lead to permanent, severe visual impairment or even total blindness.

Treatment and implications for vision: As chorioretinitis frequently represents an ocular manifestation of a systemic disease process, affected animals should be subjected to a thorough general clinical examination. The presence of other ocular, neurological or systemic signs may arouse a high degree of clinical suspicion for a particular disorder (e.g. in cases of canine distemper virus infection). Where possible, every effort should be made to investigate, identify and address any underlying systemic disorder (see Chapters 3, 14 and 20). In those rare

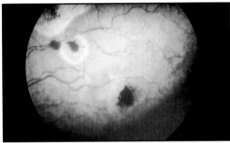

18.54 Post-inflammatory chorioretinopathy within the peripheral tapetal fundus of a Jack Russell Terrier. These well circumscribed hyper-reflective lesions surrounding foci of pigment migration were considered inactive and of unknown cause. These lesions were non-progressive but did have a modest effect on vision.

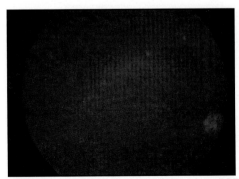

18.55 Extensive depigmentation of the RPE and choroid in a Jack Russell Terrier with chronic uveodermatological syndrome. This region had previously been densely pigmented but the choroidal vascular pattern is now visible. The tapetal reflection was also lost in this dog.

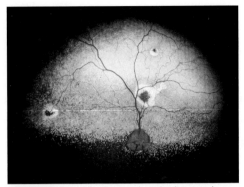

18.56 Small focal chorioretinal scars (cause unknown) were an incidental finding in this otherwise normal adult mixed-breed dog and had no demonstrable effect on vision. Note that the retinal blood vessels are not altered in their calibre or course over these lesions, which suggests that the inner retinal layers remain intact. (Courtesy of the University of California-Davis Ophthalmology Service)

cases in which mycotic disease is suspected as the cause of very severe posterior segment disease, vitreous or subretinal paracentesis may allow identification of the fungal organism. Although systemic anti-inflammatory therapy is generally warranted, systemic corticosteroids are generally contraindicated in the management of chorioretinitis associated with infectious disease processes and they should therefore be used with great caution. Systemic therapy with non-steroidal anti-inflammatory drugs (NSAIDs) may be of benefit, but topically administered medications seldom reach therapeutic concentrations in the choroid and retina. Attendant anterior uveitis should be investigated and managed appropriately (see Chapter 14).

Retinal vascular disease

The transparency of the ocular media affords the clinician an unparalleled opportunity to visualize abnormalities of the vascular system directly and non-invasively. Retinal vascular distension, tortuosity and haemorrhage are examples of relatively commonly observed abnormalities that may be noted on ophthalmoscopic examination of the fundus and which may indicate a severe underlying systemic vascular disease (Lane *et al.*, 1993).

Coagulopathies: Quantitative and qualitative disorders affecting platelet function and disorders of the intrinsic and extrinsic coagulation pathways, including inherited and immune-mediated coagulopathies and toxicity, may lead to retinal haemorrhage. The ophthalmoscopic appearance of retinal haemorrhage has previously been described in detail. In some instances, intraocular haemorrhage can be the major presenting sign of potentially life-threatening systemic bleeding disorders (see Chapter 20).

Hypertensive chorioretinopathy in cats:

Clinical and pathological features: Hypertension is a common finding in older cats. The disorder can be categorized as:

- Idiopathic systemic hypertension (in about 20% of cases), in which no underlying cause of the hypertension is found
- Secondary hypertension as a complication of another systemic disease.

Secondary systemic hypertension is most commonly a complication of renal disease and/or hyperthyroidism, diseases that frequently affect the middle-aged to older feline patient (usually 9–12 year-old cats; Jepson, 2011; Stepien, 2011). In cats with hypertension, ocular signs are prevalent as well as signs of the systemic disease, such as intracranial neurological signs (obtundation, focal facial seizures and photophobia) and auscultable cardiac abnormalities (systolic heart murmurs and gallop rhythms). Frequently, acute blindness is the first indication of systemic hypertension that is identified by cat owners.

Prolonged systemic hypertension leads to sustained vasoconstriction of the retinal arterioles through autoregulation. Beyond a certain critical pressure, this autoregulation breaks down and vascular integrity is severely compromised. There is leakage of plasma and red blood cells when the vessels become damaged and this causes retinal oedema and fluid accumulation. Retinal detachment is associated with plasma effusion from defective choroidal vasculature. In addition, RPE cells undergo ischaemic damage, contributing to retinal detachment (Crispin and Mould, 2001).

Hypertensive chorioretinopathy is observed in 40–65% of cats with systemic hypertension (Stepien, 2011). Abnormalities of the choroid and retina include (Figure 18.57):

- Arterial tortuosity
- Oedema
- Pinpoint or large areas of intraretinal, preretinal or subretinal haemorrhage
- Partial or complete serous neuroretinal detachment.

Papilloedema may be present but difficult to evaluate owing to the concurrent retinal detachment and/or hyphaema. The iris and ciliary body may also be affected, leading to bleeding into the vitreous cavity and the posterior and/or anterior chambers of the eye. Hyphaema is most often associated with posterior segment haemorrhage with blood migrating anteriorly through the pupil. Sequelae include anterior or posterior synechiae and secondary glaucoma. Vision loss is often observed by the owner as an initial sign of systemic disease, especially if there is complete retinal detachment with or without hyphaema (Sansom *et al.*, 1994; Stiles *et al.*, 1994; Maggio *et al.*, 2000).

Diagnosis of feline hypertension requires careful measurement of systolic blood pressure (SBP) using Doppler or oscillometric techniques, in conjunction with funduscopic examination, thoracic auscultation and, potentially, electrocardiography and echocardiography. Evaluation of renal and thyroid function is generally also required to determine

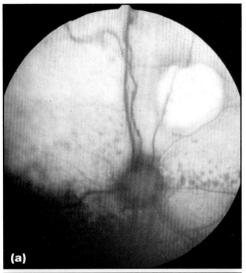

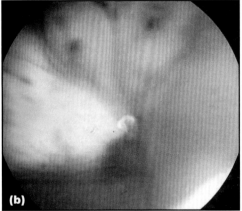

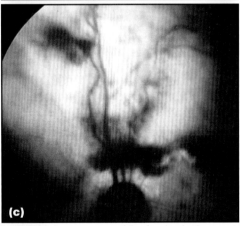

18.57 Appearance of the fundus in three cats with hypertensive chorioretinopathy. **(a)** Multiple grey lesions throughout the tapetal fundus represent areas of subretinal oedema and focal bullous retinal detachment. Note the pinpoint intraretinal haemorrhage and irregular calibre of the main retinal blood vessels. **(b)** There is extensive bullous retinal detachment with haemorrhage and oedema of the neurosensory retina. **(c)** A previously extensive retinal detachment has largely reattached but extensive subretinal haemorrhage remains, as well as intraretinal and preretinal haemorrhage.

the presence of underlying disease conditions. A diagnosis of hypertension should be strongly considered in a cat with a Doppler forelimb SBP of ≥160 mmHg or an oscillometric tail cuff SBP of ≥140–160 mmHg (Stepien, 2011).

Treatment and implications for vision: Therapy consists of treatment of the underlying cause (Brown *et al.*, 2007; Stepien, 2011). Given that the risk of organ damage is high as long as the blood pressure is above normal, antihypertensive therapy should be administered with the goal of achieving an initial SBP of <160 mmHg as soon as possible and maintenance of SBP around 140 mmHg is preferable. Most commonly, feline hypertension is treated with the calcium-channel blocker, amlodipine, together with angiotensin converting enzyme (ACE) inhibitors. Amlodipine is given at an initial dose of 0.125 mg/kg but can be increased to 0.25 mg/kg q24h. If the hypertension remains uncontrolled, benazepril is typically added, especially if proteinuria and albuminuria are present. Amlodipine has been found to be safe and effective and decreases the SBP by an average of 30–50 mmHg.

Quality of life for the cat is often improved, as well as maintenance of appetite and weight, with effective medical therapy. However, continued regular screening of blood pressure at follow-up examinations is essential in affected cats. With the successful reduction of SBP, the ophthalmic signs are often improved in the long term; partial or even complete reattachment of the neurosensory retina with subsequent chorioretinal scarring are common sequelae. Depending on the length of time for which the retina has been detached, vision may be regained, but some degree of degeneration can be expected. There is some evidence that the feline retina begins to degenerate within the first week of detachment, so prompt diagnosis and treatment of systemic hypertension is always important.

Hypertensive chorioretinopathy in dogs:
Systemic hypertension in the dog may also lead to retinal and choroidal vascular disease. In dogs, hypertension is generally secondary to other disorders (such as renal or endocrine disease), but it may be primary or idiopathic. Associated ocular abnormalities (such as visual impairment or intraocular haemorrhage) may be initial presenting signs in affected dogs (Sansom and Bodey, 1997). Fundic lesions may also be subclinical and identified only on thorough ophthalmoscopic examination of animals diagnosed with hypertension or other underlying conditions (LeBlanc *et al.*, 2011). Fundic lesions which may be observed in hypertensive dogs include:

- Narrowing of the retinal arterioles
- Retinal, subretinal and vitreal haemorrhage (Figure 18.58)
- Retinal oedema and serous detachment
- Papilloedema.

These lesions are consistent with the abnormalities found in hypertensive dogs using fluorescein angiography, which include choroidal (particularly choriocapillary) ischaemia, arteriolar vasoconstriction and subretinal oedema. The response of ocular lesions to appropriate antihypertensive therapy varies considerably and to some extent is likely to be

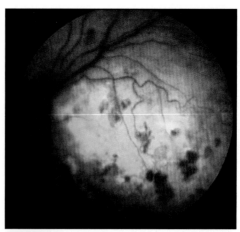

18.58 Retinal haemorrhage, subretinal oedema and multifocal areas of retinal detachment and degeneration in a 9-year-old Labrador Retriever with systemic hypertension. (Courtesy of NC Buyukmihci)

influenced by the duration and aetiopathogenesis of hypertension in individual patients (Villagrasa and Cascales, 2000).

Diabetic retinopathy: In contrast to human diabetic patients, in whom retinal vascular disease is a major cause of blindness, the most common ocular complication of diabetes mellitus in dogs is cataract formation. However, retinal vascular changes have been described in canine patients with long-standing diabetes, and it would appear that the difference in the reported incidence of diabetic retinopathy between the species reflects the difference in the longevity and the duration of the diabetes. With longer survival times post-diagnosis and cataract surgery now commonly performed, allowing visualization of the fundus in diabetic dogs, diabetic retinopathy is now recognized as being quite common in this species. Spontaneous diabetic retinopathy is seldom associated with clinically significant loss of vision in dogs. However, secondary hypertensive vasculopathy may complicate the clinical picture in some animals (see above). Retinal lesions that have been described in diabetic dogs include microaneurysms with irregular variations in the calibre of retinal blood vessels and multifocal retinal haemorrhage. Ultimately, areas of retinal degeneration with associated tapetal hyperreflectivity may become apparent (Barnett, 1981; Muñana, 1995; Landry *et al.*, 2004). The prevalence of retinopathy in diabetic cats, in the absence of systemic hypertension, has not been established or extensively studied.

Hyperviscosity syndrome: Blood or serum hyperviscosity may occur as a result of polycythaemia or hyperproteinaemia (e.g. monoclonal gammopathy related to multiple myeloma). In such cases, the retinal blood vessels may appear tortuous and distended and may demonstrate a characteristic 'sausage-link' or 'box-car' appearance with multiple sacculations due to sludging of blood and formation of aneurysms. Retinal haemorrhage and detachment and vitreal haemorrhage may also be recognized (Figures 18.59 and 18.60).

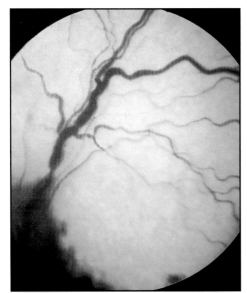

18.59 Retinal vascular changes, haemorrhage and detachment related to hyperviscosity syndrome in a dog with multiple myeloma. Note the sacculated appearance of the superior retinal venules.

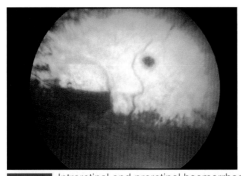

18.60 Intraretinal and preretinal haemorrhage associated with vascular disease and coagulopathy due to multiple myeloma in an adult dog.

Lipaemia retinalis: Raised serum triglycerides, in particular due to hyperchylomicronaemia, may result in the retinal vessels appearing white to pale pink, which is most readily appreciated within the peripheral blood vessels of the pigmented, non-tapetal fundus (Wyman and McKissick, 1973; Crispin, 1993) and in animals with anaemia (Gunn-Moore *et al.*, 1997; Figure 18.61). Lipaemia retinalis is not associated with impairment of vision, but in both dogs and

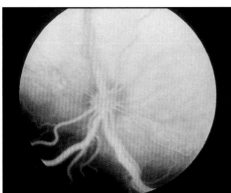

18.61 Lipaemia retinalis in a kitten with primary hyperchylomicronaemia.

cats this fundus abnormality should prompt investigation and characterization of the underlying disorder affecting systemic lipid metabolism.

Fluoroquinolone toxicity in cats
Fluoroquinolones are bactericidal antimicrobial drugs that are widely used in veterinary medicine. Quinolone carboxylic acid derivatives have a broad spectrum of activity against Gram-positive and Gram-negative bacteria, as well as *Mycoplasma* species. Fluoroquinolones are excreted by renal and hepatic routes.

Enrofloxacin: This widely used fluoroquinolone is currently approved for oral dosage in cats at 5 mg/kg/day. Historically, in the 1990s, a flexible, higher dose regimen was approved and independent veterinary surgeons reported an increased incidence of vision-related problems in cats, including blindness, partial blindness and mydriasis, following once daily oral administration of enrofloxacin (Gelatt *et al.*, 2001). In response to the increased incidence of vision-related problems reported, a specific feline safety study was designed to assess clinical and laboratory effects of high-dose oral enrofloxacin in young healthy cats (Ford *et al.*, 2007).

Dramatic changes were observed in the treated cats, with neurological, funduscopic and electroretinographic abnormalities noted in these experimental animals. Funduscopic changes were first noticed in all enrofloxacin-treated cats on or before day 3 as an increased granular appearance and greying of the area centralis, then similar changes along the visual streak. This was followed by generalized vascular attenuation (between days 2 and 4) and then generalized tapetal hyper-reflectivity (between days 5 and 7) (Figure 18.62). ERG was performed before and during the study, and decreases in b wave amplitude were found to precede the funduscopic changes. Morphological changes in the photoreceptor layers were significantly correlated with the duration of enrofloxacin administration, and retinal degenerative changes were generalized following three doses of enrofloxacin. Loss of rod photoreceptors preceded degeneration of cone photoreceptors. The study concluded that high doses of enrofloxacin (50 mg/kg/day) are acutely toxic to the outer retina of normal cats.

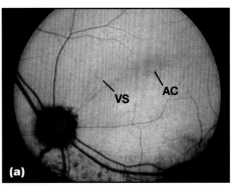

18.62 Fluoroquinolone retinotoxicity. **(a)** Image from a control cat with a normal fundus (day 1). (continues) ▶

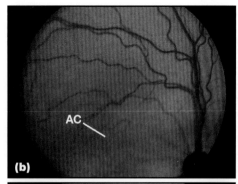

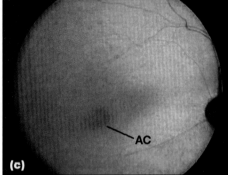

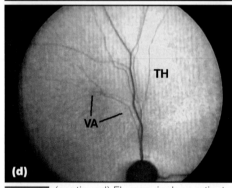

18.62 (continued) Fluoroquinolone retinotoxicity.
(b–d) Serial images of the fundus of a cat treated with enrofloxacin (days 3, 5 and 7). Note the progressive change in granularity and greying of the area centralis (AC) and visual streak (VS), respectively, observed from day 3, vascular attenuation (VA) observed from day 5, and marked tapetal hyper-reflectivity (TH) by day 7.

Although enrofloxacin has been the compound associated with feline retinal degeneration, cats have recently been shown to have a functional defect in ABCG2, a transmembrane transporter that plays a role in limiting access of compounds, including the potentially phototoxic fluoroquinolones, to the retina across the blood–retina barrier (Ramirez et al., 2011). Thus, all of the fluoroquinolones must be considered potentially retinotoxic to cats. Retinal toxicity has been observed following oral administration of very high doses of orbifloxacin to cats, and whilst recently developed fluoroquinolones such as pradofloxacin (Messias et al., 2008) have shown improved safety profiles, the limitations of studying toxic effects in healthy young cats must be borne in mind. Older cats and those with renal or hepatic disease have reduced clearance and increased plasma levels of fluoroquinolones compared with young healthy cats and are, therefore, at an increased risk

of developing adverse responses to these drugs. Other risk factors in cats include dose, duration of treatment and route of administration. Intravenous administration of fluoroquinolones was found to be a contributing factor to retinal toxicity (Wiebe and Hamilton, 2002). It is recommended that fluoro-quinolones, and particularly enrofloxacin, should only be used in cats when no alternative drugs exist. The dose of the drug should be as low as possible and care should be taken to ensure that the recommended dose is not exceeded.

Nutritional retinal degeneration

Taurine deficiency retinopathy: Taurine is an essential amino acid for cats because they have limited ability to synthesize it from cysteine (a precursor amino acid for most animals). The function of taurine is not fully understood, but dietary levels of 500–750 ppm have been suggested for normal retinal function (Sturman, 1978). Normally, taurine is obtained from milk products, liver, shellfish and fish products, and sufficient amounts are usually available for cats in the wild. However, cats that spend their entire lives indoors need daily supplementation. Dietary levels of taurine have been increased in commercial cat food in recent years, making taurine deficiency unusual, but, on occasion, cats may still be presented with a nutritional retinopathy due to taurine deficiency when fed vegetarian or home-made non-commercial diets. It is also conceivable that some cats may have a lower capacity for absorption of dietary taurine.

Taurine deficiency retinopathy (also called feline central retinal degeneration, FCRD) has a characteristic appearance (Leon et al., 1995). Early changes are most often observed in the area centralis, which develops a greyish discoloration (Figure 18.63a). Later in the disease process, this colour change becomes more pronounced and turns into an elliptical area of hyper-reflectivity (Figure 18.63b). Over time, if the deficiency lasts for several months, changes also occur on the nasal side of the ONH. These two areas coalesce with progression into a

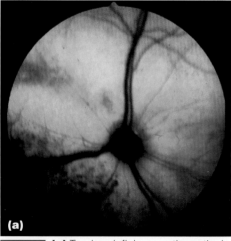

18.63 **(a)** Taurine deficiency retinopathy in a 2-year-old cat. Note the greyish discoloration along the visual streak. (continues) ▶

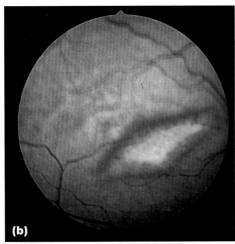

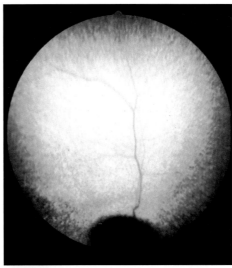

18.63 (continued) **(b)** Taurine deficiency retinopathy in a 3-year-old cat. Note that the area centralis region is hyper-reflective and bordered by greyish discoloration.

18.65 End-stage retinal degeneration in a 10-year-old European Shorthaired cat.

hyper-reflective band with greyish borders (Figure 18.64). Later, these changes spread superiorly and inferiorly from the hyper-reflective band until the entire fundus becomes hyper-reflective/atrophic. End-stage retinopathy due to taurine deficiency is difficult to differentiate from end-stage hereditary retinal degeneration (Figure 18.65).

Whilst ophthalmoscopic signs of retinopathy do not appear until after 3–7 months of dietary deficiency, electroretinographic changes in cone responses have been described early in the deficiency state (within 5 weeks) with increased implicit time and decreased amplitude of the a and b waves. Both cone and rod function deteriorates over about 10 weeks of deficiency. These deficits are associated with histological changes, which are more severe in the outer retina first. The retinal effects of taurine deficiency are only partially reversible. The degenerative changes in the photoreceptor outer segments may be reversed, especially in rods, although, when there is degeneration of large areas of photoreceptor cells, such as in the atrophic areas

with hyper-reflectivity, these changes are permanent. Thus, suspicion of retinal degeneration in the cat warrants thorough assessment of the dietary history and evaluation of blood taurine levels. Taurine deficiency has been linked with feline cardiomyopathy and it is important, therefore, that cardiac function is also evaluated in cats with signs of this retinopathy (Hayes and Trautwein, 1989).

Vitamin E deficiency: The long-term feeding of vitamin E-deficient diets to dogs leads to the development of a pigmentary retinopathy which is clinically and pathologically indistinguishable from retinal pigment epithelial dystrophy (RPED; see below) (Riis *et al.*, 1981). A relative deficiency of vitamin E may be encountered in dogs that have severe fat malabsorption syndromes associated with exocrine pancreatic, hepatobiliary or gastrointestinal disease, or are fed poor quality, high fat diets (Davidson *et al.*, 1998), particularly those diets that have a high content of polyunsaturated fatty acids.

Retinal pigment epithelial dystrophy
RPED is a progressive retinal degeneration, previously known as central progressive retinal atrophy (CPRA), which has been described in several breeds of dog in the UK. Breeds in which the condition has been reported include the Cocker Spaniel, Border Collie, Golden and Labrador Retriever, Smooth and Rough Collie, Briard (Barnett, 1969, 1976; Bedford, 1984) and the Polish Lowland Sheepdog or Nizzini (Watson *et al.*, 1993). Although this breed predisposition implies an inherited basis for the disease, a specific mode of inheritance has not yet been elucidated.

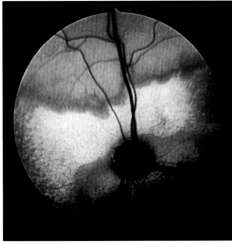

18.64 Taurine deficiency retinopathy in a 5-year-old cat. A hyper-reflective/atrophic band is seen, spanning the area of the visual streak.

Clinical and pathological features: Typically, animals affected with RPED suffer a slowly progressive loss of central vision. The age of onset and rate of progression of this disease are variable and complete blindness may or may not result. Clinical signs are generally not apparent until affected animals are 2–6 years of age. However, as the early stages of

RPED are not associated with significant visual impairment, it is likely that the disease is frequently overlooked until later in its course (Parry, 1954). In some cases, the disease may become stationary, with no progression from mid-stage for several years, whilst in others complete blindness may result within 12 months.

RPED is characterized ophthalmoscopically by the appearance of light brown pigment spots and patches within the central tapetal fundus (Figure 18.66), which progressively increase in number, coalesce and become associated with patchy areas of tapetal hyper-reflectivity and vascular attenuation. Lesions are initially more severe within the central, temporal region of the tapetal fundus, becoming more widespread across the whole tapetal fundus as the disease progresses. Optic nerve atrophy, pigmentary disturbances within the non-tapetal fundus and the development of secondary cortical cataract are inconsistent findings in RPED and, if they occur, are generally only recognized in advanced stages of the disease process.

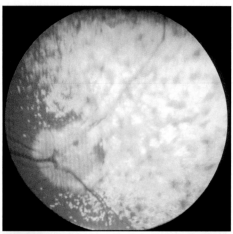

18.66 RPED in an English Cocker Spaniel with hypovitaminosis E. Multiple foci of light brown pigment are visible throughout the tapetal fundus and are associated with retinal degeneration (signalled by attenuation of the retinal blood vessels and mottled tapetal hyper-reflectivity).

Characteristic histopathological findings in this disease include an accumulation of autofluorescent lipopigment within the cells of the RPE (Lightfoot *et al.*, 1996). It is thought that auto-oxidative processes may play a role in the accumulation of this lipopigment. The pronounced clinical and pathological similarities that exist between canine RPED and the retinopathy associated with deficiency of the antioxidant vitamin E are consistent with this hypothesis. RPED-affected Cocker Spaniels have been found to have extremely low plasma levels of vitamin E, and a characteristic neurological syndrome, including ataxia and proprioceptive deficits particularly affecting the hindlimbs, has been demonstrated in a number of these dogs (McLellan *et al.*, 2002, 2003).

Treatment and implications for vision: An ophthalmoscopic diagnosis of RPED warrants measurement of fasting plasma vitamin E values. Should a

diagnosis of vitamin E deficiency be made, high-dose oral supplementation with 600–900 IU of natural source vitamin E (alpha tocopherol) administered twice daily with food is recommended (McLellan and Bedford, 2012). Plasma levels should be rechecked after a few weeks of supplementation. Although supplementation may arrest the progression of retinal and neurological lesions in clinically affected animals, this is unlikely to be accompanied by an improvement in vision.

Neuronal ceroid lipofuscinoses
The neuronal ceroid lipofuscinoses (NCLs) are a group of inherited storage diseases which are well recognized in domestic animals and humans; in the latter, NCL is often referred to as Batten's disease (Jolly *et al.*, 1992). These diseases are characterized by an intracellular accumulation of autofluorescent lipopigment within many tissues throughout the body, in particular the nervous system and retina. Within this heterogeneous group of related disorders, various clinical syndromes with differing ages of onset and clinical course are recognized.

Clinical manifestations of NCL include multifocal nervous signs such as tremors and seizures (due to brain atrophy) and loss of vision (due to retinal changes as well as degenerative changes within the CNS). Ophthalmoscopic evidence of retinal degeneration is not a consistent or prominent feature of NCL in dog breeds such as the English Setter, Border Collie or Dalmatian, in which marked funduscopic changes have not been described. Severe retinal degeneration associated with canine NCL has been described in the Miniature Schnauzer (Smith *et al.*, 1996). Early onset NCL in Miniature Longhaired Dachshunds reaches end-stage by 10–11 months of age, manifest clinically by seizures and blindness (Whiting *et al.*, 2013). It is important to distinguish NCL from GPRA in Tibetan Terriers, particularly because the neurological signs associated with NCL may be relatively mild in this breed, with nyctalopia (night blindness) being a prominent clinical sign (Cummings *et al.*, 1990; Riis *et al.*, 1992). In the Polish Lowland Sheepdog, the clinical appearance of NCL is similar to that of vitamin E deficiency (see above), which has also been identified in this breed (Narfström *et al.*, 2007). However, the relationship between NCL and vitamin E status in the Polish Lowland Sheepdog remains unclear.

Photic retinopathy
Retinal damage resulting from exposure to intense light has been well documented in a number of species and should be considered in patients exposed to the light of an indirect ophthalmoscope or operating microscope for prolonged periods. Ophthalmoscopic and histopathological evidence of degeneration of the outer retina has been described in the tapetal region of dogs subjected to illumination from the light source of an indirect ophthalmoscope for 1 hour (Buyukmihci, 1981). Use of a yellow-tinted, rather than clear glass, condensing lens to focus light on the retina prevented the development of retinal lesions.

Neoplasia

Secondary neoplastic involvement of the fundus, specifically the choroid, appears to be less common than that of the anterior uvea. However, this may reflect the presence of concurrent anterior and posterior uveitis, with the former obscuring the fundus from view. On the other hand, it may reflect the fact that fundic lesions that do not significantly impact vision go unnoticed unless ophthalmoscopy is performed. Neoplasms such as lymphoma (Figure 18.67), carcinoma, melanoma and haemangiosarcoma have all been reported at this site. In particular, the metastasis of feline carcinomas has a characteristic appearance associated with sectoral infarction within the choroid (Figure 18.68).

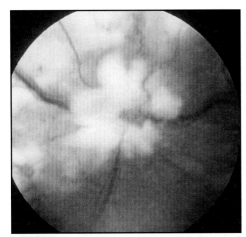

18.67 Multicentric lymphoma in a 7-year-old Domestic Shorthaired cat. There is presumed neoplastic infiltration in the ONH and peripapillary region with detachment of the surrounding retina. (Courtesy of S Crispin)

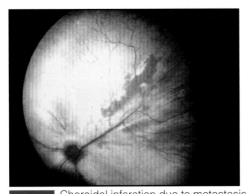

18.68 Choroidal infarction due to metastasis of a pulmonary carcinoma has resulted in a wedge-shaped area of tapetal discoloration in a 13-year-old cat.

Primary tumours rarely affect the canine posterior segment, with choroidal melanoma (Figure 18.69) being the most frequently reported primary neoplasm of the canine fundus. In contrast to the situation in humans, canine choroidal melanoma appears to be relatively benign, with most reported cases considered to be melanocytomas (Collinson and Peiffer, 1993). Primary retinal neoplasia is particularly rare in dogs and cats with sporadic reports documenting gliomas and primitive neurectodermal tumours (Dubielzig *et al.*, 2010a).

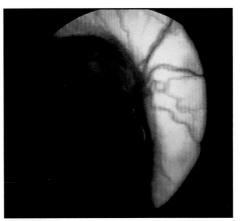

18.69 An extensive choroidal melanoma in an adult dog. (Courtesy of N Wallin-Håkansson)

The optic nerve and optic nerve head

Congenital conditions

Optic nerve hypoplasia

Optic nerve hypoplasia refers to a marked reduction in the number of optic nerve axons, as a result of reduced numbers of retinal ganglion cells. Characteristically, there is an abnormally small, dark ONH within an otherwise relatively normal fundus (Figure 18.70). Optic nerve hypoplasia is associated with impaired vision in the affected eye and reduced PLRs with a relative mydriasis (Kern and Riis, 1981). Patients with bilateral optic nerve hypoplasia may be totally blind. The condition has been reported in a number of breeds and may be inherited in the Miniature Longhaired Dachshund and Miniature and Toy Poodle. Optic nerve hypoplasia should be differentiated from micropapilla (see Figure 18.21), in which a small ONH is also visible ophthalmoscopically, but which is associated with normal PLRs and apparently normal functional vision.

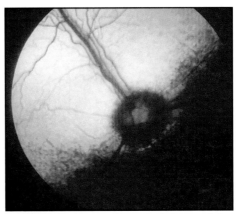

18.70 Optic nerve hypoplasia in an adult crossbreed dog. (Courtesy of SR Hollingsworth)

Optic nerve coloboma

Optic nerve colobomas represent a focal absence of ocular tissue in the region of the optic nerve, which may be related to failure of, or incomplete, closure of the ventral fetal fissure during ocular development. Although colobomas may be observed sporadically as congenital lesions in any breed, they are most commonly recognized in dogs affected by CEA (see above), in which they are seen in conjunction with lesions of choroidal hypoplasia. Optic nerve coloboma is also considered to be inherited in the Basenji (Rubin, 1989).

Colobomas of the optic nerve range in ophthalmoscopic appearance from small greyish pits to deep excavations within the ONH, into which vessels may be seen to plunge at the margins of the lesion (see Figures 18.28 and 18.29). 'Typical' colobomas are located in a ventral midline position (i.e. in the location of the fetal fissure) and 'atypical' colobomas are located at, or near, the temporal or nasal margins of the disc. Colobomas frequently have little or no appreciable effect on vision, although large defects may be associated with severe visual impairment. The presence of optic nerve coloboma has been implicated in the development of retinal detachment as a complication of CEA (Vainisi et al., 1989).

Acquired conditions

Papilloedema
Papilloedema is a term that refers to swelling of the ONH as a result of elevated intracranial and/or cerebrospinal fluid (CSF) pressure. Oedema of the ONH may also reflect primary optic nerve neoplasia (see below), may result from compression of the retrobulbar optic nerve by orbital space-occupying lesions, or may accompany systemic hypertension, acute glaucoma (dogs) or uveitis. The ONH appears 'fluffy' and swollen with deviation of the retinal blood vessels as they cross the margins of the ONH. Papilloedema recognized on ophthalmoscopy may be associated with PLR deficits or loss of vision, depending on the nature and duration of any underlying disease process (Palmer et al., 1974).

Optic neuritis
Optic neuritis has many potential causes, including (Figure 18.71):

- Viral, bacterial, parasitic and fungal infectious disease processes

Underlying disease process	Examples
Infectious	Canine distemper virus Feline infectious peritonitis (caused by feline coronavirus) Toxoplasmosis Neosporosis Extension of local or systemic bacterial infection Cryptococcosis
Immune-mediated	Granulomatous meningoencephalitis Chorioretinitis
Neoplastic infiltration	Lymphoma Feline ocular post-traumatic sarcoma
Trauma	Penetrating or blunt trauma Proptosis

18.71 Major causes of optic neuritis.

- Extension of local disease processes (such as orbital cellulitis)
- Granulomatous or neoplastic infiltration (e.g. in cases of granulomatous meningoencephalitis (GME) or lymphoma).

In many dogs with optic neuritis, the inflammatory process is deemed to be idiopathic and is assumed to be immune-mediated on the basis of the clinical response to immunosuppression.

Clinical features: Inflammation of the optic nerve usually leads to a sudden loss of the afferent PLR in association with visual impairment or blindness. Optic neuritis, with involvement of the ONH, may lead to ophthalmoscopically visible changes such as ONH congestion and swelling; the latter is recognized by the absence of a normal physiological pit. The surface of an enlarged or swollen ONH will be raised and no longer in focus in the same plane as the rest of the fundus on direct ophthalmoscopy. In addition, cellular infiltrates within the posterior vitreous, haemorrhage within or surrounding the ONH and peripapillary retinal oedema and/or detachment may also be seen (Figures 18.72 and 18.73).

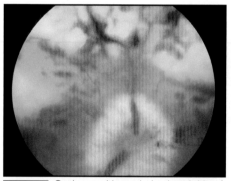

18.72 Optic neuritis and chorioretinitis of undetermined cause in an adult dog. Note the radiating, flame-like haemorrhages within the nerve fibre layer of the retina.

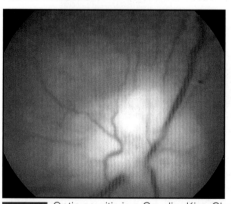

18.73 Optic neuritis in a Cavalier King Charles Spaniel with granulomatous meningoencephalitis.

Inflammation of the retrobulbar portion of the optic nerve may lead to PLR deficits and visual impairment in the absence of funduscopic abnormalities. Bilateral retrobulbar optic neuritis should therefore be an important differential diagnosis consideration, along with SARDS (see above) and CNS disorders (see Chapter 19), in those patients that present with a history of blindness of acute onset and widely dilated pupils, and which have a normal fundus appearance on ophthalmoscopy. Normal electroretinographic responses are maintained in patients with retrobulbar optic neuritis, a feature which distinguishes this condition from SARDS. A thorough neurological examination is warranted in order to detect other neurological abnormalities that might be consistent with the presence of CNS disease (see Chapter 19). Use of cross-sectional imaging techniques (such as computed tomography and magnetic resonance imaging) is recommended (see Chapter 2) and may clearly demonstrate optic nerve swelling or contrast enhancement. Although less sensitive, orbital ultrasonography may aid in the detection, and/or biopsy, of suspected optic nerve neoplasms or other orbital disease processes that have extended to involve the optic nerve. CSF analysis may be valuable, particularly in those cases in which optic neuritis is a manifestation of a more diffuse CNS inflammatory disease, such as GME (in which the CSF typically displays a mononuclear pleiocytosis and elevation in protein concentration) or neoplasia, such as lymphoma (Thomas and Eger, 1989). Samples of CSF may also be subjected to serological testing for infectious diseases such as canine distemper, toxoplasmosis or cryptococcosis.

Treatment and implications for vision: Underlying infectious or neoplastic disease should be addressed by specific, appropriate therapy. In cases of idiopathic optic neuritis, or of suspected GME, the response to systemic, immunosuppressive doses of corticosteroids may be encouraging with initial restoration of vision. However, the long-term prognosis for maintenance of vision is guarded because recurrence of active inflammation is common and optic atrophy frequently follows initial or repeated bouts of optic neuritis. Prednisolone should be administered orally at a rate of 2 mg/kg/day (divided q12h) for 10–14 days, with the dosage being gradually reduced by half at 2-weekly intervals until an alternate day maintenance dose is reached. Patients should be monitored throughout the treatment period to ensure that signs of improvement, such as resolution of ONH swelling and/or restoration of vision and PLRs, are achieved and maintained (Figure 18.74; Nafe and Carter, 1981). The prognosis in those cases of optic neuritis related to GME is extremely guarded, as ultimately other manifestations of CNS disease occur. However, remission may be achieved in response to systemic, immunosuppressive doses of corticosteroids (Thomas and Eger, 1989) and/or other systemic immunosuppressive drugs such as ciclosporin or cytosine arabinoside (Nell, 2008).

Neoplasia

Optic nerve tumours are uncommon in the dog and rare in the cat, with meningioma being the most frequently reported optic nerve tumour in dogs and lymphoma, possibly, the most common optic nerve tumour in cats (see Figure 18.67). The optic nerve

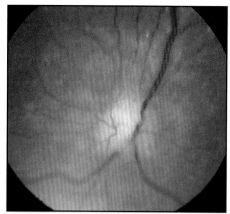

18.74 Appearance of the fundus in the same dog as in Figure 18.73 following immunosuppressive therapy with an oral corticosteroid.

may be involved secondarily by local extension or metastasis from other sites (see Chapter 8). Meningioma may involve the optic nerve by secondary extension of intracranial neoplasia or by primary neoplastic transformation of cells within the optic nerve sheath (Mauldin *et al.*, 2000). Dogs with optic nerve or orbital meningioma may present with slowly progressive exophthalmos, accompanied by loss of vision and PLR deficits. Orbital exenteration may be curative, although intracranial and chiasmal extension and pulmonary metastasis of primary optic nerve meningiomas have been reported (Barnett and Singleton, 1967; Paulsen *et al.*, 1989; Dugan *et al.*, 1993; Mauldin *et al.*, 2000).

Optic atrophy

Optic atrophy may occur as a result of a previous episode of optic nerve inflammation, a traumatic incident (particularly as a common sequel to prolapse/proptosis of the globe), previous optic nerve compression (e.g. by space-occupying lesions within the orbit or calvarium) or as a result of an elevation in intraocular pressure associated with glaucoma (which leads to ONH 'cupping'; see Chapter 15). The atrophic ONH appears grey and dark, with loss of myelin leading to an irregular crenated appearance, and loss of blood vessels (Figure 18.75). Optic atrophy is more challenging to diagnose on ophthalmoscopy in cats than in dogs owing to the normal absence of myelin from the feline ONH.

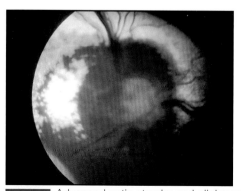

18.75 Advanced optic atrophy and glial scarring in an adult dog following orbital penetrating trauma (a bite wound) sustained within the first few months of life.

References and further reading

Acland GM, Aguirre GD, Bennett J *et al.* (2005) Long-term restoration of rod and cone vision by single dose rAAV-mediated gene transfer to the retina in a canine model of childhood blindness. *Molecular Therapy* **12**, 1072–1082

Aguirre GD and Acland GM (1988) Variation in retinal degeneration phenotype inherited at the *prcd* locus. *Experimental Eye Research* **46**, 663–687

Andrew SE, Abrams KL, Brooks DE and Kubilis PS (1997) Clinical features of steroid-responsive retinal detachments in twenty-two dogs. *Veterinary and Comparative Ophthalmology* **7**, 82–87

Barnett KC (1965a) Canine retinopathies – II. The Miniature and Toy Poodle. *Journal of Small Animal Practice* **6**, 93–109

Barnett KC (1965b) Canine retinopathies – III. The other breeds. *Journal of Small Animal Practice* **6**, 185–196

Barnett KC (1969) Primary retinal dystrophies in the dog. *Journal of the American Veterinary Medical Association* **154**, 804–808

Barnett KC (1976) Central progressive retinal atrophy in the Labrador Retriever. *Veterinary Annual* **17**, 142–144

Barnett KC (1981) Diabetic retinopathy in the dog. *British Journal of Ophthalmology* **65**, 312–314

Barnett KC and Curtis R (1985) Autosomal dominant progressive retinal atrophy in Abyssinian cats. *Journal of Heredity* **76**, 168–170

Barnett KC and Singleton WB (1967) Retrobulbar and chiasmal meningioma in a dog. *Journal of Small Animal Practice* **8**, 391–394

Bedford PGC (1982a) Collie eye anomaly in the Border Collie. *Veterinary Record* **111**, 34–35

Bedford PGC (1982b) Collie eye anomaly in the United Kingdom. *Veterinary Record* **111**, 263–270

Bedford PGC (1984) Retinal pigment epithelial dystrophy (CPRA). a study of the disease in the Briard. *Journal of Small Animal Practice* **25**, 129–138

Bedford PGC (1998) Collie eye anomaly in the Lancashire Heeler. *Veterinary Record* **143**, 354–356

Bjerkås E (1991) Collie eye anomaly in the Rough Collie in Norway. *Journal of Small Animal Practice* **32**, 89–92

Bjerkås E and Narfström K (1994) Progressive retinal atrophy in the Tibetan Spaniel in Norway and Sweden. *Veterinary Record* **134**, 377–379

Braus BK, Hauck SM, Amann B *et al.* (2008) Neuron-specific enolase antibodies in patients with sudden acquired retinal degeneration syndrome. *Veterinary Immunology and Immunopathology* **124**, 177–183

Braus BK, Rhodes M, Featherstone HJ, Renwick PW and Heinrich CL (2012) Cataracts are not associated with retinal detachment in the Bichon Frise in the UK – a retrospective study of preoperative findings and outcomes in 40 eyes. *Veterinary Ophthalmology* **15**, 98–101

Brown S, Atkins C, Bagley R *et al.* (2007) Guidelines for the identification, evaluation and management of systemic hypertension in dogs and cats. *Journal of Veterinary Internal Medicine* **21**, 542–558

Buyukmihci N (1981) Photic retinopathy in the dog. *Experimental Eye Research* **33**, 95–109

Carrig CB, MacMillan A, Brundage S, Pool RR and Morgan JP (1977) Retinal dysplasia associated with skeletal abnormalities in Labrador Retrievers. *Journal of the American Veterinary Medical Association* **170**, 49–57

Carrig CB, Sponenberg DP, Schmidt GM and Tvedten HW (1988) Inheritance of associated ocular and skeletal dysplasia in Labrador Retrievers. *Journal of the American Veterinary Medical Association* **193**, 1269–1272

Carter RT, Oliver JW, Stepien RL and Bentley E (2009) Elevations in sex hormones in dogs with sudden acquired retinal degeneration syndrome (SARDS). *Journal of the American Animal Hospital Association* **45**, 207–214

Clements PJM, Sargan DR, Gould DJ and Petersen-Jones SM (1996) Recent advances in understanding the spectrum of canine generalized progressive retinal atrophy. *Journal of Small Animal Practice* **37**, 155–162

Collinson PN and Peiffer RL (1993) Clinical presentation, morphology and behavior of primary choroidal melanomas in eight dogs. *Progress in Veterinary and Comparative Ophthalmology* **3**, 158–164

Crispin C and Mould JR (2001) Systemic hypertensive disease and the feline fundus. *Veterinary Ophthalmology* **4**, 131–140

Crispin SM (1993) Ocular manifestations of hyperlipoproteinaemia. *Journal of Small Animal Practice* **34**, 500–506

Crispin SM, Long SE and Wheeler CA (1999) Incidence and ocular manifestations of multifocal retinal dysplasia in the Golden Retriever in the UK. *Veterinary Record* **145**, 669–672

Cullen CL and Webb AA (2007a) Ocular manifestations of systemic diseases. Part 1: the dog. In: *Veterinary Ophthalmology, vol. II, 4th edn*, ed. KN Gelatt, pp.1470–1537. Blackwell Publishing, Oxford

Cullen CL and Webb AA (2007b) Ocular manifestations of systemic diseases. Part 2: the cat. In: *Veterinary Ophthalmology, vol. II, 4th edn*, ed. KN Gelatt, pp.1538–1587. Blackwell Publishing, Oxford

Cummings JF, De Lahunta A, Riis RC and Loew ER (1990) Neuropathologic changes in a young adult Tibetan Terrier with subclinical neuronal ceroid lipofuscinosis. *Progress in Veterinary Neurology* **1**, 301–309

Curtis R (1988) Retinal diseases in the dog and cat: an overview and update. *Journal of Small Animal Practice* **29**, 397–415

Davidson MG, Geoly FJ, McLellan GJ, Gilger BC and Whitley W (1998) Retinal degeneration associated with vitamin E deficiency in a group of hunting dogs. *Journal of the American Veterinary Medical Association* **213**, 645–651

Dubielzig RR, Ketring KL, McLellan GJ and Albert DM (2010a) The retina. In: *Veterinary Ocular Pathology: a Comparative Review*, ed. RR Dubielzig *et al.*, pp.349–397. Saunders Elsevier Ltd, Oxford

Dubielzig RR, Ketring KL, McLellan GJ and Albert DM (2010b) The optic nerve. In: *Veterinary Ocular Pathology: a Comparative Review*, ed. RR Dubielzig *et al.*, pp.399–417. Saunders Elsevier Ltd, Oxford

Dugan SJ, Schwarz PD, Roberts SM and Ching SV (1993) Primary optic nerve meningioma and pulmonary metastasis in a dog. *Journal of the American Animal Hospital Association* **29**, 11–16

Ekesten B (2007) Ophthalmic examination and diagnostics. Part 4: The electrodiagnostic evaluation of vision. In: *Veterinary Ophthalmology, vol. 1, 4th edn*, ed. KN Gelatt, pp.520–535. Blackwell Publishing, Oxford

Ekesten B, Komáromy AM, Ofri R, Petersen-Jones SM and Narfström K (2013) Guidelines for clinical electroretinography in the dog: 2012 update. *Documenta Ophthalmologica* **127**, 79–87

Ford MM, Dubielzig RR, Guiliano EA, Moore CP and Narfström K (2007) Ocular and systemic manifestations after oral administration of a high dose of enrofloxacin in cats. *American Journal of Veterinary Research* **68**, 190–202

Gelatt KN, van der Woerdt A, Ketring KL *et al.* (2001) Enrofloxacin associated retinal degeneration in cats. *Veterinary Ophthalmology* **4**, 99–106

Gilmour MA, Cardenas MR, Blaik MA, Bahr RJ and McGinnis JF (2006) Evaluation of a comparative pathogenesis between cancer-associated retinopathy in humans and sudden acquired retinal degeneration syndrome in dogs via diagnostic imaging and western blot analysis. *American Journal of Veterinary Research* **67**, 877–881

Goldstein O, Guyon R, Kukekova A *et al.* (2010) COL9A2 and COL9A3 mutations in canine autosomal recessive oculoskeletal dysplasia. *Mammalian Genome* **21**(7–8), 398–408

Grahn BH and Cullen CL (2001) Retinopathy of Great Pyrenees dogs: fluorescein angiography, light microscopy and transmitting and scanning electron microscopy. *Veterinary Ophthalmology* **4**, 191–199

Grahn BH, Sandmeyer LL and Breaux C (2008) Retinopathy of Coton de Tulear dogs: clinical manifestations, electroretinographic, ultrasonographic, fluorescein and indocyanine green angiographic, and optical coherence tomographic findings. *Veterinary Ophthalmology* **11**, 242–249

Grahn BH, Storey ES and McMillan C (2004) Inherited retinal dysplasia and persistent hyperplastic primary vitreous in Miniature Schnauzer dogs. *Veterinary Ophthalmology* **7**, 151–158

Grozdanic SD, Matic M, Sakaguchi DS *et al.* (2007) Evaluation of retinal status using chromatic pupil light reflex activity in healthy and diseased canine eyes. *Investigative Ophthalmology and Visual Science* **48**, 5178–5183

Gunn-Moore DA, Watson TD, Dodkin SJ *et al.* (1997) Transient hyperlipidaemia and anaemia in kittens. *Veterinary Record* **140**(14), 355–359

Hayes KC and Trautwein EA (1989) Taurine deficiency syndrome in cats. *Veterinary Clinics of North America: Small Animal Practice* **19**, 403–413

Hendrix DV, Nasisse MP, Cowen P and Davidson MG (1993) Clinical signs, concurrent diseases and risk factors associated with retinal detachment in dogs. *Progress in Veterinary and Comparative Ophthalmology* **3**, 87–91

Holle DM, Stankovics ME, Sarna CS and Aguirre GD (1999). The geographic form of retinal dysplasia in dogs is not always a congenital abnormality. *Veterinary Ophthalmology* **2**, 61–66

Holt E, Feldman EC and Buyukmihci N (1999) The prevalence of hyperadrenocorticism (Cushing's syndrome) in dogs with sudden acquired retinal degeneration (SARD). *Proceedings of the 30th Annual Meeting of the American College of Veterinary Ophthalmologists*, Chicago, Illinois, p. 35.

Itoh Y, Maehara S, Yamasaki A, Tsuzuki K and Izumisawa Y (2010) Investigation of fellow eye of unilateral retinal detachment in the Shih-Tzu. *Veterinary Ophthalmology* **13**, 289–293

Jepson RE (2011) Feline systemic hypertension: classification and pathogenesis. *Journal of Feline Medicine and Surgery* **13**(1), 25–34

Jolly RD, Martinus RD and Palmer DN (1992) Sheep and other animals with ceroid lipofuscinoses: their relevance to Batten disease. *American Journal of Medical Genetics* **42**, 609–614

Kang-Derwent JJ, Padnick-Silver L, McRipley M *et al.* (2006) The electroretinogram components in Abyssinian cats with hereditary retinal degeneration. *Investigative Ophthalmology and Visual Science* **47**, 3673–3682

Keller RL, Kania SA, Hendrix DV, Ward DA and Abrams K (2006) Evaluation of canine serum for the presence of antiretinal autoantibodies in sudden acquired retinal degeneration syndrome. *Veterinary Ophthalmology* **9**, 195–200

Kern TJ and Riis RC (1981) Optic nerve hypoplasia in three Miniature Poodles. *Journal of the American Veterinary Medical Association* **178**, 49–54

Komaromy AM, Books DE, Dawson WW *et al.* (2002) Technical issues in electrodiagnostic recording. *Veterinary Ophthalmology* **5**, 85–91

Landry MP, Herring IP and Panciera DL (2004) Funduscopic findings following cataract extraction by means of phacoemulsification in diabetic dogs: 52 cases (1993–2003). *Journal of the American Veterinary Medical Association* **225**, 709–716

Lane IF, Roberts SM and Lappin MR (1993) Ocular manifestations of vascular disease: hypertension, hyperviscosity and hyperlipidemia. *Journal of the American Animal Hospital Association* **29**, 28–36

Latshaw WK, Wyman M and Venzke WG (1969) Embryologic development of an anomaly of ocular fundus in the collie dog. *American Journal of Veterinary Research* **30**, 211–217

Lavach JD, Murphy JJ and Severin GA (1978) Retinal dysplasia in the English Springer Spaniel. *Journal of the American Animal Hospital Association* **14**, 192–199

Leblanc NL, Stepien RL and Bentley E (2011) Ocular lesions associated with systemic hypertension in dogs: 65 cases (2005–2007). *Journal of the American Veterinary Medical Association* **238**, 915–921

Leon A and Curtis R (1990) Autosomal dominant rod–cone dysplasia in the *RDY* cat: 1. Light and electron microscopic findings. *Experimental Eye Research* **51**, 361–381

Leon A, Levick WR and Sarossy MG (1995) Lesion topography and new histological features in feline taurine deficiency retinopathy. *Experimental Eye Research* **61**, 731–741

Lightfoot RM, Cabral L, Gooch L, Bedford PGC and Boulton ME (1996) Retinal pigment epithelial dystrophy in Briard dogs. *Research in Veterinary Science* **60**, 17–23

Long SE and Crispin SM (1999) Inheritance of multifocal retinal dysplasia in the Golden Retriever in the UK. *Veterinary Record* **145**, 702–704

MacMillan AD and Lipton DE (1978) Heritability of multifocal retinal dysplasia in American Cocker Spaniels. *Journal of the American Veterinary Medical Association* **172**, 568–572

Maggio F, DeFrancesco TC, Atkins CE *et al.* (2000) Ocular lesions associated with systemic hypertension in cats: 69 cases (1985–1998). *Journal of the American Veterinary Medical Association* **217**(5), 695–702

Mauldin EA, Deehr AJ, Hertzke D and Dubielzig RR (2000) Canine orbital meningiomas: a review of 22 cases. *Veterinary Ophthalmology* **3**, 11–16

McLellan GJ and Bedford PGC (2012) Oral vitamin E absorption in English Cocker Spaniels with familial vitamin E deficiency and retinal pigment epithelial dystrophy. *Veterinary Ophthalmology* **15**(Suppl. 2), 48–56

McLellan GJ, Cappello R, Mayhew IG *et al.* (2003) Clinical and pathological observations in English Cocker Spaniels with primary metabolic vitamin E deficiency and retinal pigment epithelial dystrophy. *Veterinary Record* **153**, 287–292

McLellan GJ, Elks R, Lybaert P *et al.* (2002) Vitamin E deficiency in dogs with retinal pigment epithelial dystrophy. *Veterinary Record* **151**, 663–667

Menotti-Raymond M, David VA, Pflueger S *et al.* (2010a) Widespread retina degenerative disease mutation (*rdAc*) discovered among a large number of popular cat breeds. *The Veterinary Journal* **186**, 32–38

Menotti-Raymond M, David VA, Schäffer A *et al.* (2007) Mutation in *CEP290* discovered for cat model of human retinal degeneration. *Journal of Heredity* **98**(3), 211–220

Menotti-Raymond M, Holland Deckman K, David V *et al.* (2010b) Mutation discovered in a feline model of human congenital retina blinding disease. *Investigative Ophthalmology and Visual Science* 51, 2852–2859

Messias A, Gekeler F, Wegener A *et al.* (2008) Retinal safety of a new fluoroquinolone, pradofloxacin, in cats: assessment with electroretinography. *Documenta Ophthalmologica* 116, 177–191

Meyers VN, Jezyk PF, Aguirre GD and Patterson DF (1983) Short-limbed dwarfism and ocular defects in the Samoyed dog. *Journal of the American Veterinary Medical Association* **183**, 975–979

Miller PE, Galbreath EJ, Kehren JC, Steinberg H and Dubielzig RR (1998) Photoreceptor cell death by apoptosis in dogs with sudden acquired retinal degeneration syndrome. *American Journal of Veterinary Research* **59**,149–152

Millichamp NJ (1990) Retinal degeneration in the dog and cat. *Veterinary Clinics of North America: Small Animal Practice* **20**, 799–835

Millichamp NJ, Curtis R and Barnett KC (1988) Progressive retinal atrophy in Tibetan Terriers. *Journal of the American Veterinary Medical Association* **192**, 769–776

Montgomery KW, van der Woerdt A and Cottrill NB (2008) Acute blindness in dogs: sudden acquired retinal degeneration syndrome *versus* neurological disease (140 cases: 2000–2006). *Veterinary* Ophthalmology **11**(5), 314–320

Muñana KR (1995) Long-term complications of diabetes mellitus, part 1: retinopathy, nephropathy, neuropathy. *Veterinary Clinics of North America: Small Animal Practice* **25**, 715–730

Nafe LA and Carter JD (1981) Canine optic neuritis. *Compendium on Continuing Education for the Practicing Veterinarian* **3**, 978–981

Narfström K (1985) Progressive retinal atrophy in the Abyssinian cat: clinical characteristics. *Investigative Ophthalmology and Visual Science* **26**, 193–200

Narfström K (1999) Retinal dystrophy or 'congenital stationary night blindness' in the Briard dog. *Veterinary Ophthalmology* **2**, 75–76

Narfström K, David V, Jarrete O *et al.* (2009) Retinal degeneration in the Abyssinian and Somali cat (*rdAc*): correlation between genotype and phenotype and the *rdAc* allele frequency in two continents. *Veterinary Ophthalmology* **12**(5), 285–291

Narfström K, Katz ML, Ford M *et al.* (2003) *In vivo* gene therapy in young and adult RPE65-/- dogs produces long-term visual improvement. *Journal of Heredity* **94**, 31–37

Narfström K, Maggs DJ, Garland J *et al.* (2010) A novel retinal degenerative disease of Bengal cats. *Conference Proceedings: European College of Veterinary Ophthalmologists 2010 Annual Scientific Meeting*, Berlin, Germany, p. 62

Narfström K, Menotti-Raymond M and Seeliger M (2011) Characterization of feline hereditary retinal dystrophies using clinical, functional, structural and molecular genetic studies. *Veterinary Ophthalmology* **14** (Suppl 1), 30–36

Narfström K and Nilsson SEG (1989) Morphological findings during retinal development and maturation in hereditary rod–cone degeneration of Abyssinian cats. *Experimental Eye Research* **49**, 611–628

Narfström K and Petersen-Jones S (2007) Diseases of the canine ocular fundus. In: *Veterinary Ophthalmology, vol. II 4th edn*, ed. KN Gelatt, pp. 944–1025. Blackwell Publishing, Oxford

Narfström K, Wrigstad A, Ekesten B and Berg AL (2007) Neuronal ceroid lipofuscinosis: clinical and morphologic findings in nine affected Polish Owczarek Nizinny (PON) dogs. *Veterinary Ophthalmology* **10**(2), 111–120

Narfström K, Wrigstad A, Ekesten B and Nilsson SEG (1994) Hereditary retinal dystrophy in the Briard dog: clinical and hereditary characteristics. *Veterinary and Comparative Ophthalmology* **4**, 85–92

Nell B (2008) Optic neuritis in dogs and cats. *Veterinary Clinics of North America: Small Animal Practice* **38**, 403–415

Nelson DL and MacMillan AD (1983) Multifocal retinal dysplasia in field trial Labrador Retrievers. *Journal of the American Animal Hospital Association* **19**, 388–392

O'Toole D, Young S, Severin GA and Neuman S (1983) Retinal dysplasia of English Springer Spaniel dogs: light microscopy of the postnatal lesions. *Veterinary Pathology* **20**, 298–311

Padnick-Silver L, Kang-Derwent JJ, Guiliano E *et al.* (2006) Retinal oxygenation and oxygen metabolism in Abyssinian cats with a hereditary retinal degeneration. *Investigative Ophthalmology and Visual Science* **47**, 3683–3689

Palmer AC, Malinowski W and Barnett KC (1974) Clinical signs including papilloedema associated with brain tumours in twenty-one dogs. *Journal of Small Animal Practice* **15**, 359–386

Parker HG, Kukekova AV, Akey DT *et al.* (2007) Breed relationships facilitate fine-mapping studies: a 7.8-kb deletion cosegregates with Collie eye anomaly across multiple dog breeds. *Genome Research* **17**, 1562–1571

Parry HB (1953) Degenerations of the dog retina. II. Generalized progressive retinal atrophy of hereditary origin. *British Journal of Ophthalmology* **37**, 487–502

Parry HB (1954) Degenerations of the dog retina VI. Central progressive atrophy with pigment epithelial dystrophy. *British Journal of Ophthalmology* **38**, 653–668

Paulsen ME, Severin GA, Lecouteur RA and Young S (1989) Primary optic nerve meningioma in a dog. *Journal of the American Animal Hospital Association* **25**, 147–152

Percy DH, Carmichael LE, Albert DM, King JM and Jonas AM (1971) Lesions in puppies surviving infection with canine herpesvirus. *Veterinary Pathology* **8**, 37–53

Petersen-Jones SM (1998) A review of research to elucidate the causes of the generalized progressive retinal atrophies. *The Veterinary Journal* **155**, 5–18

Rah H, Maggs DJ, Blankenship TN, Narfström K and Lyons LA (2005)

Early-onset, autosomal recessive, progressive retinal atrophy in Persian cats. *Investigative Ophthalmology and Visual Science* **46**, 1742–1747

Ramirez CJ, Minch JD, Gay JM *et al.* (2011) Molecular genetic basis for fluoroquinolone-induced retinal degeneration in cats. *Pharmacogenetic Genomics* **21**, 66–75

Riis RC, Cummings JF, Loew ER and De Lahunta A (1992) A Tibetan Terrier model of canine ceroid lipofuscinosis. *American Journal of Medical Genetics* **42**, 615–621

Riis RC, Sheffy BE, Loew E, Kern TJ and Smith JS (1981) Vitamin E deficiency retinopathy in dogs. *American Journal of Veterinary Research* **42**, 74–86

Roberts SM (1969) The collie eye anomaly. *Journal of the American Veterinary Medical Association* **155**, 859–878

Ropstad EO and Narfström K (2007) The obvious and the more hidden components of the electroretinogram *European Journal of Companion Animal Practice* **17**, 290–296

Rubin LF (1968) Heredity of retinal dysplasia in Bedlington Terriers. *Journal of the American Veterinary Medical Association* **152**, 260–262

Rubin LF (1989) *Inherited Eye Diseases in Purebred Dogs.* Williams and Wilkins, Baltimore

Rubin LF, Nelson EJ and Sharp CA (1991) Collie eye anomaly in Australian Shepherd dogs. *Progress in Veterinary and Comparative Ophthalmology* **1**, 105–108

Samuelson DA (2007) Ophthalmic anatomy. In: *Veterinary Ophthalmology, vol. I, 4th edition,* ed. KN Gelatt, pp.37–148. Blackwell Publishing, Oxford

Sansom J, Barnett KC, Dunn KA, Smith KC and Dennis R (1994) Ocular disease associated with hypertension in 16 cats. *Journal of Small Animal Practice* **35**, 604–611

Sansom J and Bodey A (1997) Ocular signs in four dogs with hypertension. *Veterinary Record* **140**, 593–598

Schmidt GM, Ellersieck MR, Wheeler CA, Blanchard GL and Keller WF (1979) Inheritance of retinal dysplasia in the English Springer Spaniel. *Journal of the American Veterinary Medical Association* **174**, 1089–1090

Schmidt GM and Vainisi SJ (2004) Retrospective study of prophylactic random transscleral retinopexy in the Bichon Frise with cataract. *Veterinary Ophthalmology* **7**, 307–310

Smith PJ, Mames RN, Samuelson DA *et al.* (1997) Photoreceptor outer segments in aqueous humor from dogs with rhegmatogenous retinal detachments. *Journal of the American Veterinary Medical Association* **21**, 1254–1256

Smith RIE, Sutton RH, Jolly RD and Smith KR (1996) A retinal degeneration associated with ceroid lipofuscinosis in adult Miniature Schnauzers. *Veterinary and Comparative Ophthalmology* **6**, 187–191

Spurlock NK and Prittie JE (2011) A review of current indications, adverse effects, and administration recommendations for intravenous immunoglobulin. *Veterinary Emergency and Critical Care* **21**(5), 471–483

Stepien RL (2011) Feline systemic hypertension: diagnosis and management. *Journal of Feline Medicine and Surgery* **13**(1), 35–43

Stiles J, Polzin DJ and Bistner SI (1994) The prevalence of retinopathy in cats with systemic hypertension and chronic renal failure or hyperthyroidism. *Journal of the American Animal Hospital Association* **30**, 564–572

Stiles J and Townsend WM (2007) Feline ophthalmology. In: *Veterinary Ophthalmology, vol. II, 4th edn* ed. KN Gelatt, p. 1140. Blackwell Publishing, Oxford

Sturman JA (1978) Taurine deficiency in the kitten: exchange and turnover of [35S] taurine in brain, retina and other tissues. *Journal of Nutrition* **108**, 1462–1476

Sullivan TC (1997) Surgery for retinal detachment. *Veterinary Clinics of North America: Small Animal Practice* **27**, 1193–1214

Thomas JB and Eger C (1989) Granulomatous meningoencephalomyelitis in 21 dogs. *Journal of Small Animal Practice* **30**, 287–293

Tofflemire K and Betbeze C (2010) Three cases of feline ocular coccidioidomycosis: presentation, clinical features, diagnosis and treatment. *Veterinary Ophthalmology* **13**(3), 166–172

Vainisi SJ and Packo KH (1995) Management of giant retinal tears in dogs. *Journal of the American Veterinary Medical Association* **206**, 491–495

Vainisi SJ, Peyman GA, Wolf ED and West CS (1989) Treatment of serous retinal detachments associated with optic disk pits in dogs. *Journal of the American Veterinary Medical Association* **195**, 1233–1236

Vainisi SJ, Wolfer JC and Smith PJ (2007) Surgery of the canine posterior segment. In: *Veterinary Ophthalmology, vol. II, 4th edn,* ed. KN Gelatt, pp.1026–1058. Blackwell, Oxford

van der Woerdt A, Nasisse MP and Davidson MG (1991) Sudden acquired retinal degeneration in the dog: clinical and laboratory findings in 36 cases. *Progress in Veterinary and Comparative Ophthalmology* **1**, 11–18

Veske A, Nilsson SE, Narfström K and Gal A (1999) Retinal dystrophy of Swedish Briard/Briard-beagle dogs is due to a 4-bp deletion in *RPE65. Genomics* **57**, 57–61

Villagrasa M and Cascales MJ (2000) Arterial hypertension: angiographic aspects of the ocular fundus in dogs. A study of 24 cases. *European Journal of Companion Animal Practice* **10**, 177–190

Wallin-Håkanson B, Wallin-Håkanson N and Hedhammar Å (2000a) Collie eye anomaly in the rough collie in Sweden: genetic transmission and influence on offspring vitality. *Journal of Small Animal Practice* **41**, 254–258

Wallin-Håkanson B, Wallin-Håkanson N and Hedhammar Å (2000b) Influence of selective breeding on the prevalence of chorioretinal dysplasia and coloboma in the rough collie in Sweden. *Journal of Small Animal Practice* **41**, 56–59

Watson P, Narfström K and Bedford PGC (1993) Retinal pigment epithelial dystrophy (RPED) in Polish Lowland Sheepdogs. *Proceedings of the British Small Animal Veterinary Association Congress,* Birmingham, p. 231

Wiebe V and Hamilton P (2002) Fluoroquinolone-induced retinal degeneration in cats. *Journal of the American Veterinary Medical Association* **221**, 1568–1571

Whiting REH, Narfström K, Yao G *et al.* (2013) Pupillary light reflex deficits in a canine model of late infantile neuronal ceroid lipofuscinosis. *Experimental Eye Research* **116**, 402–410

Wolf ED, Vainisi SJ and Santos-Anderson R (1978) Rod–cone dysplasia in the collie. *Journal of the American Veterinary Medical Association* **173**, 1331–1333

Wyman M and McKissick GE (1973) Lipemia retinalis in a dog and cat: case reports. *Journal of the American Animal Hospital Association* **9**, 288–291

Yakely WL, Wyman M, Donovan EF and Fechheimer NS (1968) Genetic transmission of an ocular fundus anomaly in Collies. *Journal of the American Veterinary Medical Association* **152**, 457–461

Zangerl B, Wickström K, Slavik J *et al.* (2010) Assessment of canine *BEST1* variations identifies new mutations and establishes an independent bestrophinopathy model (cmr3). *Molecular Vision* **16**, 2791–2804

19

Neuro-ophthalmology

Laurent Garosi and Mark Lowrie

This chapter considers disorders of vision, pupillary size, position and movement of the eyelids and globe, and lacrimation. The anatomical and physiological importance of these functions is presented alongside the principles and methods involved in their clinical assessment. This is followed by a discussion of the diseases and syndromes in which these manifestations occur.

Vision

Clinical evaluation of a suspected blind animal consists of an obstacle course evaluation, testing the menace response, visual tracking and visual placing (see Chapter 1). In addition, whilst pupillary light reflexes (PLRs) and dazzle reflexes do not specifically assess vision, they may provide useful localizing information.

Relevant neuroanatomy

The pathways involved in the conscious perception of vision are outlined in Figure 19.1. Each cerebral hemisphere receives information from the contralateral visual field. The first neuron in the visual pathway is the bipolar cell of the retina, which receives input from the photoreceptor cells of the retina (i.e. the rods and cones). These cells synapse with a second neuron called the retinal ganglion cell. Unmyelinated nerve fibres from this neuron then course centripetally along the internal retinal surface, and leave the eye via the lamina cribrosa (a perforated region of the sclera) at the optic nerve head (optic disc) to form the optic nerve, where they gain myelin and a meningeal covering. The optic nerve courses caudally in the orbit, where it is surrounded by the extraocular muscles and periorbital structures, until it enters the calvarium at the optic foramen. At the optic chiasm, the majority of axons in each optic nerve cross (75% in the dog; 66% in the cat) to form the contralateral optic tract.

Following the optic chiasm, the axons course caudodorsolaterally over the side of the diencephalon to follow one of two main pathways (note that a small proportion also project to the suprachiasmatic nucleus to influence circadian rhythms):

- Conscious perception of vision – 80% of the optic tract fibres terminate in the lateral geniculate nucleus of the thalamus. Fibres then project to the visual area of the cerebral cortex (occipital lobe) in a band of fibres called the optic radiation

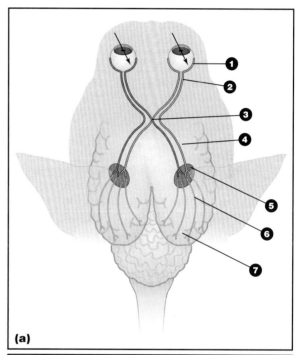

(a)

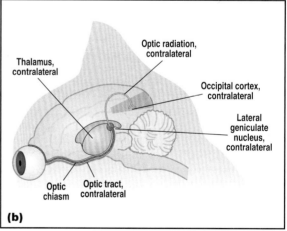

Thalamus, contralateral

Optic radiation, contralateral

Occipital cortex, contralateral

Lateral geniculate nucleus, contralateral

Optic tract, contralateral

Optic chiasm

(b)

19.1 (a) Dorsal and (b) sagittal views of the neuroanatomical pathway for conscious vision. The visual stimulus (here the left visual field is arrowed) is initiated in the retina of both eyes (1) and travels through the optic nerve (2) and optic chiasm (3) – where the majority of the fibres (65–75%) cross over – and continues along the optic tract (4). The stimulus is relayed from here to the lateral geniculate nucleus of the thalamus (5), then travels through the optic radiations (6), synapsing in the occipital cortex (7). A lesion in any part of this pathway can affect conscious vision. (Redrawn after Platt and Garosi (2012) with permission from the publisher)

- Reflex activity – the remaining 20% of the optic tract fibres are involved in two possible pathways:
  - Parasympathetic pathway – these fibres are involved in the afferent arm of the PLR (see below)
  - Somatic motor responses to retinal activity – these fibres synapse in the rostral colliculi of the midbrain, where they are important in the reflex movements of the head and eyeball in response to visual stimuli.

Clinical evaluation

Obstacle course

Assessment of the ability to navigate around objects in unfamiliar surroundings may reveal visual deficits. This assessment should be performed in photopic (light) and scotopic (dim) conditions, as well as binocularly and monocularly. Unfortunately, the latter can be very difficult to apply practically in small animals, making this test a poorly sensitive, as well as a subjective, method to assess subtle or unilateral visual impairment.

Menace response

The menace response is evoked by making a threatening gesture of the hand at each eye in turn. The expected response is rapid closure of the eyelids. The contralateral eye must be covered with the other hand to assess each eye separately. Care must be taken not to touch the patient or create air currents that might stimulate sensation of the face (cranial nerve (CN) V; the trigeminal nerve), which could elicit a palpebral or corneal reflex (see below). The postulated pathway for the menace response is illustrated in Figure 19.2.

The menace response is not considered a true reflex because it is a learned response that may not be fully developed until 10–12 weeks of age in dogs and cats. The afferent arm of this response is dependent on the degree of clarity of the ocular media (cornea, anterior chamber, lens and vitreous) and intact visual pathways (retina, optic nerves, optic chiasm, optic tracts, lateral geniculate nuclei, optic radiations and the visual cortices). The efferent arm of this response is not well understood. The information generated in the occipital cortex (contralateral to the eye stimulated) is forwarded to the motor cortex via association fibres. The motor cortex then projects to the facial nerve (CN VII) nucleus, as well as the abducens nerve (CN VI) nucleus. The motor responses mediated by these cranial nerves are the closure of the eyelid (CN VII) and retraction of the globe (CN VI), which in turn causes passive third eyelid protrusion. This response requires intact facial nerve function, so it is important to evaluate the palpebral reflex separately (see below) to ensure normal function. In animals with facial nerve paralysis, a normal menace response can be assessed by observing retraction of the globe and passive protrusion of the third eyelid. There is some experimental and clinical evidence for cerebellar involvement in the efferent pathways of the menace response: unilateral cerebellar lesions can lead to an ipsilateral

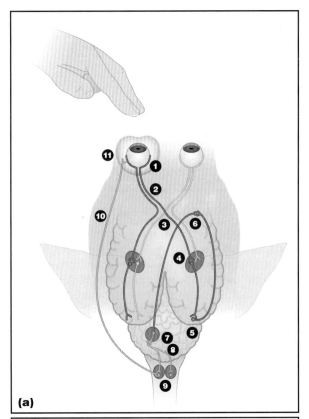

(a)

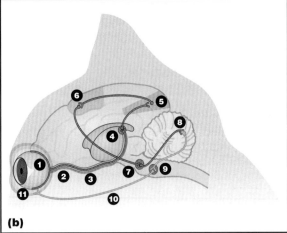

(b)

19.2 **(a)** Dorsal and **(b)** sagittal views of the neuroanatomical pathway for the menace response. The menacing stimulus is detected by the retina (1) and a resulting impulse travels through the optic nerve (2) and optic chiasm (3) to the contralateral optic tract. The stimulus is then relayed to the lateral geniculate nucleus of the thalamus (4), travels through the optic radiation and synapses in the occipital cortex (5). The signal then travels rostrally in association with interneurons and synapses in the motor cortex (6) and continues within projection fibres through the internal capsule, crus cerebri and longitudinal fibres of the pons and synapses in the pontine nucleus (7). The signal then proceeds within the transverse fibres of the pons, through the middle cerebellar peduncle and synapses in the cerebellar cortex (8). The signal then travels through the efferent cerebellar pathway and synapses on both facial nuclei (9). The signal is finally relayed through the left and right facial nerves (10; only one shown here), synapsing on the facial muscles (orbicularis oculi; 11) to cause muscular contraction and closure of the eyelids. A lesion in any part of the pathway can disrupt this response. (Redrawn after Platt and Garosi (2012) with permission from the publisher)

loss of the menace response with retention of normal vision. The neuronal pathways through the cerebellum have not been defined.

Visual tracking
Visual tracking involves the patient visually following an object (such as a dropped cotton wool ball or a light from a laser pointer) and is a useful test of vision in both dogs and cats.

Visual placing response
The placing reaction can only be tested in smaller patients. The animal is picked up and carried towards a flat surface, such as a table top. On approaching the surface, the animal will reach out to support itself on the table (Figure 19.3). Each eye can be tested separately by covering the contralateral eye. This response requires intact visual pathways, mentation and postural control of the thoracic limbs. It can be used to assess visual function in an animal where the menace response is ambiguous.

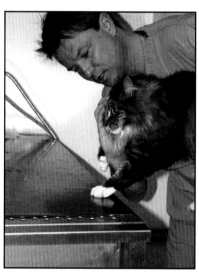

19.3
Visual placing response in a cat. On approaching the surface of the table, the cat will reach out to support itself before the paw touches the table.

Pupils

Relevant neuroanatomy
The resting pupil size is determined by two antagonistic forces:

- The parasympathetic component, which regulates the amount of light stimulating the retina by constricting the pupil
- The sympathetic component, which causes pupillary dilatation and regulates the response of the pupil to environmental factors that elicit stress, such as fear, anger or excitement.

The resultant tone, therefore, dictates the resting pupil size. The size of the pupil is in a constant state of flux owing to the dynamic equilibrium between the sympathetic and parasympathetic systems.

The ocular parasympathetic tract is a two-neuron pathway mediated by the parasympathetic component of the oculomotor nerve (CN III). It is involved in the control of pupillary constriction. The somatic efferent component of the oculomotor nerve is responsible for the motor innervation of the levator palpebrae superioris muscle (elevation of the upper eyelid) and the ipsilateral dorsal, ventral and medial recti extraocular muscles, as well as the ventral oblique muscles (movement of the globe).

The ocular sympathetic tract is a three-neuron pathway (Figure 19.4). The cell bodies of the first order neuron (or upper motor neuron, UMN) are situated in the hypothalamus and rostral midbrain. These fibres descend the cervical spinal cord in the lateral tectotegmentospinal tract to reach the first three thoracic spinal cord segments (T1 to T3). The first order neuron then synapses on the cell bodies of the lower motor neuron (LMN). The LMN is divided into the preganglionic (second order) and postganglionic (third order) neuron. The preganglionic axons leave the vertebral canal via the spinal nerve in the segmental

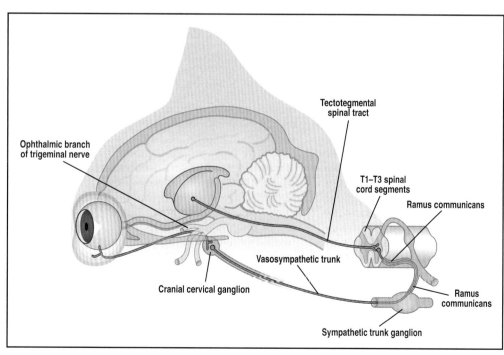

19.4
Sagittal view of the neuroanatomical pathway for sympathetic innervation to the eye. (Redrawn after Platt and Garosi (2012) with permission from the publisher)

Tectotegmental spinal tract

Ophthalmic branch of trigeminal nerve

T1–T3 spinal cord segments

Ramus communicans

Vasosympathetic trunk

Cranial cervical ganglion

Ramus communicans

Sympathetic trunk ganglion

ramus communicans, which joins the thoracic sympathetic trunk. The thoracic sympathetic trunk courses inside the thorax ventrolateral to the vertebral column and continues cranially as the cervical sympathetic trunk and vagosympathetic trunk within the carotid sheath. The fibres then synapse with the bodies of the postganglionic cells in the cranial cervical ganglion, which lies caudal to the tympanic bulla. The postganglionic axons enter the middle ear and then pass through the middle cranial fossa, where they join the ophthalmic branch of the trigeminal nerve running to the orbit. The sympathetic nervous system (SNS) innervates and provides tone to the smooth muscle of the eyes and eyelids. This tone keeps the eyeball protruded and the upper, lower and third eyelids retracted, causing the palpebral fissure to widen and the third eyelid to be pulled ventrally. The tone of the iris dilator muscle is also maintained by the SNS, which keeps the pupil partially dilated under normal circumstances and dilates it further during periods of darkness, stress, fear and painful stimuli.

Clinical evaluation

Immediately after testing the menace response, the size and symmetry of the pupils should be evaluated along with their response to light and darkness. Normally, the pupils should be symmetrical in shape and equal in size. In animals with pupils of unequal size (anisocoria) or irregular shape (dyscoria), primary and secondary anatomical and mechanical abnormalities affecting the iris (e.g. iris atrophy, hypoplasia, neoplasia, uveitis and glaucoma) must be excluded before consideration is given to neurological dysfunction. Determining which pupil is abnormal is achieved by checking the PLR and assessing whether the degree of asymmetry in pupil size is greater in bright light or in complete darkness.

Pupillary light reflex

The PLR is tested by shining a bright light into the pupil and assessing for pupillary constriction (direct reflex). The opposite pupil should constrict at the same time (consensual or indirect reflex). A slight dilatation usually follows the initial pupillary constriction (pupillary escape) as a consequence of the light adaptation of the photoreceptors. There is a rapid response mediated by photoreceptors that generates an afferent impulse, as well as slower response mediated by intrinsically photosensitive retinal ganglion cells.

The PLR involves an afferent arm and an efferent arm. The neuroanatomy of the afferent and efferent pathways of the PLR is shown in Figure 19.5. The afferent arm of this reflex shares some common pathways (ipsilateral retina, optic nerve, optic chiasm and contralateral proximal optic tract) with part of the afferent arm of the menace response and visual placing response. These tests use different integration centres within the brain and different efferent pathways. The efferent arm of the PLR is mediated by the parasympathetic portion of the oculomotor nerve. The PLR does not test vision because the cerebrum is not involved in the PLR pathway. Axons involved in vision reach the consciousness after synapsing in the lateral geniculate nucleus, but the axons involved with

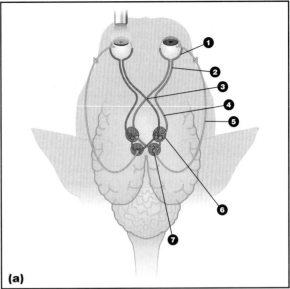

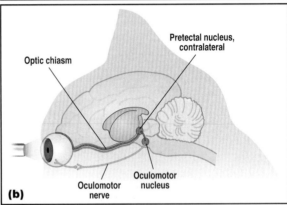

19.5 **(a)** Dorsal and **(b)** sagittal views of the neuroanatomical pathway for the PLR. A bright light stimulus enters the retina and initiates an impulse (1) that travels through the optic nerve (2), optic chiasm (3) and optic tract (4). The stimulus is relayed to the pretectal nucleus within the rostral colliculus (6). The parasympathetic nucleus of the oculomotor nerve (7) is stimulated and the signal is transmitted through its parasympathetic branch (5), resulting in contraction of the iris sphincter muscle and constriction of the pupil. A lesion in any part of the pathway can disrupt the PLR. (Redrawn after Platt and Garosi (2012) with permission from the publisher)

the PLR synapse with a third neuron in the pretectal nucleus and never reach the consciousness. Most of the axons arising from the pretectal nucleus decussate again and synapse on the parasympathetic component of the oculomotor nucleus (ipsilateral to the stimulated eye) in the mesencephalon. There are also neurons that do not decussate and project to the oculomotor nucleus on the contralateral side to the stimulated eye. The proportion of axons that decussate is higher than the proportion of axons that do not decussate, explaining why the direct response (constriction in the eye receiving the light stimulus) is greater than the consensual response (constriction in the eye not receiving the light stimulus). By combining the results of vision testing, the dazzle reflex and the PLR, it is possible to determine whether the lesion is located within a pathway shared by these tests or within a pathway that is independent.

Dark adaptation test

Assessment of pupil size and symmetry should also be conducted in darkness to evaluate sympathetic function. The dark adaptation test involves assessment of the pupils after a few minutes in complete darkness (as this allows complete relaxation of the pupillary sphincter muscle).

Swinging flashlight test

The swinging flashlight test assesses the integrity of the entire PLR pathway. It is best conducted in a darkened room because the extent of the iris constriction will be greater and more easily observed. A strong light is swung from one eye to the other. If pupillary dilatation is observed during direct light stimulation, instead of the expected pupil constriction, the swinging flashlight test is said to be positive for the eye with the dilating pupil. The explanation for this is that the direct stimulus is no longer sufficient to maintain the previously evoked degree of pupil constriction, so both pupils dilate, whilst maintaining the relative anisocoria. A positive swinging flashlight test indicates an ipsilateral, unilateral, prechiasmal optic nerve lesion and/or unilateral retinal disease.

Eyelids

Relevant neuroanatomy

The levator palpebrae superioris muscle is the main muscle responsible for the elevation and retraction of the upper eyelid and is innervated by the motor part of the oculomotor nerve. The smooth muscles of the upper and lower eyelid, innervated by the oculosympathetic nerves, also participate in eyelid opening and third eyelid retraction. The eyelids are closed by the orbicularis oculi muscle, which is innervated by the palpebral branch of the auriculopalpebral nerve (a branch of the facial nerve). The protrusion of the third eyelid is generally a passive, non-neurological process (except in the cat, where it is mediated by the abducens and oculomotor nerves), whilst its retraction is an active involuntary process associated with tonic contraction of the smooth muscles controlled by the sympathetic supply of the eye.

Clinical evaluation

Eyelid closure can be evaluated via the following tests:

- Menace response (see above)
- Dazzle reflex
- Corneal and palpebral reflexes.

Dazzle reflex

If the PLR cannot be elicited, the dazzle reflex is often helpful in lesion localization (Figure 19.6). The dazzle reflex is a subcortical reflex characterized by a bilateral partial eyelid blink in response to a very bright light illuminating one eye at a time. As this is a subcortical reflex, it may be present in a blind animal and does not evaluate the cortical component of

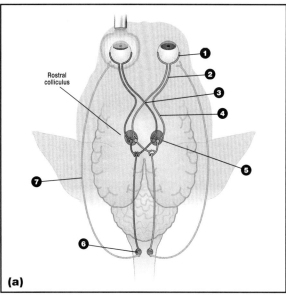

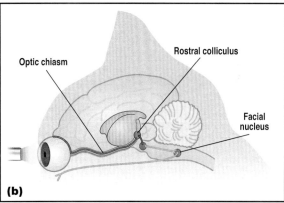

19.6 **(a)** Dorsal and **(b)** sagittal views of the proposed neuroanatomical pathway for the dazzle reflex. This reflex is similar to the PLR but differs in that the efferent pathway is mediated by the oculomotor nerve in the PLR pathway, whereas it is the facial nerve that carries the efferent information for the dazzle reflex. A very bright light stimulus enters the retina (1) and travels through the optic nerve (2), optic chiasm (3) and optic tract (4). The stimulus is relayed to the pretectal nucleus within the rostral colliculus (5). From here, the signal is transmitted to the ipsilateral facial nucleus in the brainstem (6). The facial nerve (7) then carries the efferent stimulus to the orbicularis oculi muscles of the eyelids, resulting in a reflex blink.

the visual pathway. The afferent arm of this reflex is the same as the afferent arm of the PLR, mediated by the optic nerve up to the level of the midbrain (i.e. the subcortical portion of the visual pathway), whilst the efferent arm of the dazzle reflex is mediated by the facial nerve.

Corneal and palpebral reflexes

Closure of the eyelid is the expected motor response of both the corneal and palpebral reflex. The trigeminal nerve provides sensory innervation of the face (cutaneous elements of the face as well as the cornea, mucosa of the nasal septum and mucosa of the oral cavity) and motor innervation to the masticatory muscles (temporalis, masseter, medial and lateral pterygoid and rostral part of the digastric muscles). The motor function of the trigeminal nerve is assessed by evaluating the size and symmetry of the masticatory muscles and testing the resistance of the jaw when opening the mouth. The sensory function of the trigeminal nerve (sensation of the ocular surface and face) can be tested by the corneal reflex (ophthalmic branch) and the palpebral reflex (ophthalmic or maxillary branch when touching the medial or lateral canthus of the eye, respectively). The corneal reflex is a subcortical reflex involving closure of the eyelid in response to a tactile or painful stimulus to a non-anaesthetized cornea.

The lateral and medial canthus of each eye should be evaluated separately. A blink response with complete closure of the palpebral fissures, as well as retraction of the globe with passive protrusion of the third eyelid, should be expected. The final common neurological pathways for eyelid closure and globe retraction in the corneal and palpebral reflexes are mediated by the facial nerve and abducens nerve, respectively. Intact facial and abducens nerves are required for the menace response, palpebral reflex and dazzle reflex because they are responsible for orbicularis oculi muscle contraction, closing the palpebral fissures, and globe retraction.

Globe

Relevant neuroanatomy

The oculomotor nerve (CN III) innervates the ipsilateral dorsal, ventral and medial recti muscles, as well as the ventral oblique muscle. This nerve also mediates pupillary constriction and is involved in the retraction of the upper eyelid (levator palpebrae superioris) via its parasympathetic component (see above). Thus, it plays an important role in the efferent arm of the PLR and eyelid position. The oculomotor nuclei are located in the rostral mesencephalon. The axons exit the brainstem and traverse the cavernous sinus lateral to the hypophysis before exiting the skull through the orbital fissure.

The trochlear nerve (CN IV) innervates the contralateral dorsal oblique muscle. This muscle is responsible for inward turning of the eye. The trochlear nucleus is located in the caudal mesencephalon. After exiting the brainstem, its axons decussate on the dorsal surface of the brainstem and course rostrally through the cavernous sinus before exiting the skull via the orbital fissure. The abducens nerve (CN VI) innervates the ipsilateral lateral rectus and retractor bulbi muscles. Its nucleus is located in the rostral medulla oblongata and its axons follow the same pathway as those of the oculomotor and trochlear nerves.

Clinical examination

During examination of the eyes, the globes should be assessed to determine whether they are positioned normally within the orbits. The normal position of the globe is dependent on the innervation of the extraocular muscles by the oculomotor, trochlear and abducens nerves (Figure 19.7). The function of these cranial nerves can be tested by assessing vestibular eye movements (see below) and evaluating the degree of abduction (CN VI) and adduction (CN III).

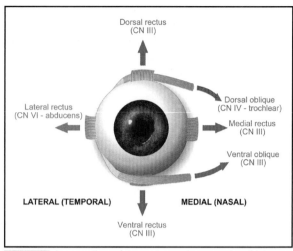

19.7 Innervation of the extraocular muscles. Note that the retractor bulbi muscle is also innervated by the abducens nerve. (© Jacques Penderis and reproduced from the *BSAVA Manual of Canine and Feline Neurology, 4th edition*)

Nystagmus

Nystagmus is an involuntary rhythmic movement of the eyeballs. Vestibular nystagmus has a slow and a fast phase (i.e. jerk nystagmus), whilst pendular nystagmus is characterized by a continuous oscillation of both globes without slow or fast components. There are two major categories of vestibular nystagmus:

- Physiological nystagmus – this occurs in healthy animals. It can be induced by turning the head from side to side and this test is sometimes referred to as assessment of 'vestibular eye movements'. This physiological nystagmus stabilizes images on the retina during head movement. It is always observed in the plane of rotation of the head and consists of a slow phase in the direction opposite to that of the head rotation and a fast phase in the same direction as the head rotation. In the absence of any head movement, nystagmus should never be present in a normal animal. This reflex evaluates the vestibular system (sensory arm of the reflex), as well as the medial longitudinal fasciculus in the brainstem and cranial nerves controlling the extraocular muscles (CN III, IV and VI). The fast phase of the nystagmus is always in the direction of head movement. By convention, the direction of the jerk nystagmus is determined by the direction of the fast phase. It is best tested in a cat or small dog by holding the animal at arm's length and rotating its head from side to side. A reduction or absence of vestibular eye movements is considered abnormal
- Pathological nystagmus – this generally reflects an underlying vestibular disorder and its presence is always indicative of a pathological process. The eyes have a tendency to drift spontaneously in the direction of the lesion (slow phase), and via a brainstem mechanism (involving the medial longitudinal fasciculus) the eyes are quickly returned to their initial location (fast phase). This type of abnormal nystagmus

can be seen at rest (i.e. spontaneous nystagmus) or with abnormal head positions (i.e. positional nystagmus). Horizontal, vertical and rotary nystagmus may be present (Figure 19.8). Nystagmus may also be observed in clinically blind animals.

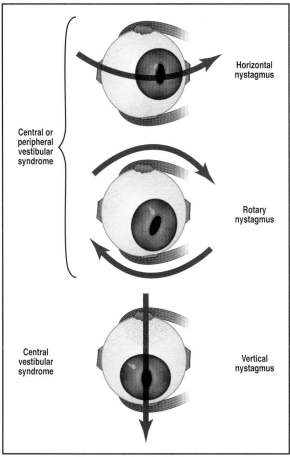

19.8 The directions of pathological nystagmus. (Redrawn after Platt and Garosi (2012) with permission from the publisher)

Lacrimal gland

Relevant neuroanatomy

The lacrimal gland is innervated by the parasympathetic portion of the facial nerve (CN VII), which also innervates the lateral nasal gland and the mandibular and sublingual salivary glands. Lacrimation can be the result of basal tear secretion, reflex tear production or tears induced by a variety of drugs. The afferent arm of reflex tear production (trigeminal–lacrimal reflex) is the ophthalmic branch of the trigeminal nerve (CN V). The efferent arm is the parasympathetic portion of the facial nerve. Dysfunction of the parasympathetic supply to the lacrimal gland results in neurogenic keratoconjunctivitis sicca (KCS). This is mainly seen with lesions of the portion of the facial nerve located between the medulla and middle ear. Lesions distal to the facial canal in the temporal bone will not affect the parasympathetic division of the facial nerve. Increased reflex tear production occurs in response to sensory

stimuli such as direct corneal stimulation and exposure to cold or irritants.

Clinical evaluation

Schirmer tear test

Schirmer tear tests measure the basal and reflex tear production of the eyes. Placing paper test strips in each eye in the conscious patient stimulates the cornea, resulting in reflex tear production. This is called Schirmer tear test 1 (STT-1). When this test is performed following the application of topical anaesthesia to the eye, it is assessing basal tear production because the afferent arm of the lacrimal reflex has been removed by the anaesthetic. This is called Schirmer tear test 2 (STT-2). Schirmer tear tests are discussed in greater detail in Chapters 1 and 10.

Investigation of disease

Fundic examination

The retina and optic nerve head have a unique position within the central nervous system (CNS) in that they are directly visible on clinical examination in normal animals. This feature is particularly useful in patients with suspected neuro-ophthalmological disease and patients with other clinical manifestations of CNS disease (see Chapters 1 and 18 for detailed descriptions of ophthalmoscopic examination and the normal and pathological appearance of the retina and optic nerve head, respectively).

Electroretinography

Electroretinography evaluates retinal function, particularly of the photoreceptors (rods and cones) and bipolar cells, but not visual function. In clinical practice, it is primarily used to differentiate photoreceptor diseases (such as progressive retinal atrophy (PRA) and sudden acquired retinal degeneration syndrome (SARDS)) from more central causes of blindness (see Chapters 1 and 18).

Visual evoked potentials

Visual evoked potentials (VEPs) are stimulus-locked recordings of brain activity in response to a light flashing on the retina. Recordings are obtained from electrodes placed in the skin overlying the occipital cortex. They provide a functional assessment of the central visual pathways (i.e. the optic nerve, optic tracts and visual cortex) but also rely on normal retinal function for signal generation. VEPs are largely a research tool and have not yet found widespread use in veterinary practice due to their variability and requirement for general anaesthesia.

Common conditions

Blindness

Blindness can be partial or complete, unilateral or bilateral. The presentation depends on the aetiology and as such the general physical, ophthalmic and neurological examinations provide important clues as to the likely underlying problem. The main goals are to establish whether the blindness is the result of an ophthalmological or a neurological disease and, in the event of a neurological condition being suspected, to accurately localize the lesion within the visual pathways. Having determined the neurological localization, a list of possible causes can be formulated. After this, it is important to proceed through a systematic investigation, selecting appropriate tests to diagnose and implement treatment for the underlying condition.

Traditionally, blindness is divided into central and peripheral components, although this terminology can cause confusion. For the purposes of this text:

- Peripheral blindness results from a lesion located in the visual pathway shared with the PLR pathway (i.e. a lesion situated rostral to the thalamus, e.g. in the eye, optic nerve, optic chiasm or proximal optic tract) (Figure 19.9a)
- Central blindness results from a lesion located in the visual pathway not shared with the PLR pathway (i.e. a lesion situated caudal to the thalamus, e.g. in the distal optic tract, lateral geniculate nucleus, optic radiation or occipital cortex) (Figure 19.9b).

Stepwise approach to blindness

The approach to blindness involves the following steps:

- Step 1 – is the animal unilaterally or bilaterally blind?
  This question is primarily answered by evaluating the menace response in each eye separately. If the menace response is absent or delayed, the eyelids must be assessed for their ability to close by eliciting the palpebral reflex. If facial paralysis is present, eyeball retraction, elevation of the third eyelid and head retraction may help in the assessment of vision. If facial paralysis is present, or if there is doubt about the result of the menace response test, then the ability of the patient to navigate an obstacle course, visual tracking testing and/or the visual placing response should be evaluated (if the size of the animal allows them to be lifted)
- Step 2 – is the blindness peripheral or central?
  Following assessment of the menace response, the clinician should evaluate pupil size and the PLR to determine whether the lesion is affecting the peripheral or central visual pathway. The PLR is expected to be absent with a lesion in the peripheral visual pathway, whereas the PLR is not affected with a lesion in the central visual pathway. It should be noted that the PLR requires fewer intact axons than the conscious perception of vision and, therefore, partial lesions of the peripheral visual pathway may cause loss of vision whilst sparing the PLR, creating the illusion of a lesion affecting the central visual pathway. It should be noted that the PLR can be preserved in animals with retinal diseases that spare the inner retina (e.g. SARDS or PRA) due to preservation of slower PLRs mediated by photosensitive ganglion cells in the inner retina.

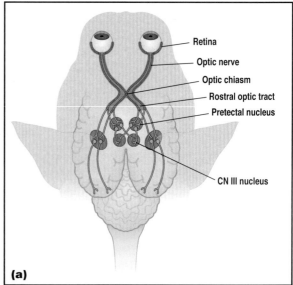

(a)

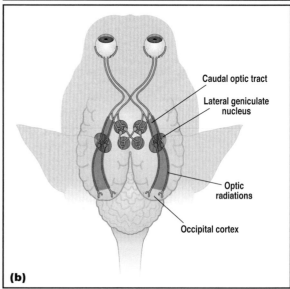

(b)

19.9 **(a)** Peripheral visual pathway (outlined in red). This includes the retina, optic nerve, optic chiasm and the rostral portion of the optic tract. Lesions in the peripheral visual pathway generally affect the PLR. **(b)** Central visual pathway (outlined in red). This includes the caudal portion of the optic tract, the lateral geniculate nucleus and the occipital cortex. Lesions in the central visual pathway typically spare the PLR. (Redrawn after Platt and Garosi (2012) with permission from the publisher)

Central blindness may be accompanied by other forebrain signs such as abnormal behaviour, seizures, sensory deficits (facial/nasal hypalgesia) and postural reaction deficits. These sensory and postural reaction deficits, as for the visual deficits, are all contralateral to the side of the forebrain lesion. Thus, careful attention should be paid to cranial nerve function, mentation and postural reaction evaluation (i.e. proprioceptive placing and hopping)
- Step 3 – is the lesion focal, multifocal or diffuse?

The lesion localization for unilateral and bilateral blindness is detailed in Figure 19.10 with examples provided in Figures 19.11 and 19.12.

The next diagnostic step depends on whether central or peripheral blindness is suspected. If this has been difficult to ascertain, then the full repertoire of investigations should be performed, starting with the least invasive. The tests below are listed in the order in which they should be performed and an assumption has been made that a complete ophthalmic and general physical examination has been undertaken.

Unilateral or bilateral blindness?	Intact direct PLR?	Peripheral or central blindness?	Lesion distribution within the visual pathways
Unilateral	No	Peripheral	Retina or optic nerve lesion (ipsilateral)
Unilateral	Yes	Central	Focal lesion in the contralateral distal portion of the optic tract, lateral geniculate nucleus, optic radiation or visual cortex (i.e. contralateral forebrain)
Bilateral	No	Peripheral	Bilateral disease affecting retina and/or optic nerves or focal lesion of the optic chiasm
Bilateral	Yes	Central	Multifocal or diffuse lesion in the distal part of the optic tracts, lateral geniculate nuclei, optic radiations or visual cortices (i.e. bilateral forebrain)

19.10 Lesion localization for unilateral and bilateral blindness.

19.11

Approach to a case with unilateral blindness in the left eye, using the PLR and an ophthalmoscopic examination to determine lesion localization. The red shading depicts the possible locations of the lesion along the visual pathways. (Redrawn after Platt and Garosi (2012) with permission from the publisher)

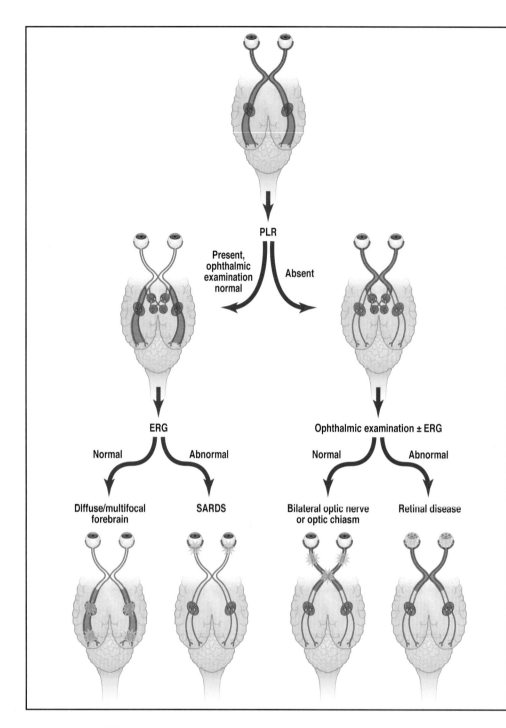

19.12

Approach to a case with sudden-onset bilateral blindness, using the PLR, an ophthalmic examination and, if indicated, electroretinography to determine lesion localization. The red shading represents possible locations of lesions along the visual pathways. Note that retinal disease may be primary or secondary to, for example, uveitis or glaucoma. ERG = electroretinogram; SARDS = sudden acquired retinal degeneration syndrome. (Redrawn after Platt and Garosi (2012) with permission from the publisher)

- Peripheral blindness:
  - Electroretinography – this is used to assess the retinal response to light (see Chapters 1 and 18). A non-recordable trace is indicative of loss of photoreceptor function. If the fundus appears ophthalmoscopically normal, a diagnosis of SARDS can be made
  - Advanced imaging – magnetic resonance imaging (MRI) is preferred as it allows visualization of the retrobulbar space, optic nerve and chiasm
  - Cerebrospinal fluid (CSF) collection and analysis – the optic nerve is surrounded by meninges and CSF. Thus, even in the presence of a normal MRI study, CSF analysis may reveal evidence of an inflammatory

disease process (e.g. optic neuritis) (for further information on CSF collection and analysis, the reader is referred to the *BSAVA Manual of Canine and Feline Neurology*)
  - Serology and polymerase chain reaction (PCR) on serum and/or CSF samples for infectious diseases as indicated based on history, clinical features and conditions known to be prevalent within the geographical region.
- Central blindness:
  - Blood profile – including haematology, biochemistry, electrolytes, ammonia and bile acid stimulation test (especially with bilateral blindness)
  - Advanced imaging

- CSF collection
- Serology/PCR on serum and/or CSF for geographically relevant infectious diseases.

Differential diagnosis

The differential diagnoses for patients with unilateral and bilateral blindness are listed in Figures 19.13 and 19.14, respectively.

Diseases associated with blindness

Advanced retinal degeneration: For detailed information on conditions such as PRA and other causes of retinal degeneration, the reader is referred to Chapter 18.

Retinal detachment: This is an important cause of sudden-onset blindness and can be diagnosed by ophthalmic examination (Figure 19.15). The reader is referred to Chapter 18 for further details.

Sudden acquired retinal degeneration syndrome: The typical presentation of SARDS is acute blindness with dilated pupils. Affected patients are usually middle-aged and show concurrent systemic clinical signs of polyuria/polydipsia, lethargy and weight gain. The ocular examination commonly reveals bilateral mydriasis and decreased to absent PLRs bilaterally. It should be noted that the PLR can initially be relatively normal, but slow, creating the illusion of a more central lesion. Initially, the fundus appears normal, although ophthalmoscopic signs of progressive retinal degeneration may develop over the following months. Electroretinography is required to distinguish SARDS from other lesions responsible for acute blindness. There is no treatment and the blindness is permanent. Concurrent clinical signs may mimic hyperadrenocorticism but usually resolve within a few months. The reader is referred to Chapter 18 for further information on SARDS.

Disease	Peripheral blindness	Central blindness
Vascular	Hyphaema Vitreal haemorrhage Hypertensive chorioretinopathy	Brain infarct Brain haemorrhage
Inflammatory	Keratitis Anterior uveitis Chorioretinitis Optic neuritis Retrobulbar abscess/ cellulitis	Infectious encephalitis (viral, protozoal, fungal, bacterial) Meningoencephalitis of unknown origin (granulomatous, necrotizing, idiopathic)
Traumatic	Globe and orbit trauma	Head trauma
Neoplastic	Tumour of (or compressing) the optic nerve Primary or secondary intraocular tumour	Primary or secondary brain tumour
Other	Corneal oedema Glaucoma Lens luxation Cataract Retinal detachment Retinal degeneration Optic nerve hypoplasia	Intracranial intra-arachnoid cyst Porencephaly/ hydranencephaly

19.13 Causes of unilateral blindness.

Disease	Peripheral blindness	Central blindness
Vascular	Hyphaema Vitreal haemorrhage Hypertensive chorioretinopathy	Brain haemorrhage Global brain ischaemia (post-anaesthetic blindness)
Inflammatory	Keratitis Anterior uveitis Chorioretinitis Optic neuritis	Infectious encephalitis (viral, protozoal, fungal, bacterial) Meningoencephalitis of unknown aetiology (granulomatous, necrotizing, idiopathic)
Traumatic	Globe and orbit trauma	Head trauma
Toxic	Ivermectin toxicity (dogs) Fluoroquinolone toxicity (cats)	Lead poisoning
Anomalous/ other	Corneal oedema Glaucoma Lens luxation Cataracts Retinal detachment Retinal degeneration (especially progressive retinal atrophy) Optic nerve hypoplasia	Intracranial intra-arachnoid cyst Porencephaly/ hydranencephaly Hydrocephalus
Metabolic	Diabetic cataracts	Hypoxia/ischaemia/ excitotoxicity (e.g. post-anaesthesia, post-ictal) Hepatic encephalopathy Osmotic abnormalities (sodium imbalance) Hypoglycaemia Ketoacidosis
Neoplastic	Tumour of the optic chiasm or in the vicinity of the optic chiasm (meningioma, pituitary macroadenoma)	Primary or secondary brain tumour
Degenerative	Sudden acquired retinal degeneration syndrome Corneal oedema Cataracts Retinal degeneration Retinal detachment	

19.14 Causes of bilateral blindness (see also Chapter 21).

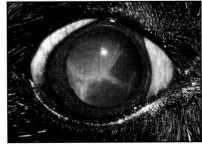

19.15 Retinal detachment visible through the pupil on direct illumination in a dog. (Courtesy of D Gould)

Optic neuritis: The optic nerves are essentially white matter tracts surrounded by meninges and, therefore, are affected by similar disease processes to those that affect the CNS. Optic neuritis is an acute, progressive inflammation of the optic nerves and can be the result of a number of different diseases, including meningoencephalitis of unknown aetiology (MUA) and infection (e.g. viral, rickettsial or fungal). Fundic examination reveals loss of visualization of the optic nerve head margins, dilatation of the

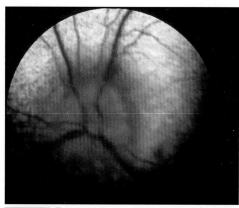

19.16 Fundus of a dog with optic neuritis. Note the poor optic nerve head demarcation associated with the peripapillary oedema, the pink discoloration of the optic nerve head caused by inflammation, and the change in direction of the superficial retinal blood vessels as they course over the elevated optic nerve head. (Courtesy of D Gould)

retinal venules, elevation of the optic nerve head(s) and/or haemorrhage and/or changes in tapetal reflectivity (Figure 19.16). Diagnosis is only presumptive and is confirmed by performing advanced orbital and brain imaging, CSF analysis and serological testing for infectious diseases. The treatment depends upon the underlying cause and many cases represent MUA, which responds to immunosuppressive doses of corticosteroids. Relapse is a common feature and the prognosis is guarded. Optic neuritis is discussed in greater detail in Chapter 18.

Global brain ischaemia: This is most commonly due to cardiac or pulmonary insufficiency secondary to cardiopulmonary arrest or anaesthetic complications (e.g. hypotension and hypoxia). Suspected risk factors for the development of global brain ischaemia during anaesthesia include brachycephalic conformation and the use of ketamine for the induction and maintenance of anaesthesia. The use of mouth gags was also recently identified as a potential risk factor for cerebral ischaemia and blindness in cats (Stiles *et al.*, 2012). Certain areas of the brain are more susceptible to ischaemia than others (hippocampus, cerebral and cerebellar cortex, basal nuclei). Clinically, global brain ischaemia is characterized by a number of neurological deficits (blindness, compulsive walking, ataxia, seizures) that have a peracute onset and can progress over the first 24 hours (Palmer and Walker, 1970; Jurk *et al.*, 2001; Panarello *et al.*, 2004; Timm *et al.*, 2008). MRI can be used to identify an underlying ischaemic encephalopathy with the distribution of lesions reflecting areas with a particular susceptibility to hypoxia. Generally, treatment of these patients aims to provide supportive care, maintain adequate tissue oxygenation and manage neurological and non-neurological complications. In a study in cats with post-anaesthetic cortical blindness, 70% had documented recovery of vision within a 6-week period (Stiles *et al.*, 2012). Such information in dogs is lacking, although the prognosis for recovery of vision is generally considered guarded.

Anisocoria
The size of the pupils represents a dynamic equilibrium between the parasympathetic nervous system (PNS), which is responsive to the amount of light entering the eye, and the SNS, which is responsive to the emotional state of the animal.

Clinical signs
Anisocoria, when caused by a neurological problem, may result from any one of the following neurological lesions:

- A unilateral lesion of the parasympathetic component of the oculomotor nerve
- A unilateral lesion of the sympathetic supply to the eye (Horner's syndrome)
- A unilateral retinal or optic nerve lesion
- A cerebellar lesion
- An acute brain disorder (resulting in severe midbrain damage).

Parasympathetic denervation of the eye: Efferent parasympathetic denervation of the pupil (internal ophthalmoplegia) can occur with or without disrupting the motor innervation of the extraocular muscles by the oculomotor nerve (external ophthalmoplegia).

- Internal ophthalmoplegia – clinical signs manifest as a markedly dilated pupil that is non-reactive to direct and indirect light stimulation. The anisocoria is particularly obvious in ambient light and maximal and equal dilatation of both pupils should occur on dark adaptation testing.
- External ophthalmoplegia – characterized by ptosis (drooping of the upper eyelid), lateral strabismus, inability to direct the globe dorsally, ventrally or medially ± signs of internal ophthalmoplegia.

Differential diagnoses for internal ophthalmoplegia to be aware of during an examination include pharmacological blockade with atropine or atropine-like compounds. Prior use of these topical drugs can confuse the results of the neuro-ophthalmological examination.

Sympathetic denervation of the eye: The loss of sympathetic innervation to the eye causes a combination of clinical signs, which are collectively termed Horner's syndrome (Figure 19.17). This syndrome manifests as a constellation of clinical signs:

- Miosis
- Drooping of the upper eyelid (ptosis) due to the loss of smooth muscle tone affecting Müller's muscle
- Enophthalmos, which is the result of:
  - Denervation and lack of tone of the orbital smooth muscles within the periorbita
  - The unopposed antagonistic action of the extraocular muscles (especially the retractor bulbi muscles) that retract the eyeball.
- Protrusion of the third eyelid – denervation of the smooth muscle of the third eyelid and concurrent enophthalmos result in passive protrusion of the third eyelid.

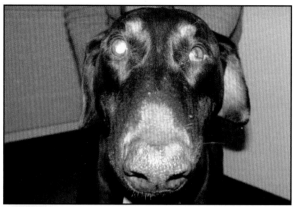

19.17 Idiopathic left-sided Horner's syndrome. Note the miosis, ptosis and protrusion of the third eyelid. (Courtesy of D Gould)

A lesion anywhere along the sympathetic pathway can cause Horner's syndrome. The syndrome is classified according to the level of the lesion along the sympathetic pathway: first order (UMN), second order (preganglionic fibres) or third order (postganglionic fibres). Thus, lesions causing Horner's syndrome tend to affect a region, as opposed to a specific nucleus or nerve, and therefore accompanying neurological and other clinical signs are useful to further localize the lesion within the sympathetic pathway. This syndrome is most commonly seen with second order lesions affecting the preganglionic fibres located within the intermediate grey matter of the T1–T3 spinal cord segments to the tympanic bulla, and the third order lesions affecting postganglionic fibres located between the tympanic bulla and the eye.

Unilateral retinal or optic nerve lesion: Severe unilateral retinal or optic nerve lesions may result in a slight ipsilateral mydriasis, which responds only to light directed into the normal contralateral eye (i.e. an abnormal direct PLR and normal indirect PLR). Such lesions result in the absence of vision and menace response in the affected eye, as well as a positive swinging flashlight test (see Figure 19.13 for causes of unilateral blindness).

Cerebellar lesion: Unilateral mydriasis with a pupil that is slowly responsive to light has been reported as an occasional finding with unilateral lesions of the cerebellum involving the fastigial or interpositial nuclei. The third eyelid may protrude and the palpebral fissure may be enlarged. These changes are usually observed in the eye that is ipsilateral to an interpositial nucleus lesion and in the eye that is contralateral to a fastigial nucleus lesion. A partial protrusion of the third eyelid and mild enlargement of the palpebral fissure may also occur (deLahunta and Glass, 2008).

Acute traumatic brain lesion: Pupillary abnormalities are frequently seen following raised intracranial pressure (ICP), which occurs either as a result of a mass lesion or trauma to the head. Pupillary size, symmetry and reactivity can provide valuable information about the severity of the brain injury and the likely prognosis. Following head trauma, these parameters are important indicators to monitor neurological status.

In the trauma patient, before consideration is given to primary neurological disease, it is important to rule out ocular disease as a cause of the anisocoria. For example, an acute ocular injury can cause uveitis with spasm of the ciliary muscle and pupillary sphincter muscle of the iris, resulting in unilateral miosis; whereas, a long-standing ocular injury to the iris, traumatic injury of the retina or orbital structures may result in unilateral mydriasis.

A wide array of pupillary abnormalities is possible following head trauma. The presence of miosis may indicate a lesion resulting from disruption of the sympathetic innervation to the eye. This may be due to a lesion within the diencephalon or brainstem (i.e. a first order lesion) or an injury anywhere along the pathway through the brachial plexus, cranial mediastinum, cervical soft tissues and tympanic bulla. Lesions affecting sympathetic innervation to the eye may also be associated with third eyelid elevation, enophthalmos and ptosis as part of Horner's syndrome. The presence of mydriasis may indicate brain herniation and/or a progressive brainstem lesion and is an indication for immediate, aggressive therapy. Bilateral mydriasis with no response to light is considered to be indicative of an irreversible injury to the oculomotor nuclei in the midbrain and is associated with a poor prognosis. Fixed, unresponsive and mid-range pupils are usually seen with cerebellar herniation (deLahunta and Glass, 2008). Traditionally, it has been reported that brain herniation and severe midbrain lesions cause miotic pupils that slowly become mydriatic with no response to light. However, in practice, this progression may be so rapid that neither the miosis, nor the transition period to mydriasis, is observed.

Stepwise approach to anisocoria

The approach to anisocoria involves the following steps:

- Step 1 – perform an ophthalmological examination to rule-out non-neurological causes for the asymmetry (primary or secondary anatomical or mechanical pupil/iris abnormalities)
- Step 2 – determine which pupil is abnormal by checking the PLR and whether the asymmetry in pupil size increases in bright light or darkness (Figure 19.18)
- Step 3 – if the PLR is abnormal and the pupil is relatively dilated, then a parasympathetic lesion should be considered. To determine whether the lesion is pre- or postganglionic, pharmacological testing should be performed (see Figure 19.19)
- Step 4 – if the PLR is normal and the pupil is relatively constricted, then a sympathetic or cerebellar lesion should be considered. In the absence of cerebellar signs on neurological examination, pharmacological testing should be performed to determine whether the lesion is pre- or postganglionic and the patient should be assessed for other neurological signs (see Figures 19.20 and 19.21).

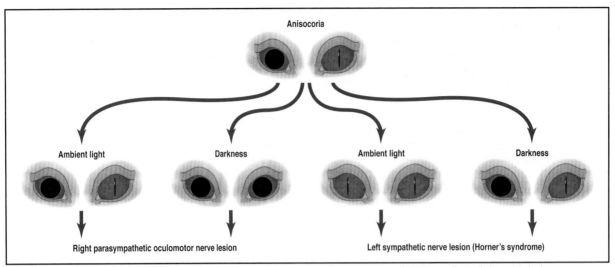

19.18 A stepwise approach to localizing anisocoria based on the response of both pupils to light and darkness. Determining which pupil is abnormal can be achieved by checking the PLR and assessing whether the asymmetry in pupil size increases in bright light (suggesting parasympathetic dysfunction in the larger pupil) or in darkness (suggesting sympathetic dysfunction in the smaller pupil).

Pharmacological localization: Pharmacological tests should be conducted on both eyes using the normal eye as a control.

Parasympathetic denervation of the eye: Topical application of a diluted direct-acting cholinergic parasympathomimetic drug (e.g. 0.1% pilocarpine) to the affected and control eyes tests the ability of the pupil to constrict (Figure 19.19).

- If the affected pupil remains dilated and the control pupil constricts, then unilateral or asymmetrical iris disease (e.g. iris atrophy) or

prior application of a mydriatic drug (e.g. atropine or atropine-like drugs) should be suspected.
- If the affected pupil constricts before the control pupil, a postganglionic lesion of the oculomotor nerve (i.e. the ciliary ganglion or short ciliary nerves) should be suspected. This is because of denervation hypersensitivity, whereby the denervated effector cells are more responsive to pilocarpine than the control eye due to receptor upregulation.
- A preganglionic lesion (parasympathetic nucleus of the oculomotor nerve, or the oculomotor

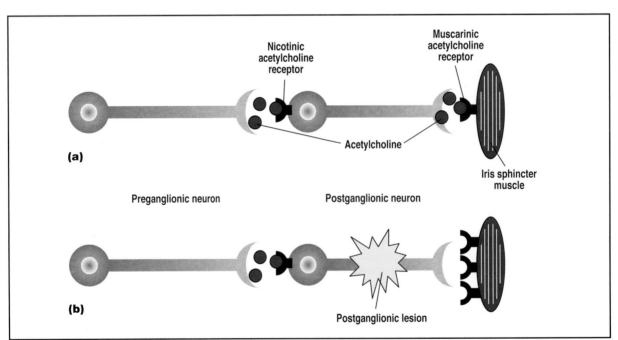

19.19 Evaluation of parasympathetic denervation using 0.1% pilocarpine. Rapid constriction of the pupil compared with **(a)** the normal eye is observed with **(b)** a postganglionic lesion due to denervation hypersensitivity. With a preganglionic lesion, constriction occurs more slowly, similar to the normal eye (20–30 minutes). A complete absence of pupillary response following administration of 0.1% pilocarpine to the affected eye probably suggests a non-neurological cause (e.g. iris atrophy)

nerve) can be evaluated by the topical administration of 0.5% physostigmine (an indirect-acting parasympathomimetic) into each eye. If the affected pupil constricts before the control pupil, a preganglionic lesion is present. If a postganglionic lesion is present, then the affected pupil will not constrict.

Sympathetic denervation of the eye: Pharmacological testing using topical phenylephrine can be used to determine the site of the lesion in Horner's syndrome (i.e. first, second or third order) (Figure 19.20). For this test, 1% phenylephrine (a direct-acting sympathomimetic drug) is administered topically to both eyes and the time taken for the pupils to dilate is noted. This test is based on the principle of denervation hypersensitivity, whereby the innervated effector cells (i.e. iris dilator muscle) increase their sensitivity to direct-acting sympathomimetics following denervation. This phenomenon usually takes up to 2 weeks to develop. The general rule to remember when testing is that the closer the lesion is to the iris, the less time it takes for the pupil to dilate. A common mistake when conducting pharmacological testing is to misinterpret retraction of the third eyelid as a positive response to phenylephrine application, instead of assessing time to pupil dilation.

- With postganglionic lesions (i.e. third order Horner's syndrome), the sympathetically innervated effector cells become supersensitive to direct-acting sympathomimetics and thus respond to weak and ordinarily ineffective concentrations of this drug. On this basis, topical administration of 1 drop of 1% phenylephrine leads to mydriasis in the affected eye within 20 minutes, with no response in the control eye.
- The ability of this pharmacological test to differentiate a first order (UMN) from a second order (preganglionic) lesion remains controversial and hence it is recommended to use this test in conjunction with a neurological examination or imaging studies as indicated.
- When performing this pharmacological test, it is important to ensure that the same volume and concentration of the drug is delivered to the contralateral eye and that the corneal epithelium is intact in both eyes. Thus, pharmacological testing should be conducted before topical anaesthetics are applied or tonometry is performed.

Diseases associated with anisocoria
The criteria for differentiating the various causes of anisocoria are summarized in Figure 19.21. Pupil abnormalities are common with acute brain disorders such as head trauma and other conditions that cause a rapid change in ICP (intracranial bleed, decompensation from brain tumour or inflammatory/infectious brain diseases). In the absence of concurrent ocular trauma, miotic pupils may indicate loss of cortical input or direct damage to the sympathetic centres in the diencephalon, allowing unopposed oculomotor pupillary constriction. Pupils that are initially miotic and then become mydriatic and unresponsive to light are indicative of a progressive severe brainstem lesion (mostly seen with raised ICP and caudal subtentorial herniation) (Figures 19.22 and 19.23). Extensive lesions that affect sympathetic innervation as well as the oculomotor nerve result in mid-position fixed pupils.

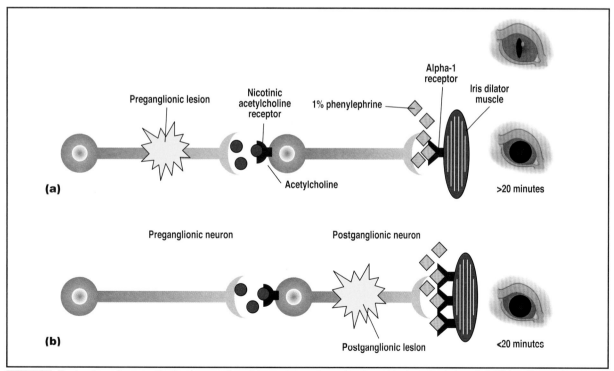

19.20 Evaluation of sympathetic denervation (Horner's syndrome) using 1% phenylephrine. **(a)** With a first order (upper motor neuron) or second order (preganglionic neuron) lesion, dilation occurs slowly or not at all. **(b)** Rapid dilation of the pupil (within 20 minutes) is observed with a third order (postganglionic neuron) lesion due to denervation hypersensitivity.

Pupil abnormality	Lesion localization	Associated signs	Differential diagnosis	Diagnostic tests
Unilateral mydriasis, direct PLR absent and indirect PLR present OR with lateral strabismus	Parasympathetic component of oculomotor nerve (CN III) or iris abnormality (such as iris atrophy or drug-induced, e.g. prior use of topical atropine) (lower image shows both internal and external ophthalmoplegia)	The pupil remains mydriatic in light with constriction of the unaffected pupil and normal vision. Other signs that may be present if the motor component of CN III is involved include narrowing of the palpebral fissure due to upper eyelid ptosis, ventrolateral strabismus and reduced ocular movements	Inflammatory or neoplastic disease affecting ipsilateral oculomotor nucleus or efferent pathway; iris abnormality	Pharmacological test with pilocarpine or physostigmine; CT/MRI of the brain
Unilateral mydriasis, direct and indirect PLR absent	Unilateral retinal or optic nerve	Pupils are equally dilated in darkness, vision is abnormal and fundoscopic examination may also be abnormal. Swinging flashlight test is positive in the affected eye	Inflammatory, traumatic, degenerative or neoplastic disease affecting the ipsilateral retina or optic nerve; congenital abnormalities (e.g. optic nerve hypoplasia); retrobulbar mass (e.g. abscess or tumour)	Fundoscopic examination; electroretinography; ultrasonography of the eye and orbit; CT/MRI of the orbit and brain; CSF analysis
Unilateral mydriasis, direct and indirect PLR present	Contralateral cerebellar lesion (fastigial nucleus)	Menace deficit with normal vision and PLR. Other cerebellar signs may be present on the contralateral side to the mydriatic pupil (e.g. hypermetria, vestibular signs, coarse tremor of the head and body)	Cerebrovascular accident; inflammatory disease; anomaly; neoplastic disease	CT/MRI of the brain; CSF analysis
	Ipsilateral cerebellar lesion (interposital nucleus)	Menace deficit with normal vision and PLR. Other cerebellar signs may be present (e.g. hypermetria, vestibular signs, increase in extensor tone)	Cerebrovascular accident; inflammatory disease; anomaly; neoplastic disease	CT/MRI of the brain; CSF analysis
Unilateral miosis OR	Sympathetic supply to the eye (Horner's syndrome)	Anisocoria may be more pronounced in the dark. Vision is unaffected. Other signs that may be present include third eyelid protrusion, enophthalmos and upper eyelid ptosis. Can be seen with paralysis of the mandibular branch of the trigeminal nerve (CN V), resulting in a 'dropped jaw'	**First order lesions:** neoplastic disease; inflammatory disease; vascular accident affecting the brain or spinal cord **Second order lesions:** rostral thoracic spinal lesions; brachial plexus lesions; injuries to the soft tissues of the neck; thoracic cavity pathology **Third order lesions:** middle ear disease; idiopathic; skull fractures; retrobulbar lesions	Pharmacological test with phenylephrine **First order lesions:** CT/MRI of the brain and cervical area **Second order lesions:** CT/MRI of the cervical area and brachial plexus; thoracic radiography **Third order lesions:** otoscopic examination; radiography or, preferably, CT/MRI of the bullae
	Reflex uveitis/ anterior uveitis	Reflex uveitis (an axonal reflex resulting from painful stimuli to the trigeminal nerve (CN V)) and anterior uveitis cause pupil constriction	Ulcerative keratitis; all causes of anterior uveitis including blunt trauma	Thorough general physical and ocular examination and further systemic evaluation as indicated by the clinical history and findings
Miosis and mydriasis in opposite eyes	Acute brain disorder	Compression of the midbrain causes miotic pupils, whereas compression of CN III or its nucleus results in a fixed, dilated, non-responsive pupil. NB. A patient is expected to be comatose or stuporous for this localization to apply	Raised intracranial pressure due to a mass lesion or swelling (e.g. head trauma, neoplasia, inflammatory disease)	CT/MRI of the brain following stabilization of the patient

19.21 Lesion localization, differential diagnoses and diagnostic tests to perform in patients with anisocoria. CSF = cerebrospinal fluid; CT = computed tomography; MRI = magnetic resonance imaging; PLR = pupillary light reflex.

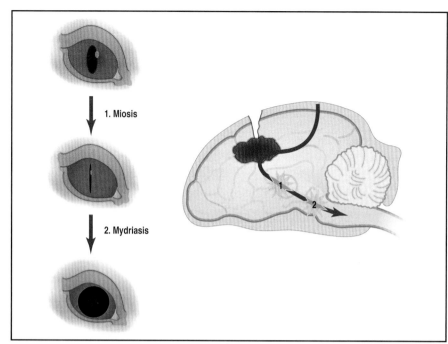

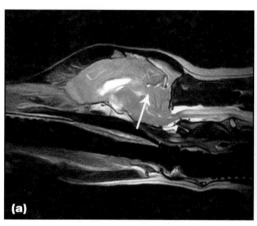

19.22 Pupil size following head trauma can progress from normal and reactive to light (top), through miotic and pinpoint (middle) to dilated and unresponsive (bottom) as the pathology progresses. The onset of miosis is related to a brain injury that has caused damage to the sympathetic system responsible for pupil dilatation. As the injury progresses and causes transtentorial herniation, the oculomotor nucleus is affected and results in pupil dilatation.

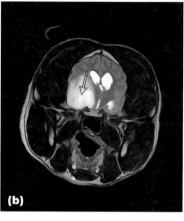

19.23

MR images showing **(a)** caudal transtentorial herniation (arrowed) in a dog with **(b)** a brain tumour (arrowed). The miosis is progressing to mydriasis.

Horner's syndrome: This can result from lesions anywhere along the sympathetic pathway. Having determined the likely location of the lesion (from the accompanying neurological signs and pharmacological testing), it should be possible to formulate a list of differential diagnoses (Figure 19.24). Diseases commonly associated with second order Horner's syndrome include brachial plexus lesions (e.g. traumatic or neoplastic), cranial mediastinal masses and neck injuries (e.g. iatrogenic venepuncture). Conditions causing third order Horner's syndrome include otitis media, middle ear neoplasia, orbital disease and idiopathic Horner's syndrome. First order lesions are very rare and invariably accompanied by profound neurological abnormalities attributable to a midbrain, brainstem or spinal cord lesion (e.g. severe mentation changes and postural reaction deficits).

Lesion localization	Associated signs	Differential diagnoses	Diagnostic tests
First order Horner's syndrome			
Brainstem	Mentation change, other cranial nerve signs, tetraparesis and ataxia or tetraplegia with increased tone to all four limbs	Cerebrovascular accident; neoplastic disease; inflammatory disease; trauma	CT/MRI of the brain; CSF analysis
Cervical spinal cord	Tetraparesis and ataxia or tetraplegia with normal or increased tone to all four limbs and normal segmental spinal reflexes	Intervertebral disc disease; fibrocartilaginous emboli; neoplasia; discospondylitis; trauma; inflammatory disease	CT/MRI of the neck; CSF analysis

19.24 Lesion localization, differential diagnoses and diagnostic tests to perform in patients with Horner's syndrome. CSF = cerebrospinal fluid; CT = computed tomography; MRI = magnetic resonance imaging. (continues) ▶

Lesion localization	Associated signs	Differential diagnoses	Diagnostic tests
Second order Horner's syndrome			
T1–T3 spinal cord segments	Tetraparesis and ataxia or tetraplegia with decreased tone in the thoracic limbs and reduced to absent reflexes, possibly some muscle atrophy of the forelimbs	Intervertebral disc disease; neoplasia; fibrocartilaginous emboli; discospondylitis; myelomalacia; trauma	Radiography; CT/MRI of the neck
T1–T3 ventral roots and proximal nerves	Ipsilateral thoracic limb lameness or monoparesis with decreased tone in the thoracic limbs and reduced to absent reflexes, some muscle atrophy and an absent or decreased cutaneous trunci reflex ipsilateral to the Horner's syndrome.	Brachial plexus tumour or tumour compressing the brachial plexus; brachial plexus neuritis or avulsion	Nerve conduction studies; electromyography; radiography; CT/MRI of the neck
Cranial thoracic sympathetic trunk	None	Trauma; neoplasia; infection	Radiography; CT/MRI of the neck and thorax
Cervical sympathetic trunk	Laryngeal and oesophageal signs may occur if the lesion is bilateral	Trauma; neoplasia; infection; iatrogenic (venepuncture)	Radiography; CT/MRI of the neck
Third order Horner's syndrome			
Cranial cervical ganglion	Dysphagia, laryngeal paralysis (CN X), facial paresis/paralysis (CN VII)	Iatrogenic (venepuncture); trauma; neoplasia; infection	Radiography; CT/MRI of the neck
Middle ear cavity	Facial nerve (CN VII) and vestibular (CN VIII) signs may be present	Otitis media; neoplasia; trauma	CT/MRI of the ears
Retrobulbar	Disorders of pupillary size and vision (CN II and/or CN III)	Trauma; infection/abscess; neoplasia	CT/MRI of the orbit

19.24 (continued) Lesion localization, differential diagnoses and diagnostic tests to perform in patients with Horner's syndrome. CSF = cerebrospinal fluid; CT = computed tomography; MRI = magnetic resonance imaging.

Cavernous sinus syndrome: The cavernous sinus is a paired venous sinus that runs along the floor of the middle cranial fossa, extending from the orbital fissure to the petro-occipital canal. Cavernous sinus syndrome (CSS) or middle cranial fossa syndrome is characterized by variable involvement of multiple cranial nerves, including the oculomotor nerve (CN III), the trochlear nerve (CN IV), the abducens nerve (CN VI), the maxillary and ophthalmic branches of the trigeminal nerve (CN V) as well as the sympathetic supply to the eye. Internal ophthalmoplegia is the most common presentation of CSS. However, other signs that may be associated with this syndrome include decreased corneal sensation (ophthalmic branch of CN V), ptosis (CN III), absent retractor oculi reflex (CN VI) and ophthalmoplegia/paresis (CNs III, IV and VI). Horner's syndrome is less frequently seen. Vision is not affected unless the underlying disease process extends rostrally to affect the optic chiasm. Malignant metastatic CNS neoplasia may result in CSS (due to haematogenous spread or intravascular tumour proliferation), as can primary tumours surrounding the cavernous sinus (e.g. meningiomas, pituitary tumours, germ cell tumours, oligodendrogliomas) (Lewis *et al.*, 1984; Theisen *et al.*, 1996; Rossmeisl *et al.*, 2005). Subsequent growth of these primary and secondary tumours results in obliteration of the sinus and surrounding structures. Other reported causes of CSS include granulomatous meningoencephalitis, vascular malformations, primary intracranial infectious disease and systemic infectious disease. Computed tomography (CT) or MRI of the brain is required for diagnosis (Figure 19.25).

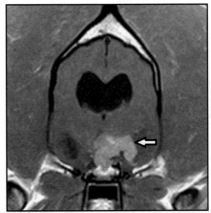

19.25 Post-contrast transverse T1-weighted MR image of a meningioma (arrowed) within the left middle cranial fossa causing cavernous sinus syndrome (middle cranial fossa syndrome) in a dog.

Feline spastic pupil syndrome: The postganglionic fibres of the oculomotor nerve that form the efferent arm of the PLR are termed the short ciliary nerves. In the dog, this represents 5–8 short ciliary nerves. However, in the cat, there are only two short ciliary nerves (the malar and nasal). This anatomical difference may result in the characteristic D-shaped (Figure 19.26) or reverse D-shaped pupil seen in cats with lesions in only one of the two ciliary nerves. When both ciliary nerves are affected, the result is static anisocoria with relative mydriasis. Clinical signs have been ascribed to a viral neuritis (e.g. feline leukaemia virus and feline immunodeficiency virus) or lymphosarcoma infiltration (Brightman *et al.*, 1977, 1991).

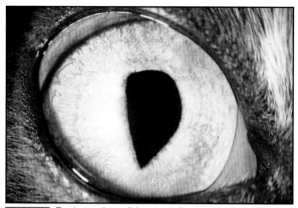

19.26 D-shaped pupil in a cat due to a lesion affecting the nasal ciliary nerve. (Courtesy of the Animal Health Trust)

Primary dysautonomia: This is a rare idiopathic neurodegenerative disorder characterized by chromatolytic degeneration of neurons in the autonomic ganglia, resulting in clinical signs attributable to failure of the SNS and PNS (O'Brien and Johnson, 2002). Mydriasis (Figure 19.27) with absent PLRs is a common finding and can be associated with other signs of autonomic dysfunction such as dysuria (with a distended urinary bladder), xerostomia, decreased tear production and additional signs of somatic motor system involvement (e.g. decreased anal tone, vomiting or regurgitation). Degeneration of the postganglionic neuron results in a hypersensitivity of the denervated muscle to cholinergic drugs. Dogs and cats with dysautonomia generally show rapid constriction of the pupils following the administration of 0.1% pilocarpine ophthalmic solution. The prognosis is typically grave.

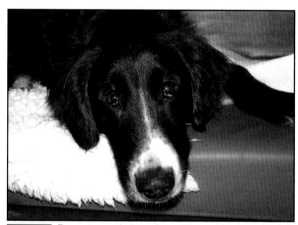

19.27 Dysautonomia in a dog with mydriasis in the left eye, bilateral mild third eyelid protrusion and xeromycteria (dry nose).

Eye position and movement abnormalities

Strabismus

Strabismus refers to a deviation of the eyeball within the orbit that the patient cannot overcome. The strabismus may be present at rest (resting strabismus) or may be evident only on provocation (e.g. by moving the head into an abnormal position; positional strabismus). Resting strabismus can be the result of

a lesion within the nuclei or nerves innervating the extraocular muscles (CNs III, IV and VI) or a lesion of the extraocular muscles themselves. It can also be associated with non-neurological conditions causing a mass effect in the orbit (retrobulbar tumour or abscess). Positional strabismus results from a loss of vestibular control over maintenance of the normal eye position within the orbit. Vestibular information is projected through the medial longitudinal fasciculus to the oculomotor, trochlear and abducens nerves. If this input is abnormal, a strabismus may be seen when the head position is perturbed. A ventral or ventrolateral strabismus is most commonly observed.

Clinical signs:

Oculomotor nerve lesion: Paralysis of the oculomotor nerve results in a resting ventrolateral strabismus and an inability to rotate the eye upwards, downwards or inwards during vestibular eye movement testing (external ophthalmoplegia). This type of strabismus must be differentiated from a vestibular strabismus that only occurs when the position of the head is altered. The clinical signs can also be associated with a dilated unresponsive pupil (referred to as internal ophthalmoplegia) and/or narrowing of the palpebral fissure (due to upper eyelid ptosis) (see above).

Trochlear nerve lesion: Lesions of the trochlear nerve result in a dorsolateral strabismus (extorsion, i.e. rotation of the dorsal portion of the eye laterally) of the ipsilateral eye. In dogs, this is best evaluated by fundoscopic examination, observing temporal deviation of the dorsal retinal vessels. In cats, it can be seen by an alteration in the orientation of the pupil. This is a very rare isolated finding because a lesion of this nerve usually occurs in combination with lesions of the oculomotor and abducens nerves, resulting in complete ophthalmoplegia (i.e. internal and external ophthalmoplegia).

Abducens nerve lesion: A lesion of the abducens nerve results in an ipsilateral convergent strabismus (Figure 19.28), an inability to retract the eyeball and an inability of the eye to move laterally when evaluating the horizontal physiological nystagmus induced

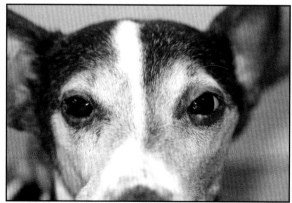

19.28 Medial strabismus in the left eye of a dog with abducens nerve paralysis.

by vestibular eye movements. As with lesions of the trochlear nerve, it is rare to see an isolated abducens nerve lesion.

Vestibular lesion: A positional strabismus can be seen with lesions of the vestibular system or medial longitudinal fasciculus. The strabismus is provoked when the head is placed in an abnormal position (extended dorsally or with the animal placed in dorsal recumbency). Vestibular dysfunction often causes a ventral or ventrolateral positional strabismus in the eye on the same side as the vestibular lesion.

Other causes: Fibrosing esotropia, congenital esotropia and hydrocephalus may all lead to a strabismus (see below).

Stepwise approach to strabismus: The approach to strabismus involves the following steps:

- Step 1 – assess eye movement (vestibular eye movements, see below) to ascertain that there is paralysis of the extraocular muscles
- Step 2 – determine whether the strabismus is resting or positional
  - Resting strabismus – the disorder may be affecting the nuclei and cranial nerves of the oculomotor, trochlear and abducens nerves or the extraocular muscles
  - Positional strabismus – a lesion of the vestibular system or medial longitudinal fasciculus should be suspected. Thus, it is important to assess for other signs of vestibular dysfunction (head tilt, loss of balance, ataxia) and to try to determine whether the vestibular disorder is central (within the brainstem or cerebellum) or peripheral (within the vestibulocochlear nerve (CN VIII) or structures of the ear) (Figure 19.29)

Clinical sign	Peripheral vestibular disease	Central vestibular disease
Head tilt	Towards the lesion	Towards the lesion (away from the lesion if central vestibular disease with a paradoxical head tilt)
Pathological nystagmus	Horizontal or rotary	Horizontal, vertical or rotary
Postural reaction deficits	Normal	Deficits on the same side as the lesion
Horner's syndrome	Possible (on the side of the lesion)	Very rare
Consciousness	Normal mentation (disorientation possible)	Altered mentation
Other cranial nerve deficits	Facial nerve (CN VII) (on the side of the lesion)	Trigeminal (CN V) to hypoglossal (CN XII) nerves may be affected
Cerebellar signs	No	On the same side as the lesion

19.29 Clinical signs of central and peripheral vestibular disease.

- Step 3 – carefully evaluate the oculomotor, trochlear and abducens nerves as part of the clinical assessment. The parasympathetic function of the oculomotor nerve (ability to constrict the pupil) should also be tested via PLR evaluation as part of this assessment
- Step 4 – perform a corneal reflex test. This test is used to assess the integrity of the trigeminal and abducens nerves. It is performed by touching the central portion of the cornea with a blunt object, such as a moistened cotton bud or wisp of cotton wool, whilst avoiding contact with the eyelids. Reflex retraction of the globe with passive protrusion of the third eyelid is seen in the normal patient when the eyelids are held open. Sensation is mediated via the ophthalmic branch of the trigeminal nerve and retraction of the globe is mediated via the abducens nerve
- Step 5 – retropulse the globe to assess for the presence of a retrobulbar mass.

Once these tests have been performed, it should be possible to localize the problem more precisely and determine what further diagnostic tests are required.

Diseases associated with strabismus:

Cavernous sinus syndrome: This can cause complete loss of eye movement (external ophthalmoplegia; see above).

Fibrosing extraocular muscle myositis: This is a severe fibrosing myositis, primarily affecting the medial rectus muscle; reported most frequently, but not exclusively, in young Shar Pei dogs. The disease can be unilateral or bilateral and progresses to cause permanent fibrosis of the affected extraocular muscles. The most common clinical sign is a medial strabismus (esotropia; Figure 19.30) due to the preferential involvement of the medial rectus muscle, and in the chronic stage enophthalmos is noted. This condition has been treated with immunosuppressive doses of prednisolone, but in severe cases surgical resection of the affected muscles may be necessary. For further information on extraocular muscle myositis with axial exophthalmos, see Exophthalmos below.

Congenital hydrocephalus: Congenital hydrocephalus is most commonly associated with disorders of vision, mentation and gait abnormalities. However, a positional or resting lateral or ventrolateral strabismus can be observed in these patients (Figure 19.31). It is believed that the strabismus is the result of compression of the oculomotor nerve or nucleus secondary to hydrocephalus. Affected animals usually have a domed head with an open fontanelle palpable on examination. However, the presence of an open fontanelle should not cause concern in asymptomatic patients.

Vestibular disorders: For information on vestibular disorders, see the section on Nystagmus below.

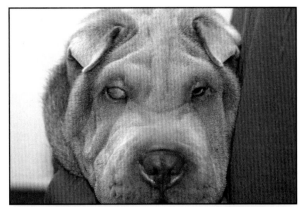

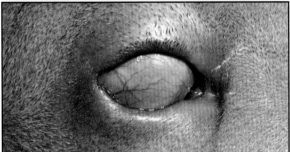

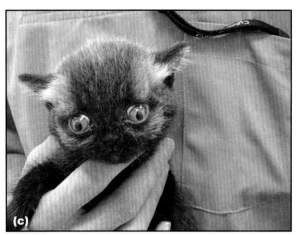

19.30 Strabismus in a Shar Pei due to fibrosing extraocular muscle myositis. In this case, the condition was unilateral and led to severe esotropia and functional blindness in the right eye. (Courtesy of C Heinrich)

19.31 (continued) Bilateral divergent strabismus in a kitten with congenital hydrocephalus. **(c)** Bilateral exotropia is present. Note the bilateral scleral show. (Courtesy of P Oliveira)

Congenital strabismus: Congenital strabismus (usually an esotropia) has been reported in association with albinism (primarily in Siamese, Himalayan and Birman cats with developmental abnormalities of the visual pathways; Cucchiaro, 1985; Bacon *et al.*, 1999) and as a 'normal' finding in brachycephalic breeds. These disorders are non-progressive and generally cause few problems. Brachycephalic dogs and cats may show apparent exotropia.

Orbital lesions: Any mass within the orbit can interfere with normal globe movement (Figure 19.32). Exophthalmos is the most common presentation of this condition, but abnormal globe position may precede this clinical sign (see Chapter 8 for further information on orbital disease causing strabismus).

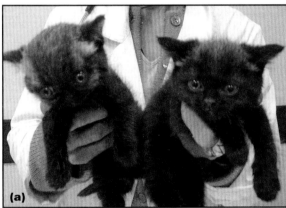

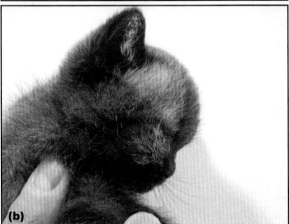

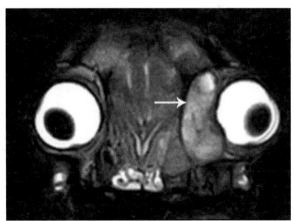

19.32 Transverse T2-weighted MR image of a retrobulbar mass (arrowed) within the left orbit causing lateral strabismus and exophthalmos in the left eye.

Exophthalmos

Exophthalmos can be seen in animals with:

- Masticatory myositis (usually bilateral)
- Extraocular muscle myositis (usually bilateral)
- Orbital space-occupying lesions such as abscesses or tumours (usually unilateral)
- Orbital cellulitis (unilateral or bilateral).

19.31 Bilateral divergent strabismus in a kitten with congenital hydrocephalus. **(a)** Affected kitten (left) with a normal littermate for comparison. **(b)** Side view showing the domed appearance of the head due to the hydrocephalus. (Courtesy of P Oliveira) (continues) ▶

These conditions may also cause mechanical strabismus and interfere with normal globe movement. Readers are referred to Chapter 8 for further information on these conditions.

Masticatory muscle myositis: Masticatory muscle myositis (MMM) is an autoimmune, focal, inflammatory myopathy of young dogs. The clinical signs are restricted to the muscles of mastication (masseter, temporalis, pterygoid and rostral digastricus), which are innervated by the mandibular branch of the trigeminal nerve. The reason for such selective inflammation is that the masticatory muscles have a unique fibre type called type 2M, which differs from the typical type 1A and 2A fibres found in the muscles of the limbs. These type 2M fibres are targeted by the immune system of the dog, resulting in the production of type 2M antibodies and the subsequent inflammatory myositis. Two forms of the disease are recognized:

- Acute MMM – common clinical signs include bilateral masticatory muscle swelling, pyrexia, mandibular lymphadenopathy, inability to open the mouth (usually due to pain) and exophthalmos due to swelling of the pterygoid muscles (Figure 19.33)

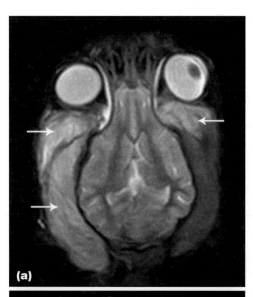

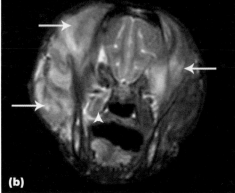

19.33 **(a)** Dorsal and **(b)** transverse STIR MR images of a dog with masticatory muscle myositis. Note the areas of diffuse hyperintensity within the temporalis, masseter (arrowed) and pterygoid (arrowhead) muscles.

- Chronic MMM – common clinical signs include bilateral masticatory muscle atrophy with fibrosis and an inability to open the mouth (Figure 19.34), often accompanied by enophthalmos. In severe cases, pain may be elicited on jaw movement.

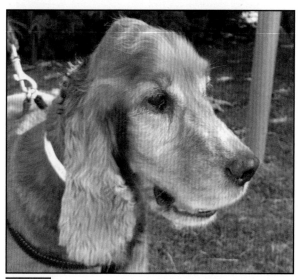

19.34 Chronic masticatory muscle myositis.

Circulating anti-type 2M autoantibodies can be detected in >80% of dogs with MMM and this forms the basis for the diagnosis of this condition (Shelton *et al.*, 1987). False-negative results may occur owing to the previous administration of corticosteroids or in end-stage disease, in which fibrosis and scarring have replaced the normal type 2M fibres, resulting in the reduction of anti-type 2M antibody production. Serum creatine kinase levels are modestly elevated in some dogs during the acute phase of MMM. Electromyography can help confirm the selective involvement of the masticatory muscles and differentiate MMM from polymyositis. However, electromyography may be unrewarding in dogs with end-stage disease because of the severe fibrosis and myofibre depletion. Evaluation of a muscle biopsy sample taken from the masticatory muscles can also provide diagnostic confirmation of the disease, as well as prognostic information, by determining the stage of the disease (Taylor, 2000).

Immunosuppressive doses of corticosteroids (prednisolone at a dosage of 1–2 mg/kg orally q12h) comprise the cornerstone of treatment for MMM (Gilmour *et al.*, 1992). This therapy should be continued until jaw function and serum creatine kinase levels (when initially elevated) have both returned to normal. The dosage of prednisolone is then slowly decreased over a few months to the lowest alternate day dose necessary to maintain the remission of clinical signs. Other immunosuppressive agents, such as azathioprine (1–2 mg/kg orally q24h) are indicated in dogs that fail to respond to corticosteroid treatment or that relapse when the dose is tapered.

Extraocular muscle myositis: Extraocular muscle myositis (EOM) is a focal inflammatory myopathy with clinical signs restricted to the extraocular muscles, sparing the masticatory and limb muscles (Carpenter *et al.*, 1989). A presumed underlying immune-mediated aetiology, similar to that of MMM, is suspected, but directed specifically against the extraocular muscle fibres. Vision may be impaired as a result of compression of the optic nerve. Bilateral axial exophthalmos from swelling of the extraocular muscles is the most consistent clinical sign associated with this type of inflammatory myopathy. However, extraocular muscle fibrosis, leading to unilateral or bilateral restrictive strabismus (Allgower *et al.*, 2000) and enophthalmos in the affected eyes, has also been recognized in the chronic stage of the disease. Serum creatine kinase levels are usually normal or mildly elevated. The absence of masticatory muscle swelling and circulating antibodies directed against type 2M fibres, helps differentiate EOM from the acute phase of MMM (Taylor, 2000). The suspicion of EOM can be reinforced by demonstrating the enlargement of the extraocular muscles on orbital ultrasonography or MRI. Although difficult to perform, biopsy of the extraocular muscles can be used to confirm the diagnosis. Due to the presumed underlying immune-mediated aetiology, immunosuppressive treatment with prednisolone is indicated as for MMM. However, the response to corticosteroids is not favourable during the chronic phase of the disease when fibrosis is predominant. See Chapter 8 for more information on this condition.

Enophthalmos

Enophthalmos can be seen with Horner's syndrome, secondary to disruption of the sympathetic supply to the eye and with conditions causing atrophy of the masticatory muscles. Unilateral masticatory muscle atrophy is commonly seen with trigeminal nerve sheath tumours or neuritis of the trigeminal nerve (Figures 19.35 and 19.36). Bilateral masticatory muscle atrophy can be caused by:

- Bilateral involvement of the motor branch of the trigeminal nerve (idiopathic trigeminal neuropathy, chronic polyradiculoneuritis, idiopathic hypertrophic chronic pachymeningitis or neoplastic cell infiltration of the trigeminal nerve)

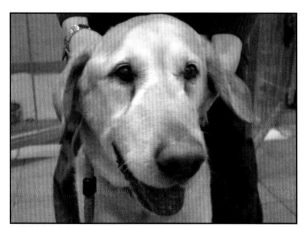

19.35 Unilateral right-sided masticatory muscle atrophy secondary to a trigeminal nerve sheath tumour.

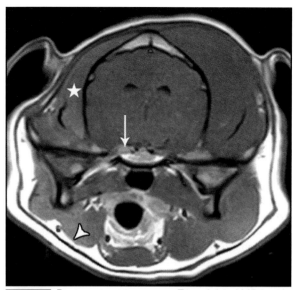

19.36 Post-contrast transverse T1-weighted MR image showing a trigeminal nerve sheath tumour (arrowed), which has caused atrophy of the temporalis (∗) and masseter (arrowhead) muscles on the affected side.

- Systemic disorders (cachexia, hyperadrenocorticism or chronic exogenous corticosteroid administration)
- Chronic masticatory muscle myositis.

Nystagmus

Nystagmus is a characteristic eye movement. There are two types of nystagmus:

- Jerk nystagmus – characterized by a fast and slow phase
- Pendular nystagmus – characterized by continuous oscillations of the eye with no slow or fast phase.

Jerk nystagmus: Two types of pathological jerk nystagmus are observed and both are seen with vestibular disease. Pathological nystagmus can be either spontaneous (observed when the head is in a normal position at rest) and/or positional, which occurs when the head is held in different positions. With disorders of the peripheral components of the vestibular system in the inner ear, the fast phase of the nystagmus is always opposite to the side of the lesion and the nystagmus is usually horizontal or rotary. Lesions of the central components of the vestibular system (i.e. the brainstem and cerebellum) can cause a pathological nystagmus in any direction and, occasionally, it changes direction with different positions of the head (variable nystagmus). A vertical nystagmus is more commonly due to a central lesion.

The primary goal of the clinician when examining a patient with jerk nystagmus is to determine whether the patient has evidence of peripheral or central vestibular disease. The differential diagnoses, diagnostic and treatment considerations, and prognoses differ according to the localization. Both peripheral and central vestibular diseases can cause nystagmus, as well as other neurological signs such as head tilt, positional strabismus, falling and ataxia.

Most lesions causing vestibular disease affect a region, rather than a specific nerve or nucleus, so accompanying neurological abnormalities can often be used to localize the lesion to the peripheral or central vestibular system (see Figure 19.29).

The identification of ear disease, facial nerve paralysis and/or Horner's syndrome is suggestive of peripheral vestibular disease, owing to the proximity of the facial nerve and the sympathetic nerve supply to the eye to the vestibular nerve in the region of the petrous temporal bone and tympanic bulla. The identification of central vestibular disease requires the recognition of clinical signs that cannot be attributed to diseases of the peripheral vestibular system. The absence of these specific central signs does not rule out a central vestibular lesion, but the presence of them makes central disease far more likely. Lesions affecting the central vestibular system typically result in additional clinical signs suggestive of brainstem and/or cerebellar involvement. The reticular formation is integrally associated with the brainstem, as are the ascending and descending motor and sensory pathways (i.e. the long tracts) to the limbs. Deficits of the trigeminal to hypoglossal (CN XII) nerves (with the exception of the facial and vestibulocochlear nerves) can also be associated with central vestibular disease.

Pendular nystagmus: This type of nystagmus is not associated with vestibular dysfunction and may occur secondary to congenital abnormalities of the visual pathways in Siamese, Birman and Himalayan cats, as well as in the Belgian Sheepdog (Cucchiaro, 1985; Hogan and Williams, 1995; Bacon *et al.*, 1999). No obvious vision impairment is noted, the disease is non-progressive and the signs are usually so mild that the owner fails to notice them.

Diseases associated with nystagmus: The common causes of peripheral and central vestibular disease in dogs and cats are detailed in Figure 19.37. This list is not exhaustive and readers are referred to the *BSAVA Manual of Canine and Feline Neurology* for specific details.

Blink disorders and eyelid opening abnormalities

Inability to blink
Disorders of the blink reflex can occur with lesions affecting the afferent or efferent arm of the palpebral reflex.

Clinical signs and associated diseases:

Trigeminal nerve lesion: The sensory component of the trigeminal nerve represents the afferent arm of the blink or palpebral reflex. Animals that lose the blink reflex as a result of a lesion of the trigeminal nerve can still show spontaneous blinking, an intact menace response and an intact dazzle reflex. Loss of innervation of the cornea due to a lesion within the ophthalmic branch of the trigeminal nerve can also result in neurotrophic keratitis. This innervation is necessary for the normal maintenance and integrity

Type of disease	Peripheral vestibular disease	Central vestibular disease
Vascular		*Brain infarct* Brain haemorrhage Feline ischaemic encephalopathy
Idiopathic	*Acute idiopathic peripheral vestibular disease*	
Traumatic	Head trauma	Head trauma
Toxic	Systemic aminoglycosides Topical chlorhexidine	Metronidazole Lead
Anomalous	Congenital vestibular disease	Cystic formation Hydrocephalus
Metabolic	Hypothyroidism (dogs)	
Inflammatory/ infectious	*Otitis media/interna* Nasopharyngeal polyps (cats)	*Meningoencephalitides of unknown aetiology* (e.g. granulomatous meningoencephalitis; dogs) Infectious encephalitis (canine distemper virus, toxoplasmosis, neosporosis, bacterial, *feline infectious peritonitis, which is caused by feline coronavirus*)
Neoplastic	Middle or inner ear tumour Peripheral nerve tumour	*Caudal fossa tumours* (*primary or metastatic*)
Nutritional		Thiamine deficiency
Degenerative		Lysosomal storage diseases Abiotrophies

19.37 Diseases causing vestibular signs in dogs and cats (the more common diseases are in *italics*).

of the cornea as well as reflex tear production (see Chapters 10 and 12 for further information).

A pure sensory neuropathy of the trigeminal nerve is rare, but has been reported in a case of sensory polyganglioradiculoneuritis (Chrisman *et al.*, 1999) and as a focal sensory neuropathy in a young Border Collie (Carmichael and Griffiths, 1981). Loss of the sensory portion of the trigeminal nerve is usually seen with conditions that also affect the motor function of the trigeminal nerve (e.g. idiopathic trigeminal neuropathy, chronic polyradiculoneuritis, neoplastic infiltration of the trigeminal nerve, malignant peripheral nerve sheath tumour and trigeminal neuritis).

Facial nerve lesion: The major function of the facial nerve is to supply the muscles of facial expression. Thus, its primary role involves motor function, although it also has a sensory role in providing taste to the rostral two-thirds of the tongue and hard palate. The facial nerve also has a parasympathetic component, which innervates the lacrimal gland, lateral nasal glands and the mandibular and sublingual salivary glands.

The most common clinical sign associated with facial nerve dysfunction is paresis or paralysis of the face. This can manifest as a drooping face either unilaterally (Figure 19.38) or bilaterally. More subtle cases may show a drooping of the ear and/or lip, drooling, difficulty chewing food, a decreased blink reflex and deviation of the nasal planum towards the unaffected side. Involvement of the parasympathetic supply to the lacrimal and nasal glands may occur concurrently, causing dry eye (KCS) and a dry nose (xeromycteria). An STT should be performed to determine whether dry eye is present.

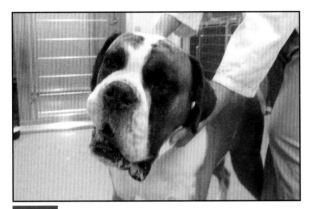

19.38 A dog with left-sided facial paralysis.

Anatomically, the facial nerve is closely associated with the vestibulocochlear nerve. Thus, many of the diseases that affect the facial nerve can also affect the vestibulocochlear nerve. With this in mind, it is not unusual to see a patient present with concurrent facial nerve paralysis and a head tilt. However, this presentation is not pathognomonic for any particular condition. Facial nerve paralysis can be associated with middle ear disease (e.g. infection, polyps, tumours) (Figure 19.39), head/peripheral nerve trauma, iatrogenic damage following bulla osteotomy, hypothyroidism and the use of potentiated sulphonamides (hypersensitivity), it can also occur as part of a neuropathy, or may be an idiopathic

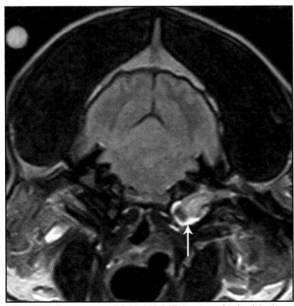

19.39 Transverse T2 FLAIR MR image of left-sided otitis media (arrowed) causing facial nerve paralysis.

condition. The latter is the most common 'cause' of facial nerve paralysis in dogs (75%) and cats (25%) (Braund et al., 1979). It can be seen unilaterally or bilaterally. Cocker Spaniels and Boxers are predisposed and the aetiology is unknown.

Diagnosis of idiopathic disease is made by excluding other possible causes and no specific treatment exists. Even though tear production is expected to be normal with idiopathic facial paresis/paralysis, corneal lesions may occur as a result of exposure due to reduced eyelid closure, and this should be addressed by application of ocular lubricants and, if necessary, temporary tarsorrhaphy. The prognosis for a complete recovery is guarded; recovery can take weeks to months, but may not occur at all. Chronicity may result in muscle contracture and deform the facial expression permanently (Figure 19.40).

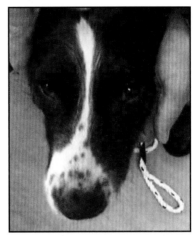

19.40 Deviation of the nose to the left-hand side in a Springer Spaniel with chronic left-sided facial nerve paralysis. Chronicity results in muscle contracture and pulling of the nose to the affected side.

Hemifacial spasm

Primary irritation of the facial nerve nucleus, irritation of the LMN or increased excitability of the facial nerve nucleus as a result of UMN dysfunction may cause a constant state of contraction of the ipsilateral facial muscles, described as a hemifacial spasm (Figure 19.41). This type of spasm has been reported in dogs with chronic otitis media (Roberts and Vainisi, 1967; Parker et al., 1973) and in two dogs with intracranial mass lesions (Van Meervenne et al., 2008).

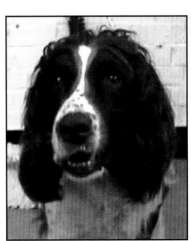

19.41 Hemifacial spasm affecting the left side of the face in a dog with otitis media.

Ptosis

Ptosis refers to drooping of the upper eyelid. This can result from oculomotor nerve lesions or sympathetic denervation of the eye.

Oculomotor ptosis: This is the result of denervation of the levator palpebrae superioris muscle and is usually seen in association with other signs of oculomotor dysfunction (see above).

Sympathetic ptosis: This is the result of denervation of the smooth muscles of the eyelids anywhere along the efferent sympathetic pathway that supplies the eye (see section on Horner's syndrome above).

Stepwise approach to blink disorders and eyelid opening abnormalities

- Blink disorders – perform an otoscopic evaluation and a thyroid panel consisting of total thyroxine (T4) and endogenous thyroid-stimulating hormone (TSH). This should be completed in all cases of facial nerve disease. If ear disease is suspected, then imaging of the tympanic bullae using radiography, CT or MRI is required. Samples for culture (obtained via myringotomy under general anaesthesia or by swabbing the purulent material if the tympanic membrane is ruptured) should be submitted if ear disease is present.
- Eyelid opening abnormalities – conduct a neurological examination to determine whether an oculomotor nerve lesion (resulting in concurrent anisocoria with mydriasis and/or eye movement disorders) or sympathetic denervation of the eye (resulting in miosis) is present. Tests of oculomotor function (e.g. PLR, resting or positional strabismus and vestibular eye movements) and an assessment of sympathetic nerve lesions (e.g. presence of Horner's syndrome and pharmacological testing) are required (see above).

Third eyelid disorders

Protrusion of the third eyelid can occur with sympathetic denervation of the eye (see sections on Horner's syndrome and Dysautonomia above) or may be secondary to atrophy of the masticatory muscles (see Enophthalmos above). It can be seen to protrude intermittently in animals with tetanus, secondary to tetany of the extraocular muscles, resulting in retraction of the eyeball. Patients with facial nerve paralysis may also have partial or full protrusion of the third eyelid that appears more prominent due to lower lid drooping which increases exposure of the third eyelid.

Haw's syndrome

This syndrome of bilateral protrusion of the third eyelid has been reported in young cats (Figure 19.42), often following a period of diarrhoea, and a torovirus aetiology has been proposed (Muir *et al.*, 1990). It usually resolves with time and treatment is not necessary.

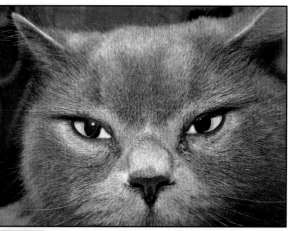

19.42 Haw's syndrome. (Courtesy of C Heinrich)

Lacrimation disorders

Decreased tear production

Neurogenic keratoconjunctivitis sicca: Neurogenic KCS can result from a lesion affecting the parasympathetic nucleus of the facial nerve, pterygo-palatine ganglion and/or the preganglionic or post-ganglionic parasympathetic fibres anywhere along their efferent pathway. This includes lesions of (petrositis, head trauma) or within (otitis media/interna) the petrous temporal bone (see Chapter 10 for further information).

Sjögren's-like syndrome: Sjögren's syndrome (SS) is a condition in humans characterized by xerophthalmia and xerostomia that results from a lymphocyte-mediated destruction of the exocrine glands. This syndrome may be a primary autoimmune disease or part of another immune-mediated connective tissue disorder. A similar syndrome has been described in cats (Canapp *et al.*, 2001) and dogs (Quimby *et al.*, 1979). Treatment is aimed at alleviating the clinical signs. Pharmacological immunosuppression has not been reported to alleviate the xerophthalmia or xerostomia.

Other causes: Dysautonomia (see above) may lead to a reduction in tear production due to dysfunction of the parasympathetic nerve supply to the lacrimal glands.

Increased tear production

Increased tear production may simply be due to stimulation of the trigeminal–lacrimal reflex by direct corneal contact, exposure to cold or irritants.

References and further reading

Allgoewer I, Blair M, Basher T *et al.* (2000) Extraocular muscle myositis and restrictive strabismus in 10 dogs. *Veterinary Ophthalmology* 3, 21–26

Bacon BA, Lepore F and Guillemot JP (1999) Binocular interactions and spatial disparity sensitivity in the superior colliculus of the Siamese cat. *Experimental Brain Research* 124, 181–192

Braund KG, Luttgen PJ, Sorjonen DC and Redding RW (1979) Idiopathic facial paralysis in the dog. *Veterinary Record* 105,

297–299

Brightman AH, Macy DW and Gosselin Y (1977) Pupillary abnormalities associated with the feline leukaemia complex. *Feline Practice* **7**, 23–27

Brightman AH, Ogilvie GK and Tompkins M (1991) Ocular disease in FeLV positive cats: 11 cases (1981–1986). *Journal of the American Veterinary Medical Association* **198**, 1049–1051

Canapp SO, Cohn LA, Maggs DJ *et al.* (2001) Xerostomia, xerophthalmia, and plasmacytic infiltrates of the salivary glands (Sjögren's-like syndrome) in a cat. *Journal of the American Veterinary Medical Association* **218**, 59–65

Carmichael S and Griffiths IR (1981) Case of isolated sensory trigeminal neuropathy in a dog. *Veterinary Record* **107**, 280

Carpenter JL, Schmidt GM, Moore FM *et al.* (1989) Canine bilateral extraocular polymyositis. *Veterinary Pathology* **26**, 510–512

Chrisman CL, Platt SR, Chandra AM *et al.* (1999) Sensory polyganglioradiculoneuritis in a dog. *Journal of the American Animal Hospital Association* **35**, 232–235

Cucchiaro J (1985) Visual abnormalities in albino mammals. In: *Hereditary and Visual Development*, ed. JB Sheffield and SR Hilfer, pp. 63–83. Springer-Verlag, New York

deLahunta A and Glass E (2008) *Veterinary Neuroanatomy and Clinical Neurology, 3rd edn.* WB Saunders, Missouri

Gilmour MA, Morgan RV and Moore FM (1992) Masticatory myopathy in the dog: a retrospective study of 18 cases. *Journal of the American Animal Hospital Association* **28**, 300–306

Hogan D and Williams RW (1995) Analysis of the retinas and optic nerves of achiasmatic Belgian Sheepdogs. *Journal of Comparative Neurology* **352**, 367–380

Jurk IR, Thibodeau MS, Whitney K *et al.* (2001) Acute vision loss after general anesthesia in a cat. *Veterinary Ophthalmology* **2**, 155–158

Lewis GT, Blanchard GL, Trapp AL et al. (1984) Ophthalmoplegia caused by thyroid adenocarcinoma invasion of the cavernous sinuses in the dog. *Journal of the American Animal Hospital Association* **20**, 805–812

Muir P, Harbour DA, Gruffydd-Jones TJ *et al.* (1990) A clinical and microbiological study of cats with protruding nictitating membranes and diarrhoea: isolation of a novel virus. *Veterinary Record* **127**, 324–330

O'Brien DP and Johnson GC (2002) Dysautonomia and autonomic neuropathies. *Veterinary Clinics of North America: Small Animal Practice* **32**, 251–265

Palmer AC and Walker RG (1970) The neuropathological effects of cardiac arrest in animals: a study of five cases. Journal of Small Animal Practice **11**, 779–790

Panarello GL, Dewey CW, Barone G *et al.* (2004) Magnetic resonance imaging of two suspected cases of global brain ischemia. *Journal of Veterinary Emergency and Critical Care* **14**, 269–277

Parker AJ, Cusick PK, Park RD *et al.* (1973) Hemifacial spasms in a dog. *Veterinary Record* **93**, 514–516

Platt S and Garosi L (2012) *Small Animal Neurological Emergencies.* Manson Publishing, London

Platt S and Olby N (2013) *BSAVA Manual of Canine and Feline Neurology, 4th edn.* BSAVA Publications, Gloucester

Quimby FW, Schwartz RS, Poskitt T *et al.* (1979) A disorder of dogs resembling Sjögren's syndrome. *Clinical Immunology and Immunopathology* **12**, 471–476

Roberts SR and Vainisi SJ (1967) Hemifacial spasm in dogs. *Journal of the American Veterinary Medical Association* **150**, 381–385

Rossmeisl JH Jr, Higgins MA, Inzana KD *et al.* (2005) Bilateral cavernous sinus syndrome in dogs: 6 cases (1999–2004). *Journal of the American Veterinary Medical Association* **226**, 1105–1111

Shelton GD, Cardinet GH 3rd and Bandman E (1987) Canine masticatory muscle disorders: a study of 29 cases. *Muscle Nerve* **10**, 753–766

Stiles J, Weil AB, Packer RA and Lantz GC (2012) Post-anesthetic cortical blindness in cats: twenty cases. *The Veterinary Journal* **193**, 367–373

Taylor SM (2000) Selected disorders of muscle and the neuromuscular junction. *Veterinary Clinics of North America: Small Animal Practice* **30**, 59–75

Theisen SK, Podell M, Schneider T *et al.* (1996) A retrospective study of cavernous sinus syndrome in 4 dogs and 8 cats. *Journal of Veterinary Internal Medicine* **10**, 65–71

Timm K, Flegel T and Oechtering G (2008) Sequential magnetic resonance imaging changes after suspected global brain ischaemia in a dog. *Journal of Small Animal Practice* **49**, 408–412

Troxel MT, Drobatz KJ and Vite CH (2005) Signs of neurological dysfunction in dogs with central versus peripheral vestibular disease. *Journal of the American Veterinary Medical Association* **227**, 570–574

Van Meervenne SAE, Bhatti SFM and Martlé V (2008) Hemifacial spasm associated with an intracranial mass in two dogs. *Journal of Small Animal Practice* **49**, 472–475

20

Ophthalmic manifestations of systemic disease

David Gould and Jim Carter

An ophthalmic examination can provide useful information about the nature and extent of systemic diseases. Systemic hypertension, for example, is often first recognized by ophthalmoscopy, and its response to treatment may be followed by regular ophthalmic examinations alongside repeated blood pressure measurements. Systemic infections, such as distemper and feline coronavirus, commonly have characteristic ophthalmic manifestations that may aid diagnosis. With lymphoma and other neoplasms, neoplastic cellular infiltrates within the eye may be a first manifestation of disease or an indicator of metastatic spread. In addition to these examples, a wide range of other systemic diseases, including metabolic and nutritional disorders, may involve the eye. As such, an ophthalmic examination should always be included in the diagnostic work-up of patients showing signs of systemic disease and, arguably, should be included as part of any general physical examination.

This chapter provides an overview of those systemic diseases that commonly produce ophthalmic manifestations. The reader is directed to other chapters and texts for further specific information on the diagnosis and treatment of these diseases.

Infectious diseases

Viral infections

Canine distemper virus

Canine distemper virus (CDV) causes acute conjunctivitis, keratoconjunctivitis sicca (KCS), chorioretinitis and optic neuritis (Willis, 2000a). Mild asymptomatic anterior uveitis has been described in experimental infections, but is seldom a significant problem in natural infections.

- Acute conjunctivitis is seen in the early stages of distemper infection, as the virus targets the mucous membranes. Initially, the conjunctival discharge is serous in nature but becomes mucopurulent over 7–10 days owing to secondary bacterial infection.
- KCS occurs as the virus directly targets the lacrimal glandular tissue causing dacryoadenitis (Sansom and Barnett, 1985; Willis, 2000a). In most dogs, spontaneous recovery of tear production occurs over the course of 4–8 weeks, but chronic keratoconjunctivitis may result,

presumably depending on the degree of lacrimal gland damage inflicted during the course of the infection (see Chapter 10).

- Chorioretinitis is characterized by multifocal areas of active inflammation visible across the tapetal and non-tapetal fundus. The lesions are not usually severe enough to cause blindness. Post-inflammatory chorioretinitis lesions appear as hyper-reflective areas that persist for life (see Chapter 18).
- Optic neuritis presents as sudden-onset blindness, which may be unilateral or bilateral. If the optic nerve head is involved, it appears swollen, sometimes with associated haemorrhage. Optic neuritis has been reported as the only clinical sign of CDV, but is more commonly associated with encephalomyelitis (Richards et al., 2011; see also Chapter 18).

Canine adenovirus

The cause of infectious canine hepatitis, canine adenovirus-1 (CAV-1), causes an acute anterior uveitis with corneal oedema ('blue eye'), which usually resolves over a period of weeks. Unilateral ocular signs are most common, but bilateral disease may also occur (Willis, 2000a). The corneal oedema is due to antigen–antibody complex deposition on the corneal endothelium, resulting in an inflammatory response which blocks the endothelial Na$^+$/K$^+$ ATPase pump mechanism that usually removes water from the corneal stroma to maintain its clarity (Curtis and Barnett, 1983). The condition is now uncommon as a consequence of widespread vaccination (see Chapter 14).

CAV-2 is one of the agents implicated in canine infectious laryngotracheobronchitis ('kennel cough'). It has been isolated from cases of idiopathic canine conjunctivitis, which suggests that it may be a causal agent (Ledbetter et al., 2009b; see also Chapter 11). Live CAV-2 vaccines (which confer protection against both CAV-1 and CAV-2) are occasionally reported to cause acute unilateral or bilateral 'blue eye' (Figure 20.1). Symptomatic treatment for anterior uveitis usually leads to resolution over a period of 2–3 weeks.

Canine herpesvirus

Canine herpesvirus-1 (CHV-1) infection of puppies in utero or in the early neonatal period may result in fatal disseminated viral disease, but in older dogs it tends to cause only mild clinical illness such as transient upper respiratory disease or vaginitis. Ocular

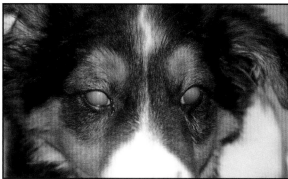

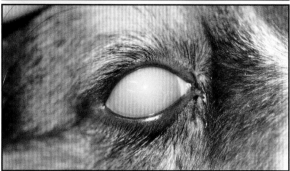

20.1 Bilateral corneal oedema in a 12-week-old puppy that developed 3 weeks after live CAV-2 vaccination. The condition resolved following a 2-week course of topical corticosteroids.

signs of CHV-1 infection in newborn puppies include keratitis, panuveitis, retinal necrosis and optic neuritis (Albert *et al.*, 1976). In adult dogs, CHV-1 has been associated with self-limiting conjunctivitis (Ledbetter *et al.*, 2009a). Dendritic, punctate and geographical corneal ulceration has also been reported in naturally acquired CHV-1 disease (Ledbetter *et al.*, 2006, 2009c; see also Chapter 11).

Feline herpesvirus

Feline herpesvirus-1 (FHV-1) is a widespread cause of feline morbidity worldwide. In addition to its role as a major upper respiratory tract pathogen, it is a significant cause of feline ocular disease (see Chapters 11 and 12). Primary FHV-1 infection causes conjunctivitis in association with upper respiratory tract disease, usually in young cats (Thiry *et al.*, 2009). FHV-1 is a common cause of corneal ulceration, which may develop during primary infection or during bouts of recrudescent disease. Dendritic corneal ulceration is considered pathognomonic for FHV-1 disease (Figure 20.2).

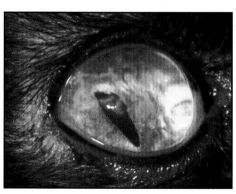

20.2

Dendritic corneal ulceration associated with FHV-1 infection.

Chronic stromal keratitis may develop in cats with recurrent recrudescent disease. This is thought to represent an immune-mediated response to viral antigens sequestered within the cornea. In addition to conjunctivitis and keratitis, FHV-1 has also been linked to a multitude of other ocular abnormalities, including ophthalmia neonatorum, symblepharon, KCS, tear film instability, eosinophilic keratitis, corneal sequestration, calcific band keratopathy, periocular dermatitis and anterior uveitis (Gould, 2011).

Feline infectious peritonitis

Feline infectious peritonitis (FIP) is caused by feline coronavirus. The signs are classically described as effusive ('wet' FIP, characterized by polyserositis causing abdominal and thoracic effusions) or non-effusive ('dry' FIP, characterized by widespread pyogranulomatous lesions in various organs). However, these really reflect the two extremes of a wide clinical spectrum and mixed signs may be commonly encountered. The disease is almost always fatal, although cats suffering from non-effusive FIP tend to have a more chronic disease course than cats with effusive FIP. Ocular signs are more common in non-effusive FIP than in effusive FIP, being reported in 36% of the former and <5% of the latter (Andrew, 2000). The disease is usually bilateral but not symmetrical.

Anterior uveitis is the most common ocular manifestation of FIP, occurring in around 30% of non-effusive FIP cases. Vasculitis due to immune complex deposition within the blood vessel walls of the iris allows breakdown of the blood–ocular barrier, resulting in uveitis (Addie *et al.*, 2009) (Figure 20.3). FIP can also affect the posterior segment, causing chorioretinitis (Doherty, 1971; Slauson and Finn, 1972; Gelatt, 1973; Peiffer and Wilcock, 1991) (Figure 20.4). Retinal blood vessel changes, particularly those affecting the retinal venules, may be marked in FIP. Immune complex deposition induces vasculitis, whilst chronic antigenic stimulation may also lead to hyperglobulinaemia and hyperviscosity syndrome (Figure 20.5).

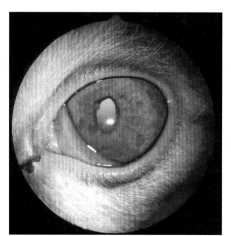

20.3 Anterior uveitis in a cat with FIP. Clinical signs include mucoid ocular discharge, miosis, iris thickening, diffuse corneal oedema and 'mutton fat' endothelial precipitates (also known as keratic precipitates). (Courtesy of G McLellan)

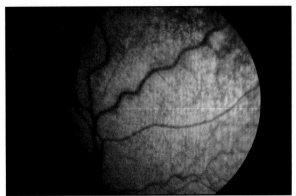

20.4 Active chorioretinitis in a cat with FIP. The condition was bilateral. The retinal venules are mildly thickened and tortuous, and multiple hyporeflective inflammatory foci are evident within the retina.

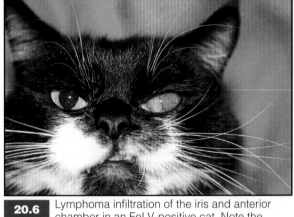

20.6 Lymphoma infiltration of the iris and anterior chamber in an FeLV-positive cat. Note the marked pupil asymmetry.

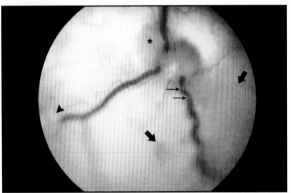

20.5 Fundus of a cat with FIP. The condition was bilateral. The retinal venules are markedly thickened and tortuous with segmentation or 'box-carring' due to serum hyperviscosity (thin arrows). The inferior retinal blood vessels appear out of focus owing to retinal detachment (thick arrows). A large white perivascular effusion is visible overlying a retinal venule (arrowhead). Areas of subretinal effusion are visible adjacent to the optic nerve head (*).

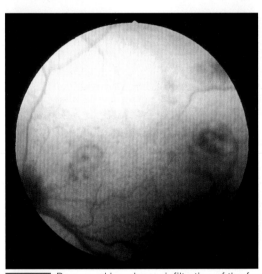

20.7 Presumed lymphoma infiltration of the fundus in a cat diagnosed with ocular and CNS lymphoma.

Feline leukaemia virus

Feline leukaemia virus (FeLV) infection of fetal and newborn kittens may cause retinal dysplasia with diffuse intraocular inflammation, leading to progressive retinal disorganization and necrosis (Albert *et al.*, 1977). In adult cats, the only ocular signs attributed directly to FeLV are pupillary abnormalities, such as hemi-dilated pupils, which are a consequence of viral infiltration of the malar or nasal branches of the short ciliary nerves (Willis, 2000b). Additional ophthalmic signs associated with FeLV infection are primarily related to co-infections, neoplasia or disease of the haemopoietic system.

FeLV-induced lymphoma can affect any ocular structure but the anterior segment is the most common ocular target, where it may present as a focal anterior uveal mass or as a diffuse infiltrative lesion within the iris, often with associated anterior uveitis (Corcoran and Koch, 1995; Figure 20.6). Secondary glaucoma may occur as a result of obstruction of the aqueous humour outflow pathway. Lymphoma may also affect the posterior segment with neoplastic infiltration of the fundus (Figure 20.7). FeLV-induced anaemia and thrombocytopenia may cause pallor of the superficial retinal blood vessels, hyphaema or posterior segment haemorrhage (Brightman *et al.*, 1991).

Feline immunodeficiency virus

A large number of ocular signs have been reported in feline immunodeficiency virus (FIV) infection. Experimental FIV infection in cats causes a self-resolving acute conjunctivitis shortly after virus challenge (Callanan *et al.*, 1992). The virus has also been linked to chronic conjunctivitis, although it is unclear whether this is a direct effect or due to secondary infection.

Anterior uveitis develops in 15% of experimentally infected cats. The mechanism involves immune complex deposition within the anterior uvea. In addition, as FIV infection predisposes to secondary infection with organisms such as *Toxoplasma gondii*, many clinical cases of anterior uveitis in FIV-infected cats may represent such opportunistic infections (English *et al.*, 1990; Davidson *et al.*, 1993a). FIV has also been associated with intermediate uveitis (pars planitis), which is inflammation of the posterior ciliary body. This manifests as white opacities within the anterior vitreous, just behind the lens (Willis, 2000b; Hosie *et al.*, 2009; see also Chapter 17). Glaucoma has also been reported in FIV-infected cats, but is likely to be secondary to chronic uveitis rather than a primary manifestation of FIV (Willis, 2000b).

An FIV retinopathy, manifest as large geographical areas of retinal degeneration, has been described in both experimentally and naturally infected cats. Retinal perivasculitis and haemorrhage have also been reported. These may well represent primary FIV pathology, as similar findings are reported in human immunodeficiency virus (HIV) infection (English *et al.*, 1990; Willis, 2000b). Neuro-ophthalmic abnormalities reported in FIV-infected cats, such as anisocoria and nystagmus, are likely to be ocular manifestations of central nervous system (CNS) disease (English *et al.*, 1994).

FIV-infected cats are at higher risk of developing lymphoma than non-infected cats. Given that FIV provirus is rarely detected in tumour cells, the link is likely to be indirect, most probably as a result of FIV-associated immunosuppression and resultant reduced immune surveillance (English *et al.*, 1994; Sellon and Hartmann, 2006). During the terminal phase of FIV disease, cats are at an increased risk of a variety of opportunistic infections. FIV has been shown to prolong or worsen clinical signs in cats experimentally infected with *Toxoplasma gondii* or *Chlamydophila felis* (Davidson *et al.*, 1993a; O'Dair *et al.*, 1994).

Feline panleucopenia
In utero or early neonatal infection with feline parvovirus may lead to retinal necrosis and dysplasia and optic nerve hypoplasia, as well as non-ocular diseases such as cerebellar hypoplasia and immunosuppression (Percy *et al.*, 1975; Truyen *et al.*, 2009).

Feline poxvirus
Feline poxvirus can cause eyelid lesions in association with generalized skin disease (Martland *et al.*, 1985; see Chapter 9).

Bacterial infections

Chlamydophila
Chlamydophila felis is an important cause of acute and chronic conjunctivitis in cats (see Chapter 11). It is primarily a local pathogen, with most infected cats displaying no systemic signs of disease. However, some cases are associated with mild upper respiratory tract signs. Furthermore, the organism is excreted in the urogenital and gastrointestinal tracts, which may act as a source of infection for other cats (Gruffydd-Jones *et al.*, 2009).

Tick-borne bacteria
Ehrlichia canis, which is transmitted by the tick vector *Rhipicephalus sanguineus*, causes canine monocytic ehrlichiosis. It is not endemic in the UK, but the condition may be seen in imported animals. Acute, subclinical and chronic phases of disease exist.

- In acute ehrlichiosis, systemic signs of fever, lethargy, anorexia and lymphadenopathy may be accompanied by ophthalmological signs, including conjunctival hyperaemia, anterior uveitis, chorioretinitis, retinal haemorrhage and optic neuritis (Leiva *et al.*, 2005b).
- In chronic ehrlichiosis, ocular signs are due to haematological abnormalities such as thrombocytopenia and monoclonal gammopathy, leading to hyperviscosity syndrome. Episcleral congestion, anterior uveitis, uveal and retinal haemorrhage, retinal blood vessel thickening and retinal detachment may develop (Leiva *et al.*, 2005b; Komnenou *et al.*, 2007).

Other *Ehrlichia* species and tick-borne diseases, such as Rocky Mountain spotted fever (caused by *Rickettsia rickettsii*) or infectious cyclic thrombocytopenia (caused by *Anaplasma platys*), may be transmitted by a range of different tick vectors but are very unlikely to be seen in the UK. In endemic areas, co-infections with more than one tick-borne bacterium may occasionally be recognized.

Borrelia burgdorferi is a tick-transmitted spirochaete that causes Lyme disease in humans, dogs, horses and cats. The infection in dogs is often asymptomatic, but a wide range of signs have been reported, including fever, polyarthropathy, protein-losing nephropathy, cardiac disease and neurological abnormalities. Ocular signs in dogs include anterior uveitis, chorioretinitis and orbital myositis (Raya *et al.*, 2010).

Brucella canis
Brucella canis is a Gram-negative bacterium most commonly associated with epididymitis in dogs and with abortion/stillbirth in bitches. However, it can also infect other tissues, including the eye, where it may cause chronic and recurrent anterior uveitis. It is not currently seen in the UK.

Leptospira
Leptospira interrogans is a spirochaete that causes disease in a number of veterinary species. A wide range of serovars exist, of which *L. icterohaemorrhagiae* and *L. canicola* are the most important canine pathogens (Andre-Fontaine, 2006). The serovars are maintained in nature by a wide range of subclinically infected wild and domestic animal reservoir hosts, which act as a source of infection for incidental hosts via contact with contaminated urine. Clinical effects vary from peracute infection with severe renal and/or hepatic disease, which may be fatal, to chronic or subclinical disease. Vaccination may not be fully protective against chronic infections. Uveitis is the most common ocular sign.

Bartonella henselae
The cause of cat scratch fever in humans has been isolated from the anterior chamber of cats with anterior uveitis in the USA (Lappin and Black, 1999; Powell *et al.*, 2010). However, more recent larger studies have shown no difference in *Bartonella* seroprevalence rates between cats with uveitis and healthy cats, and a study of 104 cats with naturally occurring uveitis failed to identify *B. henselae* DNA

within any aqueous humour samples (Fontenelle *et al.*, 2008; Powell *et al.*, 2010). The significance of *B. henselae* in the aetiology of feline uveitis is therefore debatable (Stiles, 2011).

Mycobacteria

In cats, the non-tuberculous mycobacteria *M. malmoense* (Figure 20.8), *M. simiae* and a novel species closely related to *M. simiae* have been isolated from cases of conjunctival, corneal and intraocular disease. Other mycobacterial species, including *M. tuberculosis* and *M. bovis*, are much less common ocular pathogens in cats but are of zoonotic and public health significance (Dietrich *et al.*, 2003; Fyfe *et al.*, 2008; Gunn-Moore *et al.*, 2010).

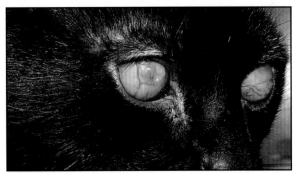

20.8 *Mycobacterium malmoense* infection in a cat, which involves the cornea and anterior chamber of both eyes.

Protozoal diseases

Toxoplasma gondii

In transplacentally or neonatally infected kittens, chorioretinitis is the most common ocular manifestation of toxoplasmosis, frequently seen in association with severe and often fatal systemic disease. In adult cats, signs may develop as a result of tachyzoite spread following acute primary infection, or via reactivation of latent tissue cysts following immunosuppression. Anterior uveitis and chorioretinitis are the principal ocular manifestations (Davidson *et al.*, 1993b). In dogs, ocular signs include chorioretinitis, anterior uveitis and optic neuritis (Davidson, 2000; Dubey *et al.*, 2009).

Neospora caninum

Ocular signs of neosporosis in dogs are associated with neurological disease and include blindness, anisocoria, optic neuritis, chorioretinitis, anterior uveitis and extraocular myositis (Dubey *et al.*, 1990, 2007; Dubey and Lappin, 2006).

Leishmania

Leishmania infection is not endemic in the UK, but may be present in imported animals. Around 25% of *Leishmania*-infected dogs develop ocular or periocular signs, most frequently anterior uveitis, periocular dermatitis and keratoconjunctivitis (Peña *et al.*, 2000). Histopathological examination shows granulomatous inflammatory lesions developing in the conjunctiva, cornea, sclera, limbus, ciliary body, iridocorneal drainage angle, iris, choroid and optic nerve (Peña *et al.*, 2008). Chronic leishmaniosis may cause hyperglobulinaemia, leading to serum hyperviscosity, and systemic hypertension is not uncommon. Signs include retinal blood vessel tortuosity and thickening, retinal haemorrhage and retinal detachment. Feline ocular leishmaniosis is rare, but has been associated with anterior uveitis, panuveitis and corneal ulceration (Hervás *et al.*, 2001; Leiva *et al.*, 2005a).

Mycotic and algal diseases

In the UK, ocular fungal infections are rare and, with the exception of uncommon cases of cryptococcosis and disseminated aspergillosis, are usually only encountered in imported animals. Blastomycosis, coccidiomycosis, histoplasmosis and prototothecosis have all been reported to cause ocular disease, which may be the presenting complaint (Gionfriddo, 2000; Krohne, 2000). Systemic mycoses typically cause a pyogranulomatous uveitis with signs of chorioretinitis predominating over those associated with anterior uveitis, and are occasionally associated with optic neuritis.

- *Cryptococcus* spp. have a worldwide distribution in the environment, but ocular infection is not common in the UK (Figure 20.9).

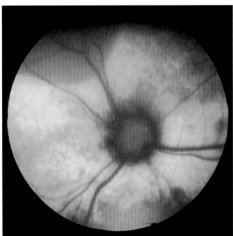
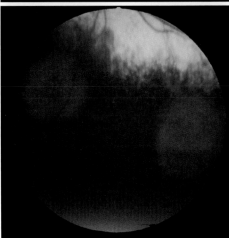

20.9 Cryptococcosis in a cat. Bilateral fundus changes, consisting of multiple subretinal pyogranulomatous infiltrates and partial retinal detachment, are present.

- The German Shepherd Dog appears to be predisposed to disseminated aspergillosis. Ocular involvement is generally accompanied by clinical signs of very serious systemic illness (Day, 2006; Schultz *et al.*, 2008). In cats, aspergillosis has been identified as a rare but increasingly reported cause of orbital disease, with retrobulbar granuloma formation reported (Barrs *et al.*, 2012).

Parasitic diseases

Migrating parasitic larvae may gain access to the anterior or posterior segment of the eye, where they can induce anterior or posterior uveitis. *Angiostrongylus vasorum* is an increasing clinical problem in dogs in the UK (Chapman *et al.*, 2004; Manning, 2007). Subconjunctival haemorrhage is an early presenting sign and develops secondary to the parasite-induced coagulopathy (Figure 20.10). Aberrant migration of L3 larvae to the anterior or posterior segment can induce a severe granulomatous uveitis (Figure 20.11; see also Chapter 17).

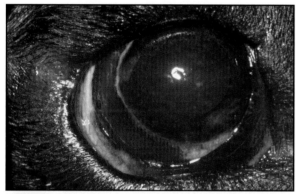

20.10 Extensive subconjunctival haemorrhage in a Staffordshire Bull Terrier with *Angiostrongylus vasorum* infestation.

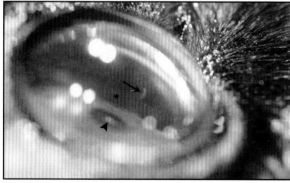

20.11 *Angiostrongylus vasorum* larva (arrowed) within the anterior chamber of a Cocker Spaniel presenting with severe anterior uveitis. A goniolens has been placed on the cornea to allow visualization of the iridocorneal drainage angle, from which the parasite is seen emerging. The iris (*) and pupil (arrowhead) are shown for orientation.

Aberrant migration of *Toxocara canis* L2 larvae has been reported to cause focal granulomatous lesions within the fundus and has also been suggested to cause more extensive retinal degeneration (Rubin and Saunders, 1965; Hughes *et al.*, 1987;

Johnson *et al.*, 1989). *Dirofilaria immitis* is not endemic in the UK but may be encountered in imported dogs, in which it causes anterior uveitis (Dantas-Torres *et al.*, 2009). *Onchocerca* spp. have been reported to cause canine and, more recently, feline ocular disease, although to date no cases have been described in the UK (Sréter *et al.*, 2002; Labelle *et al.*, 2011). Aberrant migration of Dipteran larvae such as *Cuterebra* spp. may rarely affect ocular tissues, although no UK cases have yet been reported.

Non-infectious diseases

Lysosomal storage diseases

These rare, recessively inherited diseases, are due to a deficiency of specific degradative enzymes with resultant accumulation of their substrates. Diffuse corneal clouding has been observed in alpha-mannosidosis, GM1 gangliosidosis, mucopolysaccharidosis (MPS) I, MPS II, MPS VI and MPS VII. Retinal lesions have been identified in ceroid lipofuscinosis, GM1 gangliosidosis and mucolipidosis II. Fucosidosis, globoid cell leucodystrophy (Krabbe's disease), GM2 gangliosidosis and Niemann–Pick disease may produce progressive blindness or nystagmus secondary to neurological disease (Cullen and Webb, 2007ab).

Chediak–Higashi syndrome

This autosomal recessive disease of cats affects cytoplasmic granules in a wide range of cell types, including platelets, neutrophils and melanin-containing cells, and is characterized by bleeding tendency, increased susceptibility to infection and partial albinism. Ophthalmic signs include pale irides, retinal hypopigmentation, degeneration and absence of the tapetum, cataracts and nystagmus (Collier *et al.*, 1979).

Ehlers–Danlos syndrome

This autosomal dominant disease of connective tissue causes fragile skin and increased joint laxity in dogs. Ophthalmic signs include an abnormal limbus, corneal clouding, lens luxation and cataract (Gething, 1971).

Oculoskeletal dysplasia

Oculoskeletal dysplasia (OSD) describes an autosomal dominant disease with incomplete penetrance, which causes short-limbed dwarfism and retinal dysplasia in dogs. The condition has been reported in the Labrador Retriever and Samoyed (Meyers *et al.*, 1983; see Chapters 17 and 18).

Nutritional diseases

Taurine deficiency

Dietary taurine deficiency in cats causes feline central retinal degeneration (FCRD; as discussed in Chapter 18), in addition to dilated cardiomyopathy. FCRD initially manifests as a focal area of retinal degeneration affecting the area centralis. Over time this progresses to diffuse retinal degeneration, resulting in irreversible blindness (Bellhorn *et al.*, 1974; Cullen and Webb, 2007b) (Figure 20.12.).

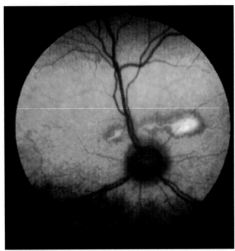

20.12 FCRD presumed to be due to taurine deficiency. (Courtesy of S Crispin)

Thiamine deficiency

This is rare and is usually due to long-term ingestion of thiaminase-rich foods (e.g. raw fish) or thiamine-deficient foods. In addition to progressive neurological defects, it causes fixed and dilated pupils (Loew *et al.*, 1970). Other ophthalmic signs reported in cats include peripapillary retinal haemorrhage, papilloedema and optic nerve head neovascularization (Barnett and Crispin, 1998) (Figure 20.13).

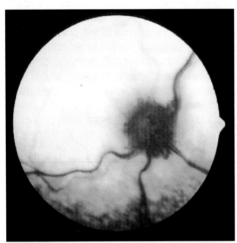

20.13 Papilloedema, neovascularization of the optic nerve head and blood vessel tortuosity in a cat affected with thiamine deficiency. (Courtesy of S Crispin)

Zinc deficiency

Zinc-responsive dermatosis is an uncommon disease of dogs resulting from an absolute or relative deficiency in zinc. Alaskan Malamutes and Siberian Huskies are predisposed. The condition causes periocular alopecia, scaling and crusting (Colombini, 1999; see Chapter 9).

Vitamin E deficiency

Deficiency of this fat-soluble vitamin may result in characteristic retinal degeneration in dogs, in addition to signs of neurological disease in some affected animals. English Cocker Spaniels have been reported to have a familial form of vitamin E deficiency due to abnormal metabolism of vitamin E, but deficiency can also occasionally be recognized in association with lipid malabsorption (e.g. due to exocrine pancreatic insufficiency) or as a result of malnutrition (see Chapter 18).

Hypocalcaemia

In addition to systemic signs, hypocalcaemic cataract may occur as a result of perturbations in the complex metabolism of calcium and vitamin D. In young, growing animals, nutritional causes should be considered. Eclampsia may be recognized in lactating bitches and in older animals renal disease or primary hypoparathyroidism may lead to cataract in addition to other systemic signs. This has a characteristic punctate appearance within the anterior and posterior cortices of the lens (Figure 20.14).

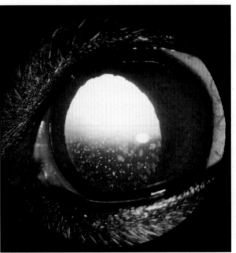

20.14 Punctate hypocalcaemic cataract in a hypoparathyroid dog.

Vascular diseases

Haemorrhage

Any systemic bleeding disorder predisposes to sub-conjunctival and intraocular haemorrhage. Causes include systemic hypertension, thrombocytopenia, clotting factor defects, vasculitis and hyperviscosity.

Anaemia

Anaemic retinal vessels appear pale and narrowed. Increased blood vessel fragility associated with chronic anaemia may lead to retinal haemorrhage.

Hyperviscosity

Highly elevated serum protein levels may lead to serum hyperviscosity, manifest as retinal blood vessel tortuosity, retinal haemorrhage and, in severe cases, retinal detachment, intraocular haemorrhage and/or glaucoma (see also Chapter 18). Causes of hyperviscosity include hyperglobulinaemia (due to multiple myeloma, chronic infection or inflammatory conditions) and polycythaemia (Figure 20.15). Ocular abnormalities may be the presenting complaint in hyperviscosity syndrome.

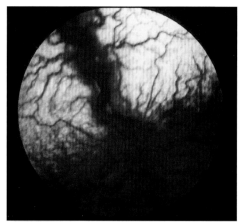

20.15 Hyperviscosity syndrome in a dog with polycythaemia. Note the pronounced thickening, tortuosity and darkening of the retinal blood vessels. (Courtesy of S Crispin)

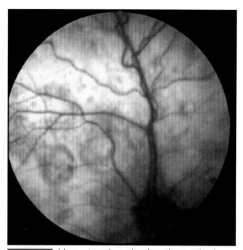

20.17 Hypertensive chorioretinopathy in a cat. Note the multiple bullous retinal detachments and mild tortuosity of the superficial arterioles.

Hyperlipidaemia

Elevated blood triglyceride levels, particularly hyper-chylomicronaemia, may give the blood a milky appearance that can be visualized within the retinal vessels (lipaemia retinalis). If there is underlying anterior uveitis, triglycerides may leak through the iridal blood vessels to cause lipid-laden aqueous, giving a milky appearance to the anterior chamber (Figure 20.16). Primary hyperlipidaemia is inherited in the Miniature Schnauzer (Whitney *et al.*, 1993). Secondary disease may occur in animals fed lipid-rich diets or in animals with raised triglyceride levels due to systemic disease such as diabetes mellitus, pancreatitis, hypothyroidism or liver disease. Hyperchylomicronaemia may contribute to corneal lipid deposition (see Chapter 12).

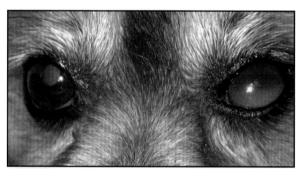

20.16 Hyperlipidaemia in association with cataract and lens-induced uveitis in a mixed-breed dog. In the left eye, lipid within the aqueous humour has settled in the inferior anterior chamber. (Courtesy of G McLellan)

Systemic hypertension

The eye is a major target organ for systemic hypertension (Crispin and Mould, 2001). The most common ophthalmic lesions in both dogs and cats are retinal blood vessel tortuosity, focal retinal oedema and bullous retinal detachment and retinal haemorrhage (Figure 20.17). As the disease progresses, total retinal detachment and intravitreal haemorrhage may develop. The anterior segment is less commonly affected that the posterior segment, but hyphaema is not uncommon. For further

information on the clinical features, diagnosis and management of hypertensive chorioretinopathy, the reader is referred to Chapter 18.

Metabolic diseases

Diabetes mellitus

Cataracts are a very common complication of diabetes mellitus in dogs, with one study reporting that 80% of diabetic dogs develop cataracts within 16 months of diagnosis (Beam *et al.*, 1999). Cataract development occurs as a result of changes in osmotic potential within the lens as it becomes saturated with glucose. Glucose is converted to sorbitol, which attracts water into the lens, leading to osmotic disruption and cataract formation (see Chapter 16). Oxidative stress also plays an important role. Cataract is not commonly encountered in diabetic cats owing to the lower capacity for conversion of glucose to sorbitol in older adults of this species (Richter *et al.*, 2002). Chronic hyperglycaemia may also lead to damage of the retinal blood vessels, and diabetic retinopathy may develop in some affected dogs (see Chapter 18).

Hyperadrenocorticism and hypothyroidism

There is little evidence that hyperadrenocorticism or hypothyroidism is a direct cause of ocular disease, but dogs affected with these conditions are commonly noted to have concurrent ophthalmic disease such as KCS, corneal lipidosis, corneal ulceration, cataracts, lipaemia retinalis and hypertensive retinopathy (Cullen and Webb, 2007a).

Hyperthyroidism

Hypertensive retinopathy is seen relatively frequently in hyperthyroid cats but it is unclear whether there is a direct link between hyperthyroidism and hypertension, or whether a degree of renal compromise is required.

Hypoparathyroidism

Primary or secondary hypoparathyroidism may lead to hypocalcaemic cataract (see above).

Systemic neoplasia

Uveitis may be seen with a variety of systemic neoplasms, particularly lymphoma. In most cases, this is due to tumour infiltration into the eye (Figure 20.18; see also Chapter 14). Brain tumours may cause blindness, visual deficits or ocular cranial nerve abnormalities, depending on their location. Brain tumours may also be associated with papilloedema, presumably due to raised intracranial pressure. Papilloedema may be seen with orbital tumours, as a consequence of compression of the optic nerve sheath (see Chapters 18 and 19). Primary lung carcinoma in cats has been reported to metastasize preferentially to the eye to cause an ischaemic chorioretinopathy, which gives a characteristic appearance of wedge-shaped areas of tan discoloration in the tapetal fundus with retinal blood vessel attenuation (Cassotis *et al.*, 1999; see Chapter 18).

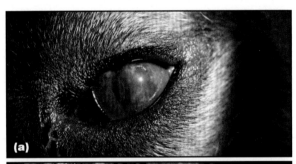
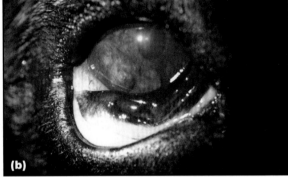

20.18 **(a)** Left eye and **(b)** right eye of a dog showing lymphoma infiltrating the iris and anterior chamber with secondary uveitis and hyphaema.

Dermatological diseases

Atopy

Periocular and ocular signs were present in 60% of dogs with atopy in one reported study. The ocular signs of allergic conjunctivitis included conjunctival hyperaemia, chemosis, excessive lacrimation, mucoid ocular discharge, pruritus and possible keratitis, and even corneal ulceration in extreme cases (Lourenco-Martins *et al.*, 2011).

Infectious and parasitic skin disease

Mite infestations involving the eyelids are usually due to *Demodex* spp., but *Sarcoptes scabiei* may also affect the eyelids (see Chapter 9 for further details). *Demodex* is considered to be a normal inhabitant of the hair follicles, sebaceous glands and sweat glands, with associated disease developing only when there are large numbers present and some degree of immunocompromise. *Sarcoptes* infection tends to cause intense pruritus with other parts of the body being classically involved along with the eyelids.

Dermatophytosis (most commonly *Microsporum canis* but also *Trichophyton mentagrophytes* and *M. gypseum*) may affect the eyelids, but is typically seen as part of a generalized problem. The typical clinical presentation is expanding alopecia, scaling and cutaneous erythema. Juvenile pyoderma/cellulitis is typically caused by *Staphylococcus* spp. with resultant abscess formation within the meibomian glands and the potential for marked ocular surface or self-trauma. Oedema, pustules, papules or crusts are noticed periorally, periocularly, on the chin or muzzle or in the ears of those dogs with skin lesions (White *et al.*, 1989).

Immune-mediated diseases

Uveodermatological syndrome

Uveodermatological syndrome (UVD; Vogt–Koyanagi–Harada-like syndrome) is an autoimmune disease that targets melanocytes. The Alaskan Malamute, Siberian Husky and Japanese Akita breeds are predisposed. Anterior and posterior uveitis may be the earliest presenting sign, and secondary glaucoma and retinal detachment are common sequelae. Associated skin changes (poliosis, vitiligo and ulceration of the mucocutaneous junctions) may precede or follow the ocular signs (Figure 20.19; see also Chapters 9 and 14). Other autoimmune skin diseases, including pemphigus and lupus erythematosus, may cause erosive periocular disease (see Chapter 9).

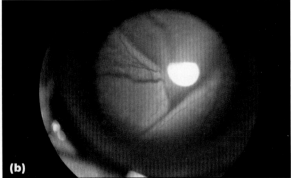
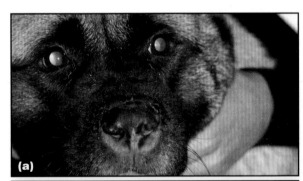

20.19 UVD in a 2-year-old Akita. **(a)** Depigmentation and erosive lesions of the planum nasale and eyelid margins are evident, along with **(b)** bilateral retinal detachment.

Granulomatous meningoencephalomyelitis

Granulomatous meningoencephalomyelitis (GME) is a non-suppurative inflammatory disease of unknown origin that affects the CNS of dogs. Ophthalmic signs include optic neuritis, chorioretinitis, anterior uveitis and retinal detachment (Adamo *et al.*, 2007; Kidder *et al.*, 2008; see also Chapter 14).

Miscellaneous diseases

Histiocytosis

Systemic histiocytosis in the Bernese Mountain Dog is a non-neoplastic histiocytic proliferative disease that may involve the eyes with signs including eyelid masses, episcleral nodules and anterior and posterior uveitis. Systemic lesions include nodules and plaques affecting the head/face, trunk and limbs, as well as erythema, swelling and depigmentation of the nasal planum/nares. This condition should be differentiated from malignant histiocytosis, which carries a much more guarded prognosis (Rosin *et al.*, 1986; Palmeiro *et al.*, 2007).

Dysautonomia

Dysautonomia has been recognized in both cats and dogs and is characterized by degeneration of neurons within the autonomic ganglia, resulting in clinical signs related to dysfunction of the sympathetic and parasympathetic nervous systems. Signs include vomiting, anorexia, weight loss, depression, gastrointestinal disturbances and dysuria. Ocular signs include reduced or absent pupillary light reflexes and elevated nictitating membranes. There may also be a reduction in tear production due to loss of parasympathetic innervation to the lacrimal glands (Harkin *et al.*, 2002; Kidder *et al.*, 2008).

References and further reading

Adamo PF, Adams WM and Steinberg H (2007) Granulomatous meningoencephalomyelitis in dogs. *Compendium (Yardley, PA)* **29**, 678–690

Addie D, Belak S, Boucraut-Baralon C *et al.* (2009) Feline infectious peritonitis. ABCD guidelines on prevention and management. *Journal of Feline Medicine and Surgery* **11**, 594–604

Albert DM, Lahav M, Carmichael LE *et al.* (1976) Canine herpes-induced retinal dysplasia and associated ocular anomalies. *Investigative Ophthalmology and Visual Sciences* **15**, 267–278

Albert DM, Lahav M, Colby ED *et al.* (1977) Retinal neoplasia and dysplasia. I. Induction by feline leukemia virus. *Investigative Ophthalmology and Visual Sciences* **16**, 325–337

Andre-Fontaine G (2006) Canine leptospirosis – do we have a problem? *Veterinary Microbiology* **117**, 19–24

Andrew SE (2000) Feline infectious peritonitis. *Veterinary Clinics of North America: Small Animal Practice* **30**, 987–1000

Barnett KC and Crispin SM (1998) Fundus. In: *Feline Ophthalmology: An Atlas & Text*, pp.146 168. WB Saunders Co. Ltd, London

Barrs VR, Halliday C, Martin P *et al.* (2012) Sinonasal and sino-orbital aspergillosis in 23 cats: aetiology, clinicopathological features and treatment outcomes. *Veterinary Journal* **191**, 58–64

Beam S, Correa MT and Davidson MG (1999) A retrospective-cohort study on the development of cataracts in dogs with diabetes mellitus: 200 cases. *Veterinary Ophthalmology* **2**, 169–172

Bellhorn RW, Aguirre GD and Bellhorn MB (1974) Feline central retinal degeneration. *Investigative Ophthalmology* **13**, 608–616

Brightman AH, Ogilvie GK and Tompkins M (1991) Ocular disease in FeLV-positive cats: 11 cases (1981–1986). *Journal of the American Veterinary Medical Association* **198**, 1049–1051

Callanan JJ, Thompson H, Toth SR *et al.* (1992) Clinical and pathological findings in feline immunodeficiency virus experimental infection. *Veterinary Immunology and Immunopathology* **35**, 3–13

Cassotis NJ, Dubielzig RR, Gilger BC *et al.* (1999) Angioinvasive

pulmonary carcinoma with posterior segment metastasis in four cats. *Veterinary Ophthalmology* **2**, 125–131

Chapman PS, Boag AK, Guitian J *et al.* (2004) *Angiostrongylus vasorum* infection in 23 dogs (1999–2002). *Journal of Small Animal Practice* **45**, 435–440

Collier LL, Bryan GM and Prieur DJ (1979) Ocular manifestations of the Chédiak–Higashi syndrome in four species of animals. *Journal of the American Veterinary Medical Association* **175**(6), 587–590

Colombini S (1999) Canine zinc-responsive dermatosis. *Veterinary Clinics of North America: Small Animal Practice* **29**, 1373–1383

Corcoran KPR and Koch S (1995) Histopathology of feline ocular lymphosarcoma: 49 cases. *Veterinary Comparative Ophthalmology* **5**, 35–41

Crispin SM and Mould JR (2001) Systemic hypertensive disease and the feline fundus. *Veterinary Ophthalmology* **4**, 131–140

Cullen CL and Webb AA (2007a) Ocular manifestations of systemic diseases. Part 1: The Dog. In: *Veterinary Ophthalmology, 4th edn*, ed. KN Gelatt, pp.1470–1537. Blackwell Publishing, Iowa

Cullen CL and Webb AA (2007b) Ocular manifestations of systemic diseases. Part 2: The Cat. In: *Veterinary Ophthalmology, 4th edn*, ed. KN Gelatt, pp.1538–1587. Blackwell Publishing, Iowa

Curtis R and Barnett KC (1983) The 'blue eye' phenomenon. *Veterinary Record* **112**, 347–353

Dantas-Torres F, Lia RP, Barbuto M *et al.* (2009) Ocular dirofilariosis caused by *Dirofilaria immitis* in a dog: first case report from Europe. *Journal of Small Animal Practice* **50**, 667–669

Davidson MG (2000) Toxoplasmosis. *Veterinary Clinics of North America: Small Animal Practice* **30**, 1051–1062

Davidson MG, Lappin MR, English RV *et al.* (1993b) A feline model of ocular toxoplasmosis. *Investigative Ophthalmology and Visual Sciences* **34**, 3653–3660

Davidson MG, Rottman JB, English RV *et al.* (1993a) Feline immunodeficiency virus predisposes cats to acute generalized toxoplasmosis. *American Journal of Pathology* **143**, 1486–1497

Day MJ (2006) Canine disseminated aspergillosis. In: *Infectious Diseases of the Dog and Cat, 3rd edn*, ed. CE Greene, pp. 610–627. Saunders Elsevier, Missouri

Dietrich U, Arnold P, Guscetti F *et al.* (2003) Ocular manifestation of disseminated *Mycobacterium simiae* infection in a cat. *Journal of Small Animal Practice* **44**, 121–125

Doherty MJ (1971) Ocular manifestations of feline infectious peritonitis. *Journal of the American Veterinary Medical Association* **159**, 417–424

Dubey JP, Koestner A and Piper RC (1990) Repeated transplacental transmission of *Neospora caninum* in dogs. *Journal of the American Veterinary Medical Association* **197**, 857–860

Dubey JP and Lappin MR (2006) Toxoplasmosis and neosporosis. In: *Infectious Diseases of the Dog and Cat, 3rd edn*, ed. CE Greene, pp. 754–775. Saunders Elsevier, Missouri

Dubey JP, Lindsay DS and Lappin MR (2009) Toxoplasmosis and other intestinal coccidial infections in cats and dogs. *Veterinary Clinics of North America: Small Animal Practice* **39**, 1009–1034

Dubey JP, Schares G and Ortega-Mora LM (2007) Epidemiology and control of neosporosis and *Neospora caninum*. *Clinical Microbiology Reviews* **20**, 323–367

English RV, Davidson MG, Nasisse MP *et al.* (1990) Intraocular disease associated with feline immunodeficiency virus infection in cats. *Journal of the American Veterinary Medical Association* **196**, 1116–1119

English RV, Nelson P, Johnson CM *et al.* (1994) Development of clinical disease in cats experimentally infected with feline immunodeficiency virus infection. *Journal of Infectious Diseases* **170**, 543–552

Fontenelle JP, Powell CC, Hill AE *et al.* (2008) Prevalence of serum antibodies against *Bartonella* species in the serum of cats with or without uveitis. *Journal of Feline Medicine and Surgery* **10**, 41–46

Fyfe JA, McCowan C, O'Brien CR *et al.* (2008) Molecular characterization of a novel fastidious *Mycobacterium* causing lepromatous lesions of the skin, subcutis, cornea and conjunctiva of cats living in Victoria, Australia. *Journal of Clinical Microbiology* **46**, 618–626

Gelatt KN (1973) Iridocyclitis-panophthalmitis associated with feline infectious peritonitis. *Veterinary Medicine, Small Animal Clinician* **68**, 56–57

Gething MA (1971) Suspected Ehlers–Danlos syndrome in the dog. *Veterinary Record* **89**, 638–641

Gionfriddo JR (2000) Feline systemic fungal infections. *Veterinary Clinics of North America: Small Animal Practice* **30**, 1029–1050

Gould D (2011) Feline herpesvirus-1: ocular manifestations, diagnosis and treatment options. *Journal of Feline Medicine and Surgery* **13**, 333–346

Gruffydd-Jones T, Addie D, Belak S *et al.* (2009) *Chlamydophila felis* infection. ABCD guidelines on prevention and management. *Journal of Feline Medicine and Surgery* **11**, 605–609

Gunn-Moore D, Dean R and Shaw S (2010) Mycobacterial infections in cats and dogs. *In Practice* **32**, 444–452

Harkin KR, Andrews GA and Nietfeld JC (2002) Dysautonomia in dogs: 65 cases (1993–2000). *Journal of the American Veterinary Medical Association* **220**, 633–639

Hervás J, Chacón-Manrique de Lara F, López J *et al.* (2001) Granulomatous (pseudotumoral) iridociclitis associated with leishmaniasis in a cat. *Veterinary Record* **149**, 624–625

Hosie MJ, Addie D, Belak S *et al.* (2009) Feline immunodeficiency. ABCD guidelines on prevention and management. *Journal of Feline Medicine and Surgery* **11**, 575–584

Hughes PL, Dubielzig RR and Kazacos KR (1987) Multifocal retinitis in New Zealand sheepdogs. *Veterinary Pathology* **24**, 22–27

Johnson BW, Kirkpatrick CE, Whiteley HE *et al.* (1989) Retinitis and intraocular larval migration in a group of Border Collies. *Journal of the American Animal Hospital Association* **25**, 623–629

Kidder AC, Johannes C, O'Brien DP *et al.* (2008) Feline dysautonomia in the Midwestern United States: a retrospective study of nine cases. *Journal of Feline Medicine and Surgery* **10**, 130–136

Komnenou AA, Mylonakis ME, Kouti V *et al.* (2007). Ocular manifestations of natural canine monocytic ehrlichiosis (*Ehrlichia canis*): a retrospective study of 90 cases. *Veterinary Ophthalmology* **10**, 137–142

Krohne SG (2000) Canine systemic fungal infections. *Veterinary Clinics of North America: Small Animal Practice* **30**, 1063–1090

Krupka I and Straubinger RK (2010) Lyme borreliosis in dogs and cats: background, diagnosis, treatment and prevention of infections with *Borrelia burgdorferi sensu stricto*. *Veterinary Clinics of North America: Small Animal Practice* **40**, 1103–1119

Labelle AL, Daniels JB, Dix M *et al.* (2011) *Onchocerca lupi* causing ocular disease in two cats. *Veterinary Ophthalmology* **14**(Suppl.), 105–110

Lappin MR and Black JC (1999) *Bartonella* spp. infection as a possible cause of uveitis in a cat. *Journal of the American Veterinary Medical Association* **214**, 1205–1207

Ledbetter EC, Dubovi EJ, Kim SG *et al.* (2009a) Experimental primary ocular canine herpesvirus-1 infection in adult dogs. *American Journal of Veterinary Research* **70**, 513–521

Ledbetter EC, Hornbuckle WE and Dubovi EJ (2009b) Virological survey of dogs with naturally acquired idiopathic conjunctivitis. *Journal of the American Veterinary Medical Association* **235**, 954–959

Ledbetter EC, Kim SG and Dubovi EJ (2009c) Outbreak of ocular disease associated with naturally-acquired canine herpesvirus-1 infection in a closed domestic dog colony. *Veterinary Ophthalmology* **12**, 242–247

Ledbetter EC, Riis RC, Kern TJ *et al.* (2006) Corneal ulceration associated with naturally occurring canine herpesvirus-1 infection in two adult dogs. *Journal of the American Veterinary Medical Association* **229**, 376–384

Leiva M, Lloret A, Peña T *et al.* (2005a) Therapy of ocular and visceral leishmaniasis in a cat. *Veterinary Ophthalmology* **8**, 71–75

Leiva M, Naranjo C and Pena MT (2005b) Ocular signs of canine monocytic ehrlichiosis: a retrospective study in dogs from Barcelona, Spain. *Veterinary Ophthalmology* **8**, 387–393

Littman MP (2003) Canine borreliosis. *Veterinary Clinics of North America: Small Animal Practice* **33**, 827–862

Loew FM, Martin CL, Dunlop RH *et al.* (1970) Naturally-occurring and experimental thiamine deficiency in cats receiving commercial cat food. *Canadian Veterinary Journal* **11**, 109–113

Lourenco-Martins AM, Delgado E, Neto I *et al.* (2011) Allergic conjunctivitis and conjunctival provocation tests in atopic dogs. *Veterinary Ophthalmology* **14**, 248–256

Manning SP (2007) Ocular examination in the diagnosis of angiostrongylosis in dogs. *Veterinary Record* **160**, 625–627

Martland MF, Poulton GJ and Done RA (1985) Three cases of cowpox infection of domestic cats. *Veterinary Record* **117**, 231–233

Meyers VN, Jezyk PF, Aguirre GD and Patterson DF (1983) Short-limbed dwarfism and ocular defects in the Samoyed dog. *Journal of the American Veterinary Medical Association* **183**, 975–979

O'Dair HA, Hopper CD, Gruffydd-Jones TJ *et al.* (1994) Clinical aspects of *Chlamydia psittaci* infection in cats infected with feline immunodeficiency virus. *Veterinary Record* **134**, 365–368

Palmeiro BS, Morris DO, Goldschmidt MH *et al.* (2007) Cutaneous reactive histiocytosis in dogs: a retrospective evaluation of 32 cases. *Veterinary Dermatology* **18**, 332–340

Peiffer RL, Jr. and Wilcock BP (1991) Histopathologic study of uveitis in cats: 139 cases (1978–1988). *Journal of the American Veterinary Medical Association* **198**, 135–138

Peña MT, Naranjo C, Klauss G *et al.* (2008) Histopathological features of ocular leishmaniosis in the dog. *Journal of Comparative Pathology* **138**, 32–39

Peña MT, Roura X and Davidson MG (2000) Ocular and periocular manifestations of leishmaniosis in dogs: 105 cases (1993–1998). *Veterinary Ophthalmology* **3**, 35–41

Percy DH, Scott FW and Albert DM (1975) Retinal dysplasia due to feline panleukopenia virus infection. *Journal of the American Veterinary Medical Association* **167**, 935–937

Powell CC, Mcinnis CL, Fontenelle JP *et al.* (2010) *Bartonella* species, feline herpesvirus-1, and *Toxoplasma gondii* PCR assay results from blood and aqueous humor samples from 104 cats with naturally occurring endogenous uveitis. *Journal of Feline Medicine and Surgery* **12**, 923–928

Raya AI, Afonso JC, Perez-Ecija RA *et al.* (2010) Orbital myositis associated with Lyme disease in a dog. *Veterinary Record* **167**, 663–664

Richards TR, Whelan NC, Pinard CL *et al.* (2011). Optic neuritis caused by canine distemper virus in a Jack Russell terrier. *The Canadian Veterinary Journal* **52**, 398–402

Richter M, Guscetti F and Spiess B (2002) Aldose reductase activity and glucose-related opacities in incubated lenses from dogs and cats. *American Journal of Veterinary Research* **63**, 1591–1197

Rosin A, Moore P and Dubielzig R (1986) Malignant histiocytosis in Bernese Mountain Dogs. *Journal of the American Veterinary Medical Association* **188**, 1041–1045

Rubin LF and Saunders LZ (1965) Intraocular larva migrans in dogs. *Pathologia Veterinaria* **2**, 566–573

Sansom J and Barnett KC (1985) Keratoconjunctivitis sicca in the dog: a review of two hundred cases. *Journal of Small Animal Practice* **26**, 121–131

Schultz RM, Johnson EG, Wisner ER *et al.* (2008) Clinicopathologic and diagnostic imaging characteristics of systemic aspergillosis in 30 dogs. *Journal of Veterinary Internal Medicine* **22**, 851–859

Sellon RK and Hartmann K (2006) Feline immunodeficiency virus. In: *Infectious Diseases of the Dog and Cat*, 3rd edn, ed. CE Greene, pp.131–143. Saunders Elsevier, Missouri

Slauson DO and Finn JP (1972) Meningoencephalitis and panophthalmitis in feline infectious peritonitis. *Journal of the American Veterinary Medical Association* **160**, 729–734

Sréter T, Széll Z, Egyed Z and Varga I (2002) Ocular onchocercosis in dogs: a review. *Veterinary Record* **151**, 176–180

Stiles J (1995) Treatment of cats with ocular disease attributable to herpesvirus infection: 17 cases (1983–1993). *Journal of the American Veterinary Medical Association* **207**, 599–603

Stiles J (2000) Infectious disease and the eye. *Veterinary Clinics of North America: Small Animal Practice* **30**(5)

Stiles J (2011) Bartonellosis in cats: a role in uveitis? *Veterinary Ophthalmology* **14**(suppl. 1), 9–14

Thiry E, Addie D, Belak S *et al.* (2009) Feline herpesvirus infection. ABCD guidelines on prevention and management. *Journal of Feline Medicine and Surgery* **11**, 547–555

Truyen U, Addie D, Belak S *et al.* (2009) Feline panleukopenia. ABCD guidelines on prevention and management. *Journal of Feline Medicine and Surgery* **11**, 538–546

White SD, Rosychuk RA, Stewart LJ *et al.* (1989) Juvenile cellulitis in dogs: 15 cases (1979–1988). *Journal of the American Veterinary Medical Association* **195**, 1609–1611

Whitney MS, Boon GD, Rebar AH *et al.* (1993) Ultracentrifugal and electrophoretic characteristics of the plasma lipoproteins of Miniature Schnauzer dogs with idiopathic hyperlipoproteinemia. *Journal of Veterinary Internal Medicine* **7**, 253–260

Williams DL (2008) Ophthalmic immunology and immune-mediated disease. *Veterinary Clinics of North America: Small Animal Practice* **38**(2)

Willis AM (2000a) Canine viral infections. *Veterinary Clinics of North America: Small Animal Practice* **30**, 1119–1133

Willis AM (2000b) Feline leukemia virus and feline immunodeficiency virus. *Veterinary Clinics of North America: Small Animal Practice* **30**, 971–986

21

A problem-oriented approach to common ophthalmic presentations

Natasha Mitchell

This chapter presents a series of algorithms intended to allow a structured approach to the work-up of some commonly encountered ophthalmic presentations. Given the broad nature of the presenting signs and the long potential differential diagnosis list, the reader should bear in mind that these algorithms are intended to act as a guide rather than a prescribed protocol, and that some presentations may require a different approach depending on additional findings from the signalment, history and ophthalmic examination.

The presentations included are:

- The bulging eye (Figure 21.1)
- Abnormal blink
- Anisocoria
- Blindness
- Hyphaema
- The cloudy eye (cornea, anterior chamber, lens, and vitreous)
- The red and painful eye
- The watery eye.

Clinical sign	Buphthalmos	Exophthalmos
Visible conjunctiva	Minimal	Red congested conjunctiva
Third eyelid	Not protruding	Usually protruding, unless axial retrobulbar space-occupying lesion such as extraocular myositis
Corneal diameter (measure with STT strip)	>2 mm larger than the other eye	No difference between eyes
Retropulsion	No resistance	Resistance ± pain
View from top of head	Eye variably protrudes	Eye more notably protrudes
Pain opening the mouth	None	Yes if retrobulbar abscess, and some tumours and sialoceles
Ocular signs	Corneal oedema, Haab's striae, mydriasis	Eye difficult to examine because of third eyelid protrusion and chemosis, may have exposure keratitis
Submandibular lymph nodes	Normal	May be enlarged with abscess or neoplasia
Intraocular pressure	High: >25 mmHg	Likely to be high end of normal or slightly increased, as a result of increased episcleral pressure
Main differential diagnoses	Chronic glaucoma; intraocular tumour	Retrobulbar abscess/cellulitis; retrobulbar tumour; retrobulbar sialocele; skull fractures; proptosis if eyelids trapped behind globe
Plan	Examine the other eye; establish whether primary or secondary glaucoma	Ocular ultrasonography; further diagnostic imaging, including MRI and CT, can give very valuable information, e.g. extension into adjacent structures; lancing behind the last molar tooth under general anaesthetic is appropriate if retrobulbar abscess (painful, confirmed with ultrasonography and FNA); ultrasound-guided FNA or Trucut biopsy

21.1 An enlarged globe (buphthalmos) must be distinguished from a globe in a forward position (exophthalmos) based on the clinical signs. CT = computed tomography; FNA = fine-needle aspiration; MRI = magnetic resonance imaging; STT = Schirmer tear test.

Key for algorithms

CN = cranial nerve; CNS = central nervous system; CSF = cerebrospinal fluid; FeLV = feline leukaemia virus;
FIV = feline immunodeficiency virus; IOP = intraocular pressure; KCS = keratoconjunctivitis sicca;
MRI = magnetic resonance imaging; PLR = pupillary light reflex; PRA = progressive retinal atrophy;
RPED = retinal pigment epithelial dystrophy; SARDS = sudden acquired retinal degeneration syndrome;
STT = Schirmer tear test.

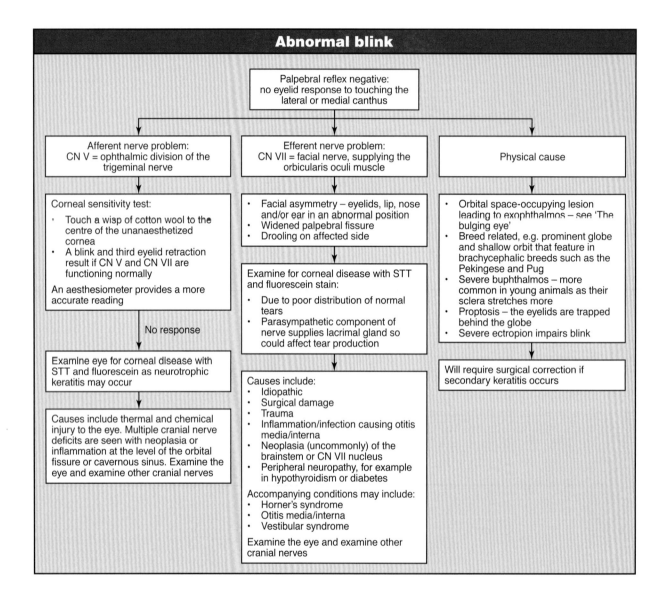

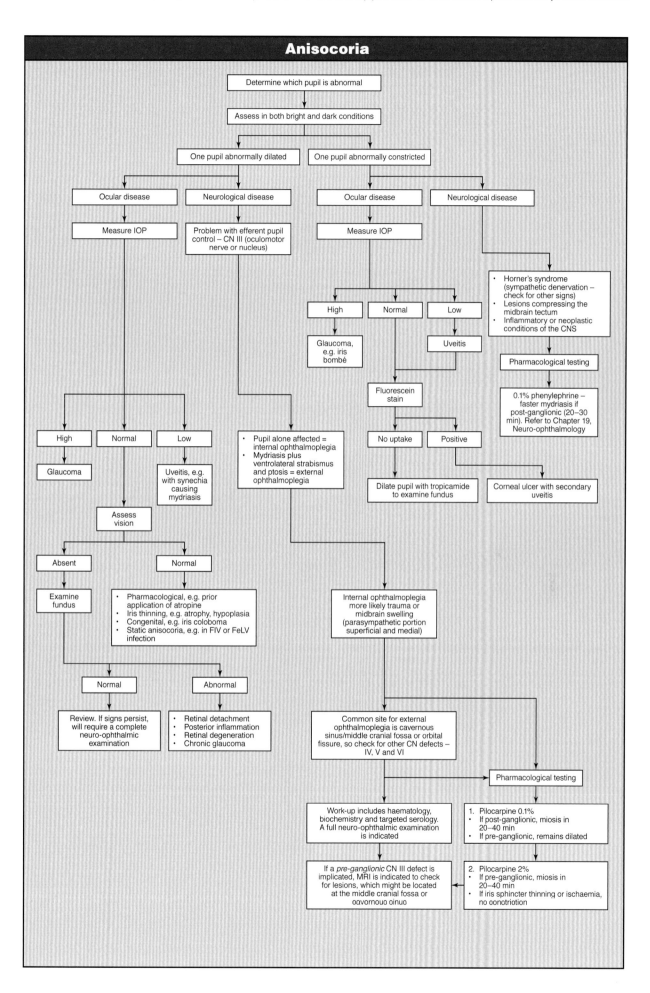

Anisocoria

Determine which pupil is abnormal

Assess in both bright and dark conditions

One pupil abnormally dilated | One pupil abnormally constricted

One pupil abnormally dilated:

Ocular disease → Measure IOP

Neurological disease → Problem with efferent pupil control – CN III (oculomotor nerve or nucleus)

Measure IOP → High → Glaucoma

Normal → Assess vision

Low → Uveitis, e.g. with synechia causing mydriasis

Assess vision → Absent → Examine fundus

Normal →
- Pharmacological, e.g. prior application of atropine
- Iris thinning, e.g. atrophy, hypoplasia
- Congenital, e.g. iris coloboma
- Static anisocoria, e.g. in FIV or FeLV infection

Examine fundus → Normal → Review. If signs persist, will require a complete neuro-ophthalmic examination

Abnormal →
- Retinal detachment
- Posterior inflammation
- Retinal degeneration
- Chronic glaucoma

Problem with efferent pupil control:
- Pupil alone affected = internal ophthalmoplegia
- Mydriasis plus ventrolateral strabismus and ptosis = external ophthalmoplegia

One pupil abnormally constricted:

Ocular disease → Measure IOP

Measure IOP → High → Glaucoma, e.g. iris bombé

Normal → Fluorescein stain

Low → Uveitis

Fluorescein stain → No uptake → Dilate pupil with tropicamide to examine fundus

Positive → Corneal ulcer with secondary uveitis

Neurological disease →
- Horner's syndrome (sympathetic denervation – check for other signs)
- Lesions compressing the midbrain tectum
- Inflammatory or neoplastic conditions of the CNS

Pharmacological testing → 0.1% phenylephrine – faster mydriasis if post-ganglionic (20–30 min). Refer to Chapter 19, Neuro-ophthalmology

Internal ophthalmoplegia more likely trauma or midbrain swelling (parasympathetic portion superficial and medial)

Common site for external ophthalmoplegia is cavernous sinus/middle cranial fossa or orbital fissure, so check for other CN defects – IV, V and VI

Pharmacological testing

Work-up includes haematology, biochemistry and targeted serology. A full neuro-ophthalmic examination is indicated

1. Pilocarpine 0.1%
- If post-ganglionic, miosis in 20–40 min
- If pre-ganglionic, remains dilated

2. Pilocarpine 2%
- If pre-ganglionic, miosis in 20–40 min
- If iris sphincter thinning or ischaemia, no constriction

If a *pre-ganglionic* CN III defect is implicated, MRI is indicated to check for lesions, which might be located at the middle cranial fossa or cavernous sinus

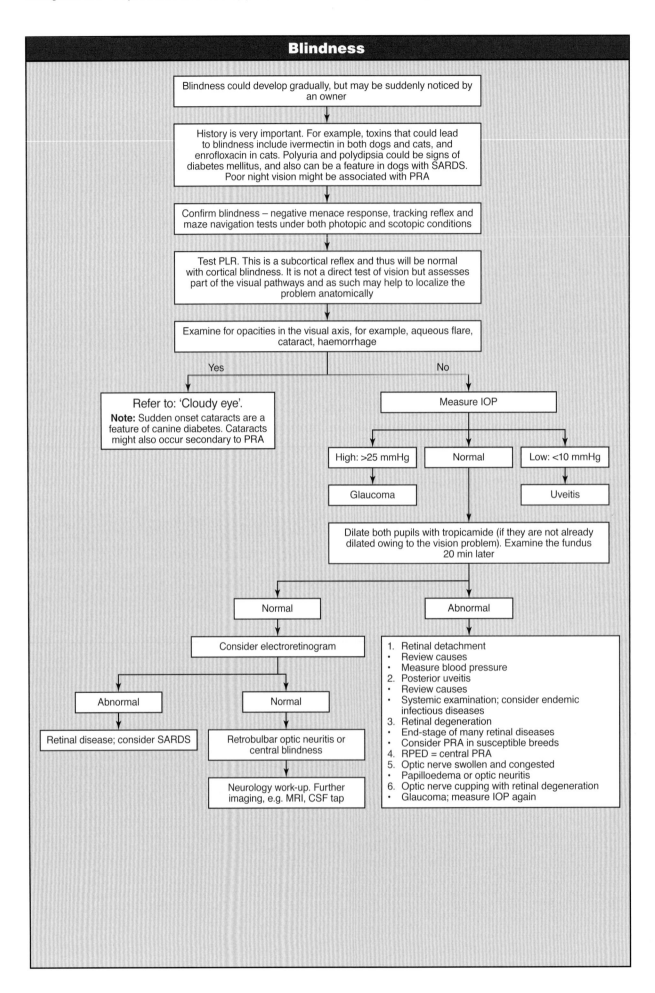

Blindness

Blindness could develop gradually, but may be suddenly noticed by an owner

History is very important. For example, toxins that could lead to blindness include ivermectin in both dogs and cats, and enrofloxacin in cats. Polyuria and polydipsia could be signs of diabetes mellitus, and also can be a feature in dogs with SARDS. Poor night vision might be associated with PRA

Confirm blindness – negative menace response, tracking reflex and maze navigation tests under both photopic and scotopic conditions

Test PLR. This is a subcortical reflex and thus will be normal with cortical blindness. It is not a direct test of vision but assesses part of the visual pathways and as such may help to localize the problem anatomically

Examine for opacities in the visual axis, for example, aqueous flare, cataract, haemorrhage

Yes → Refer to: 'Cloudy eye'.
Note: Sudden onset cataracts are a feature of canine diabetes. Cataracts might also occur secondary to PRA

No → Measure IOP

High: >25 mmHg → Glaucoma

Normal

Low: <10 mmHg → Uveitis

Dilate both pupils with tropicamide (if they are not already dilated owing to the vision problem). Examine the fundus 20 min later

Normal → Consider electroretinogram

Abnormal

Abnormal → Retinal disease; consider SARDS

Normal → Retrobulbar optic neuritis or central blindness → Neurology work-up. Further imaging, e.g. MRI, CSF tap

Abnormal:
1. Retinal detachment
   - Review causes
   - Measure blood pressure
2. Posterior uveitis
   - Review causes
   - Systemic examination; consider endemic infectious diseases
3. Retinal degeneration
   - End-stage of many retinal diseases
   - Consider PRA in susceptible breeds
4. RPED = central PRA
5. Optic nerve swollen and congested
   - Papilloedema or optic neuritis
6. Optic nerve cupping with retinal degeneration
   - Glaucoma; measure IOP again

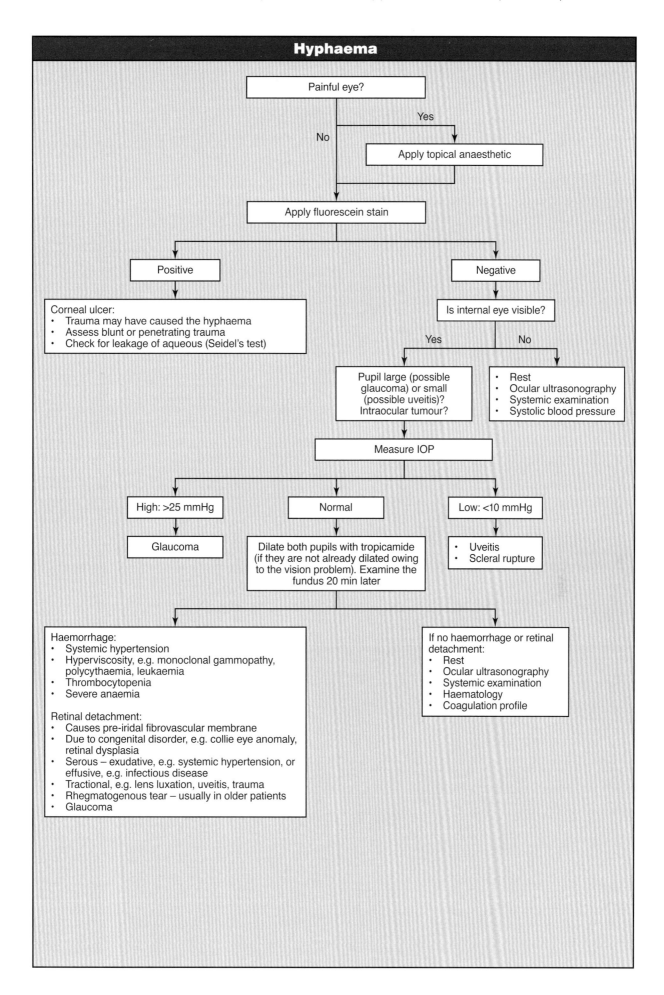

Hyphaema

Painful eye?

No / Yes

Apply topical anaesthetic

Apply fluorescein stain

Positive / Negative

Corneal ulcer:
- Trauma may have caused the hyphaema
- Assess blunt or penetrating trauma
- Check for leakage of aqueous (Seidel's test)

Is internal eye visible?

Yes / No

Pupil large (possible glaucoma) or small (possible uveitis)? Intraocular tumour?

- Rest
- Ocular ultrasonography
- Systemic examination
- Systolic blood pressure

Measure IOP

High: >25 mmHg / Normal / Low: <10 mmHg

Glaucoma

Dilate both pupils with tropicamide (if they are not already dilated owing to the vision problem). Examine the fundus 20 min later

- Uveitis
- Scleral rupture

Haemorrhage:
- Systemic hypertension
- Hyperviscosity, e.g. monoclonal gammopathy, polycythaemia, leukaemia
- Thrombocytopenia
- Severe anaemia

Retinal detachment:
- Causes pre-iridal fibrovascular membrane
- Due to congenital disorder, e.g. collie eye anomaly, retinal dysplasia
- Serous – exudative, e.g. systemic hypertension, or effusive, e.g. infectious disease
- Tractional, e.g. lens luxation, uveitis, trauma
- Rhegmatogenous tear – usually in older patients
- Glaucoma

If no haemorrhage or retinal detachment:
- Rest
- Ocular ultrasonography
- Systemic examination
- Haematology
- Coagulation profile

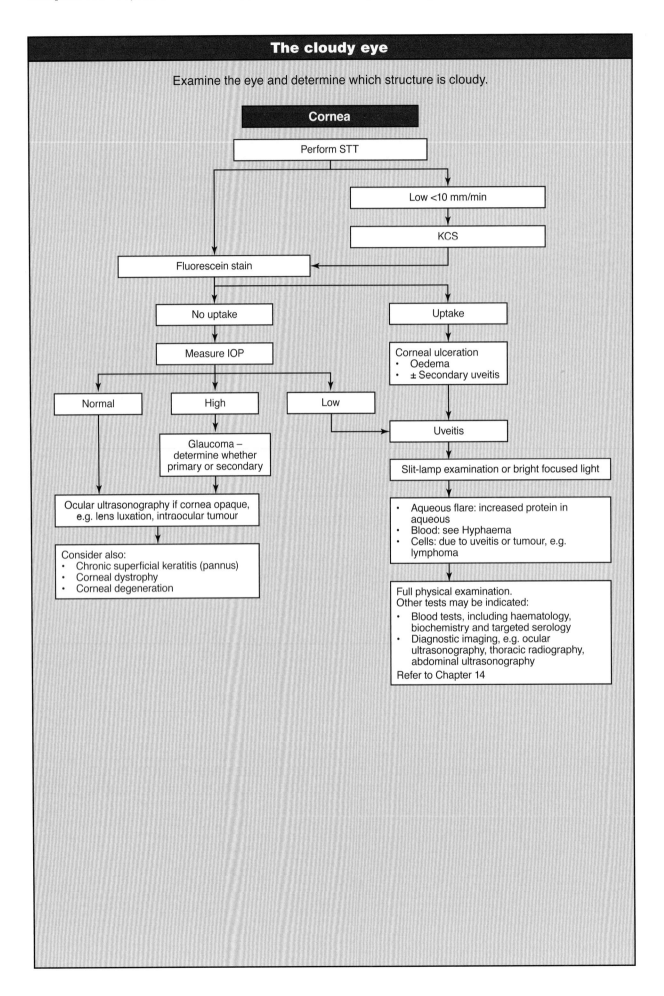

The cloudy eye

Examine the eye and determine which structure is cloudy.

Cornea

Perform STT

Low <10 mm/min

KCS

Fluorescein stain

No uptake

Uptake

Measure IOP

Corneal ulceration
- Oedema
- ± Secondary uveitis

Normal

High

Low

Uveitis

Glaucoma –
determine whether
primary or secondary

Slit-lamp examination or bright focused light

Ocular ultrasonography if cornea opaque,
e.g. lens luxation, intraocular tumour

- Aqueous flare: increased protein in
  aqueous
- Blood: see Hyphaema
- Cells: due to uveitis or tumour, e.g.
  lymphoma

Consider also:
- Chronic superficial keratitis (pannus)
- Corneal dystrophy
- Corneal degeneration

Full physical examination.
Other tests may be indicated:
- Blood tests, including haematology,
  biochemistry and targeted serology
- Diagnostic imaging, e.g. ocular
  ultrasonography, thoracic radiography,
  abdominal ultrasonography
Refer to Chapter 14

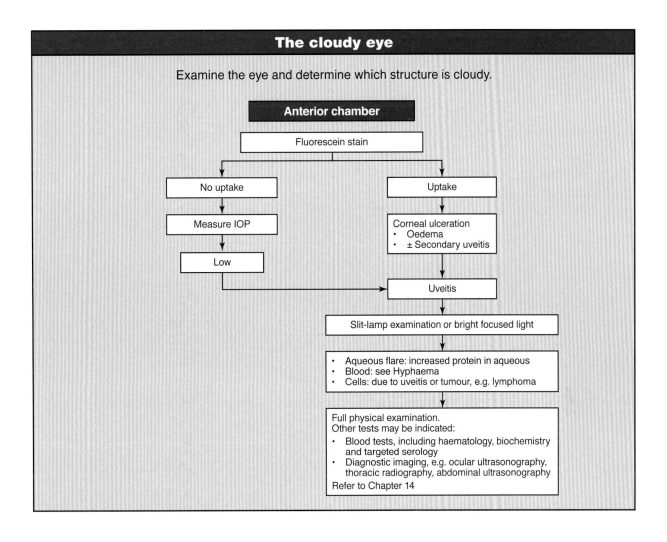

The cloudy eye

Examine the eye and determine which structure is cloudy.

Anterior chamber

Fluorescein stain

→ No uptake → Measure IOP → Low

→ Uptake → Corneal ulceration
- Oedema
- ± Secondary uveitis

→ Uveitis

Slit-lamp examination or bright focused light

- Aqueous flare: increased protein in aqueous
- Blood: see Hyphaema
- Cells: due to uveitis or tumour, e.g. lymphoma

Full physical examination.
Other tests may be indicated:
- Blood tests, including haematology, biochemistry and targeted serology
- Diagnostic imaging, e.g. ocular ultrasonography, thoracic radiography, abdominal ultrasonography
Refer to Chapter 14

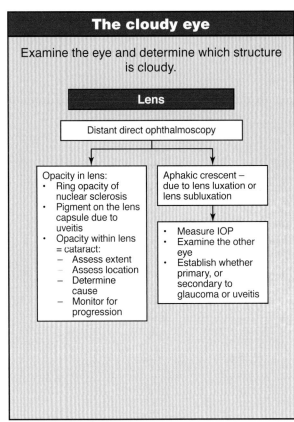

The cloudy eye

Examine the eye and determine which structure is cloudy.

Lens

Distant direct ophthalmoscopy

Opacity in lens:
- Ring opacity of nuclear sclerosis
- Pigment on the lens capsule due to uveitis
- Opacity within lens = cataract:
  - Assess extent
  - Assess location
  - Determine cause
  - Monitor for progression

Aphakic crescent – due to lens luxation or lens subluxation

- Measure IOP
- Examine the other eye
- Establish whether primary, or secondary to glaucoma or uveitis

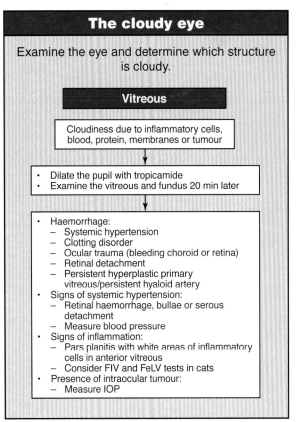

The cloudy eye

Examine the eye and determine which structure is cloudy.

Vitreous

Cloudiness due to inflammatory cells, blood, protein, membranes or tumour

- Dilate the pupil with tropicamide
- Examine the vitreous and fundus 20 min later

- Haemorrhage:
  - Systemic hypertension
  - Clotting disorder
  - Ocular trauma (bleeding choroid or retina)
  - Retinal detachment
  - Persistent hyperplastic primary vitreous/persistent hyaloid artery
- Signs of systemic hypertension:
  - Retinal haemorrhage, bullae or serous detachment
  - Measure blood pressure
- Signs of inflammation:
  - Pars planitis with white areas of inflammatory cells in anterior vitreous
  - Consider FIV and FeLV tests in cats
- Presence of intraocular tumour:
  - Measure IOP

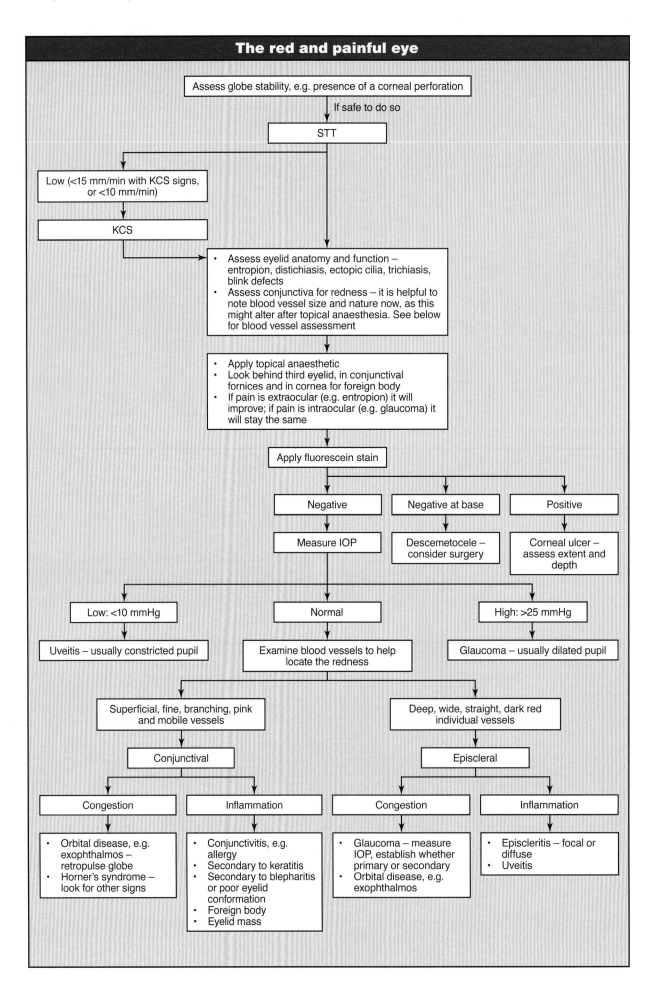

The red and painful eye

Assess globe stability, e.g. presence of a corneal perforation

If safe to do so

STT

Low (<15 mm/min with KCS signs, or <10 mm/min)

KCS

- Assess eyelid anatomy and function – entropion, distichiasis, ectopic cilia, trichiasis, blink defects
- Assess conjunctiva for redness – it is helpful to note blood vessel size and nature now, as this might alter after topical anaesthesia. See below for blood vessel assessment

- Apply topical anaesthetic
- Look behind third eyelid, in conjunctival fornices and in cornea for foreign body
- If pain is extraocular (e.g. entropion) it will improve; if pain is intraocular (e.g. glaucoma) it will stay the same

Apply fluorescein stain

Negative	Negative at base	Positive
Measure IOP	Descemetocele – consider surgery	Corneal ulcer – assess extent and depth

Low: <10 mmHg	Normal	High: >25 mmHg
Uveitis – usually constricted pupil	Examine blood vessels to help locate the redness	Glaucoma – usually dilated pupil

Superficial, fine, branching, pink and mobile vessels

Deep, wide, straight, dark red individual vessels

Conjunctival

Episcleral

Congestion	Inflammation	Congestion	Inflammation
• Orbital disease, e.g. exophthalmos – retropulse globe • Horner's syndrome – look for other signs	• Conjunctivitis, e.g. allergy • Secondary to keratitis • Secondary to blepharitis or poor eyelid conformation • Foreign body • Eyelid mass	• Glaucoma – measure IOP, establish whether primary or secondary • Orbital disease, e.g. exophthalmos	• Episcleritis – focal or diffuse • Uveitis

The watery eye

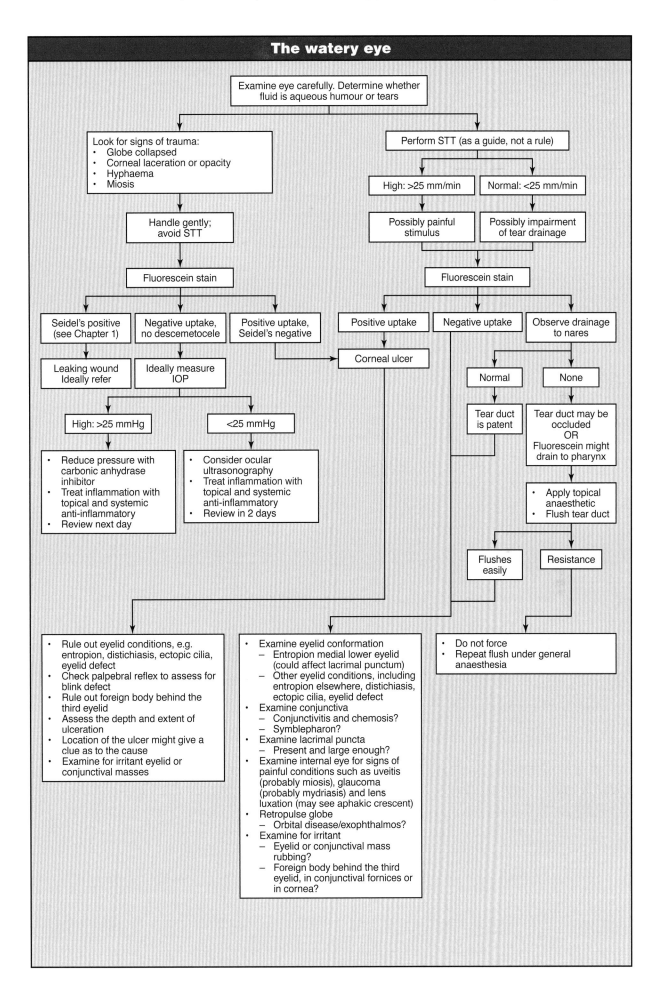

Examine eye carefully. Determine whether fluid is aqueous humour or tears

Look for signs of trauma:
- Globe collapsed
- Corneal laceration or opacity
- Hyphaema
- Miosis

Perform STT (as a guide, not a rule)

High: >25 mm/min

Normal: <25 mm/min

Possibly painful stimulus

Possibly impairment of tear drainage

Handle gently; avoid STT

Fluorescein stain

Fluorescein stain

Seidel's positive (see Chapter 1)

Negative uptake, no descemetocele

Positive uptake, Seidel's negative

Positive uptake

Negative uptake

Observe drainage to nares

Leaking wound Ideally refer

Ideally measure IOP

Corneal ulcer

Normal

None

High: >25 mmHg

<25 mmHg

Tear duct is patent

Tear duct may be occluded OR Fluorescein might drain to pharynx

- Reduce pressure with carbonic anhydrase inhibitor
- Treat inflammation with topical and systemic anti-inflammatory
- Review next day

- Consider ocular ultrasonography
- Treat inflammation with topical and systemic anti-inflammatory
- Review in 2 days

- Apply topical anaesthetic
- Flush tear duct

Flushes easily

Resistance

- Rule out eyelid conditions, e.g. entropion, distichiasis, ectopic cilia, eyelid defect
- Check palpebral reflex to assess for blink defect
- Rule out foreign body behind the third eyelid
- Assess the depth and extent of ulceration
- Location of the ulcer might give a clue as to the cause
- Examine for irritant eyelid or conjunctival masses

- Examine eyelid conformation
  - Entropion medial lower eyelid (could affect lacrimal punctum)
  - Other eyelid conditions, including entropion elsewhere, distichiasis, ectopic cilia, eyelid defect
- Examine conjunctiva
  - Conjunctivitis and chemosis?
  - Symblepharon?
- Examine lacrimal puncta
  - Present and large enough?
- Examine internal eye for signs of painful conditions such as uveitis (probably miosis), glaucoma (probably mydriasis) and lens luxation (may see aphakic crescent)
- Retropulse globe
  - Orbital disease/exophthalmos?
- Examine for irritant
  - Eyelid or conjunctival mass rubbing?
  - Foreign body behind the third eyelid, in conjunctival fornices or in cornea?

- Do not force
- Repeat flush under general anaesthesia

Index

Page numbers in *italic* indicate figures.

Index

Index

Iris
  anatomy and physiology 241–2
  aniridia 244
  anterior uveitis 37, 247–60, 265–9
  atrophy 246
  bombé *251, 256*, 284
  cysts *31*, 37, 246–7, 265, 286
  heterochromia 243
  hypoplasia/coloboma 244
  melanosis 246, 265
  merle ocular dysgensis 244
  neoplasia *15*, 37, 263, 269–70, 271, *386*
  rests *300, 305*
  subalbinism 243
  trauma 261, 269
Irish Red and White Setter
  cataract *303*
  genetic testing *66*
Irish Setter
  genetic testing *66*
  progressive retinal atrophy 64
Ischaemia, and blindness 368
Italian Spinone, entropion *144*
Itraconazole 101, 256

Jack Russell Terrier
  follicular conjunctivitis *183*
  genetic testing *66*
Jaeger lid plate *89*
Jagdterrier, genetic testing *66*
Japanese Akita, uveodermatological syndrome *154*, 392
Japanese Shiba Inu, primary glaucoma *282*
Jones test 17, 175
Joseph implant *292*
Juvenile cellulitis *155*

Karelian Bear Dog, genetic testing *66*
Keratectomy 208, 213, *227*
Keratitis
  in cats
    ulcerative/non-ulcerative
      acute bullous keratopathy 229
      corneal sequestrum 226–7
      eosinophilic 227–8
      eyelid/adnexal disease 224
      feline herpesvirus 224–5
      Florida spots 228
      infectious 227
      keratoconjunctivitis sicca 227
      lipid/calcium keratopathy 228
      neuroparalytic/neurotrophic keratopathy 229
      pigmentary 228
      superficial chronic corneal epithelial defects 227
      symblepharon 225–6
      trauma 228
  chronic superficial *53, 207*, 219–20
  in dogs
    non-ulcerative
      calcium degeneration 222
      chronic superficial 219–20
      corneal lipidosis 221–2
      pigmentary 220–1
    ulcerative
      acute stromal collagenolysis 214–15
      causes 208–9
      chemical/thermal burns 217
      degeneration 217
      eyelid/adnexal disease 212
      foreign bodies 216–17
      neurological disease 217–18
      superficial chronic corneal epithelial defects 212–14
      tear film disorders 212
      trauma 215–16
      treatment 209–12
  eosinophilic *56, 207*, 227–8
  septic 253–4
Keratoconjunctivitis sicca (KCS)
  and canine distemper virus 384
  in cats 174, 227
  in dogs
    congenital 172
    drug-induced 171–2
    immunogenic 170
    neurogenic 170–1, 382
    parotid duct transposition 173

and traumatic proptosis 127
  trimethoprim/sulphonamide 100
Keratomalacia *see* Acute stromal collagenolysis
Keratomycosis 101
Keratopathy
  acute bullous 229
  calcium 222, 228
  lipid 221, 228
  neuroparalytic 218
  neurotrophic 217–18
Keratotomy 213
Ketamine 71
Ketoconazole 101
Kühnt–Szymanowski procedure (modified) *145*
Kuvasz, genetic testing *66*

Laboratory investigation
  cytology 53–6
  histopathology 56–60
  microbiology investigation 51–3
  sampling 51
Labrador Retriever
  cataract *303*
  conjunctivitis, radiation-induced *185*
  dermoid *137*
  entropion *144*
  genetic testing *66*
  haemorrhage *187*
  histiocytic neoplasia 258
  juvenile cellulitis *155*
  mast cell tumour *186*
  primary glaucoma *282*
  pyogranulomatous blepharoconjunctivitis *185*
  uveodermatological syndrome *258*
  vitreoretinal dysplasia *317*
Lacrimal dilators *89*
Lacrimal excretory system
  canine conditions
    atresia 177–8
    cysts 178–9
    dacryocystitis 177
    laceration 179–80
    malpositioned lower lacrimal punctum 178
    micropunctum 178
    obstruction 179
  embryology, anatomy and physiology 175
  feline conditions
    atresia 181
    dacrocystitis 180
    laceration 181
    malpositioned lower lacrimal punctum 180
    obstruction 180
  investigation of disease 175–7
Lacrimal gland
  clinical evaluation 363
  disorders of tear production 382
  neuroanatomy 363
Lacrimal secretory system
  canine conditions
    cysts 174
    goblet cell dysfunction 174
    keratoconjuntivitis sicca 169–73
    meibomianitis 173
    neoplasia 174
  embryology, anatomy and physiology 167–8
  feline conditions
    keratoconjunctivitis sicca 174
  investigation of disease 168–9
Lacrimostimulants 106–7
  (see also specific agents)
Lagophthalmos
  in cats 161
  in dogs *126*, 127 138
Lancashire Heeler, genetic testing *67*
Lapponian Herder, genetic testing *67*
Large Munsterlander, cataract *303*
Latanoprost *103*, 104, *287*
Lateral canthoplasty, sliding *157*
Leishmania 101, 153, 184, 219, 235, 255, 268, 388
Lens
  canine conditions
    aphakia 301
    anterior segment dysgenesis 302
    cataracts 301, 302–6
    coloboma 302

Index

Neoplasia *continued*
   imaging 44–7
   intraocular *30*
   iridociliary 247, 264, 271
   lacrimal gland 174
   optic nerve 42, 353
   orbit *30*, *45*, 46, *58*, *115*, 124–6, *196*
   sclera, episclera and limbus 237–8, 239–40
   systemic 392
   third eyelid 197
   types 46–7
   uveal tract 263–4, 269–70
   vitreous 319
   (*see also individual neoplasms*)
Neopolitan Mastiff
   entropion *144*
   macropalpepral fissure *137*
   multifocal retinopathy 339
Neospora caninum 255, 388
Neotrombicula autumnalis 153
Nerve stimulator 77
Nettleship lacrimal dilator *89*
Neuromuscular blockade *75*, 77–8
Neuronal ceroid lipofuscinoses 350
Neuro-ophthalmology
   anatomy
      eyelids 361
      globe 362
      lacrimal gland 363
      pupils 359–60
      vision 357–8
   anisocoria
      and associated diseases 371–5
      clinical signs 368–9
      stepwise approach 369–71
   blindness
      and associated diseases 367–8
      causes *367*
      lesion localization *365*
      stepwise approach 364–7
   clinical evaluation 6–7
      eyelids 361–2
      globe 362–3
      lacrimal gland 363
      pupils 360–1
      vision 358–9
   eye position/movement abnormalities
      enophthalmos 379
      exophthalmos 377–9
      nystagmus 379–80
      strabismus 375–7
   eyelid opening/blink abnormalities
      hemifacial spasm 381
      nerve lesions 380–1
      ptosis 382
   investigation of disease 363
   lacrimation disorders 382
   third eyelid disorders 382
Neuroparalytic keratopathy 218
Neurotrophic keratopathy 217–18
Newfoundland, entropion *144*
Niacinamide 236
Nictitating membrane
   acquired abnormalities
      cysts 196
      inflammation 197–8
      neoplasia 197
      protrusion 196
      trauma 198
   developmental abnormalities
      scrolled cartilage 194
      prolapse 194–6
      protrusion 196
   embryology, anatomy and physiology 193–4
   surgical procedures
      flap surgery 198, *210*, *214*
      principles 80
      for prolapse *195*
Nodular fasciitis 198
Nodular granulomatous episcleritis 235
Nodular granulomatous episclerokeratitis 198
Non-steroidal anti-inflammatory drugs 70–1, 101–3, 209, 259
   (*see also specific agents*)
Non-ulcerative keratitis *see* Keratitis
Norwegian Buhund, cataract *303*
Norwegian Elkhound
   genetic testing *67*
   primary glaucoma *282*

Notoedres cati 162
Nova Scotia Duck Tolling Retriever, genetic testing *67*
Nuclear sclerosis *11*, 306–7
Nutritional diseases 389–90
Nystagmus
   clinical examination 362–3
   jerk 379–80
   pendular 380

Ocicat, genetic testing *65*
Ocular centesis *see* Aqueocentesis, Vitreocentesis
Ocular melanosis 238, 263, 265, 286
Oculocardiac reflex 72
Oculomotor nerve, lesion 375
Ofloxacin *99*
Old English Mastiff
   genetic testing *67*
   multifocal retinopathy 339
Old English Sheepdog
   cataract *303*
   merle ocular dysgenesis 244
Onchocerca 235, 257, 389
Operating microscope 83–4
Ophthalmia neonatorum
   in cats *160*
   in dogs 136
Ophthalmic examination
   with ambient illumination 3–4
   aqueocentesis/vitrocentesis 21–2, 54–5
   chart *12*
   electroretinography 21, 330–2
   equipment 2–3
   external staining 15–18
   eyelids 135–6
   fluorescein angiography 18
   with focal illumination 7–8
   gonioscopy 20
   neuro-ophthalmic reflexes 6, 7
   ophthalmoscopy
      direct 8–11
      indirect 13–14
   orbit/globe 115
   patient restraint 1–2
   retinoscopy 20
   sample collection 5, 21–2
   Schirmer tear test 4–5
   signalment and history 3
   slit-lamp examination 14–15
   tonometry 18–20
   vision testing 6–7
Ophthalmomyiasis interna 253, 256–7
Ophthalmoscopes *2*, *13*
Ophthalmoscopy
   direct 8–11
   of the fundus 324–30
   indirect 13–14
   of the lens 299–300
Opioids 69–70
   (*see also specific agents*)
Optical coherence tomography (OCT) 48
Optic cup 322, *323*
Optic nerve/nerve head
   atrophy 353
   coloboma 351–2
   cupping 280–1
   hypoplasia 351
   imaging 29, *30*, *42*
   neoplasia 42, 353
   neuritis 352–3
   papilloedema 352
   and vision testing 6
Optic neuritis
   and blindness 367–8
   and canine distemper virus 384
   causes *352*
   clinical features 352–3
   imaging 41–2
   treatment 353
Oral examination 115
Orbit
   acquired abnormalities
      abscess/cellulitis 42–3, 121–3
      cysts 128–9
      fat/muscle atrophy 129
      foreign bodies *30*, 43–4
      myositis 44, 123–4
      neoplasia *30*, *45*, 46, *58*, *115*, 124–6, *196*
      trauma 47, 126–8

Index